Fit & Well:
Core Concepts and Labs in
Physical Fitness and Wellness

WEL 1600 / 1700

13th edition

BELMONT UNIVERSITY

Fahey, Insel, Roth, and Insel

create.mheducation.com

ISBN-13:   9781307351033

ISBN-10:   1307351034

Contents

Online Supplements 369

Introduction to Wellness, Fitness, and Lifestyle Management

1

LOOKING AHEAD...

After reading this chapter, you should be able to

- Describe the dimensions of wellness.
- Identify the major health and lifestyle problems in the United States today.
- Describe the behaviors that are part of a wellness lifestyle.
- Explain the steps in creating a behavior management plan.
- Evaluate some of the available sources of wellness information.

TEST YOUR KNOWLEDGE

1. Which of the following lifestyle factors is the leading preventable cause of death for Americans?
   a. excess alcohol consumption
   b. cigarette smoking
   c. obesity

2. The terms *health* and *wellness* mean the same thing. True or false?

3. A person's genetic makeup determines whether he or she will develop certain diseases (such as breast cancer), regardless of that person's health habits. True or false?

   See answers on the next page.

© Hero Images/Getty Images RF

Acollege sophomore sets the following goals for herself:

- Join new social circles and make new friends whenever possible.
- Exercise every day.
- Clean up trash and plant trees in blighted neighborhoods in her community.

These goals may seem unrelated, but they have one thing in common. Each contributes, in its own way, to this student's health and well-being. Not satisfied merely to be free of illness, she wants more. She has decided to live actively and fully—not just to be healthy, but to pursue a state of overall wellness.

WELLNESS: NEW HEALTH GOALS

Generations of people have viewed health simply as the absence of disease, and that view largely prevails today. The word **health** typically refers to the overall condition of a person's body or mind and to the presence or absence of illness or injury. **Wellness** expands this idea of health to include our ability to achieve optimal health. Beyond the simple presence or absence of disease, wellness refers to optimal health and vitality—to living life to its fullest. Although we use the terms *health* and *wellness* interchangeably, they differ in two important ways:

Answers (Test Your Knowledge)

1. **b.** Smoking causes about 480,000 deaths per year. Obesity is responsible for as many as 400,000 premature deaths, and alcohol is a factor in 90,000 deaths per year.
2. **False.** Although the words are used interchangeably, they have different meanings. The term *health* refers to the overall condition of the body or mind and to the presence or absence of illness or injury. The term *wellness* refers to optimal health and vitality, encompassing all the dimensions of well-being.
3. **False.** In many cases, behavior can tip the balance toward good health even when heredity or environment is a negative factor.

- Health—or some aspects of it—can be determined or influenced by factors beyond your control, such as your genes, age, and family history. For example, a man with a family history of prostate cancer will have a higher-than-average risk for developing prostate cancer.
- Wellness is largely determined by the decisions you make about how you live. That same man can reduce his risk of cancer by eating sensibly, exercising, and having regular screening tests. Even if he develops the disease, he may still reduce its effects and live a rich, meaningful life. This means not only caring for himself physically, but also maintaining a positive outlook, keeping up his relationships with others, challenging himself intellectually, and nurturing other aspects of his life.

Wellness, therefore, involves making conscious decisions to control **risk factors** that contribute to disease or injury. Age and family history are risk factors you cannot control. Behaviors such as exercising, eating a healthy diet, and choosing not to smoke are well within your control.

The Dimensions of Wellness

Here are nine dimensions of wellness:

- Physical
- Emotional
- Intellectual
- Interpersonal
- Cultural
- Spiritual
- Environmental
- Financial
- Occupational

Each dimension affects the others. Furthermore, the process of achieving wellness is constant and dynamic (Figure 1.1), involving change and growth. Ignoring any dimension of wellness can have harmful effects on your life. The following

FIGURE 1.1   The wellness continuum.
The concept of wellness includes vitality in nine interrelated dimensions, all of which contribute to overall wellness.

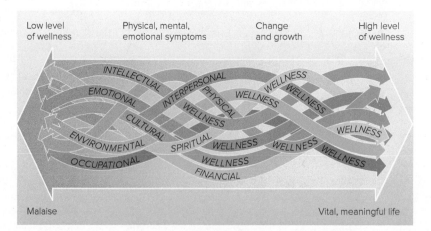

PHYSICAL WELLNESS	EMOTIONAL WELLNESS	INTELLECTUAL WELLNESS
• Eating well • Exercising • Avoiding harmful habits • Practicing safer sex • Recognizing symptoms of disease • Getting regular checkups • Avoiding injuries	• Optimism • Trust • Self-esteem • Self-acceptance • Self-confidence • Ability to understand and accept one's feelings • Ability to share feelings with others	• Openness to new ideas • Capacity to question • Ability to think critically • Motivation to master new skills • Sense of humor • Creativity • Curiosity • Lifelong learning
INTERPERSONAL WELLNESS	CULTURAL WELLNESS	SPIRITUAL WELLNESS
• Communication skills • Capacity for intimacy • Ability to establish and maintain satisfying relationships • Ability to cultivate a support system of friends and family	• Creating relationships with those who are different from you • Maintaining and valuing your own cultural identity • Avoiding stereotyping based on ethnicity, gender, religion, or sexual orientation	• Capacity for love • Compassion • Forgiveness • Altruism • Joy and fulfillment • Caring for others • Sense of meaning and purpose • Sense of belonging to something greater than oneself
ENVIRONMENTAL WELLNESS	FINANCIAL WELLNESS	OCCUPATIONAL WELLNESS
• Having abundant, clean natural resources • Maintaining sustainable development • Recycling whenever possible • Reducing pollution and waste	• Having a basic understanding of how money works • Living within one's means • Avoiding debt, especially for unnecessary items • Saving for the future and for emergencies	• Enjoying what you do • Feeling valued by your manager • Building satisfying relationships with coworkers • Taking advantage of opportunities to learn and be challenged

FIGURE 1.2 Qualities and behaviors associated with the dimensions of wellness.

sections briefly introduce the dimensions of wellness. Figure 1.2 lists specific qualities and behaviors associated with each dimension. Lab 1.1 will help you learn what wellness means to you and where you fall on the wellness continuum.

Physical Wellness Your physical wellness includes not just your body's overall condition and the absence of disease but also your fitness level and your ability to care for yourself. The higher your fitness level, the higher your level of physical wellness will be. Similarly, as you take better care of your own physical needs, you ensure greater physical wellness. To achieve optimum physical wellness, you need to make choices that help you avoid illnesses and injuries. The decisions you make now—and the habits you develop over your lifetime—will largely determine the length and quality of your life.

Emotional Wellness Your emotional wellness reflects your ability to understand and deal with your feelings. Emotional wellness involves attending to your own thoughts and feelings, monitoring your reactions, and identifying obstacles to emotional stability. *Self-acceptance* is your personal satisfaction with yourself, which might exclude society's expectations, whereas *self-esteem* relates to the way you think others perceive you. *Self-confidence* can be a part of both acceptance and esteem. Achieving this type of wellness means

finding solutions to emotional problems, with professional help if necessary.

Intellectual Wellness Those who enjoy intellectual wellness continually challenge their minds. An active mind is essential to wellness because it detects problems and finds solutions. People who enjoy intellectual wellness never stop learning. They seek out and relish new experiences and challenges.

Interpersonal Wellness Satisfying and supportive relationships are important to physical and emotional wellness. Learning good communication skills, developing the capacity for intimacy, and cultivating a supportive network are all important to interpersonal (or social) wellness. Social wellness requires participating in and contributing to your community and to society.

> **health** The overall condition of body or mind and the presence or absence of illness or injury.   TERMS
>
> **wellness** Optimal health and vitality, encompassing all dimensions of well-being.
>
> **risk factor** A condition that increases one's chances of disease or injury.

Wellness Tip Enhancing one dimension of wellness can have positive effects on others. For example, joining a meditation group can help you enhance your spiritual well-being, but it can also affect the emotional and interpersonal dimensions of wellness by enabling you to meet new people and develop new friendships.

© Jonathan Goldberg/Alamy Stock Photo

Cultural Wellness Cultural wellness refers to the way you interact with others who are different from you in terms of ethnicity, religion, gender, sexual orientation, age, and customs (practices). It involves creating relationships with others and suspending judgment on others' behavior until you have lived with them or "walked in their shoes." It also includes accepting, valuing, and even celebrating the different cultural ways people interact in the world. The extent to which you maintain and value cultural identities is one measure of cultural wellness.

---

infectious disease   A disease that can spread from person to person; caused by microorganisms such as bacteria and viruses.   TERMS

Spiritual Wellness To enjoy spiritual wellness is to possess a set of guiding beliefs, principles, or values that give meaning and purpose to your life, especially in difficult times. The well person uses spirituality to focus on positive aspects of life and to fend off negative feelings such as cynicism, anger, and pessimism. Organized religions help many people develop spiritual health. Religion, however, is not the only source or form of spiritual wellness. Many people find meaning and purpose in their lives on their own—through nature, art, meditation, or good works—or with their loved ones.

Environmental Wellness Your environmental wellness is defined by the livability of your surroundings. Personal health depends on the health of the planet—from the safety of the food supply to the degree of violence in society. To improve your environmental wellness, you can learn about and protect yourself against hazards in your surroundings and work to make your world a cleaner and safer place.

Financial Wellness Financial wellness refers to your ability to live within your means and manage your money in a way that gives you peace of mind. It includes balancing your income and expenses, staying out of debt, saving for the future, and understanding your emotions related to money. For more on this topic, see the box "Financial Wellness".

Occupational Wellness Occupational wellness refers to the level of happiness and fulfillment you gain through your work. Although high salaries and prestigious titles are gratifying, they alone do not bring about occupational wellness. An occupationally well person likes his or her work, feels a connection with others in the workplace, and takes advantage of opportunities to learn and be challenged. Another important aspect of occupational wellness is recognition from managers and colleagues. An ideal job draws on your interests and passions, as well as your vocational skills, and allows you to feel that you are making a contribution.

New Opportunities for Taking Charge

One hundred and sixty-five years ago, Americans considered themselves lucky just to survive to adulthood. A boy born in 1850, for example, could expect to live only about 38 years, and a girl, 40 years. Many people died from common **infectious diseases** (such as pneumonia, tuberculosis, or diarrhea) and poor environmental conditions (such as water pollution and poor sanitation).

By 2015, however, life expectancy nearly doubled, to 78.8 years (Figure 1.3). This increase in life span is due largely to the development of vaccines and antibiotics to fight infections, and to public health measures to improve living conditions. But even though life expectancy has increased, poor health limits most Americans' activities during the last

Researchers surveyed nearly 90,000 college students about their financial behaviors and attitudes. According to results released in 2016, a large percentage of students feel less prepared to manage their money than to handle almost any other aspect of college life. They also express distress over their current and future financial decisions. Front and center in their minds is how to manage student loan debt. Financial wellness means having a healthy relationship with money. Here are strategies for establishing that relationship:

Follow a Budget

A budget is a way of tracking where your money goes and making sure you're spending it on the things that are most important to you. To start one, list your monthly income and your expenditures. If you aren't sure where you spend your money, track your expenses for a few weeks or a month. Then organize them into categories, such as housing, food, transportation, entertainment, services, personal care, clothes, books and school supplies, health care, credit card and loan payments, and miscellaneous. Knowing where your money goes is the first step in gaining control of it.

Be Wary of Credit Cards

Students have easy access to credit but little training in finances. The percentage of students who have access to credit cards has increased from 28% in 2012 to 41% in 2015. This increase in credit card use has also correlated with an increase in paying credit card bills late, paying only the minimum amount, and having larger total outstanding credit balances.

Shifting away from using credit cards and toward using debit cards is a good strategy for staying out of debt. Familiarity with financial terminology helps as well. Basic financial literacy with using credit cards involves understanding terms like APR (annual percentage rate—the interest you're charged on your balance), credit limit (the maximum amount you can borrow), minimum monthly payment (the smallest payment your creditor will accept each month), grace period (the number of days you have to pay your bill before interest or penalties are charged), and over-the-limit and late fees (the amounts you'll be charged if you go over your credit limit or your payment is late).

Manage Your Debt and Get Politically Active

A 2016 study indicated that the average student loan debt was $37,000—and this number is expected to rise. When it comes to student loans, having a personal plan for repayment can save time and money, reduce stress, and help you prepare for the future. However, only about 10% of students surveyed feel they have all the information needed to pay off their loans. Work with your lender and make sure you know how to access your balance, when to start repayment, how to make payments, what your repayment plan options are, and what to do if you have trouble making payments. Information on managing federal student loans is available from (https://studentaid.ed.gov/sa/).

Your student debt may reflect circumstances beyond your control. For example, financial aid programs may require students to hold down jobs while also maintaining certain grade point averages. Consider contacting policymakers and asking them to pass measures to help students in need. One suggestion is for the Free Application for Federal Student Aid (FAFSA) to take into account how much debt a family or student already has when determining how much aid to grant.

Start Saving

If you start saving early, the same miracle of compound interest that locks you into years of credit card debt can work to your benefit (for an online compound interest calculator, visit http://www.interestcalc.org). Experts recommend "paying yourself first" every month—that is, putting some money into savings before you start paying your bills, depending on what your budget allows. You may want to save for a large purchase, or you may even be looking ahead to retirement. If you work for a company with a 401(k) retirement plan, contribute as much as you can every pay period.

Become Financially Literate

Most Americans have not received basic financial training. For this reason, the U.S. government has established the Financial Literacy and Education Commission (MyMoney.gov) to help Americans learn how to save, invest, and manage money better. Developing lifelong financial skills should begin in early adulthood, during the college years, if not earlier, as money-management experience appears to have a more direct effect on financial knowledge than does education. For example, when tested on their basic financial literacy, students who had checking accounts had higher scores than those who did not.

© Robin Lund/Alamy Stock photo RF

SOURCES: Smith, C., & G. A. Barboza. 2013. *The role of trans-generational financial knowledge and self-reported financial literacy on borrowing practices and debt accumulation of college students.* Social Science Electronic Publishing, Inc. (http://ssrn.com/abstract=2342168); Plymouth State University. 2013. *Student Monetary Awareness and Responsibility Today!* Plymouth State University. (http://www.plymouth.edu/office/financial-aid/smart/); U.S. Financial Literacy and Education Commission, MyMoney.gov, 2013. (http://www.mymoney.gov); Mitchell, J., "Student Debt Is About to Set Another Record, But the Picture Isn't All Bad," *Wall Street Journal,* May 2, 2016. (https://blogs.wsj.com/economics/2016/05/02/student-debt-is-about-to-set-another-record-but-the-picture-isnt-all-bad/); and EverFi, *Money Matters on Campus: Examining Financial Attitudes and Behaviors of Two-Year and Four-Year College Students.* www.moneymattersoncampus.org.

Box icon: © VisualCommunications/Getty Images RF

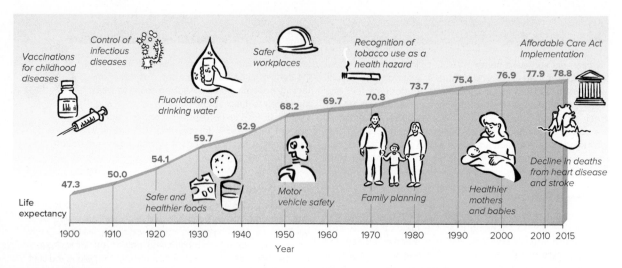

FIGURE 1.3   Public health and life expectancy of Americans from birth, 1900–2015. Public health achievements during the 20th century are credited with adding more than 25 years to life expectancy for Americans, greatly improving quality of life, and dramatically reducing deaths from infectious diseases. Public health improvements continue into the 21st century, including greater roadway safety, a steep decline in childhood lead poisoning, and an expansion of health insurance coverage.

SOURCES: Xu, J., et al. 2016. "Mortality in the United States, 2015," *NCHS Data Brief*, No. 267; Centers for Disease Control and Prevention. "Ten great public health achievements—United States, 2001–2010," *MMWR* 60(19): 619–623; Centers for Disease Control and Prevention 1999. "Ten great public health achievements—United States, 1900–1999," *MMWR* 48(50): 1141.

10–15% of their lives, resulting in some sort of impaired life (Figure 1.4).

Today, a different set of diseases has emerged as our major health threat: Heart disease, cancer, and chronic lower respiratory diseases are now the three leading causes of death for Americans (Table 1.1). While life expectancy has consistently increased each decade in the United States since 1850, the rate of improvement has slowed (and as of 2015 actually dropped for the first time in decades). A recent increase in deaths from heart disease, stroke, and diabetes may be linked to the obesity epidemic that began in the late 1970s. Medical treatments may be reaching their limits in treating heart disease and in preventing other early deaths related to obesity. Moreover, people are becoming obese at earlier ages, exposing them to the adverse effects of excess body fat over a longer period of time. Obesity and poor eating habits can lead to all the major **chronic diseases**.

The good news is that people have some control over whether they develop chronic diseases. Every day people can make choices that increase or decrease their risks. These **lifestyle choices** include decisions regarding smoking, diet, exercise, sleep, and alcohol use. Table 1.2 shows the estimated number of annual deaths tied to selected underlying causes. For example, the estimated 90,000 deaths due to alcohol include deaths due directly to alcohol poisoning as well as alcohol-related deaths from liver cancer and accidents. As Table 1.2 makes clear, lifestyle factors contribute to many deaths in the United States, and people can influence their own health risks. The need to make good choices is especially true for teens and young adults. For Americans aged 15–24, for example, the leading cause of death is unintentional injuries (accidents), with the greatest number of deaths linked to car crashes (Table 1.3).

chronic diseases   A disease that develops and continues over a long period of time, such as heart disease or cancer.

TERMS

lifestyle choice   A conscious behavior that can increase or decrease a person's risk of disease or injury; such behaviors include decisions regarding smoking, eating a healthy diet, exercising, and using alcohol.

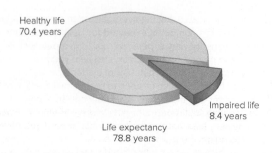

FIGURE 1.4   Quantity of life versus quality of life. Years of healthy life as a proportion of life expectancy in the U.S. population.

SOURCE: National Center for Health Statistics, 2016. "Healthy People 2020," *Midcourse Review,* Hyattsville, MD.

Table 1.1   Leading Causes of Death in the United States, 2015

RANK	CAUSE OF DEATH	NUMBER OF DEATHS	PERCENTAGE OF TOTAL DEATHS	LIFESTYLE FACTORS
1	Heart disease	633,842	23.4	D I S A O
2	Cancer	595,930	22.0	D I S A O
3	Chronic lower respiratory diseases	155,041	5.7	D I S O
4	Unintentional injuries (accidents)	146,571	5.4	I S A
5	Stroke	140,323	5.2	D I S A O
6	Alzheimer's disease	110,561	4.1	I S
7	Diabetes mellitus	79,535	2.9	D I S A O
8	Influenza and pneumonia	57,062	2.1	S A
9	Kidney disease	49,959	1.8	D S A O
10	Intentional self-harm (suicide)	44,193	1.6	A
	All causes	2,712,630	100.0	

Key
- D Diet plays a part
- I Inactive lifestyle plays a part
- S Smoking plays a part
- A Excessive alcohol use plays a part
- O Obesity is a contributing factor

NOTE: Although not among the overall top 10 causes of death, HIV/AIDS (6,465 deaths in 2015) is a major killer. In 2015, HIV/AIDS was the 13th leading cause of death for Americans aged 15–24 years and the 9th leading cause of death for those aged 25–34 years.

SOURCE: Centers for Disease Control and Prevention. 2017. *10 Leading Causes of Death by Age Group, United States, 2015.* Web-based Injury Statistics Query and Reporting System (www.cdc.gov/injury/wisqars); *Centers for Disease Control and Prevention. 2016. Cause of Death 1999-2015 on CDC WONDER Online Database* (http://wonder.cdc.gov/ucd-icd10.html).

National Health

Wellness is a personal concern, but the U.S. government has financial and humanitarian interests in it, too. A healthy population is the nation's source of vitality, creativity, and wealth. Poor health drains the nation's resources and raises health care costs for all.

A Plan for National Health Care Total health care expenditures in the United States are the highest in the world and growing; by 2016, they exceeded $10,000 per person each year, including both out-of-pocket payments by individuals and costs paid by private and government health insurance. These costs are not distributed evenly across individuals, and people's healthcare costs may vary significantly from year to year. Health insurance helps people pay for routine preventive care and protects them financially in the event of a serious and expensive illness or injury. Many people obtain health insurance through an employer, while others qualify for government-sponsored programs, such as Medicare, which covers nearly all adults age 65 and older. Still, the United States over time has had a high number of people who lacked insurance, peaking at approximately 50 million (16% of the population) in 2010. People without insurance are less likely to receive preventive care or treatment for major health problems.

The 2010 Affordable Care Act (ACA), also called "Obamacare," aimed to both reduce the number of uninsured and control the rise in healthcare costs. It mandated that most people obtain health insurance or pay a federal penalty. It provided financial assistance for people with low incomes by expanding Medicaid (a joint federal/state insurance program) and by providing tax credits and income-based subsidies for people who obtained insurance through newly established insurance exchanges. The ACA also broadened requirements for all health insurance plans, including those offered by employers; these provisions allowed young adults to stay on their parents' plans until age 26, eliminated annual and lifetime coverage limits, capped annual out-of-pocket payments, and provided protections for people with pre-existing conditions.

According to the National Center for Health Statistics, between 2010 and 2016, the overall number of Americans without insurance dropped by 20 million, down to 9% of the population, the lowest rate in decades. In 2016, among adults age 18-64 years, about 12% were uninsured (down from 22% in 2010), 20% were covered under a government-sponsored health plan, and 69% were covered by private insurance, including about 5% using an ACA insurance exchange. Defenders of the ACA argue that in addition to reducing the number of people without insurance, the act slowed the rise in health care costs and increased quality of care through changes in payment structures and delivery methods. Detractors of the law cite higher premiums and fewer insurance options as reasons to repeal and replace some or all of the law.

At this writing, major changes to the law have been proposed by Congress, and debate is ongoing about the costs and benefits of key ACA provisions. The ACA insurance requirements and expansion set new benchmarks for this debate over national health care policy.

VITAL STATISTICS

Table 1.2	Key Contributors to Death among Americans	
	NUMBER OF DEATHS PER YEAR	PERCENTAGE OF TOTAL DEATHS PER YEAR
Tobacco	480,000	18.3
Diet/activity patterns (obesity)*	400,000	15.2
Alcohol consumption	90,000	3.4
Microbial agents**	80,000	3.0
Firearms	30,000	1.1
Illicit drug use***	25,000+	1.0
Motor vehicles	20,000	0.8
Sexual behavior****	15,000	0.6

*The number of deaths due to obesity is an area of ongoing controversy and research. Recent estimates have ranged from 112,000 to 400,000.

**Microbial agents include bacterial and viral infections, such as influenza, pneumonia, and hepatitis. Infections transmitted sexually are counted in the "sexual behavior" category, including a proportion of deaths related to hepatitis, which can be transmitted both sexually and nonsexually.

***Drug overdose deaths have increased rapidly in recent years, making it likely that this estimate will rise.

****Estimated deaths linked to sexual behavior include deaths from cervical cancer and sexually acquired HIV, hepatitis B, and hepatitis C.

SOURCES: Kochanek, K. D., et al. 2016. "Deaths: Final data for 2014," *National Vital Statistics Reports* 65(4).; National Research Council, Institute of Medicine, *Measuring the Risks and Causes of Premature Death: Summary of Workshops*, 2015. Washington, DC: National Academies Press; Stahre, M., et al. 2014. "Contribution of excessive alcohol consumption to deaths and years of potential life lost in the United States," *Preventing Chronic Disease: Research, Practice, and Policy* 11: 130293; U.S. Department of Health and Human Services. *The Health Consequences of Smoking—50 Years of Progress: A Report of the Surgeon General*. Atlanta, GA: U.S. Department of Health and Human Services, Centers for Disease Control and Prevention.

VITAL STATISTICS

Table 1.3	Leading Causes of Death among Americans Aged 15–24, 2015		
RANK	CAUSE OF DEATH	NUMBER OF DEATHS	PERCENTAGE OF TOTAL DEATHS
1	Unintentional injuries (accidents)	12,514	41.0
	Motor vehicle	6,787	22.3
	Poisoning*	3,920	12.9
	All other unintentional injuries	1,807	5.9
2	Suicide	5,491	18.0
3	Homicide	4,733	15.5
4	Cancer	1,469	4.8
5	Heart disease	997	3.3
	All causes	30,494	100.0

*Poisoning deaths in this age group are primarily due to drug and alcohol overdose.

SOURCE: Centers for Disease Control and Prevention. 2017. *10 Leading Causes of Death by Age Group, United States, 2015*. Web-based Injury Statistics Query and Reporting System (www.cdc.gov/injury/wisqars).

The Healthy People Initiative The national Healthy People initiative aims to prevent disease and improve Americans' quality of life. Healthy People reports, published each decade since 1980, set national health goals based on 10-year agendas. The initiative's most recent iteration, *Healthy People 2020*, was released to the public in 2010. *Healthy People 2020* envisions "a society in which all people live long, healthy lives" and proposes the eventual achievement of the following broad national health objectives:

- *Eliminate preventable disease, disability, injury, and premature death.* This objective involves taking more concrete steps to prevent diseases and injuries, promoting healthy lifestyle choices, improving the nation's preparedness for emergencies, and strengthening the public health infrastructure.

- *Achieve health equity, eliminate disparities, and improve the health of all groups.* This objective involves identifying, measuring, and addressing health differences between individuals or groups that result from social or economic disadvantage. (See the box "Wellness Issues for Diverse Populations.")

- *Create social and physical environments that promote good health for all.* This objective involves the use of health interventions at many levels (such as anti-smoking campaigns by schools, workplaces, and local agencies), providing a broader array of educational and job opportunities for undereducated and poor Americans, and actively developing healthier living and natural environments for everyone.

- *Promote healthy development and healthy behaviors across every stage of life.* This goal involves taking a cradle-to-grave approach to health promotion by encouraging disease prevention and healthy behaviors in Americans of all ages.

In a shift from the past, *Healthy People 2020* emphasizes the importance of health determinants—factors that affect the health of individuals, demographic groups, or entire populations. Health determinants are social (including factors such as ethnicity, education level, and economic status) and environmental (including natural and human-made environments). Thus, one goal is to improve living conditions in ways that reduce the impact of negative health determinants.

Table 1.4 shows examples of individual health promotion goals from *Healthy People 2020*, as well as estimates of how well Americans are achieving those goals. To gain an idea of

DIVERSITY MATTERS
Wellness Issues for Diverse Populations

We all need to exercise, eat well, manage stress, and cultivate positive relationships. Protecting ourselves from disease and injuries is important, too. But some of our differences—both as individuals and as members of groups—have important implications for wellness. These differences can be biological (determined genetically) or cultural (acquired as patterns of behavior through daily interactions with family, community, and society). Many health conditions are a function of biology and culture combined. You share patterns of influences with others; and information about groups can be useful in identifying areas that may be of concern to you and your family. Wellness-related differences among groups can be described in terms of a number of characteristics, including the following:

Sex and Gender. *Sex* represents the biological and physiological characteristics that define men, women, and intersex people. In contrast, *gender* refers to how people identify themselves and also the roles, behaviors, activities, and attributes that a given society considers appropriate. A person's gender is rooted in biology and physiology, but it is shaped by experience and environment—how society responds to

individuals based on their sex. Examples of gender-related characteristics that affect wellness include the higher rates of smoking and drinking found among men and the lower earnings found among women compared with men doing similar work. Although men are more biologically likely than women to suffer from certain diseases (a sex issue), men are less likely to visit their physicians for regular exams (a gender issue). Men have higher rates of death from injuries, suicide, and homicide, whereas women are at greater risk for Alzheimer's disease and depression. Men and women also differ in body composition and certain aspects of physical performance.

Race and Ethnicity. Although the concept of race is complex, with the number of people who identify themselves as biracial or multiracial growing, it is still useful to identify and track health risks among population groups. Some diseases are concentrated in certain gene pools, the result of each racial or ethnic group's relatively distinct history. Diabetes is more prevalent among individuals of Native American or Latino heritage, for example, and African Americans have higher rates of hypertension. Racial and ethnic groups may vary in their

traditional diets; their family and interpersonal relationships; their attitudes toward tobacco, alcohol, and other drugs; and their health beliefs and practices.

Income and Education. Of all the variables, inequalities in income and education are the most highly correlated to health status. Income and education are closely related, and groups with the highest poverty rates and least education have the worst health status. These Americans have higher rates of infant mortality, traumatic injury, violent death, and many diseases. They are more likely to eat poorly, be overweight, smoke, drink, and use drugs. They are exposed to more day-to-day stressors and have less access to health care services.

Disability. People with disabilities have activity limitations or need assistance due to a physical or mental impairment. About one in five people in the United States has some level of disability, and the rate is rising, especially among younger segments of the population. People with disabilities are more likely to be inactive and overweight. They report more days of depression than people without disabilities. Many also lack access to health care services.

Box icon: © Rawpixel Ltd/Getty Images RF

Table 1.4　Progress toward *Healthy People 2020* Targets

OBJECTIVE	BASELINE (% MEETING GOAL IN 2008)	MOST RECENT PROGRESS (% MEETING GOAL IN 2014–15)	TARGET (% BY 2020)	PROGRESS TOWARD GOAL
Increase proportion of people with health insurance	83.2	89.4	100.0	○
Help adults with hypertension get blood pressure under control	43.7	50.3	61.2	+
Reduce proportion of obese adults	33.9	37.7	30.5	−
Reduce proportion of adults who drank excessively in past 30 days	27.1	27.0	24.4	○
Increase proportion of adults who meet federal guidelines for exercise	18.2	21.4	20.1	✓
Reduce proportion of adults who use cigarettes	20.6	15.3	12.0	+

Key ✓ Target met　　+ Significant progress
○ Insignificant progress　　− Getting worse

SOURCE: U.S. Department of Health and Human Services. *Healthy People 2020* data search (https://www.healthypeople.gov/2020/data-search/Search-the-Data).

Wellness Tip In Table 1.1, notice how many causes of death are related to lifestyle. This is an excellent motivator for adopting healthy habits and staying in good condition. Maintaining physical fitness and a healthy diet can lead to a longer life. It's a fact!
© Pablo Hidalgo/123RF

how you can make these national goals your own, visit www .healthypeople.gov. There you can find organizations that have affiliated themselves with *Healthy People 2020*, as well as publications and other resources detailing what it takes to get healthy.

Behaviors That Contribute to Wellness

A lifestyle based on good choices and healthy behaviors maximizes quality of life. It helps people avoid disease, remain strong and fit, and maintain their physical and mental health as long as they live.

Be Physically Active The human body is designed to be active. It readily adapts to nearly any level of activity and exertion. **Physical fitness** is a set of physical attributes that allows

the body to respond or adapt to the demands and stress of physical effort. The more we ask of our bodies, the stronger and more fit they become. When our bodies are not kept active, they deteriorate: Bones lose density, joints stiffen, muscles become weak, and cellular energy systems degenerate. To be truly well, human beings must be active.

Unfortunately, a **sedentary** lifestyle is common among Americans. According to a 2013 survey, only about half of adult Americans met the federal physical activity guidelines in 2013 (150 minutes or more per week of moderate aerobic exercise or 75 minutes per week of vigorous aerobic exercise). The older the adults, the less likely they were to meet the guidelines.

The benefits of physical activity are both physical and mental, immediate and long term (Figure 1.5). In the short term, being physically fit makes it easier to do everyday tasks, such as lifting; it provides reserve strength for emergencies; and it helps people look and feel good. In the long term, being physically fit confers protection against chronic diseases and lowers the risk of dying prematurely. (See the box "Does Being Physically Active Make a Difference in How Long You Live?") Physically active people are less likely to develop or die from heart disease, respiratory disease, high blood pressure, cancer, osteoporosis, and type 2 diabetes (the most common form of diabetes). As they get older, they may be able to avoid weight gain, muscle and bone loss, fatigue, and other problems associated with aging.

Choose a Healthy Diet In addition to being sedentary, many Americans have a diet that is too high in calories, unhealthy fats, and added sugars, as well as too low in fiber, complex carbohydrates, fruits, and vegetables. Like physical inactivity, this diet is linked to a number of chronic diseases. A healthy diet provides necessary nutrients and sufficient energy without also providing too much of the dietary substances linked to diseases.

Maintain a Healthy Body Weight Overweight and obesity are associated with a number of disabling and potentially fatal conditions and diseases, including heart disease, cancer, and type 2 diabetes. Researchers estimate that obesity kills between 112,000 and 400,000 Americans each year. Healthy body weight is an important part of wellness—but short-term dieting is not part of fitness or wellness. Maintaining a healthy body weight requires a lifelong commitment to regular exercise, a healthy diet, and effective stress management.

Manage Stress Effectively Many people cope with stress by eating, drinking, or smoking too much. Others don't deal with it at all. In the short term, inappropriate stress management can

> **physical fitness**   A set of physical attributes that   TERMS
> allows the body to respond or adapt to the demands
> and stress of physical effort.
>
> **sedentary**   Physically inactive; literally, "sitting."

lead to fatigue, sleep disturbances, and other symptoms. Over longer periods of time, poor stress management can lead to less efficient functioning of the immune system and increased susceptibility to disease. Learning to incorporate effective stress management techniques into daily life is an important part of a fit and well lifestyle.

Avoid Tobacco and Drug Use and Limit Alcohol Consumption Tobacco use is associated with 9 of the top 10 causes of death in the United States; personal tobacco use and secondhand smoke kill nearly 500,000 Americans each year, more than any other behavioral or environmental factor. In 2015, 15% of adult Americans described themselves as current smokers. Lung cancer is the most common cause of cancer death among both men and women and one of the leading causes of death overall. On average, the direct health care costs associated with smoking exceed $170 billion per year. If the cost of lost productivity from sickness, disability, and premature death is included, the total exceeds $300 billion.

Excessive alcohol consumption is linked to 8 of the top 10 causes of death and results in about 90,000 deaths a year in the United States. The social, economic, and medical costs of alcohol abuse are estimated at more than $250 billion per year. Alcohol or drug intoxication is an especially notable factor in the death and disability of young people, particularly through **unintentional injuries** (such as drownings and car crashes caused by drunken driving) and violence.

Protect Yourself from Disease and Injury The most effective way of dealing with disease and injury is to prevent them. Many of the lifestyle strategies discussed here help protect you against chronic illnesses. In addition, you can take specific steps to avoid infectious diseases, particularly those that are sexually transmitted.

Take Other Steps toward Wellness Other important behaviors contribute to wellness, including these:

- *Developing meaningful relationships*—for example, learning to communicate and dealing with anger
- *Planning for successful aging*—for example, anticipating physical challenges and maintaining hobbies
- *Learning about the health care system*—for example, knowing what treatment options are available to you
- *Acting responsibly toward the environment*—for example, helping to reduce pollution and encouraging sustainable practices

Wellness Factors That Seem Outside Our Control

Heredity, the environment, and adequate health care are other important influences on health and wellness. These factors can interact in ways that raise or lower the quality of a person's life and the risk of developing particular diseases. For example, a sedentary lifestyle combined with a genetic predisposition for diabetes can greatly increase a person's risk of developing the disease. If this sedentary, genetically predisposed person also lacks adequate health care, he or she is much more likely to suffer dangerous complications from diabetes.

But in many cases, behavior can tip the balance toward health even if heredity or environment is a negative factor. Breast cancer, for example, can run in families, but it is also associated with overweight and a sedentary lifestyle. A woman with a family history of breast cancer is less likely to die from the disease if she controls her weight, exercises, and has regular mammograms to help detect the disease in its early, most treatable stage.

College Students and Wellness

Each year, thousands of students lose productive academic time to activities causing stress and other physical and emotional health problems—some of which can continue for a lifetime. According to the fall 2016 American College Health Association National College Health Assessment II, the following were commonly reported factors affecting academic performance:

- Stress (32.2% of students affected)
- Anxiety (24.9%)
- Sleep difficulties (20.6%)
- Depression (15.4%)
- Work (14.2%)
- Cold/flu/sore throat (13.0%)
- Concern for a troubled friend/family member (10.1%)
- Internet use/computer games (9.0%)

• Increased endurance, strength, and flexibility	• Reduced risk of dying prematurely from all causes
• Healthier muscles, bones, and joints	• Reduced risk of developing and/or dying from heart disease, diabetes, high blood pressure, and colon cancer
• Increased energy (calorie) expenditure	
• Improved body composition	
• More energy	• Reduced risk of becoming obese
• Improved ability to cope with stress	• Reduced anxiety, tension, and depression
• Improved mood, higher self-esteem, and a greater sense of well-being	• Reduced risk of falls and fractures
• Improved ability to fall asleep and sleep well	• Reduced spending for health care

FIGURE 1.5 Benefits of regular physical activity.

unintentional injury An injury that occurs without harm being intended.   TERMS

THE EVIDENCE FOR EXERCISE
Does Being Physically Active Make a Difference in How Long You Live?

How can we be sure that physical activity and exercise are good for our health? To answer this question, the U.S. Department of Health and Human Services asked a committee to review scientific literature. The committee's mission was to determine if enough evidence exists to warrant the government making physical activity recommendations to the public. The committee's report, the *Physical Activity Guidelines Advisory Committee Report, 2008,* summarizes the scientific evidence for the health benefits of regular physical activity and the risks of sedentary behavior. The report provides the rationale for the federal government's physical activity guidelines, and its findings were confirmed in the *Scientific Report of the 2015 Dietary Guidelines Committee.*

The Physical Activity Guidelines Advisory Committee started by asking whether physical activity actually helps people live longer. The committee investigated the link between physical activity and all-cause mortality—deaths from all causes—by looking at 73 studies dating from 1995 to 2008. The studies included men and women from all age groups (16 to 65+) and from different racial and ethnic groups.

The data from these studies strongly support an *inverse relation* between physical activity and all-cause mortality; that is, physically active people were less likely to die during a study's follow-up period (ranging from 10 months to 28 years). The review found that active people have about a 30% lower risk of dying compared with inactive people. These inverse associations were found not just for healthy adults but also for older adults (age 65 and older); for people with coronary artery disease, diabetes, or impaired mobility; and for people who were overweight or obese. Poor fitness and low physical activity levels were found to be better predictors of premature death than smoking, diabetes, or obesity. Based on the evidence, the committee determined that about 150 minutes (2.5 hours) of physical activity per week is enough to reduce all-cause mortality (see Chapter 2 for more details). It appears that it is the overall volume of energy expended, no matter which kinds of activities are done, that makes a difference in risk of premature death.

The committee also looked at whether there is a *dose-response* relation between physical activity and all-cause mortality—that is, whether more activity reduces death rates even further. Again, the studies showed an inverse relation between these two variables. So, more activity above and beyond 150 minutes per week produces greater benefits. Surprisingly, for inactive people, benefits are seen at levels below 150 minutes per week. In fact, *any* increase in physical activity resulted in reduced risk of death. The committee refers to this as the "some is good; more is better" message. A target of 150 minutes per week is recommended, but any level of activity below the target is encouraged for inactive people.

Looking more closely at this relationship, the committee found that the greatest risk reduction is seen at the lower end of the physical activity spectrum (30–90 minutes per week). In fact, sedentary people who become more active have the greatest potential for improving health and reducing the risk of premature death. Additional risk reduction occurs as physical activity increases, but at a slower rate. For example, people who engaged in physical activity 90 minutes per week had a 20% reduction in mortality risk compared with inactive people, and those who were active 150 minutes per week, as noted earlier, had a 30% reduction in risk. But to achieve a 40% reduction in mortality risk, study participants had to be physically active 420 minutes per week (7 hours).

A 2017 American Heart Association report projected that cardiovascular disease costs in the United States will exceed $1 trillion by 2035. Regular exercise reduces the risk of cardiovascular disease and related health problems such as hypertension, high cholesterol, and diabetes. The message from the research is clear: It doesn't matter what activity you choose or even how much time you can devote to it per week, as long as you get moving!

SOURCE: American Heart Association. 2017. *Cardiovascular Disease: A Costly Burden for America; Projections through 2035.* Dallas, TX: American Heart Association; 2015 Dietary Guidelines Advisory Committee. 2015. *Scientific Report of the 2015 Dietary Guidelines Advisory Committee.* Washington, DC: U.S. Department of Health and Human Services; Physical Activity Guidelines Advisory Committee, *Physical Activity Guidelines Advisory Committee Report, 2008.* Washington, DC: U.S. Department of Health and Human Services.

© yellowdog/Getty Images RF

Box Icon: © Vstock LLC/Getty Images RF

Each of these factors is related to one or more dimensions of wellness, and most can be influenced by choices students make daily. For example, there are many ways to manage stress: By reducing unhealthy choices, such as using alcohol to relax, and by increasing healthy choices, such as using time-management techniques, even busy students can reduce the impact of stress.

What about wellness choices in other areas? The American College Health Association survey found the following:

Ask Yourself

QUESTIONS FOR CRITICAL THINKING AND REFLECTION

How often do you feel exuberant? Vital? Joyful? What makes you feel that way? Conversely, how often do you feel downhearted, de-energized, or depressed? What makes you feel that way? Have you ever thought about how you might increase experiences of vitality and decrease experiences of discouragement?

- Only 48.4% of sexually active students reported that they used a condom mostly or always during vaginal intercourse in the past 30 days.
- About 18.3% of students had seven or more drinks the last time they partied.
- About 11.7% of students used one or more prescription drugs that were not prescribed to them within the past year.
- About 10.1% of students smoked cigarettes, and 4.3% used e-cigarettes, at least once during the past month.

How do your daily wellness choices compare to those of other students? What is recommended to promote wellness? Remember: The sooner you trade an unhealthy behavior for a healthier one, the longer you'll be around to enjoy the benefits.

REACHING WELLNESS THROUGH LIFESTYLE MANAGEMENT

Moving in the direction of wellness means cultivating healthy behaviors and working to overcome unhealthy ones. This approach to lifestyle management is called **behavior change**. As you may already know from experience, changing an unhealthy habit can be harder than it sounds. When you embark on a behavior change plan, it may seem like too much work at first. But as you make progress, you will gain confidence in your ability to take charge of your life. You will also experience the benefits of wellness—more energy, greater vitality, deeper feelings of appreciation and curiosity, and a higher quality of life.

The rest of this chapter outlines a general process for changing unhealthy behaviors that is backed by research and has worked for many people. You will also find many specific strategies and tips for change. For additional support, work through the activities in the Behavior Change Workbook at the end of the text.

Getting Serious about Your Health

Before you can start changing a wellness-related behavior, you have to know that the behavior is problematic and that you *can* change it. To make good decisions, you need information about relevant topics and issues, including what resources are available to help you change.

Examine Your Current Health Habits Consider how your current lifestyle is affecting your health today. How will it affect your health in the future? Do you know which of your current habits enhance your health and which ones may be harmful? Begin your journey toward wellness with self-assessment: Think about your own behavior, complete the self-assessment in Lab 1.2, and talk with friends and family members about what they've noticed about your lifestyle and your health. Digital trackers can also help with your self-assessment; see the box "Quantify Yourself."

Choose a Target Behavior Changing any behavior can be demanding. This is why it's a good idea to start small, by choosing one behavior you want to change—called a **target behavior**—and working on it until you succeed. Your chances of success will be greater if your first goal is simple, such as resisting the urge to snack between classes. As you change one behavior, make your next goal a little more significant, and build on your success over time.

Learn about Your Target Behavior After you've chosen a target behavior, you need to learn its risks and benefits for you—both now and in the future. As a starting point, use this text and the resources listed in the For Further Exploration section at the end of each chapter; see the box "Evaluating Sources of Health Information" for additional guidelines. Ask these questions:

- How is your target behavior affecting your level of wellness today?
- Which diseases or conditions does this behavior place you at risk for?
- What effect would changing your behavior have on your health?

Find Help Have you identified a particularly challenging target behavior or mood—something like overuse of alcohol, binge eating, or depression—that interferes with your ability to function or places you at a serious health risk? If so, you many need help to change behaviors or conditions that are too deeply rooted or too serious for self-management. Don't be discouraged by the seriousness or extent of the problem; many resources are available to help you solve it. On campus, the student health center or campus counseling center can provide assistance. To locate community resources, consult yellowpages.com, your physician, or the Internet.

Building Motivation to Change

Knowledge is necessary for behavior change, but it isn't usually enough to make people act. Millions of people have sedentary lifestyles, for example, even though they know it's bad for their health. To succeed at behavior change, you need to be motivated and to know that even though an active lifestyle may be inconvenient, it may be required.

Examine the Pros and Cons of Change Health behaviors have short-term and long-term benefits and costs. Consider the benefits and costs of an inactive lifestyle:

- *Short-term.* Such a lifestyle allows you more time to watch TV and hang out with friends, but it leaves you less fit and less able to participate in recreational activities.

---

behavior change   A lifestyle management **TERMS**
process that involves cultivating healthy behaviors
and working to overcome unhealthy ones.

target behavior   An isolated behavior selected
as the object of a behavior change program.

WELLNESS IN THE DIGITAL AGE
Quantify Yourself

You feel stressed and under the weather. How can you feel better? Do you have a habit you want to kick. Where to start?

People's increasing desire to track their moods, sleep, exercise, and diet patterns has brought about some 165,000 health-related apps and movements, like Quantified Self—a California-based company that promotes self-tracking tools among communities across the world. By giving you numerical data related to your daily behaviors, digital trackers provide objective feedback about what is going on with your health. The technology also helps you describe your behaviors to doctors and can be integrated with behavior change strategies learned through counseling. Here are three steps to making good use of technology for wellness:

1. **Monitor yourself.** How much are you smoking? Sleeping? Exercising? What are you eating? Digital trackers can help answer these questions for you. A wristband can record whether you are getting enough restful sleep. Your smartphone can tell you how many steps you took to get across campus.

2. **Analyze your data.** You've tracked your sleep, your blood pressure, and your steps. You've kept a journal related to your diet. You've taken your body measurements. What patterns do you notice? What time of day do you tend to need food? Cigarettes? Sleep? How do your patterns match up with your goals?

Standard weight-loss apps allow users to input weight goals and monitor progress toward those goals; more sophisticated apps can analyze users' data and offer daily physical-activity goals, or help them establish a regular eating schedule. You can now find advice, education, e-mail reminders, alerts for lapses in progress, motivational messages, and journals to record and track negative emotion. Many weight-loss apps also link to social media for encouragement and social support, or rewarding games and challenges. Additional features can be critical; tracking alone isn't sufficient for successful behavior change. You need to apply change strategies such as those described later in the chapter.

3. **Extend the list of behaviors you'd like to change.** You can track more than just your diet and exercise habits with digital assistance. Electronic devices and smart programs are available to help with many aspects of wellness, including the following:

- Stress management
- Meditation and spirituality
- Heart rate and respiration
- Menstrual cycles
- Family medical history
- Journaling

With so many possibilities, how do you choose what to monitor? Start with one or two variables. The interactive labs at the end of each chapter focus on aspects of fitness and wellness to get you going. Also, you'll find a variety of digital devices and apps discussed in later chapters, in "Wellness in the Digital Age" boxes. You may find one or more apps (many of which are free) that appeal to you and can help you make progress toward your fitness and wellness goals.

SOURCES: IMS Institute for Healthcare Informatics. September 17, 2015. *IMS health study: Patient options expand as mobile healthcare apps address wellness and chronic disease treatment needs.* (http://www.imshealth.com/en/about-us/news/ims-health-study:-patient-options-expand-as-mobile-healthcare-apps-address-wellness-and-chronic-disease-treatment-needs); and Schoeppe, S., et al. 2016. "Efficacy of interventions that use apps to improve diet, physical activity and sedentary behaviour: A systematic review," *International Journal of Behavioral Nutrition and Physical Activity,* 13(127).

Wellness Tip Look for behavior-change support if you need it. Certain health behaviors are exceptionally difficult to change. Some people can quit smoking on their own; others get help from a smoking cessation program or a nicotine replacement product.

- *Long-term.* This lifestyle increases the risk of heart disease, cancer, stroke, and premature death.

To successfully change your behavior, you must believe that the benefits of change outweigh the costs.

Carefully examine the pros and cons of continuing your current behavior and of changing to a healthier one. Focus on the effects that are most meaningful to you, including those tied to your personal identity and values. For example, engaging in regular physical activity and getting adequate sleep can support an image of yourself as an active person who is a good role model for others. To work toward being independent and taking control over your life, quitting smoking can be one way to eliminate a dependency. To complete your analysis, ask friends and family members about the effects of your behavior on them. For example, a younger sister may tell you that your smoking habit influenced her decision to take up smoking.

The short-term benefits of behavior change can be an important motivating force. Although some people are motivated by

CRITICAL CONSUMER
Evaluating Sources of Health Information

Surveys indicate that college students are smart about evaluating health information. They trust the health information they receive from health professionals and educators and are skeptical about popular information sources, such as magazine articles and websites.

How smart are you about evaluating health information? Here are some tips.

General Strategies

Whenever you encounter health-related information, take the following steps to make sure it is credible:

● **Go to the original source.** Media reports and social media posts often simplify the results of medical research. Find out for yourself what a study really reported, and determine whether it was based on good science. What type of study was it? Was it published in a recognized medical journal? Was it an animal study, or did it involve people? Did the study include a large number of people? What did the study's authors actually report?

● **Watch for misleading language.** Reports that tout "breakthroughs" or "dramatic proof" are probably hype. A study may state that a behavior "contributes to" or is "associated with" an outcome, but this does not prove a cause-and-effect relationship.

● **Distinguish between research reports and public health advice.** Do not change your behavior based on the results of a single report or study. If an agency such as the National Cancer Institute urges a behavior change, however, you should follow its advice. Large, publicly funded organizations issue such advice based on many studies, not a single report.

● **Remember that anecdotes are not facts.** A friend may tell you he lost weight on some new diet, but individual success stories do not mean the plan is truly safe or effective. Do any scientific studies back up the claims of the article?

● **Be skeptical.** If a report seems too good to be true, it probably is. Be wary of information contained in advertisements. An ad's goal is to sell a product, even if there is no need for it, and sometimes even if the product has not been proven to be safe or effective.

● **Make choices that are right for you.** Friends and family members can be a great source of ideas and inspiration, but you need to make health-related choices that work best for you.

Internet Resources

Online information sources pose special challenges. When reviewing a health-related website, ask these questions:

● **What is the source of the information?** Websites maintained by government agencies, professional associations, or established academic or medical institutions are likely to present trustworthy information. Many other groups and individuals post accurate information, but it is important to look at the qualifications of the people who are behind the site. (Check the home page or click the "About Us" link.) Verify information you get from social media by visiting the originating organization's website and evaluating the source.

● **How often is the site updated?** Look for sites that are updated frequently. Check the "last modified" date of any web page. Newer studies may contradict the results of earlier ones.

● **Is the site promotional?** Be wary of information from sites that sell specific products, use testimonials as evidence, appear to have a social or political agenda, or ask for money.

● **What do other sources say about a topic?** Be wary of claims and information that appear at only one site or come from a chat room, bulletin board, or blog. Do other authors cite the same studies as the ones in this article?

● **Does the site conform to any set of guidelines or criteria for quality and accuracy?** Look for sites that identify themselves as conforming to some code or set of principles, such as those set forth by the Health on the Net Foundation or the American Medical Association. Medical and health journals that have been peer reviewed (edited by experts in the field), and websites maintained by government agencies, professional associations, or established academic or medical institutions are most likely to present trustworthy information.

Box icon: © sam74100/Getty Images RF

long-term goals, such as avoiding a disease that may hit them in 30 years, most are more likely to be moved to action by shorter-term, more personal goals. Feeling better, doing better in school, improving at a sport, reducing stress, and increasing self-esteem are common short-term benefits of health behavior change. Many wellness behaviors are associated with immediate improvements in quality of life. For example, surveys of Americans have found that nonsmokers feel healthy and full of energy more days each month than do smokers, and they report fewer days of sadness and troubled sleep. The same is true when physically active people are compared with sedentary people. Over time, these types of differences add up to a substantially higher quality of life for people who engage in healthy behaviors.

Boost Self-Efficacy When you start thinking about changing a health behavior, a big factor in your eventual success is whether you have confidence in yourself and in your ability to change. **Self-efficacy** refers to your belief in your ability to successfully take action and perform a specific task. Strategies for boosting self-efficacy include developing an internal locus of control, using visualization and self-talk, and getting encouragement from supportive people.

LOCUS OF CONTROL   Who do you believe is controlling your life? Is it your parents, friends, or school? Is it "fate"? Or is it you? **Locus of control** refers to the figurative "place" a person designates as the source of responsibility for the events in his or her life. People who believe they are in control of their own lives are said to have an *internal locus of control*. Those who believe that factors beyond their control determine the course of their lives are said to have an *external locus of control*.

For lifestyle management, an internal locus of control is an advantage because it reinforces motivation and commitment. An external locus of control can sabotage efforts to change behavior. For example, if you believe that you are destined to die of breast cancer because your mother died from the disease, you may view screening mammograms as a waste of time. In contrast, if you believe that you can take action to reduce your risk of breast cancer in spite of hereditary factors, you will be motivated to follow guidelines for early detection of the disease.

If you find yourself attributing too much influence to outside forces, gather more information about your wellness-related behaviors. List all the ways that making lifestyle changes will improve your health. If you believe you'll succeed, and if you recognize that you are in charge of your life, you're on your way to wellness.

VISUALIZATION AND SELF-TALK   One of the best ways to boost your confidence and self-efficacy is to visualize yourself successfully engaging in a new, healthier behavior. Imagine yourself going for an afternoon run three days a week or no longer smoking cigarettes. Also visualize yourself enjoying all the short-term and long-term benefits that your lifestyle change will bring. Create a new self-image: What will you and your life be like when you become a regular exerciser or a nonsmoker?

You can also use **self-talk**, the internal dialogue you carry on with yourself, to increase your confidence in your ability to change. Counter any self-defeating patterns of thought with more positive or realistic thoughts: "I am a strong, capable person, and I can maintain my commitment to change." See Chapter 10 for more on self-talk.

ROLE MODELS AND OTHER SUPPORTIVE INDIVIDUALS   Social support can make a big difference in your level of

Fitness Tip   Visualization is such a powerful technique that Olympic athletes learn how to harness it for peak performance. It works for average people, too. Set a small fitness goal, then imagine yourself doing it—as clearly and as often as you can. Visualization can help you believe in yourself, and belief can be a step toward success!
© Hero Images Inc./Alamy Stock Photo RF

motivation and your chances of success. Perhaps you know people who have reached the goal you are striving for; they could be role models or mentors, providing information and support for your efforts. Gain strength from their experiences, and tell yourself, "If they can do it, so can I." In addition, find a buddy who wants to make the same changes you do and who can take an active role in your behavior change program. For example, an exercise partner can provide companionship and encouragement when you might be tempted to skip your workout.

Identify and Overcome Barriers to Change   Don't let past failures at behavior change discourage you; they can be a great source of information you can use to boost your chances of future success. Make a list of the problems and challenges you faced in any previous behavior change attempts. To this list, add the short-term costs of behavior change that you identified in your analysis of the pros and cons of change. After you've listed these key barriers to change, develop a practical plan for overcoming each one. For example, if you always smoke when you're with certain friends, decide in advance how you will turn down the next cigarette you are offered.

Enhancing Your Readiness to Change

The transtheoretical, or "stages-of-change," model is an effective approach to lifestyle self-management. According to this model, you move through distinct stages as you work to change your target behavior. It is important to determine what stage you are in now so that you can choose appropriate strategies for progressing through the cycle of change. (Figure 1.6) This

---

self-efficacy   The belief in one's ability to take action and perform a specific task.

locus of control   The figurative "place" a person designates as the source of responsibility for the events in his or her life.

self-talk   A person's internal dialogue

TERMS

approach can help you enhance your readiness and intention to change. Read the following sections to determine what stage you are in for your target behavior.

Precontemplation People at this stage do not think they have a problem and do not intend to change their behavior. They may be unaware of the risks associated with their behavior or may deny them. They may have tried unsuccessfully to change in the past and may now think the situation is hopeless. They may also blame other people or external factors for their problems. People in the precontemplation stage believe that there are more reasons or more important reasons not to change than there are reasons to change.

Contemplation People at this stage know they have a problem and intend to take action within six months. They acknowledge the benefits of behavior change but worry about the costs of changing. To be successful, people must believe that the benefits of change outweigh the costs. People in the contemplation stage wonder about possible courses of action but don't know how to proceed. There may also be specific barriers to change that appear too difficult to overcome.

Preparation People at this stage plan to take action within a month or may already have begun to make small changes in their behavior. They may be engaging in their new, healthier behavior but not yet regularly or consistently. They may have created a plan for change but may be worried about failing.

Action During the action stage, people outwardly modify their behavior and their environment. The action stage requires the greatest commitment of time and energy, and people in this stage are at risk for reverting to old, unhealthy patterns of behavior.

Maintenance People at this stage have maintained their new, healthier lifestyle for at least six months. Lapses may have occurred, but people in maintenance have been successful in quickly reestablishing the desired behavior. The maintenance stage can last for months or years.

Termination People at the termination stage have exited the cycle of change and are no longer tempted to lapse back into their old behavior. They have a new self-image and total self-efficacy with regard to their target behavior. For ideas on changing stages, see the box "Tips for Moving Forward in the Cycle of Behavior Change."

Dealing with Relapse

People seldom progress through the stages of change in a straightforward, linear way. Rather, they tend to move to a new stage and then slip back to a previous stage before resuming their forward progress. Research suggests that most people

FIGURE 1.6 **The stages of change: A spiral model.**

SOURCE: Centers for Disease Control and Prevention. (n.d.) *PEP guide: Personal empowerment plan for improving eating and increasing physical activity.* Dallas, TX: The Cooper Institute.
(bike): © Adam Brown/Getty Images RF; (desk): © Ray Kachatorian/Getty Images

make several attempts before they successfully change a behavior; four out of five people experience some degree of backsliding. For this reason, the stages of change are best conceptualized as a spiral in which people cycle back through previous stages but are further along in the process each time they renew their commitment.

If you experience a *lapse*—a single slip—or a *relapse*—a return to old habits—don't give up. Relapse can be demoralizing, but it is not the same as failure. Failure means stopping before you reach your goal and never changing your target behavior. During the early stages of the change process, it's a good idea to plan for relapse so that you can avoid guilt and self-blame and get back on track quickly. Follow these steps:

1. *Forgive yourself.* A single setback isn't the end of the world, but abandoning your efforts to change could have negative effects on your life.

2. *Give yourself credit for the progress you have already made.* You can use that success as motivation to continue.

3. *Move on.* You can learn from a relapse and use that knowledge to deal with potential setbacks in the future.

Developing Skills for Change: Creating a Personalized Plan

Once you are committed to making a change, put together a plan of action. Your key to success is a well-thought-out plan

TAKE CHARGE
Tips for Moving Forward in the Cycle of Behavior Change

Precontemplation

- **Raise your awareness.** Research your target behavior and its effects.

- **Be self-aware.** Look at the mechanisms you use to resist change, such as denial or rationalization. Find ways to counteract these mechanisms.

- **Seek social support.** Friends and family members can help you identify target behaviors and understand their impact on the people around you.

- **Identify helpful resources.** These might include exercise classes or stress-management workshops offered by your school.

Contemplation

- **Keep a journal.** A record of your target behavior and the circumstances that elicit the behavior can help you plan a change program.

- **Do a cost-benefit analysis.** Identify the costs and benefits (both current and future) of maintaining your behavior and of changing it. Costs can be monetary, social, emotional, and so on.

- **Identify barriers to change.** Knowing these obstacles can help you overcome them.

- **Engage your emotions.** Watch movies or read books about people with your target behavior. Imagine what your life will be like if you don't change.

- **Create a new self-image.** Imagine what you'll be like after changing your target behavior. Try to think of yourself in new terms right now.

- **Think before you act.** Learn why you engage in the target behavior. Determine what "sets you off" and train yourself not to act reflexively.

Preparation

- **Create a plan.** Include a start date, goals, rewards, and specific steps you will take to change your behavior.

- **Make change a priority.** Create and sign a contract with yourself.

- **Practice visualization and self-talk.** These techniques can help prepare you mentally for challenging situations.

- **Take short steps.** Successfully practicing your new behavior for a short time—even a single day—can boost your confidence and motivation.

Action

- **Monitor your progress.** Keep up with your journal entries.

- **Change your environment.** Make changes that will discourage the target behavior—for example, getting rid of snack foods or not stocking the refrigerator with beer.

- **Find alternatives to your target behavior.** Make a list of things you can do to replace the behavior.

- **Reward yourself.** Rewards should be identified in your change plan. Give yourself lots of praise, and focus on your success.

- **Involve your friends.** Tell them you want to change, and ask for their help.

- **Don't get discouraged.** Real change is difficult.

Maintenance

- **Keep going.** Continue using the positive strategies that worked in earlier stages.

- **Be prepared for lapses.** Don't let slip-ups set you back.

- **Be a role model.** After you have successfully changed your behavior, you may be able to help someone else do the same thing.

If relapses keep occurring or if you can't seem to control them, you may need to return to a previous stage of the behavior change process. If this is necessary, reevaluate your goals and your strategy. A different or less stressful approach may help you avoid setbacks when you try again.

---

that sets goals, anticipates problems, and includes rewards. This plan includes the following steps:

1. *Monitor your behavior and gather data.* Keep a record of your target behavior and the circumstances surrounding it. Record this information for at least a week or two. Keep your notes in a health journal or notebook or on your smartphone or computer (see the sample journal entries in Figure 1.7). Record each occurrence of your behavior, noting the following:

   - What the activity was

   - When and where it happened

   - What you were doing

   - How you felt at that time

   If your goal is to start an exercise program, track your activities to determine how to make time for workouts.

2. *Analyze the data and identify patterns.* After you have collected data on the behavior, analyze the data to identify patterns. When are you most likely to overeat? To skip a meal? What events trigger your appetite? Perhaps you are

| Date | November 5 | | | Day | M | **TU** | W TH F SA SU | | | | | |

Time of day	M/S	Food eaten	Cals.	H	Where did you eat?	What else were you doing?	How did someone else influence you?	What made you want to eat what you did?	Emotions and feelings?	Thoughts and concerns?
7:30	M	1 C Crispix cereal 1/2 C skim milk coffee, black 1 C orange juice	110 40 — 120	3	home	looking at news headlines on my phone	alone	I always eat cereal in the morning	a little keyed up & worried	thinking about quiz in class today
10:30	S	1 apple	90	1	hall outside classroom	studying	alone	felt tired & wanted to wake up	tired	worried about next class
12:30	M	1 C chili 1 roll 1 pat butter 1 orange 2 oatmeal cookies 1 soda	290 120 35 60 120 150	2	campus food court	talking	eating w/ friends; we decided to eat at the food court	wanted to be part of group	excited and happy	interested in hearing everyone's plans for the weekend
	M/S = Meal or snack			H = Hunger rating (0–3)						

FIGURE 1.7 Sample health journal entries.

especially hungry at midmorning or when you put off eating dinner until 9:00 P.M. Perhaps you overindulge in food and drink when you go to a particular restaurant or when you're with certain friends. Note the connections between your feelings and such external cues as time of day, location, situation, and the actions of others around you.

3. *Be "SMART" about setting goals.* If your goals are too challenging, you will have trouble making steady progress and will be more likely to give up altogether. If, for example, you are in poor physical condition, it will not make sense to set a goal of being ready to run a marathon within two months. If you set goals you can live with, it will be easier to stick with your behavior change plan and be successful.

Experts suggest that your goals meet the SMART criteria. That is, your behavior change goals should be

- *Specific.* Avoid vague goals like "eat more fruits and vegetables." Instead, state your objectives in specific terms, such as "eat two cups of fruit and three cups of vegetables every day."
- *Measurable.* Recognize that your progress will be easier to track if your goals are quantifiable, so give your goal a number. You might measure your goal in terms of time (such as "walk briskly for 20 minutes a day"), distance ("run two miles, three days per week"), or some other amount ("drink eight glasses of water every day").
- *Attainable.* Set goals that are within your physical limits. For example, if you are a poor swimmer, you might not be able to meet a short-term fitness goal by swimming laps. Walking or biking might be better options.

- *Realistic.* Manage your expectations when you set goals. For example, long-time smokers may not be able to quit cold turkey. A more realistic approach might be to use nicotine replacement patches or gum for several weeks while getting help from a support group.
- *Time frame–specific.* Give yourself a reasonable amount of time to reach your goal, state the time frame in your behavior change plan, and set your agenda to meet the goal within the given time frame.

Using these criteria, sedentary people who want to improve their health and build fitness might set a goal of being able to run three miles in 30 minutes, to be achieved within a time frame of six months. To work toward that goal, they might set a number of smaller, intermediate goals that are easier to achieve. For example, the list of goals might look like this:

WEEK	FREQUENCY	ACTIVITY	DURATION (MINUTES)
1	3	Walk < 1 mile	10–15
2	3	Walk 1 mile	15–20
3	4	Walk 1–2 miles	20–25
4	4	Walk 2–3 miles	25–30
5–7	3–4	Walk/run 1 mile	15–20
21–24	4–5	Run 2–3 miles	25–30

You may not be able to meet these goals, but you never know until you try. As you work toward meeting your long-term goal, you may find it necessary to adjust your short-term goals. For example, you may find that you can start running sooner than you thought, or you may be able to run farther than you originally estimated. In such cases, you may want to make your goals more challenging. To stay motivated, however, some people may choose to make them easier.

For some goals and situations, it may make more sense to focus on something other than your outcome goal. If your goal involves a long-term lifestyle change, such as reaching a healthy weight, focus on developing healthy habits rather than targeting a specific weight loss. Your goal in this case might be exercising 30 minutes every day, reducing portion sizes, or eliminating late-night snacks.

4. *Devise a plan of action.* Develop a strategy that will support your efforts to change. Your plan of action should include the following steps:

- *Get what you need.* Identify resources that can help you. For example, you can join a community walking club or sign up for a smoking cessation program. You may also need to buy some new running shoes or nicotine replacement patches. Get the items you need right away; waiting can delay your progress.

- *Modify your environment.* If you have cues in your environment that trigger your target behavior, try to control them. For example, if you normally have alcohol at home, getting rid of it can help prevent you from indulging. If you usually study with a group of friends in an environment that allows smoking, move to a nonsmoking area. If you always buy a snack at a certain vending machine, change your route to avoid it.

- *Control related habits.* You may have habits that contribute to your target behavior; modifying these habits can help change the behavior. For example, if you usually plop down on the sofa while watching TV, try putting an exercise bike in front of the set that so you can burn calories while watching your favorite programs.

- *Reward yourself.* Giving yourself instant, real rewards for good behavior will reinforce your efforts. Plan your rewards; decide in advance what each one will be and how you will earn it. Tie rewards to achieving specific goals or subgoals. For example, you might treat yourself to a movie after a week of avoiding snacks. Make a list of items or events to use as rewards. They should be special to you and preferably unrelated to food or alcohol.

- *Involve the people around you.* Ask family and friends to help you with your plan. To help them respond appropriately to your needs, create a specific list of dos and don'ts. For example, ask them to support you when you set aside time to exercise or when you avoid second helpings at dinner.

- *Plan for challenges.* Think about situations and people that might derail your program and develop ways to cope with them. For example, if you think it will be hard

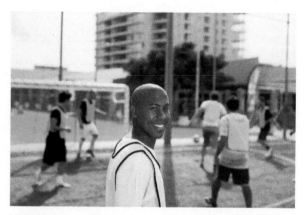

Wellness Tip Your environment contains powerful cues for both positive and negative lifestyle choices. The presence of parks and running/bike paths encourages physical activity, even in an urban setting. Examine your environment for cues that can support your behavior change efforts.
© Tony Tallec/Alamy Stock Photo RF

to stick to your usual exercise program during exams, schedule short bouts of physical activity (such as a brisk walk) as stress-reducing study breaks.

5. *Make a personal contract.* A serious personal contract—one that commits you to your word—can result in a higher chance of follow-through than a casual, offhand promise. Your contract can help prevent procrastination by specifying important dates and can also serve as a reminder of your personal commitment to change.

Your contract should include a statement of your goal and your commitment to reaching it. The contract should also include details, such as the following:

- The date you will start
- The steps you will take to measure your progress
- The strategies you plan to use to promote change
- The date you expect to reach your final goal

Have someone—preferably someone who will be actively helping you with your program—sign your contract as a witness.

Figure 1.8 shows a sample behavior change contract for someone committing to eating more fruit every day. A blank contract is included as Activity 8 in the Behavior Change Workbook at the end of this text.

Putting Your Plan into Action

The starting date has arrived, and you are ready to put your plan into action. This stage requires commitment, the resolve to stick with the plan no matter what temptations you encounter. Remember all the reasons you have to make the change—and remember that *you* are the boss. Use all your strategies to

Behavior Change Contract

1. I, _Tammy Lau_, agree to _increase my consumption of fruit from 1 cup per week to 2 cups per day._

2. I will begin on _10/5_ and plan to reach my goal of _2 cups of fruit per day_ by _12/7_

3. To reach my final goal, I have devised the following schedule of mini-goals. For each step in my program, I will give myself the reward listed.

I will begin to have ½ cup of fruit with breakfast	10/5	see movie
I will begin to have ½ cup of fruit with lunch	10/26	new video game
I will begin to substitute fruit juice for soda 1 time per day	11/16	concert

My overall reward for reaching my goal will be _trip to beach_

4. I have gathered and analyzed data on my target behavior and have identified the following strategies for changing my behavior: _Keep the fridge stocked with easy-to-carry fruit. Pack fruit in my backpack every day. Buy lunch at place that serves fruit._

5. I will use the following tools to monitor my progress toward my final goal:
   Chart on fridge door
   Diet log app

I sign this contract as an indication of my personal commitment to reach my goal: _Tammy Lau_ _9/28_

I have recruited a helper who will witness my contract and _also increase his consumption of fruit; eat lunch with me twice a week._

Eric March _9/28_

FIGURE 1.8 A sample behavior change contract.

make your plan work. Make sure your environment is change friendly, and get as much support and encouragement from others as possible. Keep track of your progress in your health journal, and give yourself regular rewards. And don't forget to give yourself a pat on the back—congratulate yourself; notice how much better you look or feel, and feel good about how far you've come and how you've gained control of your behavior.

Staying with It

As you continue with your program, don't be surprised when you run up against obstacles; they're inevitable. In fact, it's a good idea to expect problems and give yourself time to step back, see how you're doing. Feel free to make some changes before going on. If your program is grinding to a halt, identify what is blocking your progress. It may come from one of the sources described in the following sections.

Social Influences Take a hard look at the reactions of the people you're counting on, and see if they're really supporting you. If they come up short, connect with others who will be more supportive. A related trap is trying to get your friends or family members to change *their* behaviors. The decision to make a major behavior change is something people come to only after intensive self-examination. You may be able to influence someone by tactfully providing facts or support, but that's

all. Focus on yourself. When you succeed, you may become a role model for others.

Levels of Motivation and Commitment You won't make real progress until an inner drive prompts you to the stage of change at which you are ready to make a personal commitment to the goal. If commitment is your problem, you may need to wait until the behavior you're dealing with makes you unhappier or unhealthier; then your desire to change it will be stronger. Or you may find that changing your goal will inspire you to keep going. For more ideas, refer to Activity 9 in the Behavior Change Workbook.

Choice of Techniques and Level of Effort If your plan is not working as well as you thought it would, make changes where you're having the most trouble. If you've lagged on your running schedule, for example, maybe it's because you don't like running. An aerobics class might suit you better. There are many ways to move toward your goal. Or you may not be trying hard enough. Plan to push toward your goal. If it were easy, you wouldn't need a plan.

Stress Barrier If you hit a wall in your program, look at the sources of stress in your life. If the stress is temporary, such as catching a cold or having a term paper due, you may want to wait until it passes before strengthening your efforts. If the stress is ongoing, find healthy ways to manage it (see Chapter 10). You may even want to make stress management your highest priority for behavior change.

Procrastinating, Rationalizing, and Blaming Be alert to games you might be playing with yourself, so you can stop them. Such games include the following:

- *Procrastinating.* If you tell yourself, "It's Friday already; I might as well wait until Monday to start," you're procrastinating. Break your plan into smaller steps that you can accomplish one day at a time.

- *Rationalizing.* If you tell yourself, "I wanted to go swimming today but wouldn't have had time to wash my hair afterward," you're making excuses.

- *Blaming.* If you tell yourself, "I couldn't exercise because Dave was hogging the elliptical trainer," you're blaming others for your own failure to follow through. Blaming is a way of taking focus off the real problem and denying responsibility for your own actions.

Being Fit and Well for Life

Your first attempts at making behavior changes may never go beyond the contemplation or preparation stage. But as you experience some success, you'll start to have more positive feelings about yourself. You may discover new physical activities and sports you enjoy, and you may encounter new situations and meet new people. Perhaps you'll surprise yourself by

Ask Yourself

QUESTIONS FOR CRITICAL THINKING AND REFLECTION

Think about the last time you made an unhealthy choice instead of a healthy one. How could you have changed the situation, the people in the situation, or your own thoughts, feelings, or intentions to avoid making that choice? What can you do in similar situations in the future to produce a different outcome?

TIPS FOR TODAY AND THE FUTURE

You are in charge of your health. Many of the decisions you make every day have an impact on the quality of your life, both now and in the future.

RIGHT NOW YOU CAN

- Go for a 15-minute walk.
- Have a piece of fruit for a snack.
- Call a friend and arrange for a time to catch up with each other.
- Think about whether you have a health behavior you'd like to change. If you do, consider the elements of a behavior change strategy. For example, begin a mental list of the pros and cons of the behavior, or talk to someone who can support you in your attempts to change.

IN THE FUTURE YOU CAN

- Stay current on health and wellness news and issues.
- Participate in health awareness and promotion campaigns in your community—for example, support smoking restrictions in local venues.
- Be a role model for someone else who is working on a health behavior you have successfully changed.

accomplishing things you didn't think were possible—breaking a long-standing nicotine habit, competing in a race, climbing a mountain, or developing a leaner body. Most of all, you'll discover the feeling of empowerment that comes from taking charge of your health. Being healthy takes effort, but the paybacks in energy and vitality are priceless.

Once you've started, don't stop. Assume that health improvement is forever. Take on the easier problems first, and then use what you learn to tackle more difficult problems later. When you feel challenged, remind yourself that you are creating a lifestyle that minimizes your health risks and maximizes your enjoyment of life. You can take charge of your health in a dramatic and meaningful way. *Fit & Well* will show you how.

SUMMARY

- Wellness is the ability to live life fully, with vitality and meaning. Wellness is dynamic and multidimensional; it incorporates physical, emotional, intellectual, interpersonal, cultural, spiritual, environmental, financial, and occupational dimensions.

- As chronic diseases have emerged as major health threats in the United States, people must recognize that they have greater control over and greater responsibility for their health than ever before.

- Behaviors that promote wellness include being physically active, choosing a healthy diet, maintaining a healthy body weight, managing stress effectively, avoiding tobacco and limiting alcohol use, and protecting yourself from disease and injury.

- Although heredity, environment, and health care all play roles in wellness and disease, behavior can mitigate their effects.

- The national Healthy People 2020 initiative aims to prevent disease and improve Americans' quality of life. To achieve this goal, it proposes broad national health objectives, emphasizing the importance of health determinants—factors that affect the health of individuals, demographic groups, or entire populations.

- To make lifestyle changes, you need information about yourself, your health habits, and resources available to help you change.

- You can increase your motivation for behavior change by examining the benefits and costs of change, boosting self-efficacy, and identifying and overcoming key barriers to change.

- The stages-of-change model describes six stages that people may move through as they try to change their behavior: precontemplation, contemplation, preparation, action, maintenance, and termination.

- A specific plan for change can be developed by (1) collecting data on your behavior and recording it in a journal; (2) analyzing the recorded data; (3) setting specific goals; (4) devising strategies for modifying the environment, rewarding yourself, and involving others; and (5) making a personal contract.

- To start and maintain a behavior change program, you need commitment, a well-developed and manageable plan, social support, and strong stress-management techniques. You will also benefit from monitoring the progress of your program and revising it as necessary.

FOR FURTHER EXPLORATION

The Internet addresses listed here were accurate at the time of publication.

Centers for Disease Control and Prevention (CDC). Through phone, fax, and the Internet, the CDC provides a wide variety of health information.

http://www.cdc.gov

Federal Deposit Insurance Corporation: Money Smart. A free source of information, unaffiliated with commercial interests, that includes eight modules on topics such as "borrowing basics" and "paying for college and cars."

> https://www.fdic.gov/consumers/consumer/moneysmart/mscbi/mscbi.html

Federal Trade Commission: Consumer Protection—Health. Includes online brochures about a variety of consumer health topics, including fitness equipment, generic drugs, and fraudulent health claims.

> http://www.ftc.gov/bcp/menus/consumer/health.shtm

Healthfinder. A gateway to online publications, websites, support and self-help groups, and agencies and organizations that produce reliable health information.

> http://www.healthfinder.gov

Health.gov. A portal for online information from a wide variety of federal agencies.

> http://health.gov

Healthy Campus. The American College Health Association's introduction to the Healthy Campus program.

> http://www.acha.org/HealthyCampus

Healthy People. Provides information on Healthy People objectives and priority areas.

> http://www.healthypeople.gov

MedlinePlus. Provides links to news and reliable information about health from government agencies and professional associations; also includes a health encyclopedia and information on prescription and over-the-counter drugs.

> http://www.nlm.nih.gov/medlineplus/

National Health Information Center (NHIC). Puts consumers in touch with the organizations that are best able to provide answers to health-related questions.

> http://www.health.gov/nhic/

National Institutes of Health (NIH). Provides information about all NIH activities as well as consumer publications, hotline information, and an A-to-Z listing of health issues with links to the appropriate NIH institute.

> http://www.nih.gov

National Wellness Institute. Serves professionals and organizations that promote optimal health and wellness.

> http://www.nationalwellness.org

Office of Minority Health. Promotes improved health among racial and ethnic minority populations.

> http://minorityhealth.hhs.gov

Office on Women's Health. Provides information and answers to frequently asked questions.

> http://www.womenshealth.gov

Quantified Self. Offers a forum for people interested in tracking their diet, sleep, and other behaviors and activities using technology.

> http://quantifiedself.com

Surgeon General. Includes information on activities of the Surgeon General and the text of many key reports on such topics as tobacco use, physical activity, and mental health.

> http://www.surgeongeneral.gov

World Health Organization (WHO). Provides information about health topics and issues affecting people around the world.

> http://www.who.int/en

SELECTED BIBLIOGRAPHY

American Cancer Society. 2016. *Cancer Facts and Figures—2016.* Atlanta, GA: American Cancer Society.

American College Health Association. 2017. *American College Health Association—National College Health Assessment II: Reference Group Executive Summary Fall 2016.* Hanover, MD: American College Health Association.

American Heart Association. 2015. *Heart Disease and Stroke Statistics—2016 Update.* Dallas, TX: American Heart Association.

Centers for Disease Control and Prevention. 2016. *Economic Trends in Tobacco* (https://www.cdc.gov/tobacco/data_statistics/fact_sheets/economics/econ_facts/index.htm).

Centers for Disease Control and Prevention. 2013. *Racial and Ethnic Approaches to Community Health (REACH)* (http://www.cdc.gov/nccdphp/dch/programs/reach).

Centers for Medicare and Medicaid Services. 2017. *National Health Expenditure Data: Projections 2016-2025* (https://www.cms.gov/Research-Statistics-Data-and-Systems/Statistics-Trends-and-Reports/NationalHealthExpendData/NationalHealthAccountsProjected.html).

Chacko, A., et al. 2015. Early-life risk factors for chronic nonrespiratory diseases. *European Respiratory Journal* 45: 244–259.

Everett, B. G., et al. 2013. The nonlinear relationship between education and mortality: An examination of cohort, race/ethnic, and gender differences. *Population Research and Policy Review* 32(6).

Fisher, E. G., et al. 2011. Behavior matters. *American Journal of Preventive Medicine* 40(5): e15–30.

Flegal, K. M., et al. 2016. Prevalence and trends in obesity among U.S. adults, 2005–2014. *Journal of the American Medical Association* 315(21): 2284–2291.

Goldrick-Rab, S. 2016. *Paying the Price: College Costs, Financial Aid, and the Betrayal of the American Dream.* Chicago, IL: University of Chicago Press.

Hersi, M., et al. 2017. Risk factors associated with the onset and progression of Alzheimer's disease: A systematic review of the evidence. *NeuroToxicology* March 22, 2017 In press.

Jepsen, R., et al. 2015. Physical activity and quality of life in severely obese adults during a two-year lifestyle intervention programme. *Journal of Obesity* 11, Article ID 314194.

Kaiser Family Foundation. 2016. *Key Facts about the Uninsured Population* (http://kff.org/uninsured/fact-sheet/key-facts-about-the-uninsured-population).

Keehan, S. P., et al. 2017. National health expenditure projections, 2016-25: Price increases, aging push sector to 20 percent of economy. *Health Affairs* 36(3): 553–563.

Kochanek, K. D., et al. 2016. Deaths: Final data for 2014. *National Vital Statistics Reports* 65(4).

Kovesdy, C.P., S. L. Furth, C. Zoccali, on behalf of the World Kidney Day Steering Committee. 2017. Obesity and kidney disease: Hidden consequences of the epidemic. *Journal of Renal Care* 43(1): 3–10.

Mokdad, A. H., et al. 2005. Correction: Actual causes of death in the United States, 2000. *Journal of the American Medical Association* 293(3): 293–294.

Morris. J. K., et al. 2017. Aerobic exercise for Alzheimer's disease: A randomized controlled pilot trial. *PLoS ONE* 12(2): e0170547. (https://doi.org/10.1371/journal.pone.0170547).

National Center for Complementary and Integrative Health. 2014. *Finding and Evaluating Online Resources* (https://nccih.nih.gov/health/webresources).

National Center for Health Statistics. 2017. *National Health Insurance Coverage: Early Release of Estimates from the National Health Interview Survey, 2016* (https://www.cdc.gov/nchs/data/nhis/earlyrelease/insur201705.pdf).

National Center for Health Statistics. 2016. *Healthy People 2020 Midcourse Review.* Hyattsville, MD: National Center for Health Statistics.

National Center for Health Statistics. 2016. *Health, United States, 2015 with Special Feature on Racial and Ethnic Health Disparities.* Hyattsville, Md.: National Center for Health Statistics.

National Kidney Foundation. 2016. Smoking and Your Health (https://www.kidney.org/atoz/content/smoking, accessed April 27, 2017).

National Research Council, Institute of Medicine. 2015. *Measuring the Risks and Causes of Premature Death: Summary of Workshops.* Washington, DC: National Academies Press

Participants at the 6th Global Conference on Health Promotion. 2005. *The Bangkok Charter for Health Promotion in a Globalized World.* Geneva: World Health Organization.

Persky, S., et al. 2014. The role of weight, race, and health care experiences in care use among young men and women. *Obesity* 22(4): 1194–1200.

Pinkhasov, R. M., et al. 2010. Are men shortchanged on health? Perspective on health care utilization and health risk behavior in men and women in the United States. *International Journal of Clinical Practice* 64(4): 475–487.

Taksler, G., et al. 2017. "Resilience and Grit: Pursuing Organizational Change & Preventing Burnout in GIM," *Research presented at The Society of General Internal Medicine 2017 Annual Meeting,* April 19–22, 2017. Washington, DC.

University of California, Berkeley. 2010. *Evaluating Web Pages: Techniques to Apply and Questions to Ask* (http://www.lib.berkeley.edu/TeachingLib/Guides/Internet/Evaluate.html).

U.S. Department of Health and Human Services, Public Health Service, Office of the Surgeon General. 2014. *The Health Consequences of Smoking—50 Years of Progress: A Report of the Surgeon General, 2014.* Atlanta, GA: U.S. Department of Health and Human Services, Centers for Disease Control and Prevention.

Wai, S. N., et al. 2017. Dietary patterns and clinical outcomes in chronic kidney disease: The CKD.QLD nutrition study. *Journal of Renal Nutrition* 27(3): 175–182.

Williams, D. R. 2012. Miles to go before we sleep: Racial inequities in health. *Journal of Health and Social Behavior* 53(3): 279–295.

Wojno, M. A. 2013. 12 Things College Students Don't Need. *Kiplinger,* August 29.

World Health Organization. 2011. *Why Gender and Health?* (http://www.who.int/gender/genderandhealth/en).

Name _____ Section _____ Date _____

LAB 1.1   Your Wellness Profile

Consider how your lifestyle, attitudes, and characteristics relate to each of the dimensions of wellness. Fill in at least three strengths for each dimension (examples of strengths are listed with each dimension). Once you've completed your lists, choose what you believe are your five most important strengths and circle them.

Physical wellness: To maintain overall physical health and engage in appropriate physical activity (e.g., stamina, strength, flexibility, healthy body composition).

_____

_____

_____

Emotional wellness: To have a positive self-concept, deal constructively with your feelings, and develop positive qualities (e.g., optimism, trust, self-confidence, determination).

_____

_____

_____

Intellectual wellness: To pursue and retain knowledge, think critically about issues, make sound decisions, identify problems, and find solutions (e.g., common sense, creativity, curiosity).

_____

_____

_____

Interpersonal/social wellness: To develop and maintain meaningful relationships with a network of friends and family members, and to contribute to your community (e.g., friendly, good-natured, compassionate, supportive, good listener).

_____

_____

_____

Cultural wellness: To accept, value, and even celebrate personal and cultural differences (e.g., refuse to stereotype based on ethnicity, gender, religion, or sexual orientation; create relationships with those who are different from you; maintain and value your own cultural identity).

_____

_____

_____

_____

Spiritual wellness: To develop a set of beliefs, principles, or values that gives meaning or purpose to your life; to develop faith in something beyond yourself (e.g., religious faith, service to others).

_____

_____

_____

Environmental wellness: To protect yourself from environmental hazards and to minimize the negative impact of your behavior on the environment (e.g., carpooling, recycling).

_____

_____

_____

Financial wellness: To be able to live within your means and manage your money in a way that gives you peace of mind (e.g., drawing up a budget, setting up a savings account).

_____

_____

_____

Occupational Wellness: To gain a measure of happiness and fulfillment through your work (e.g., enjoy what you do, feel valued by your manager, build positive relationships with coworkers, take advantage of opportunities to learn and be challenged).

_____

_____

LABORATORY ACTIVITIES

Next, think about where you fall on the wellness continuum for each of the dimensions of wellness. Indicate your placement for each—physical, emotional, intellectual, interpersonal/social, cultural, spiritual, environmental, financial, and occupational—by placing Xs on the continuum below.

| Low level of wellness | Physical, psychological, emotional symptoms | Change and growth | High level of wellness |

Based on both your current lifestyle and your goals for the future, what do you think your placement on the wellness continuum will be in 10 years? What new health behaviors will you have to adopt to achieve your goals? Which of your current behaviors will you need to change to maintain or improve your level of wellness in the future?

_____

_____

Does the description of wellness given in this chapter encompass everything you believe to be part of wellness for you? Write your own definition of wellness, including any additional dimensions that are important to you. Then rate your level of wellness based on your own definition.

_____

_____

Using Your Results

How did you score? Are you satisfied with your current level of wellness—overall and in each dimension? In which dimension(s) would you most like to increase your level of wellness?

_____

_____

Target behavior   **Wellness Dimension**

1. _____   _____

2. _____   _____

3. _____   _____

What should you do next? As you consider possible target behaviors for a behavior change program, choose things that will maintain or increase your level of wellness in one of the dimensions you listed as an area of concern. Remember to consider health behaviors that may threaten your level of wellness in the future, such as smoking or eating a high-fat diet. Below, list several possible target behaviors and the wellness dimensions that they influence.

_____

_____

For additional guidance in choosing a target behavior, complete the lifestyle self-assessment in Lab 1.2.

Name _____ Section _____ Date _____

LAB 1.2 Lifestyle Evaluation

How does your current lifestyle compare with the lifestyle recommended for wellness? For each question, choose the answer that best describes your behavior. Then add up your score for each section.

	Almost Always	Sometimes	Never
Exercise/Fitness			
1. I engage in moderate exercise, such as brisk walking or swimming, for the equivalent of at least 150 minutes per week.	(4)	1	0
2. I do exercises to develop muscular strength and endurance at least twice a week.	(2)	1	0
3. I spend some of my leisure time participating in individual, family, or team activities, such as gardening, bowling, or softball.	(2)	1	0
4. I maintain a healthy body weight, avoiding overweight and underweight.	(2)	1	0
Exercise/Fitness Score: 10			
Nutrition			
1. I eat a variety of foods each day, including seven or more servings of fruits and/or vegetables.	3	(1)	0
2. I limit the amount of saturated and trans fat in my diet.	3	(1)	0
3. I avoid skipping meals.	(2)	1	0
4. I limit the amount of salt and added sugars I eat.	2	(1)	0
Nutrition Score: 5			
Tobacco Use			
1. I avoid smoking cigarettes.	(4)	1	0
2. I avoid using a pipe or cigars.	(3)	1	0
3. I avoid spit tobacco.	(2)	1	0
4. I limit my exposure to environmental tobacco smoke.	(2)	1	0
Tobacco Use Score: 10			
Alcohol and Drugs			
1. I avoid alcohol, or I drink no more than one (women) or two (men) drinks a day.	(4)	1	0
2. I avoid using alcohol or other drugs as a way of handling stressful situations or the problems in my life.	(3)	1	0
3. I am careful not to drink alcohol when taking medications (such as cold or allergy medications) or when pregnant.	(3)	1	0
4. I read and follow the label directions when using prescribed and over-the-counter drugs.	(2)	1	0
Alcohol and Drugs Score: 10			
Emotional Health			
1. I enjoy being a student, and I have a job or do other work that I enjoy.	(3)	1	0
2. I find it easy to relax and express my feelings freely.	2	(1)	0
3. I manage stress well.	2	(1)	0
4. I have close friends, relatives, or others whom I can talk to about personal matters and call on for help when needed.	(2)	1	0
5. I participate in group activities (such as community or church organizations) or hobbies that I enjoy.	(2)	1	0
Emotional Health Score: 8			

LABORATORY ACTIVITIES

		Almost Always	Sometimes	Never

Safety

1.	I wear a safety belt while riding in a car.	②2	1	0
2.	I avoid driving while under the influence of alcohol or other drugs.	②2	1	0
3.	I obey traffic rules and the speed limit when driving.	②2	1	0
4.	I read and follow instructions on the labels of potentially harmful products or substances, such as household cleaners, poisons, and electrical appliances.	②2	1	0
5.	I avoid using a cell phone while driving.	②2	1	0

Safety Score: _____10_____

Disease Prevention

1.	I know the warning signs of cancer, heart attack, and stroke.	②2	1	0
2.	I avoid overexposure to the sun and use sunscreen.	②2	1	0
3.	I get recommended medical screening tests (such as blood pressure and cholesterol checks and Pap tests), immunizations, and booster shots.	②2	1	0
4.	I do not share needles to inject drugs.	②2	1	0
5.	I am not sexually active, *or* I have sex with only one mutually faithful, uninfected partner, *or* I always engage in safer sex (using condoms).	②2	1	0

Disease Prevention Score: _____10_____

Scores of 9 and 10 Excellent! Your answers show that you are aware of the importance of this area to your health. More important, you are putting your knowledge to work for you by practicing good health habits. As long as you continue to do so, this area should not pose a serious health risk.
Scores of 6 to 8 Your health practices in this area are good, but there is room for improvement.
Scores of 3 to 5 Your health risks are showing.
Scores of 0 to 2 You may be taking serious and unnecessary risks with your health.

Using Your Results

How did you score? In which areas did you score the lowest? Are you satisfied with your scores in each area? In which areas would you most like to improve your scores?

_____

_____

What should you do next? To improve your scores, look closely at any item to which you answered "sometimes" or "never." Identify and list at least three possible targets for a health behavior change program. (If you are aware of other risky health behaviors you currently engage in, but that were not covered by this assessment, you may include those in your list.) For each item on your list, identify your current "stage of change" and one strategy you could adopt to move forward (see the section "Enhancing Your Readiness to Change"). Possible strategies might include obtaining information about the behavior, completing an analysis of the pros and cons of change, or beginning a written record of your target behavior.

Behavior	**Stage**	**Strategy**
1. _____	_____	_____
2. _____	_____	_____
3. _____	_____	_____

SOURCE: Adapted from *Healthstyle: A Self-Test,* developed by the U.S. Public Health Service. The behaviors covered in this test are recommended for most Americans, but some may not apply to people with certain chronic diseases or disabilities or to pregnant women, who may require special advice from their physician.

2 Principles of Physical Fitness

LOOKING AHEAD...

After reading this chapter, you should be able to

- Describe how much physical activity is recommended for developing health and fitness.
- Identify the components of physical fitness and the way each component affects wellness.
- Explain the goal and basic principles of physical training.
- Describe the principles involved in designing a well-rounded exercise program.
- List the steps for making an exercise program safe, effective, and successful.

TEST YOUR KNOWLEDGE

1. To improve your health, you must exercise vigorously for at least 30 minutes straight, 5 or more days per week. True or false?

2. Which of the following activities uses about 150 calories?
   a. washing a car for 45–60 minutes
   b. shooting a basketball for 30 minutes
   c. jumping rope for 15 minutes
   d. all three

3. Regular exercise can make a person smarter. True or false?

See answers on the next page.

© WENN Ltd/Alamy Stock Photo

ny list of the benefits of physical activity is impressive. Although people vary greatly in physical fitness and performance ability, the benefits of regular physical activity are available to everyone. Much of the increased health benefits from exercise occurs when going from no activity (sedentary) to some moderate-intensity activity (Figure 2.1). Further health benefits occur when exercising harder or longer. The relative risk of death from all causes and the risk of heart disease decrease by as much as 65% when comparing the least and most active men and women. In Figure 2.1, relative risk of death refers to the risk of death per year of sedentary people compared to people in various activity levels.

This chapter provides an overview of physical fitness. It explains how both lifestyle physical activity and more formal exercise programs contribute to wellness. It also describes the components of fitness, the basic principles of physical training, and the essential elements of a well-rounded exercise program. Chapters 3, 4, 5 and 6 provide in-depth looks at the elements of a fitness program; Chapter 7 puts these elements together in a complete, personalized program.

PHYSICAL ACTIVITY AND EXERCISE FOR HEALTH AND FITNESS

Almost any kind of physical activity promotes health. Try to be more active during the day, regardless of whether you can fit in a formal workout. Short periods of intense exercise do not compensate for hours of inactivity. So try to get up and move around each hour when you are studying, working on the computer, or watching TV (see the box "Move More, Sit Less"). Physical activity and exercise are points along a continuum.

Physical Activity on a Continuum

Physical activity is movement that is carried out by the skeletal muscles and requires energy. Different types of physical activity can vary by ease or intensity. Standing up or walking down a hallway requires little energy or effort, but each is a higher level of activity than sitting or lying down. More intense sustained activities, such as cycling five miles or running in a race, require considerably more effort.

FIGURE 2.1 Exercise promotes longevity. The risk of death each year from all causes decreases with increased amounts and intensities of weekly physical activity.

SOURCES: Adapted from a composite of 12 studies involving more than 200,000 men and women. Wen, M., et al. 2014. "Physical activity and mortality among middleaged and older adults in the United States," *Journal Physical Activity & Health* 11, 303–312; Physical Activity Guidelines Advisory Committee. *Physical Activity Guidelines Advisory Committee Report, 2008.* Washington, D.C. 2008. U.S. Department of Health and Human Services; Schnohr, P., et al. 2015. "Dose of jogging and long-term mortality: the Copenhagen City Heart Study," *Journal American College of Cardiology* 65(5), 411–419.

Exercise refers to planned, structured, repetitive movement intended specifically to improve or maintain physical fitness. As discussed in Chapter 1, physical fitness is a set of physical attributes that allows the body to respond or adapt to the demands and stress of physical effort—to perform moderate to vigorous levels of physical activity without becoming overly tired. Levels of fitness depend on such physiological factors as the heart's ability to pump blood and the energy-generating capacity of the cells. These factors in turn depend both on *genetics*—a person's inborn potential for physical fitness—and *behavior*—getting enough physical activity to stress the body and cause long-term physiological changes.

Physical activity is essential to health and confers wide-ranging health benefits, but exercise is necessary to significantly improve physical fitness. This important distinction between physical activity, which improves health and wellness, and exercise, which improves fitness, is a key concept in understanding the guidelines discussed in this section.

Increasing Physical Activity to Improve Health and Wellness According to the U.S. Surgeon General's Office, "Engaging in regular physical activity is one of the most important things that people of all ages can do to improve their health." Physical activity is central to the national prevention strategy to improve health by promoting community design to support active lifestyles, encouraging exercise in young people, providing safe and accessible places for sports and exercise, and supporting physical activity in the workplace. The U.S. Department of Health and Human Services, American College of Sports Medicine, the American Heart Association, and the Surgeon General's Office have made specific exercise

Answers (Test Your Knowledge)

1. **False.** Experts recommend 150 minutes of moderate-intensity physical activity or 75 minutes of vigorous-intensity physical activity per week. The activity can be done in short bouts—10-minute sessions, for example—spread out over the course of the day.

2. **All three.** The more intense an activity, the more calories it burns in a given amount of time. This is one reason that people who exercise vigorously can get the same benefits in less time than people who exercise longer at a moderate intensity.

3. **True.** Regular exercise (even moderate-intensity exercise) benefits the human brain and nervous system in a variety of ways. For example, exercise improves cognitive function—that is, the brain's ability to learn, remember, think, and reason.

TAKE CHARGE
Move More, Sit Less

A regular exercise program provides huge wellness benefits, but it does not cancel out all the negative effects of too much sitting during the day. Advances in technology promote sedentary behavior; we can now work or study at a desk, watch TV or play video games in our leisure time, order takeout and delivery for meals, and shop and bank online. To avoid the negative health effects of too little daily activity, you may need a plan to reduce your sitting time. Try some of the following strategies:

• Stand up and/or walk when you are on work or personal phone calls.

• Take the stairs whenever and wherever you can; walk up and down escalators instead of just riding them.

• At work, walk to a coworker's desk rather than e-mailing or calling; take the long route to the restroom; and take a walk break whenever you take a coffee or snack break. Drink plenty of water so that you'll have to take frequent restroom breaks.

• Set reminders to get up and move: Use commercial breaks while watching TV; at work or while using a digital device, use the clock function on your computer or phone to make sure you don't sit for longer than an hour at a time.

• Engage in active chores and leisure activities.

• Track your sedentary time to get a baseline, and then continue monitoring to note any improvements. You can also use a fitness tracker such as the Fitbit or step counter to track your general activity level or to set reminders to get up and move after sitting for a particular period of time.

Box Icon: ©VisualCommunications/Getty Images RF

recommendations for promoting health. Their reports stress the importance of regular physical activity and emphasize that some physical activity is better than none. They also present evidence that regular activity promotes health and prevents premature death and a variety of diseases (see Figure 2.1). The reports include the following key guidelines for adults:

• For substantial health benefits, adults should do at least 150 minutes (2 hours and 30 minutes) a week of moderate-intensity aerobic physical activity, or 75 minutes (1 hour and 15 minutes) a week of vigorous-intensity aerobic physical activity, or an equivalent combination of moderate- and vigorous-intensity aerobic activity. Activity should preferably be spread in 30-minute segments throughout the week.

• For additional and more extensive health benefits, adults should increase their aerobic physical activity to 300 minutes (5 hours) a week of moderate-intensity activity, or 150 minutes a week of vigorous-intensity activity, or an equivalent combination of moderate- and vigorous-intensity activity. Adults can enjoy additional health benefits by engaging in physical activity beyond this amount. The Health and Retirement Study—a long-term study of older adults sponsored by the National Institute on Aging—found that people who exercised vigorously had a lower death rate than those who exercised at moderate intensities or did no physical activity. After 16 years, the survival rate was 84% in those doing vigorous exercise, 78% in those doing moderate-intensity physical activity, and only 65% in those doing no physical activity.

• Adults should also do muscle-strengthening activities, such as weight training or calisthenics, that are moderate or high intensity and involve all major muscle groups on two or more days a week. These activities provide additional health benefits— for example, they prevent muscle loss and falls in older adults.

• Everyone should avoid inactivity. Spend less time in front of a television or computer screen because such inactivity decreases metabolic health, contributes to a sedentary lifestyle, and increases the risk of obesity.

The reports state that physical activity benefits people of all ages and of all racial and ethnic groups, including people with disabilities. The reports emphasize that the benefits of activity outweigh the dangers. These levels of physical activity promote health and wellness by lowering the risk of high blood pressure, stroke, heart disease, type 2 diabetes, colon cancer, and osteoporosis and by reducing feelings of mild to moderate depression and anxiety.

What is moderate physical activity? Activities such as brisk walking, dancing, swimming, cycling, and yard work can all count toward the daily total. A moderate amount of activity uses about 150 **calories** of energy and causes a noticeable increase in heart rate, such as would occur with a brisk walk. Examples of activities that use about 150 calories in 15–60 minutes are shown in Figure 2.2. You can burn the same number of calories by doing a lower-intensity activity for a longer time or a higher-intensity activity for a shorter time. People are most likely to participate in physical activities they enjoy, such as dancing.

In contrast to moderate-intensity activity, *vigorous* physical activity—such as jogging—causes rapid breathing and a substantial increase in heart rate (Table 2.1). Physical activity and exercise recommendations for promoting general health, fitness, and weight management are shown in Table 2.2.

> **TERMS**
>
> **physical activity** Body movement that is carried out by the skeletal muscles and requires energy.
>
> **exercise** Planned, structured, repetitive movement intended to improve or maintain physical fitness.
>
> **calorie** The commonly used term for *kilocalorie*, which is a measure of energy equal to the amount of heat it takes to raise the temperature of one liter of water 1°C. One kilocalorie contains 1,000 calories, but the familiar term *calorie* is often used for the larger energy unit, including on food labels.

Common Activities	Duration (min.)	
Washing and waxing a car	45–60	**Less Vigorous, More Time**
Washing windows or floors	45–60	
Gardening	30–45	
Wheeling self in wheelchair	30–40	
Pushing a stroller 1½ miles	30	
Raking leaves	30	
Walking 2 miles	30 (15 min/mile)	
Shoveling snow	15	
Stairwalking	15	

Sporting Activities		
Playing volleyball	45–60	
Playing touch football	45	
Walking 1¾ miles	35 (20 min/mile)	
Basketball (shooting baskets)	30	
Bicycling 5 miles	30	
Dancing fast (social)	30	
Water aerobics	30	
Swimming laps	20	
Basketball (playing game)	15–20	
Bicycling 4 miles	15	
Jumping rope	15	**More Vigorous, Less Time**
Running 1½ miles	15 (10 min/mile)	

FIGURE 2.2 Examples of moderate-intensity physical activity. Each example uses about 150 calories.
SOURCE: National Heart, Lung, and Blood Institute, *Why Is Exercise Important?* (www.nhlbi.nih.gov/health/public/heart/obesity/lose_wt/physical/htm; September 1, 2015).

The daily total of physical activity can be accumulated in multiple bouts of 10 or more minutes per day—for example, two 10-minute bike rides to and from class and a brisk 10-minute walk to the store. In this lifestyle approach to physical activity, people can choose activities that they find enjoyable and that fit into their daily routine; everyday tasks at school, work, and home can be structured to contribute to the daily activity total. If Americans who are currently sedentary were to increase their lifestyle physical activity to 30 minutes per day, both public health and their individual well-being would benefit enormously (see the box "Exercise Is Good for Your Brain").

Increasing Physical Activity to Manage Weight Because two-thirds of Americans are overweight, the U.S. Department of Health and Human Services has also published physical activity guidelines focusing on weight management. These guidelines recognize that for people who need to prevent weight gain, lose weight, or maintain weight loss, 150 minutes per week of physical activity may not be enough. Instead, they recommend up to 90 minutes of physical activity per day. Unfortunately, exercise alone will seldom promote long-term weight loss; but exercise has many health benefits, even in the absence of substantial weight loss.

Exercising to Improve Physical Fitness As mentioned earlier, moderate physical activity confers significant health and wellness benefits, especially for those who are currently sedentary and become moderately active. However, people

Table 2.1	Examples of Moderate- and Vigorous-Intensity Exercise

MODERATE-INTENSITY ACTIVITY	VIGOROUS-INTENSITY ACTIVITY
Uses 3.5–7 calories per minute and causes your breathing and heart rate to increase but still allows for comfortable conversation:	Uses more than 7 calories per minute and increases your heart and breathing rates considerably. These exercises cause larger increases in physical fitness:
• Actively playing with children or pets	• Group exercise: high-impact step aerobics, aerobic dance
• Archery	• Backpacking
• Ballroom dancing	• Basketball, recreational
• Bicycling or stationary bike, moderate pace	• Bicycling, high intensity
• Downhill skiing, moderate intensity	• Calisthenics, vigorous: jumping jacks, burpees, air squats
• Figure skating, recreational	• Circuit weight training
• Fly fishing or walking along stream	• Cross-country skiing or snowshoeing
• Gardening or yard work, moderate pace	• Cross-training, such as CrossFit
• Golf	• Downhill skiing, vigorous intensity
• Hiking, leisurely pace	• Football, recreational
• Horseback riding, recreational	• Gardening or yard work, shoveling heavy snow, digging ditches
• Housework, moderate intensity	• Hand cycling
• Skateboarding	• Horseback riding, galloping or jumping
• Softball	• In-line skating
• Using stair-climber, elliptical trainer, or rowing machine, moderate pace	• Interval training: running, elliptical trainer, swimming, cycling
• Table tennis	• Jogging
• Tennis, doubles	• Kayaking, whitewater
• Walking at a moderate pace: walking to school or work, walking for pleasure	• Pushing a car
• Water aerobics	• Running up stairs
• Waxing the car	• Soccer, recreational
• Weight training and bodybuilding	• Tennis, singles
• Yoga	• Wheelchair wheeling training

SOURCE: Centers for Disease Control and Prevention. 2015. (http://www.cdc.gov/nccdphp/dnpa/physical/pdf/PA_Intensity_table_2_1.pdf)

Table 2.2	Physical Activity and Exercise Recommendations for Promoting General Health, Fitness, and Weight Management

GOAL	RECOMMENDATION
General health	Perform moderate-intensity aerobic physical activity for at least 150 minutes per week (30 minutes 5 times per week) or 75 minutes of vigorous-intensity physical activity per week (25 minutes 3 times per week). Also, be more active in your daily life: Walk instead of driving, take the stairs instead of the elevator, and watch less television.
Increased health benefits	Exercise at moderate intensity for 300 minutes per week or at vigorous intensity for 150 minutes per week.
Achieve or maintain weight loss	Exercise moderately for 60–90 minutes per day on most days of the week.
Muscle strength and endurance	Perform 1 or more sets of resistance exercises that work the major muscle groups for 8–12 repetitions (10–15 reps for older adults) on at least two nonconsecutive days per week. Examples include weight training and exercises that use body weight as resistance (such as core-stabilizing exercises, pull-ups, push-ups, lunges, and squats).
Flexibility	Perform range-of-motion (stretching) exercises at least two or three days per week. Hold each stretch for 10–30 seconds.
Neuromuscular training	Older adults should do balance training at least two or three days per week. Examples include yoga, tai chi, and balance exercises (standing on one foot, step-ups, and walking lunges). These exercises are beneficial for young and middle-aged adults, as well.

SOURCES: American College of Sports Medicine. 2011. *ACSM's Guidelines for Exercise Testing and Prescription,* 10th ed. Philadelphia: Wolters Kluwer; Garber, C. E., et al. "Quantity and quality of exercise for developing and maintaining cardiorespiratory, musculoskeletal, and neuromotor fitness in apparently healthy adults: Guidance for prescribing exercise," *Medicine and Science in Sports and Exercise* 43(7), 1334–1359.

can obtain even greater health and wellness benefits by increasing the duration and intensity of physical activity. With increased activity, they will see more improvements in quality of life and greater reductions in disease and mortality risk.

More vigorous activity, as in a structured, systematic exercise program, also improves physical fitness. Moderate physical activity alone is not enough. Physical fitness requires more intense movement that poses a substantially greater challenge to the body. The American College of Sports Medicine has issued guidelines for creating a formal exercise program that will develop physical fitness. These guidelines are described in detail later in the chapter.

How Much Physical Activity Is Enough?

Some experts believe that people get most of the health benefits of physical activity simply by becoming more active over the course of the day; the amount of activity needed depends on an individual's health status and goals. Other experts believe that leisure-time physical activity is not enough; they argue that people should exercise long enough and intensely enough to improve the body's capacity for exercise—that is, to improve physical fitness. There is probably some truth in both of these positions.

Regular physical activity, regardless of the intensity, makes you healthier and can help protect you from many chronic diseases. Although you get many of the health benefits of exercise by being more active, you obtain even more benefits when you are physically fit. In addition to long-term health benefits, fitness also contributes significantly to quality of life. Fitness can give you freedom to move your body the way you want. Fit people have more energy and better body control. They can enjoy a more active lifestyle than their more sedentary

counterparts. Even if you don't like sports, you need physical energy and stamina in your daily life and for many non-sport leisure activities, such as visiting museums, playing with children, and gardening.

Where does this leave you? Most experts agree that some physical activity is better than none, but that more—as long as it does not result in injury—is better than some. To set a personal goal for physical activity and exercise, consider your current activity level, your health status, and your overall goals. At the very least, strive to become more active and do 30 minutes of moderate-intensity activity at least five days per week. Choose to be active whenever you can. If weight management is a concern for you, begin by achieving the goal of 30 minutes of activity per day and then try to raise your activity level further, to 60–90 minutes per day or more. For even better health and well-being, participate in a structured exercise program that develops physical fitness. Any increase in physical activity will contribute to your health and well-being, now and in the future.

COMPONENTS OF PHYSICAL FITNESS

Some components of fitness relate to specific skill activities, such as tennis and skiing, and others to general health. **Health-related fitness** includes the following components:

- Cardiorespiratory endurance
- Muscular strength
- Muscular endurance
- Flexibility
- Body composition

THE EVIDENCE FOR EXERCISE
Exercise Is Good for Your Brain

Some scientists call exercise the new "brain food." Studies show that even moderate physical activity can improve brain health and function and may delay the decline in cognitive function that occurs for many people as they age. Regular physical activity has the following positive effects on the brain:

- Exercise improves cognitive function—the brain's ability to learn, remember, think, and reason.

- Exercise can help overcome the negative effects of a poor diet on brain health.

- Exercise promotes the creation of new nerve cells (neurons) throughout the nervous system. By promoting this process (called *neurogenesis*), exercise provides protection against injury and degenerative conditions that destroy neurons. Physical activity is less effective for promoting brain health when exercising in polluted air.

- Exercise enhances the nervous system's *plasticity*—its ability to change and adapt. In the brain, spinal cord, and nerves, this can mean developing new pathways for transmitting sensory information or motor commands.

- Exercise appears to have a protective effect on the brain as people age, helping to delay or even prevent the onset of neurodegenerative disorders such as Alzheimer's disease.

- Exercise reduces anxiety—a consistent finding independent of culture, gender, age, education, and socioeconomic status. It promotes the release of endorphins, which in turn promotes feelings of well-being and prevents depression.

Although most people consider brain health to be a concern for the elderly, it is vital to wellness throughout life. For this reason, many studies on exercise and brain health include children as well as older adults. Targeted research has also focused on the impact of exercise on people with disorders such as cerebral palsy, multiple sclerosis, and developmental disabilities. Generally speaking, these studies all reach a similar conclusion: Exercise enhances brain health, at least to some degree, in people of all ages and a wide range of health statuses.

Along with the brain's physical health, mental health is enhanced by exercise. Even modest activity, such as taking a daily walk, can help combat a variety of mental health disorders and improve mood.

It's hard to understate the impact of physical and mental disorders related to brain health. According to the Alzheimer's Association, 5.3 million Americans currently suffer from Alzheimer's disease, and the number is increasing at a rate of 70 people per second. People with depression, anxiety, or other mental disorders are more likely to suffer from chronic physical conditions. Taken together, these and other brain-related disorders cost untold millions of dollars in health care costs and lost productivity, as well as thousands of years of productive lifetime lost.

So, for the sake of your brain—as well as your muscles, bones, and heart—start creating your exercise program soon. You'll be healthier, and you may even feel a little smarter.

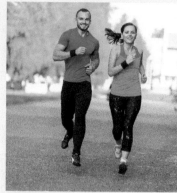

©Aleksandr Markin/123RF

SOURCES: Stubbs, B., et al. 2015. "Physical activity and anxiety," *Journal Affective Disorders* 208, 2017, 545–552; Szuhany, K. L., et al., "A meta-analytic review of the effects of exercise on brain-derived neurotrophic factor," *Journal of Psychiatric Research* 60, 56–64; Garber, C. E., et al. 2011. "Quantity and quality of exercise for developing and maintaining cardiorespiratory, musculoskeletal, and neuromotor fitness in apparently healthy adults: Guidance for prescribing exercise," *Medicine and Science in Sports and Exercise* 43(7), 1334–1359.

Box Icon: © Vstock LLC/Getty Images RF

Health-related fitness helps you withstand physical challenges and protects you from diseases.

Cardiorespiratory Endurance

Cardiorespiratory endurance is the ability to perform prolonged, large-muscle, dynamic exercise at moderate to high levels of intensity. It depends on such factors as the ability of the lungs to deliver **oxygen** from the environment to the bloodstream, the capacity of the heart to pump blood, the ability of the nervous system and blood vessels to regulate blood flow, and the capability of the cells' chemical systems to use oxygen and process fuels for exercise and rest.

When cardiorespiratory fitness is low, the heart has to work hard during normal daily activities and may not be able to work hard enough to sustain high-intensity physical activity in an emergency. As cardiorespiratory fitness improves, related physical functions also improve:

- The heart pumps more blood per heartbeat.
- The ability to consume oxygen due to adaptations in the heart, circulation, and tissues improves.
- Breathing volume decreases during daily activities and submaximal exercising—that is, when exercising at less than full intensity.
- Resting heart rate slows.
- Blood volume increases.
- Blood supply to tissues improves.
- The body can cool itself better.
- Blood vessels become more pliable.
- Resting blood pressure decreases.
- Metabolism in skeletal muscle is enhanced, which improves fuel use.
- The level of antioxidant chemicals in the body increases and oxidative stress decreases. During metabolism, the body naturally produces chemicals called free radicals (oxidative stress) that cause cell damage. Exercise training increases the production of antioxidants that help neutralize free radicals.

A healthy heart can better withstand the strains of everyday life, the stress of occasional emergencies, and the wear and tear of time.

Cardiovascular endurance training also improves the functioning of the body's chemical systems, particularly in the muscles and liver. These changes enhance the body's ability to derive energy from food, allow the body to perform more exercise with less effort, increase sensitivity to insulin, and prevent type 2 diabetes. Exercise reduces blood vessel inflammation, which is linked to coronary artery disease, heart attack, and stroke. Exercise helps maintain normal levels of water and electrolytes in the cells, which in turn preserves muscle cell function and delays fatigue.

Physically fit people also have healthier, more resilient genes. Exercise preserves gene structures called telomeres, which form the ends of the DNA strands and hold them together. Over time the telomeres shorten, reducing their effectiveness, which triggers illness and death. Exercise helps to keep them from getting too short.

Cardiorespiratory endurance is a central component of health-related fitness because heart and lung function is so essential to overall good health. A person can't live very long or very well without a healthy heart or healthy lungs. Poor cardiorespiratory fitness is linked with heart disease, type 2 diabetes, colon cancer, stroke, depression, and anxiety. A moderate level of cardiorespiratory fitness can help compensate for certain health risks, including excess body fat: People who have higher levels of body fat but who otherwise are fit have been found to have lower death rates than those who are lean but have low cardiorespiratory fitness.

You can develop cardiorespiratory endurance through activities that involve continuous, rhythmic movements of large-muscle groups, such as the legs. Such activities include walking, jogging, cycling, and group aerobics.

Ask Yourself

QUESTIONS FOR CRITICAL THINKING AND REFLECTION

Does your current lifestyle include enough physical activity—30 minutes of moderate-intensity activity five or more days a week—to support health and wellness? Does your lifestyle go beyond this level to include enough vigorous physical activity and exercise to build physical fitness? What changes could you make in your lifestyle to develop physical fitness?

Fitness Tip Cardiorespiratory endurance is a key component of health-related fitness. Like studying, you'll be more likely to exercise if you set aside blocks of time for it and make it part of your daily routine. Schedule your workouts, make them a priority, and include alternatives to account for things such as bad weather and vacations.
©John P Kelly/Getty Images

Muscular Strength

Muscular strength is the amount of force a muscle can produce with a single maximum effort. It depends on such factors as the size of muscle cells and the ability of nerves to activate muscle cells. **Relative strength** is the maximum force exerted relative to body weight, body size, and muscle size. Strong muscles are important for everyday activities, such as climbing stairs, as well as for emergency situations. They help keep the skeleton in proper alignment, preventing back and leg pain and providing the support necessary for good posture. Muscular strength has obvious importance in recreational activities. Strong people can hit a tennis ball harder, kick a soccer ball farther, and ride a bicycle uphill more easily.

TERMS

muscular strength   The amount of force a muscle can produce with a single maximum effort.

relative strength   The maximum force exerted, relative to body weight, body size, and muscle size.

Muscle tissue is an important element of overall body composition. Greater muscle mass means faster energy use and a higher rate of **metabolism**, and the sum of all the vital processes by which food energy and nutrients are made available to and used by the body. Greater muscle mass reduces markers of oxidative stress and maintains mitochondria (the "powerhouses" of the cell); both of these benefits are important for metabolic health and long life. Training to build muscular strength can also help people manage stress and boost their self-confidence.

Maintaining strength and muscle mass is vital for healthy aging. Stronger people live longer. Older people tend to experience a decrease in both number and size of muscle cells, a condition called *sarcopenia*. Many of the remaining muscle cells become slower, and some become nonfunctional because they lose their attachment to the nervous system. Strength training (also known as *resistance training* or *weight training*) increases antioxidant enzymes and lowers oxidative stress. It also helps maintain muscle mass and function and possibly helps decrease the risk of osteoporosis (bone loss) in older people, greatly enhancing their quality of life and preventing life-threatening injuries.

Muscular Endurance

Muscular endurance is the ability to resist fatigue and sustain a given level of muscle tension—that is, to hold a muscle contraction for a long time or to contract a muscle over and over again. It depends on such factors as the size of muscle cells, the ability of muscles to store fuel, blood supply, and the metabolic capacity of muscles.

Muscular endurance is important for good posture and for injury prevention. For example, if abdominal and back muscles cannot support and stabilize the spine correctly when you sit or stand for long periods, the chances of low back pain and back injury are increased. Good muscular endurance in the trunk

muscles is more important than muscular strength for preventing back pain. Muscular endurance helps people cope with daily physical demands and enhances performance in sports and work.

Flexibility

Flexibility is the ability to move the joints through their full ranges of motion. It depends on joint structure, the length and elasticity of connective tissue, and nervous system activity. Flexible, pain-free joints are important for good health and well-being. Inactivity causes the joints to become stiffer with age. Stiffness, in turn, often causes people to assume unnatural body postures that can stress joints and muscles. Stretching exercises can help ensure a healthy range of motion for all major joints.

Body Composition

Body composition refers to the proportion of fat and **fat-free mass** (muscle, bone, and water) in the body. Healthy body composition involves a high proportion of fat-free mass and an acceptably low level of body fat, adjusted for age and gender. A person with excessive body fat—especially excess fat in the abdomen—is more likely to experience health problems, including heart disease, insulin resistance, high blood pressure, stroke, joint problems, type 2 diabetes, gallbladder disease, blood vessel inflammation, some types of cancer, back pain, and premature death.

The best way to lose fat is through a lifestyle that includes a sensible diet and exercise. The best way to add muscle mass is through strength training. Large changes in body composition are not necessary to improve health; even a small increase in physical activity and a small decrease in body fat can lead to substantial health improvements.

Somatotype, or body build, affects a person's choice of exercise. *Endomorphs* are round and pear-shaped. They often excel at weight lifting and weight-supported aerobic exercises such as swimming or cycling. Conversely, they might find distance running difficult and painful. *Mesomorphs* are lean and muscular and usually excel at almost any kind of physical activity or sport. *Ectomorphs* are thin and linear. Their light frame helps them succeed in activities such as distance running and ballet. No matter what body type you have, you can benefit from some form of physical activity.

Skill (Neuromuscular)-Related Components of Fitness

In addition to the five health-related components of physical fitness, the ability to perform a particular sport or activity may depend on **skill (neuromuscular)-related fitness**. Neuromuscular refers to the complex control of muscles and movement by the brain and spinal column. The components of skill-related fitness include the following:

- *Speed*—the ability to perform a movement in a short period of time

- *Power*—the ability to exert force rapidly, based on a combination of strength and speed

---

metabolism   The sum of all the vital processes by which food energy and nutrients are made available to and used by the body.

muscular endurance   The ability of a muscle to remain contracted or to contract repeatedly for a long period of time.

flexibility   The ability to move joints through their full ranges of motion.

body composition   The proportion of fat and fat-free mass (muscle, bone, and water) in the body.

fat-free mass   The nonfat component of the human body, consisting of skeletal muscle, bone, and water.

somatotype   A body-type classification system that describes people as predominantly muscular (mesomorph), tall and thin (ectomorph), or round and heavy (endomorph).

skill (neuromuscular)-related fitness   Physical capacities that contribute to performance in a sport or an activity, including speed, power, agility, balance, coordination, and reaction time; neuromuscular fitness refers specifically to maintaining performance levels of balance, agility, and coordination through the control of muscles and movement by the brain and spinal column.

TERMS

- *Agility*—the ability to change the position of the body quickly and accurately
- *Balance*—the ability to maintain equilibrium while moving or while stationary
- *Coordination*—the ability to perform motor tasks accurately and smoothly using body movements and the senses
- *Reaction and movement time*—the ability to respond and react quickly to a stimulus

Skill-related fitness tends to be sport-specific and is best developed through practice. For example, playing basketball can develop the speed, coordination, and agility needed to engage in the sport. Participating in sports is fun, can help build fitness, and contributes to other areas of wellness. Young adults often find it easier to exercise regularly when they participate in sports and activities they enjoy, such as dancing, tennis, snowboarding, or basketball.

While not considered a health-related fitness component, neuromuscular fitness is important for healthy aging. Older adults are at risk for life-threatening falls, and development of neuromuscular fitness can reduce the risk of falls. Neuromuscular training activities such as yoga and tai chi are recommended for older adults.

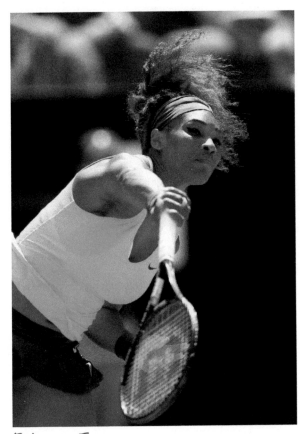

Fitness Tip You don't need to develop the skills of a professional athlete to participate in sports, but boosting sport-specific skills such as speed, power, coordination, and reaction time can make participating in sports more fun. And if you enjoy yourself, you are more likely to stick with the activity!
©Clive Mason/Getty Images

PRINCIPLES OF PHYSICAL TRAINING: ADAPTATION TO STRESS

The human body is very adaptable. The greater the demands made on it, the more it adjusts to meet those demands. Over time, immediate, short-term adjustments (**adaptations**) translate into long-term changes and improvements. When breathing and heart rate increase during exercise, for example, the heart gradually develops the ability to pump more blood with each beat. Then, during exercise, it doesn't have to beat as fast to meet the cells' demands for oxygen. The goal of **physical training** is to produce these long-term changes and improvements in the body's functioning and fitness. Although people differ in the maximum levels of physical fitness and performance they can achieve through training, the wellness benefits of exercise are available to everyone (see the box "Fitness and Disability").

Particular types and amounts of exercise are most effective in developing the various components of fitness. To put together an effective exercise program, you should first understand the basic principles of physical training, including the following:

- Specificity
- Progressive overload
- Reversibility
- Individual differences

All of these rest on the larger principle of adaptation.

Specificity—Adapting to Type of Training

To develop a particular fitness component, you must perform exercises designed specifically for that component. This is the principle of **specificity**. Weight training, for example, develops muscular strength but is less effective for developing cardiorespiratory endurance or flexibility. Specificity also applies to the skill-related fitness components (to improve at tennis, you must practice tennis) and to the different parts of the body (to develop stronger arms, you must exercise your arms). A well-rounded exercise program includes exercises geared to each component of fitness, to different parts of the body, and to specific activities or sports.

Sports science pioneer Franklin Henry from the University of California, Berkeley, developed the principle of specificity of training. His studies showed that a specific movement performed at a specific speed develops a unique skill. Motor-control studies have shown that practice reinforces motor

adaptation   The physiological changes that occur with exercise training.   TERMS

physical training   The performance of different types of activities that cause the body to adapt and improve its level of fitness.

specificity   The training principle that developing a particular fitness component requires performing exercises specifically designed for that component.

DIVERSITY MATTERS
Fitness and Disability

Physical fitness and athletic achievement are not limited to the able-bodied. People with disabilities can also attain high levels of fitness and performance. Elite athletes compete in the Paralympics, the premier event for athletes with disabilities that is held in the same year and city as the Olympics. The performance of these skilled athletes makes it clear that people with disabilities can be active, healthy, and extraordinarily fit. Just like able-bodied athletes, athletes with disabilities strive for excellence and can serve as role models.

©Boomer Jerritt/All Canada Photos/Getty Images

According to the U.S. Census Bureau, about 57 million Americans have some type of chronic disability. Some disabilities are the result of injury, such as spinal cord injuries sustained in car crashes or war. Other disabilities result from illness, such as the blindness that sometimes occurs as a complication of diabetes or the joint stiffness that accompanies arthritis. And some disabilities are present at birth, as in the case of congenital limb deformities or cerebral palsy.

Exercise and physical activity are as important for people with disabilities as for able-bodied individuals—if not more important. Being active helps prevent secondary conditions that may result from prolonged inactivity, such as circulatory or muscular problems. Currently, about 19% of people with disabilities engage in regular moderate-intensity activity.

People with disabilities don't have to be elite athletes to participate in sports and lead an active life. Some health clubs, fitness centers, city recreation centers, and universities offer activities and events geared for people of all ages and types of disabilities. They may have modified aerobics classes, special weight-training machines, classes for mild exercise in warm water, and other activities adapted for people with disabilities. Popular sports and recreational activities include adapted horseback riding, golf, swimming, and skiing. Competitive sports are also available—for example, there are wheelchair versions of billiards, tennis, weight lifting, hockey, and basketball, as well as sports for people with hearing, visual, or mental impairments. For those who prefer to get their exercise at home, special videos are geared to individuals who use wheelchairs or who have arthritis, hearing impairments, metabolic diseases, or many other disabilities.

The U.S. Department of Education's Office for Civil Rights has issued guidelines for providing equal opportunities for sports and exercise to students with disabilities. Schools and universities must make reasonable modifications to ensure that students with disabilities have equal access to sports and physical education.

If you have a disability and want to be more active, check with your physician about what's appropriate for you. Contact your local community center, university, YMCA/YWCA, hospital, independent living center, or fitness center to locate facilities. Look for a facility with experienced personnel and appropriate adaptive equipment. For specialized videos, check with hospitals and health associations that address specific disabilities, such as the Arthritis Foundation.

Box icon: © Rawpixel Ltd/Getty Images RF

patterns in the brain that are specific to a given movement. In other words, there is no general coordination, agility, balance, and accuracy. The balance required in skiing is different from the balance required to stand on one foot or do tricks on a skateboard. Each requires its own specific training.

Progressive Overload—Adapting to the Amount of Training and the FITT-VP Principle

The body adapts to the demands of exercise by improving its functioning. When the amount of exercise (also called *overload* or *stress*) is increased progressively, fitness continues to improve. This is the principle of **progressive overload**.

The amount of overload is important. Too little exercise will have no effect on fitness (although it may improve health); too much may cause injury and problems with the body's immune or endocrine (hormone) systems. The point at which exercise becomes excessive is highly individual; it occurs at a much higher level in an Olympic athlete than in a sedentary person. For every type of exercise, there is a training threshold at which fitness benefits begin to occur, a zone within which maximum fitness benefits occur, and an upper limit of safe training.

The amount of exercise needed depends on the individual's current level of fitness, the person's genetically determined capacity to adapt to training, his or her fitness goals, and the

progressive overload   The training principle that progressively increasing amounts of stress on the body causes adaptation that improves fitness.

TERMS

component being developed. A novice, for example, might experience fitness benefits from jogging a mile in 10 minutes, but this level of exercise would not benefit a trained distance runner. Beginners should start at the lower end of the fitness benefit zone; fitter individuals will make more rapid gains by exercising at the higher end of the fitness benefit zone. Progressive overload is critical. Performing the same amount of exercise during every training session will maintain fitness but will not increase it because the training stress is below the threshold required to produce adaptation. Fitness increases only if overload increases.

The amount of overload needed to maintain or improve a particular level of fitness for a particular fitness component is determined through six dimensions, represented by the acronym FITT-VP:

- *Frequency*—how often
- *Intensity*—how hard or how fast
- *Time*—how long (duration)
- *Type*—mode of activity
- *Volume*—how much (frequency × intensity × time)
- *Progression*—how a program advances over time

Chapters 3, 4, and 5 show you how to apply the FITT-VP principle to exercise programs for cardiorespiratory endurance, muscular strength and endurance, and flexibility, respectively.

Frequency Developing fitness requires regular exercise. Optimum exercise frequency, expressed in number of days per week, varies with the component being developed and the individual's fitness goals. For most people, a frequency of three to five days per week for cardiorespiratory endurance exercise and two or more days per week for resistance and flexibility training are appropriate for a general fitness program.

An important consideration in determining appropriate exercise frequency is recovery time. The amount of time required to

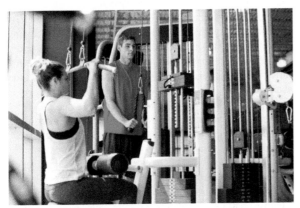

Fitness Tip Progressive overload is important because the body adapts to overload by becoming more fit. This is true even if your starting level of fitness is low. At the gym, don't be intimidated by people who seem to be in better shape than you are. Remember: They got in shape by focusing on themselves, not by worrying about what other people thought about them.
©Hero Images/Getty Images RF

recover from exercise is highly individual and depends on factors such as training experience, age, and intensity of training. For example, 24 hours of rest between highly intense workouts involving heavy weights or track sprints is not enough recovery time for safe and effective training in most cases. Intense workouts need to be spaced out during the week to allow for sufficient recovery time. On the other hand, you can exercise every day if your program consists of moderate-intensity walking or cycling. Learn to "listen to your body" to get enough rest between workouts. Chapters 3, 4, and 5 provide more detailed information about training techniques and recovery periods for workouts focused on different fitness components.

Intensity Fitness benefits occur when a person exercises harder than his or her normal level of activity. The appropriate exercise intensity varies with each fitness component. To develop cardiorespiratory endurance, for example, you must raise your heart rate above normal; you might do that by walking, swimming, or cycling faster. To develop muscular strength, you must lift a heavier weight than normal. To develop flexibility, you must stretch muscles beyond their normal length.

Time (Duration) Fitness benefits occur when you exercise for an extended period of time. For cardiorespiratory endurance exercise, 20–60 minutes per exercise session is recommended. Exercise can take place in a single session or in several sessions of 10 or more minutes. The greater the intensity of exercise, the less time needed to obtain fitness benefits. For high-intensity exercise, such as running, 20–30 minutes is appropriate. For moderate-intensity exercise, such as walking, 45–60 minutes may be needed. High-intensity exercise poses a greater risk of injury than low-intensity exercise, so if you are a nonathletic adult, it's best to first emphasize low- to moderate-intensity activity of longer duration.

To build muscular strength, muscular endurance, and flexibility, similar amounts of time are advisable, but training for these health components is more commonly organized in terms of a specific number of *repetitions* of a particular exercise. For resistance training, for example, a recommended program includes one or more sets of 8–12 repetitions of 8–10 different exercises that work the major muscle groups. Older adults should do 10–15 repetitions per set with lighter weights.

Type (Mode of Activity) The type of exercise in which you should engage varies with each fitness component and with your personal fitness goals. To develop cardiorespiratory endurance, you need to engage in continuous activities involving large-muscle groups—walking, jogging, cycling, or swimming, for example. Resistance exercises develop muscular strength and endurance, and stretching exercises build flexibility. The frequency, intensity, and time of the exercise will be different for each type of activity. (See the section "Designing Your Own Exercise Program" for more on choosing appropriate activities for your fitness program.)

Volume Volume is the product of frequency, intensity, and time—the FIT of exercise. For endurance exercise, average adults should strive to expend about 1,000 calories per week in exercise, which is the equivalent of about 150 minutes per week of moderate-intensity exercise. This same volume of exercise can be accomplished in a shorter or longer time-frame, depending on the FIT variables. For example, 75 minutes of vigorous-intensity exercise will also burn about 1,000 calories. Volume also applies to other fitness components: In weight training, lifting 10 pounds for 3 sets of 10 repetitions produces a total volume of 300 pounds ($10 \times 3 \times 10$); lifting 20 pounds in the same workout increases the volume to 600 pounds.

Progression Fitness levels off as the body adapts to exercise training, so you need to gradually increase overload over time to improve fitness. How quickly you adapt to training depends on your genetic makeup and the effort you put into your training program. To avoid injury, progress by slowly increasing the volume of exercise; for example, add 5 minutes to your jogging workout or add 10 pounds for a weight training exercise. Don't increase frequency, intensity, and time all at once. With each increase, make sure you can maintain your program before moving forward. Don't overtrain: excessive exercise can cause injury and fatigue.

Reversibility—Adapting to a Reduction in Training

Fitness is a reversible adaptation. The body adjusts to lower levels of physical activity the same way it adjusts to higher levels. This is the principle of **reversibility**. When a person stops exercising, up to 50% of fitness improvements are lost within two months. However, not all fitness levels reverse at the same rate. Strength fitness is very resilient, so a person can maintain strength fitness by doing resistance exercise as infrequently as once a week. In contrast, cardiovascular and cellular fitness reverse themselves more quickly—sometimes within just a few days or weeks. If you must temporarily reduce the frequency or duration of your training, you can maintain much of your fitness improvement by keeping the intensity of your workouts constant.

Individual Differences—Limits on Adaptability

Anyone watching the Olympics can see that, from a physical standpoint, we are not all created equal. There are large individual differences in our ability to improve fitness, achieve a desirable body composition, and learn and perform sports skills. Some people are able to run longer distances, lift more weight, or kick a soccer ball more skillfully than others will ever be able to, no matter how much they train. People respond to training at different rates, so a program that works for one person may not be right for another person.

There are limits on the adaptability—the potential for improvement—of any human body. The body's ability to transport and use oxygen, for example, can be improved by only about 5–30% through training. An endurance athlete must therefore inherit a large metabolic capacity to reach competitive performance levels. In the past few years, scientists have identified specific genes that influence body fat, strength, and endurance. For example, more than 800 genes are associated with endurance performance, and 100 of those determine individual differences in exercise capacity. However, physical training improves fitness regardless of heredity. The average person's body can improve enough to achieve reasonable fitness goals.

DESIGNING YOUR OWN EXERCISE PROGRAM

Physical training works best when you have a plan. A plan helps you make gradual but steady progress toward your goals. First, determine that exercise is safe for you (or your family members); then assess how fit you are, decide what your goals are, and choose the right activities to help you get there.

Getting Medical Clearance

Participating in exercise and sports is usually a wonderful experience that improves wellness in both the short and the long term. In rare instances, however, vigorous exertion is associated with sudden death. It may seem difficult to understand that although regular exercise protects people from heart disease, exercise also increases the risk of sudden death for some.

Exercise and Cardiac Risk Overall, the risk of death from exercise is small—and people are much safer exercising than engaging in many other common activities, including driving a car. One study of joggers found one death for every 396,000 hours of jogging; another study of men involved in a variety of physical activities found one death per 1.5 million hours of exercise.

In people under age 35, congenital heart defects (heart abnormalities present at birth) are the most common cause of exercise-related sudden death. In nearly all other cases, coronary artery disease is responsible. In this condition, fat and other substances build up in the arteries that supply blood to the heart. Death can result if an artery becomes blocked or if the heart's rhythm and pumping action are disrupted. Exercise, particularly intense exercise, may trigger a heart attack in someone with underlying heart disease. The riskiest scenario may involve the middle-aged or older individual who suddenly begins participating in a vigorous sport or activity after being sedentary for a long time. Engaging in very vigorous exercise over the long term can also be risky for some individuals, due to the stress on the cardiovascular system.

---

reversibility   The training principle that fitness improvements are lost when demands on the body are lowered.

TERMS

For example, a study of joggers in Denmark found the lowest mortality rate among those who jogged a moderate amount (2–3 workouts for a total of 60–150 minutes per week); higher rates of death were found among non-joggers and those who jogged at a very intense level and/or for long distances (even moderate jogging is high-intensity exercise). Viral, bacterial, and fungal infections can also cause heart muscle inflammation and sudden death, so don't exercise when you have a fever or flu.

Where does this leave you? Overall, exercise has enough benefits that make up for a slightly increased risk of sudden death—in healthy people as well as those with heart disease. Active people who stop exercising can expect their heart attack risk to increase by 300%. The risk of heart-related sudden death in middle-aged and older adults is lowest in people who exercise approximately 150 minutes per week—the activity level recommended by the U.S. Department of Health and Human Services.

Medical Clearance Recommendations People of any age who are not at high risk for serious health problems can safely exercise at a moderate intensity (60% or less of maximum heart rate) without a prior medical evaluation (see Chapter 3 for a discussion of maximum heart rate). Likewise, if you are male and under 40 or female and under 50 and in good health, vigorous exercise is probably safe for you. If you do not fit into these age groups, or if you have health problems—especially high blood pressure, heart disease, muscle or joint problems, or obesity—see your physician before starting a vigorous exercise program. The Physical Activity Readiness Questionnaire for Everyone (PAR-Q+) can help evaluate exercise safety; it is included in Lab 2.1. Completing it should alert you to any potential problems you may have. If a physician isn't sure whether exercise is safe for you, she or he may recommend an **exercise stress test** or a **graded exercise test (GXT)** to see whether you show symptoms of heart disease during exercise. For most people, however, it's far safer to exercise than to remain sedentary.

Assessing Yourself

The first step in creating a successful fitness program is to assess your current level of physical activity and fitness for each of the five health-related fitness components. The results of the assessment tests will help you set specific fitness goals and plan your fitness program. Lab 2.3 gives you the opportunity to assess your current overall level of activity and determine if it is appropriate. Assessment tests in Chapters 3, 4, 5 and 6 will help you evaluate your cardiorespiratory endurance, muscular strength, muscular endurance, flexibility, and body composition.

Setting Goals

The ultimate general goal of every health-related fitness program is the same—wellness that lasts a lifetime. That lifelong goal might include the specific goals of walking 30–60 minutes every day or doing a few calisthenic exercises every morning. Whatever your specific goals, they must be important enough to you to keep you motivated. Most sports psychologists believe that setting and achieving goals is the most effective way to stay motivated about exercise. (Refer to Chapter 1 for more on goal setting, as well as Common Questions Answered at the end of this chapter.) After you complete the assessment tests in Chapters 3, 4, 5, and 6, you will be able to set goals directly related to each fitness component, such as working toward a three-mile jog or doing 20 push-ups. First, though, think carefully about your overall goals, and be clear about why you are starting a program.

Choosing Activities for a Balanced Program

An ideal fitness program combines a physically active lifestyle with systematic exercise to develop and maintain physical fitness. This overall program is shown in the physical activity pyramid in Figure 2.3. If you are currently sedentary, your goal should be to focus on activities at the bottom of the pyramid and gradually increase the amount of moderate-intensity physical activity in your daily life. Appropriate activities include walking briskly, climbing stairs, doing yard work, and washing your car. You don't have to exercise vigorously, but you should experience a moderate increase in your heart and breathing rates. As described earlier, your activity time can be broken up into small blocks over the course of a day.

The next two levels of the pyramid illustrate parts of a formal exercise program. The principles of this program are consistent with those of the American College of Sports Medicine (ACSM), the professional organization for people involved in sports medicine and exercise science. The ACSM has established guidelines for creating an exercise program that will develop physical fitness (Table 2.3). A balanced program includes activities to develop all the health-related components of fitness:

- *Cardiorespiratory endurance* is developed by continuous rhythmic movements of large-muscle groups in activities such as walking, jogging, cycling, swimming, aerobic dance, and other forms of group exercise. High-intensity interval training (HIIT)—short bouts of high-intensity exercise followed by rest—also builds endurance quickly. The advantage of HIIT is that it does not take as much time as traditional endurance training. The disadvantage is that it can be painful and uncomfortable. The safety of HIIT has not been determined.

exercise stress test A test usually administered **TERMS** on a treadmill or cycle ergometer using an electrocardiogram (EKG or ECG) to analyze changes in electrical activity in the heart during exercise; used to determine if any heart disease is present and to assess current fitness level.

graded exercise test (GXT) An exercise test that starts at an easy intensity and progresses to maximum capacity.

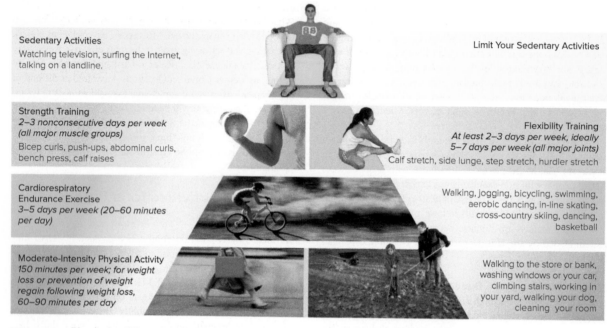

Sedentary Activities
Watching television, surfing the Internet, talking on a landline.

Limit Your Sedentary Activities

Strength Training
2–3 nonconsecutive days per week (all major muscle groups)
Bicep curls, push-ups, abdominal curls, bench press, calf raises

Flexibility Training
At least 2–3 days per week, ideally 5–7 days per week (all major joints)
Calf stretch, side lunge, step stretch, hurdler stretch

Cardiorespiratory Endurance Exercise
3–5 days per week (20–60 minutes per day)

Walking, jogging, bicycling, swimming, aerobic dancing, in-line skating, cross-country skiing, dancing, basketball

Moderate-Intensity Physical Activity
150 minutes per week; for weight loss or prevention of weight regain following weight loss, 60–90 minutes per day

Walking to the store or bank, washing windows or your car, climbing stairs, working in your yard, walking your dog, cleaning your room

FIGURE 2.3   Physical activity pyramid.
©George Doyle/Getty Images RF: ©Ryan McVay/Getty Images RF: Courtesy Shirlee Stevens: ©Westend61/Getty Images RF: ©Doug Menuez/Getty Images RF: ©UpperCut Images/Alamy Stock Photo RF

• Choose activities that you enjoy and that are convenient. Popular choices are in-line skating, skiing, dancing, cycling, and backpacking. Start-and-stop activities such as tennis, racquetball, and soccer can also develop cardiorespiratory endurance if your skill level is sufficient to enable periods of continuous play. Training for cardiorespiratory endurance is discussed in Chapter 3.

• *Muscular strength and endurance* can be developed through resistance training—training with weights or performing calisthenics such as push-ups, planks, and curl-ups. Training for muscular strength and endurance is discussed in Chapter 4.

• *Flexibility* is developed by stretching the major muscle groups regularly and with proper technique. Flexibility is discussed in Chapter 5.

• *Healthy body composition* can be developed through a sensible diet and a program of regular exercise. Cardiorespiratory endurance exercise is best for reducing body fat; resistance training builds muscle mass, which, to a small extent, helps increase metabolism. Body composition is discussed in Chapter 6.

Chapter 7 contains guidelines to help you choose activities and put together a complete exercise program that will suit your goals and preferences. (Refer to Figure 2.4 for a summary of the health and fitness benefits of different levels of physical activity and exercise programs.)

What about the tip of the activity pyramid? Although sedentary activities are often unavoidable—attending class, studying, working in an office, and so on—many people *choose* inactivity over activity during their leisure time. During sedentary activities, periodically stand, perform air squats, or walk around the room—even if only for a few minutes. Change sedentary patterns by becoming more active whenever you can.

Guidelines for Training

The following guidelines will make your exercise program more effective and successful.

Train the Way You Want Your Body to Change Stress your body so that it adapts in the desired manner. To have a more muscular build, lift weights. To be more flexible, do stretching exercises. To improve performance in a particular sport, practice that sport or its movements.

Train Regularly Consistency is the key to improving fitness. Fitness improvements are lost if too much time passes between exercise sessions. When you can't follow your regular routine, do something physical—for example, squat with rocks or soup cans, sprint in place for 20 seconds, or train at a local gym for an hour when on vacation or traveling for business. LAB 2.2, Overcoming Barriers to Being Active, will help develop strategies for exercising regularly.

Start Slowly, and Get in Shape Gradually As Figure 2.5 shows, an exercise program can be divided into three phases:

• *Beginning phase.* The body adjusts to the new type and level of activity.

Table 2.3	ACSM Exercise Recommendations for Fitness Development in Healthy Adults

EXERCISE TO DEVELOP AND MAINTAIN CARDIORESPIRATORY ENDURANCE AND BODY COMPOSITION

Frequency of training	At least five days per week for moderate-intensity exercise and at least three days per week for vigorous-intensity exercise.
Intensity of training	55/65–90% of maximum heart rate or 40/50–85% of heart rate reserve or oxygen uptake reserve. (Reserve refers to the difference between resting and maximum values of heart rate or oxygen consumption.) The lower-intensity values (55–64% of maximum heart rate and 40–49% of heart rate reserve plus rest) are most applicable to unfit individuals. For average individuals, intensities of 70–85% of maximum heart rate or 60–80% of heart rate reserve plus rest are appropriate. Well-trained people can train at near maximum intensities. These methods increase exercise intensity within the limits of each person's reserve capacity.
Time (duration) of training	20–60 total minutes per day of continuous or intermittent (in sessions lasting 10 or more minutes) aerobic activity. Duration depends on the intensity of activity; thus, low-intensity activity should be conducted over a longer period of time (30 minutes or more). Low- to moderate-intensity activity of longer duration is recommended for nonathletic adults.
Type (mode) of activity	Any activity that uses large-muscle groups, can be maintained continuously, and is rhythmic and aerobic in nature—for example, walking-hiking, running-jogging, bicycling, cross-country skiing, aerobic dancing and other forms of group exercise, rope-skipping, rowing, stair-climbing, swimming, skating, and endurance game activities.
Volume	Expend the equivalent of at least 1,000 calories per week, which is equivalent to about 150 minutes per week of moderate-intensity exercise.
Progression	Adjust frequency, intensity, and/or time until you reach your goal.

EXERCISE TO DEVELOP AND MAINTAIN MUSCULAR STRENGTH AND ENDURANCE, FLEXIBILITY, AND BODY COMPOSITION

Resistance training	One set of 8–10 exercises that condition the major muscle groups, performed two to three days per week. Most people should complete 8–12 repetitions of each exercise to the point of fatigue; practicing other repetition ranges (e.g., 3–5 or 12–15) also builds strength and endurance; for older and frailer people (approximately 50–60 and older), 10–15 repetitions with a lighter weight may be more appropriate. Multiple-set regimens will provide greater benefits if time allows. Any mode of exercise that is comfortable throughout the full range of motion is appropriate (e.g., free weights, kettlebells, calisthenics, elastic bands, or weight machines).
Flexibility training	Static stretches, performed for the major muscle groups at least two to three days per week, ideally daily. Stretch to the point of tightness, holding each stretch for 10–30 seconds; perform 2–4 repetitions of each stretch, for a total of 60 seconds of stretching time for each exercise.

*Chapter 3 provides instructions for calculating target heart rate intensity for cardiorespiratory endurance exercise.

SOURCES: American College of Sports Medicine. 2018. *ACSM's Guidelines for Exercise Testing and Prescription,* 10th ed. Philadelphia: Wolters Kluwer; Garber, C. E., et al. 2011. "Quantity and quality of exercise for developing and maintaining cardiorespiratory, musculoskeletal, and neuromotor fitness in apparently healthy adults: Guidance for prescribing exercise," *Medicine and Science in Sports and Exercise* 43(7), 1334–1359.

- *Progress phase.* Fitness increases.
- *Maintenance phase.* The targeted level of fitness is sustained over the long term.

When beginning a program, start slowly to give your body time to adapt to the stress of exercise. Choose activities carefully according to your fitness status. If you have been sedentary or are overweight, try an activity such as walking or swimming that won't jar the body or strain the joints.

As you progress, increase duration and frequency before increasing intensity. If you train too much or too intensely, you are more likely to suffer injuries or experience **overtraining**, a condition characterized by lack of energy, aching muscles and joints, depressed immune function, and decreased physical performance. Injuries and overtraining slow down an exercise program and impede motivation. The goal is not to get in shape as quickly as possible but to gradually become and then remain physically fit.

Warm Up before Exercise Warming up can decrease your chances of injury by helping your body gradually progress from rest to activity. A good warm-up can increase muscle temperature, reduce joint stiffness, bathe the joint surfaces in lubricating fluid, and increase blood flow to the muscles, including the heart. Some studies suggest that warming up may also enhance muscle metabolism and mentally prepare you for a workout.

A warm-up should include low-intensity, whole-body movements similar to those used in the activity. For example, runners may walk and jog slowly prior to running at full speed. A tennis player might hit forehands and backhands at a low intensity before playing a vigorous set of tennis. A warm-up is not the same as a stretching workout. For safety and effectiveness, it is best to stretch *after* an endurance or strength training workout, when muscles are warm—and not as part of a warm-up. (Appropriate and effective warm-ups are discussed in greater detail in Chapters 3, 4, 5 and 6.)

Cool Down after Exercise During exercise, as much as 90% of circulating blood is directed to the muscles and skin, up from as little as 20% during rest. If you stop moving suddenly

overtraining A condition caused by training too much or too intensely, characterized by lack of energy, decreased physical performance, and aching muscles and joints.

TERMS

Wellness Tip Moderation is important, especially if you're just starting to get physically active. Work at a pace that's comfortable and enjoyable, with a goal of making gradual improvements. This will help you get into the habit of being active and will help you avoid burnout.
©JoseGirarte/Getty Images RF

after exercise, the amount of blood returning to your heart and brain may be insufficient, and you may experience dizziness, a drop in blood pressure, or other problems. Cooling down at the end of a workout helps safely restore circulation to its normal resting condition. So, after you exercise, cool down before you sit or lie down or jump into the shower. Cool down by continuing to move at a slow pace—walking for 5–10 minutes, for example, as your heart and breathing rate and blood pressure slowly return to normal. At the end of the cool-down period, do stretching exercises while your muscles are still warm. Cool down longer after intense exercise sessions.

Exercise Safely Physical activity can cause injury or even death if you don't consider safety. For example, you should always do the following:

- Wear a helmet when biking, skiing, or rock climbing.
- Wear eye protection when playing racquetball or squash.
- Wear bright clothing or safety lights when exercising on a public street.

	Lifestyle physical activity	**Moderate exercise program**	**Vigorous exercise program**
Description	Moderate physical activity (150 minutes per week; muscle-strengthening exercises 2 or more days per week)	Cardiorespiratory endurance exercise (20–60 minutes, 3–5 days per week); strength training (2–3 nonconsecutive days per week); and stretching exercises (2 or more days per week)	Cardiorespiratory endurance exercise (20–60 minutes, 3–5 days per week); interval training; strength training (3–4 nonconsecutive days per week); and stretching exercises (5–7 days per week)
Sample activities or program	• Walking to and from work, 15 minutes each way • Cycling to and from class, 10 minutes each way • Doing yard work for 30 minutes • Dancing (fast) for 30 minutes • Playing basketball for 20 minutes • Muscle exercises such as push-ups, squats, or back exercises	• Jogging for 30 minutes, 3 days per week • Weight training, 1 set of 8 exercises, 2 days per week • Stretching exercises, 3 days per week	• Running for 45 minutes, 3 days per week • Intervals, running 400 m at high effort, 4 sets, 2 days per week • Weight training, 3 sets of 10 exercises, 3 days per week • Stretching exercises, 6 days per week
Health and fitness benefits	Better blood cholesterol levels, reduced body fat, better control of blood pressure, improved metabolic health, and enhanced glucose metabolism; improved quality of life; reduced risk of some chronic diseases Greater amounts of activity can help prevent weight gain and promote weight loss	All the benefits of lifestyle physical activity, plus improved physical fitness (increased cardiorespiratory endurance, muscular strength and endurance, and flexibility) and even greater improvements in health and quality of life and reductions in chronic disease risk	All the benefits of lifestyle physical activity and a moderate exercise program, with greater increases in fitness and somewhat greater reductions in chronic disease risk Participating in a vigorous exercise program may increase risk of injury and overtraining

FIGURE 2.4   Health and fitness benefits of different amounts of physical activity and exercise.
©Photodisc/Getty Images RF; ©Ijupco/123RF; ©Thinkstock Images/Getty Images RF

Beginning   Making progress   Maintaining

High

Walking
2 days/wk 60 min
Walk-jog
2 days/wk 30 min
(Progress gradually—
walk 5 min, jog 30 sec;
walk 3 min, jog 2 min;
jog 4 min; walk 1 min).
Add 1 set of 8 Resistive
exercises and stretching

Jogging
2–4 days/wk

*Interval
training*
1–2 days/wk
(if consistent
with goal)
*Resistive
exercise*
2–3 days/wk
Stretching
3–7 days/wk

Walking
3–4 days/wk
30–60 min

Jogging
3–5 days/wk
20–30 min
*Resistive
exercise*
2–3 days/wk
Stretching
3–7 days/wk

Amount of overload

Low

0   5   10   15   20   25+

Time since beginning an exercise program (in weeks)

FIGURE 2.5   Progression of an exercise program. This figure shows how you can increase the amount of overload gradually in a walking and running program. Begin with slow walking for several weeks and gradually pick up the pace. Gradually introduce short periods of running during your walks, progressively running farther and walking less until you can run continuously. Add interval training after four to six weeks of jogging—if you want to reach higher levels of fitness. Regardless of the activity and the exercise program, begin slowly and progress gradually. After you achieve the desired level of fitness, you can maintain it by exercising three to five days a week.

SOURCE: Progression data from American College of Sports Medicine. 2018. *ACSM's Guidelines for Exercise Testing and Prescription*, 10th ed. Philadelphia: Wolters Kluwer/Lippincott Williams & Wilkins Health.

- Walk or run with a partner when exercising on a deserted track or in a park.
- Give vehicles plenty of leeway, even when you have the right of way.
- In the weight room, be aware of people exercising near you, use spotters and collars when appropriate, and don't use broken equipment.
- Always use good technique. Don't put your back or joints at risk trying to lift weights or perform physical skills beyond your ability.

Overloading your muscles and joints can lead to serious injury, so train within your capacity. Use high-quality equipment and keep it in good repair. Report broken gym equipment to the health club manager or physical education instructor. (See Appendix A for more information on personal safety.)

Listen to Your Body and Get Adequate Rest Rest can be as important as exercise for improving fitness. Fitness reflects an adaptation to the stress of exercise. Building fitness involves a series of exercise stresses, recuperation, and adaptation leading to improved fitness, followed by further stresses. Build rest into your training program, and don't exercise if it

doesn't feel right. Sometimes you need a few days of rest to recover enough to train with the intensity required for improving fitness. Getting enough sleep is an important part of the recovery process. On the other hand, don't train sporadically, either. If you listen to your body and it always tells you to rest, you won't make any progress.

Cycle the Volume and Intensity of Your Workouts To add enjoyment and variety to your program and to further improve fitness, don't train at the same intensity during every workout. Train intensely on some days and train lightly on others. Proper management of workout intensity is a key to improving physical fitness. Use cycle training, also known as *periodization,* to provide enough recovery for intense training: By training lightly one workout, you can train harder the next. However, take care to increase the volume and intensity of your program gradually—never more than 10% per week.

Vary Your Activities Change your exercise program from time to time to keep things fresh and help develop a higher degree of fitness. The body adapts quickly to an exercise stress, such as walking, cycling, or swimming. Gains in fitness in a particular activity become more difficult with time. Varying the exercises in your program allows you to adapt to many types of exercise and develops fitness in a variety of activities (see the box "Vary Your Activities"). Changing activities may also help reduce your risk of injury. This is a central principle in cross-training exercise techniques such as CrossFit. CrossFit is a commercial exercise program that uses a variety of training methods to improve fitness, including running, swimming, climbing, gymnastics, functional training, Olympic weight lifting, kettlebells, rope-climbing, and calisthenics.

Train with a Partner People who train together can motivate and encourage each other through rough spots and help each other develop proper exercise techniques. Training with a partner can make exercising seem easier and more fun. It can also help you keep motivated and on track. A commitment to a friend is a powerful motivator. If you can afford it, you may benefit from a certified personal trainer who can give you instruction in exercise techniques and help provide motivation.

Train Your Mind Becoming fit requires commitment, discipline, and patience. These qualities come from understanding the importance of exercise and setting clear and reachable goals. Use the lifestyle management techniques discussed in Chapter 1 to keep your program on track. Learning about the science behind a healthy lifestyle helps keep your program relevant.

Fuel Your Activity Appropriately Good nutritional choices can help you recover from a bout of exercise and get you ready for your next workout. Consume adequate fluids to stay hydrated as well as enough calories to support your exercise program without gaining body fat. Nutrition for exercise is discussed in greater detail in Chapters 3 and 8.

TAKE CHARGE
Vary Your Activities

Do you have a hard time thinking of new activities to try? Check the boxes next to the activities listed here that interest you. Then look for resources and facilities on your campus or in your community.

OUTDOOR EXERCISES

☐ Walking	☐ In-line skating	☐ Hiking
☐ Running	☐ Skateboarding	☐ Backpacking
☐ Cycling	☐ Rowing	☐ Ice skating
☐ Swimming	☐ Horseback riding	☐ Fly fishing

SPORTS AND GAMES

☐ Basketball	☐ Softball	☐ Bowling
☐ Tennis	☐ Water skiing	☐ Surfing
☐ Volleyball	☐ Windsurfing	☐ Dancing
☐ Golf	☐ Badminton	☐ Snow skiing
☐ Soccer	☐ Ultimate Frisbee	☐ Gymnastics

EXERCISES YOU CAN DO AT HOME AND WORK

☐ Desk exercises	☐ Yard work	☐ Painting walls
☐ Calisthenics	☐ Sweeping	☐ Walking the dog
☐ Gardening	☐ Exploring on foot	☐ Shopping
☐ Housework	☐ Doing a walk-a-thon	☐ Doing errands

HEALTH CLUB EXERCISES

☐ Weight training	☐ Ski machine	☐ Elliptical trainer
☐ Circuit training	☐ Supine bike	☐ Medicine ball
☐ Group exercise	☐ Rowing machine	☐ Rope-skipping
☐ Treadmill	☐ Plyometrics	☐ Yoga/Pilates
☐ Stationary bike	☐ Water aerobics	☐ Racquetball

Have Fun You are more likely to stick with an exercise program if it's fun. Choose a variety of activities that you enjoy. Some people like to play competitive sports, such as tennis, golf, or volleyball. Competition can boost motivation, but remember: Sports are competitive, whereas training for fitness is not. Other people like more solitary activities, such as jogging, walking, or swimming. Still others like high-skill individual sports, such as snowboarding, surfing, or skateboarding. Many activities can help you get fit, so choose the ones you enjoy. You can also boost your enjoyment and build your social support network by exercising with friends and family.

Track Your Progress Monitoring the progress of your program can help keep you motivated and on track. Depending on the activities you've included in your program, you may track different measures of your program—minutes of jogging, miles of cycling, laps of swimming, number of push-ups, amount of weight lifted, and so on. If your program focuses on increasing daily physical activity, consider using an inexpensive step counter or exercise GPS app to monitor the number of steps you take each day. (See Lab 2.3 for more information on setting goals and monitoring activity with a digital tracker; see the box "Digital Workout Aids" for an introduction to products and apps that can help you track your progress.) Specific examples of program monitoring can be found in the labs for Chapters 3, 4 and 5.

Get Help and Advice If You Need It One of the best places to get help starting an exercise program is an exercise class. If you join a health club or fitness center, follow the guidelines in the box "Choosing a Fitness Center." There, expert instructors can help you learn the basics of training and answer your questions. Make sure the instructor is certified by a recognized professional organization and/or has formal training in exercise physiology. Read articles by credible

experts in fitness magazines (such as *Fitness Rx for Women* and *Fitness Rx for Men*). Many of these magazines include articles by leading experts in exercise science written at a layperson's level.

A qualified personal trainer can also help you get started in an exercise program or a new form of training. Make sure this person has proper qualifications, such as certification by the ACSM, National Strength and Conditioning Association (NSCA), or International Sports Sciences Association (ISSA). Don't seek out a person for advice simply because he or she looks fit. UCLA researchers found that 60% of the personal trainers in their study couldn't pass a basic exam on training methods, exercise physiology, or biomechanics. Trainers who performed best had college degrees in exercise physiology, physical education, or physical therapy. So choose your trainer carefully and don't get caught up with fads or appearances.

Keep Your Exercise Program in Perspective As important as physical fitness is, it is only part of a well-rounded life. You need time for work and school, family and friends, relaxation and hobbies. Some people become over-involved in exercise and neglect other parts of their lives. They think of themselves as runners, dancers, swimmers, or triathletes rather than as people who happen to participate in those activities. Balance and moderation are key ingredients of a fit and well life.

Ask Yourself

QUESTIONS FOR CRITICAL THINKING AND REFLECTION

If you were to start planning a fitness program, what would be your three most important long-term goals? What would you set as short-term goals? What rewards would be meaningful to you?

WELLNESS IN THE DIGITAL AGE
Digital Workout Aids

When you're just starting to get physically active, you can wind up with a lot of questions. How many miles did I walk? How many kettlebell swings did I do, and how explosively did I do them? How many minutes did I run? When your mind is completely focused on just *doing* an activity, it's easy to lose count of time, distance, and reps. But it's important to keep track of these things: Move too little and you won't see any progress; move too much and you run the risk of injury or burnout. Either outcome is bad news for your exercise program.

Luckily, we live in a digital age, and the fitness industry is providing an ever-growing array of high-tech tools and apps that can track your progress for you. If you like to walk or run, cell phone apps can track your distance, or the number of steps you take, and give you a detailed map of where you ran, biked, or skied. Advanced trackers can even record any hills you encounter during your workout. Heart rate monitors can help you reach and maintain the right exercise intensity. Accelerometers can measure your power output, or explosiveness, during weight lifting. If calisthenics are your choice, there are gaming systems and smartphone apps that work for specific exercises to count reps, assess your form, and challenge you to push yourself harder.

Smartphone apps, such as Coach's Eye, Hudl Technique, and Dartfish, can help you analyze your golf swing or tennis forehand in slow motion. The programs even make it possible to gauge your progress by comparing technique videos during different phases of your program (e.g., tennis technique during week 1 versus week 10).

In choosing a digital tracker, keep the following in mind:

- Consider your fitness goals and how you plan to monitor and evaluate the progress of your program.
- Look for the features you need; don't pay extra for capabilities you won't use.
- Try out a tracker before you buy it; make sure it fits and that you find it easy to use.
- Confirm that any tracker or analysis app is compatible with your smartphone or computer.

Remember, a tracker works only when you use it!

Box Icon: ©Hong Li/Getty Images

TIPS FOR TODAY AND THE FUTURE

Physical activity and exercise offer benefits in nearly every area of wellness. Even a low to moderate level of activity provides valuable health benefits. The important thing is to get moving!

RIGHT NOW YOU CAN

- Look at your calendar for the rest of the week and write in some physical activity—such as walking, running, biking, skating, swimming, hiking, or playing Frisbee—on as many days as you can. Schedule the activity for a specific time and stick to it.
- Call a friend and invite her or him to start planning a regular exercise program with you.
- Download a pedometer app on your phone and keep track of your daily activity.

IN THE FUTURE YOU CAN

- Schedule a session with a qualified personal trainer who can evaluate your current fitness level and help you set personalized fitness goals.
- Create seasonal workout programs for the spring, summer, fall, and winter. Develop programs that are varied but consistent with your overall fitness goals.

SUMMARY

- Moderate daily physical activity contributes substantially to good health. Even without a formal, vigorous exercise program, you can get many of the same health benefits just by becoming more physically active.

- If you are already active, you benefit even more by increasing the intensity or duration of your activities.

- The five components of physical fitness most important for health are cardiorespiratory endurance, muscular strength, muscular endurance, flexibility, and body composition.

- Physical training is the process of producing long-term improvements in the body's functioning through exercise. All training is based on the fact that the body adapts to physical stress.

- According to the principle of specificity, bodies change specifically in response to the type of training received.

- Bodies also adapt to progressive overload. The amount of overload needed to maintain or improve a particular level of fitness for a particular fitness component is determined through six dimensions, represented by the acronym FITT-VP: frequency, intensity, time, type, volume, and progression.

- Bodies adjust to lower levels of activity by losing fitness, a principle known as reversibility. To counter the effects of reversibility, keep training at the same intensity, even if you have to reduce the number or length of sessions.

- According to the principle of individual differences, people vary in the maximum level of fitness they can achieve and in the rate of change they can expect from an exercise program.

- When designing an exercise program, determine if you need medical clearance, assess your current level of fitness, set realistic goals, and choose activities that develop all the components of fitness.

- Train regularly, get in shape gradually, warm up and cool down, maintain a structured but flexible program, get enough rest, exercise safely, vary activities, consider training with a partner or personal trainer, train your mind, eat sensibly, have fun, monitor your progress, and keep exercise in perspective.

CRITICAL CONSUMER
Choosing a Fitness Center

Fitness centers can provide you with many benefits—motivation and companionship are among the most important. A fitness center may also offer expert instruction and supervision as well as access to better equipment than you could afford on your own. All fitness centers, however, are not of the same overall quality, and every fitness center is not for every person. If you're thinking of joining a fitness center, here are some guidelines to help you choose a club that's right for you.

Convenience

• Look for an established facility that's within 10–15 minutes of your home or work. If it's farther away, your chances of sticking to an exercise regimen start to diminish.

• Visit the facility at the time you would normally exercise. Is there adequate parking? Will you have easy access to equipment and classes at that time?

• What child care services are available, and how are they supervised?

Atmosphere

• Look around to see if there are other members who are your age and at about your fitness level. Some clubs cater to a certain age group or lifestyle, such as hard-core bodybuilders or weight lifters.

• Observe how the members dress. Will you fit in, or will you be uncomfortable?

• Observe the staff. Are they easy to identify? Are they friendly, professional, and helpful?

• Check to see that the facility is clean, including showers and lockers. Make sure the facility is climate controlled, well ventilated, and well lit.

Safety

• Find out if the facility offers some type of preactivity screening as well as basic fitness testing that includes cardiovascular screening.

• Determine if personnel are trained in CPR and if there is emergency equipment such as automated external defibrillators (AEDs) on the premises. An AED can help someone who has cardiac arrest.

• Ask if at least one staff member on each shift is trained in first aid.

Trained Personnel

• Determine if the personal trainers and fitness instructors are certified by a recognized professional association such as the ACSM, Aerobics and Fitness Association of America (AFAA), National Strength and Conditioning Association (NSCA), or International Sport Sciences Association (ISSA). All personal trainers are not equal; more than 100 organizations certify trainers, and few of these require much formal training.

• Find out if the club has a trained exercise physiologist on staff, such as someone with a degree in exercise physiology, kinesiology, or exercise science. If the facility offers nutritional counseling, it should employ someone who is a registered dietitian or has similar formal training.

• Ask how much experience the instructors have. Ideally, trainers should have both academic preparation and practical experience.

Cost

• Buy only what you need and can afford. If you want to use only workout equipment, you may not need a club that has racquetball courts and saunas.

• Check the contract. Choose the one that covers the shortest period of time possible, especially if it's your first fitness club experience. Don't feel pressured to sign a long-term contract.

• Make sure the contract permits you to extend your membership if you have a prolonged illness or go on vacation. Some clubs have exchange agreements that allow you to train in other cities while on vacation or business.

• Try out the club. Ask for a free trial workout, or a one-day pass, or an inexpensive one- or two-week trial membership.

• Find out whether there is an extra charge for the particular services you want. Get any special offers in writing.

Effectiveness

• Tour the facility. Does it offer what the brochure says it does? Does it offer the activities and equipment you want?

• Check the equipment. A good club will have treadmills, bikes, stair-climbers, resistance machines, and weights. Make sure these machines are up to date and well maintained.

• Find out if new members get a formal orientation and instruction on how to safely use the equipment. Will a staff member help you develop a program that is appropriate for your current fitness level and goals?

• Make sure the facility is certified. Look for the displayed names ACSM, American Council on Exercise (ACE), AFAA, or International Health, Racquet, and Sportsclub Association (IHRSA).

©IT Stock/PunchStock RF

Box Icon: © sam74100/Getty Images RF

COMMON QUESTIONS ANSWERED

Q **I have asthma. Is it OK for me to start an exercise program?**

A Probably, but you should see your doctor before you start exercising, especially if you have been sedentary up to this point. Your personal physician can advise you on the type of exercise program that is best for you, given the severity of your condition, and how to avoid suffering exercise-related asthma attacks.

Q **What should my fitness goals be?**

A Begin by thinking about your general overall goals—the benefits you want to obtain by increasing your activity level and/or beginning a formal exercise program. Examples of long-term goals include reducing your risk of chronic diseases, increasing your energy level, and maintaining a healthy body weight.

To help shape your fitness program, you need to set specific, short-term goals based on measurable factors. These specific goals should be an extension of your overall goals—the specific changes to your current activity and exercise habits needed to achieve your general goals. In setting short-term goals, be sure to use the SMART criteria described in Chapter 1. As noted there, your goals should be **S**pecific, **M**easurable, **A**ttainable, **R**ealistic, and **T**ime frame–specific (SMART).

You need information about your current levels of physical activity and physical fitness in order to set appropriate goals. The labs in this chapter will help you determine your physical activity level—for example, how many minutes per day you engage in moderate or vigorous activity or how many daily steps you take. Using this information, you can set goals for lifestyle physical activity to help you meet your overall goals. For example, if your general long-term goals are to reduce the risk of chronic disease and prevent weight gain, the Dietary Guidelines recommend 60 minutes of moderate physical activity daily. If you currently engage in 30 minutes of moderate activity daily, then your behavior change goal would be to add 30 minutes of daily physical activity (or an equivalent number of additional daily steps—about 3,500–4,000); your time frame for the change might be 8–12 weeks.

Labs in Chapters 3, 4, 5 and 6 provide opportunities to assess your fitness status for all the health-related components of fitness. The results of these assessments can guide you in setting specific fitness goals. For instance, if the labs in Chapter 4 indicate that you have good muscular strength and endurance in your lower body but poor strength and endurance in your upper body, then setting a specific goal for improving upper-body muscle fitness would be an appropriate goal—increasing the number of push-ups you can do from 22 to 30, for example. Chapters 3–6 include additional advice for setting appropriate goals.

After you start your behavior change program, you may discover that your goals aren't quite appropriate; perhaps you were overly optimistic, or maybe you set the bar too low. There are limits to the amount of fitness you can achieve, but within the limits of your genes, health status, and motivation, you can make significant improvements in fitness. Adjust your goals as needed.

Q **Should I follow my exercise program if I'm sick?**

A If you have a mild head cold or feel one coming on, it is probably okay to exercise moderately. Just begin slowly and see how you feel. However, if you have symptoms of a more serious illness—fever, swollen glands, nausea, extreme tiredness, muscle aches—wait until you have recovered fully before resuming your exercise program. Continuing to exercise while suffering from an illness more serious than a cold can compromise your recovery and may even be dangerous.

FOR FURTHER EXPLORATION

American College of Sports Medicine (ACSM). The principal professional organization for sports medicine and exercise science. Provides brochures, publications, and videos.
http://www.acsm.org

American Council on Exercise (ACE). Promotes exercise and fitness; the website features fact sheets on many consumer topics, including choosing shoes, cross-training, and steroids.
http://www.acefitness.org

American Heart Association: Walking 101. Provides practical advice about walking for people of all fitness levels.
http://www.heart.org/HEARTORG/HealthyLiving/PhysicalActivity/Walking/Walking-101_UCM_461766_Article.jsp#.WQkXUagrIo9

CDC Physical Activity Information. Provides information on the benefits of physical activity and suggestions for incorporating moderate physical activity into daily life.

http://www.cdc.gov/physicalactivity

CrossFit. A cross-training method involving a variety of exercises and unaccustomed physical challenges. The program includes franchised health clubs and training facilities. The website provides extensive information on cross training, nutrition, exercise techniques, and sports psychology.
http://www.crossfit.com

Disabled Sports USA. Provides sports and recreation services to people with physical or mobility disorders.

http://www.disabledsportsusa.org

Health and Retirement Study. A website describing a study of 20,000 people begun in 1992 at the University of Michigan and updated every two years. Included is an extensive reference list of published studies.
hrsonline.isr.umich.edu.

International Health, Racquet, and Sportsclub Association (IHRSA): Health Clubs. Provides guidelines for choosing a health or fitness facility and links to clubs that belong to IHRSA.
http://www.healthclubs.com

International Sports Sciences Association (ISSA). Trains and certifies personal trainers.

http://www.issaonline.com

MedlinePlus: Exercise and Physical Fitness. Provides links to news and reliable information about fitness and exercise from government agencies and professional associations.

http://www.nlm.nih.gov/medlineplus/exerciseandphysicalfitness.html

President's Council on Fitness, Sports and Nutrition. Provides information on programs and publications, including fitness guides and fact sheets.

http://www.fitness.gov

http://www.presidentschallenge.org

Shape America. A professional organization for health and physical educators.

http://www.shapeamerica.org

Shape Up America! A nonprofit organization that provides information and resources on exercise, nutrition, and weight loss.

http://www.shapeupus.org

StrongFirst. A school of strength, directed by kettlebell master Pavel Tsatsouline, that teaches men and women how to reach high levels of strength and fitness without interfering with work, school, family, or sport. The program offers clinics and web-based information.

http://www.strongfirst.com

SELECTED BIBLIOGRAPHY

Alzheimer's Association. 2016. *2016 Alzheimer's Disease Facts and Figures.* Chicago: Alzheimer's Association.

American College of Sports Medicine. 2011. *ACSM's Complete Guide to Fitness & Health.* Champaign, Ill.: Human Kinetics.

American College of Sports Medicine. 2011. The recommended quantity and quality of exercise for developing and maintaining cardiorespiratory and muscular fitness, and flexibility in healthy adults. ACSM position stand. *Medicine and Science in Sports and Exercise* 43(7): 1334–1359.

American College of Sports Medicine. 2012. *ACSM's Health/Fitness Facility Standards and Guidelines,* 4th ed. Champaign, Ill.: Human Kinetics.

American College of Sports Medicine. 2014. *ACSM's Resource Manual for Guidelines for Exercise Testing and Prescription,* 7th ed. Philadelphia: Wolters Kluwer/ Lippincott Williams & Wilkins Health.

American College of Sports Medicine. 2018. *ACSM's Guidelines for Exercise Testing and Prescription,* 10th ed. Philadelphia: Wolters Kluwer.

American Heart Association. 2017. *Cardiovascular disease: a costly burden for America. Projections through 2035.* Washington, DC: American Hearth Association.

Biswas, A., et al. 2015. Sedentary time and its association with risk for disease incidence, mortality, and hospitalization in adults: A systematic review and meta-analysis. *Annals of Internal Medicine* 162(2): 123–132.

Bouchard, C., et al. 2015. Personalized preventive medicine: Genetics and the response to regular exercise in preventive interventions. *Progress in Cardiovascular Diseases* 57(4): 337–346.

Bos, I., et al. 2013. Subclinical effects of aerobic training in urban environment. *Medicine and Science in Sports and Exercise* 45(3): 439–447.

Casazza, K., et al. 2013. Myths, presumptions, and facts about obesity. *New England Journal of Medicine* 368(5): 446–454.

Centers for Disease Control and Prevention. 2014. *State Indicator Report on Physical Activity, 2014.* Atlanta, GA: U.S. Department of Health and Human Services.

Dietary Guidelines Advisory Committee. 2015. *Scientific Report of the 2015 Dietary Advisory Committee.* Washington, DC: U.S. Department of Agriculture, Agricultural Research Service.

Donnelly, J. E., et al. 2009. Appropriate physical activity intervention strategies for weight loss and prevention of weight regain for adults (ACSM position stand). *Medicine and Science in Sports and Exercise* 41(2): 459–471.

Ekblom-Bak, E., et al. 2014. The importance of non-exercise physical activity for cardiovascular health and longevity. *British Journal of Sports Medicine* 48(3): 233–238.

Fahey, T., and M. Fahey. 2014. Nutrition, physical activity, and the obesity epidemic: Issues, policies, and solutions (1960s–present). In T. Oliver (Ed.), *The Guide to U.S. Health and Health Care Policy,* pp. 363–374. New York, DWJ Books.

Fontes, E. B., et al. 2015. Brain activity and perceived exertion during cycling exercise: An fMRI study. *British Journal of Sports Medicine* 49(8): 556–560.

Gordon, B. A., et al. 2016. Physical activity intensity can be accurately monitored by smartphone global positioning system "app." *European Journal of Sport Science* 16(5): 624–631.

Hampton, T. 2016. Experts ponder whether too much exercise can compromise cardiovascular health and longevity. *Circulation* 134: 833–834.

Howley, E., and D. Thompson. 2012. *Fitness Professional's Handbook,* 6th ed. Champaign, Ill.: Human Kinetics.

John, D. 2013. *Intervention: Course Correction for the Athlete and Trainer.* Santa Cruz, CA: On Target.

Katz, P. P., and R. Pate. 2016. Exercise as medicine. *Annals of Internal Medicine.* 165(12): 880–881.

Leifer, E. S., et al. 2016. Adverse cardiovascular response to aerobic exercise training: is this a concern. *Medicine and Science in Sports and Exercise* 48(1): 20–25.

McArdle, W. D., et al. 2014. *Exercise Physiology: Nutrition, Energy, and Human Performance.* Philadelphia: Wolters Kluwer.

Park, S. Y., et al. 2016. Exercise training improves vascular mitochondrial function. *American Journal of Physiology: Heart and Circulatory Physiology* 310(7): H821–H829.

Pate, R., and D. Buchner. 2014. *Implementing Physical Activity Strategies.* Champaign, IL: Human Kinetics.

Physical Activity Guidelines Advisory Committee. 2008. *Physical Activity Guidelines Advisory Committee Report, 2008.* Washington, DC: U.S. Department of Health and Human Services.

Puterman, E., et al. 2015. Determinants of telomere attrition over 1 year in healthy older women: Stress and health behaviors matter. *Molecular Psychiatry* 20(4): 529–535.

Song, J., et al. 2017. Do inactive older adults who increase physical activity experience less disability: Evidence from the osteoarthritis initiative. *Journal of Clinical Rheumatology* 23(1): 26–32.

Szuhany, K. L., et al. 2015. A meta-analytic review of the effects of exercise on brain-derived neurotrophic factor. *Journal of Psychiatric Research* 60: 56–64.

Thompson, W. R. 2016. Worldwide survey of fitness: Trends for 2017. *ACSM's Health & Fitness Journal* 20(6): 8–17.

U.S. Department of Health and Human Services. 1996. *Physical Activity and Health: A Report of the Surgeon General.* Atlanta, GA: U.S. Department of Health and Human Services.

U.S. Department of Health and Human Services. 2008. *Physical Activity Guidelines for Americans.* Washington, DC: U.S. Department of Health and Human Services.

U.S. Department of Health and Human Services. 2010. *The Surgeon General's Vision for a Healthy and Fit Nation.* Rockville, MD: U.S. Department of Health and Human Services, Office of the Surgeon General.

U.S. Department of Health and Human Services. 2013. *Physical Activity Guidelines for Americans Midcourse Report.* Washington, DC: U.S. Department of Health and Human Services.

Zhu, W., and N. Owen. 2018. *Sedentary Behavior and Health: Concepts, Assessments, and Interventions.* Champaign, Ill.: Human Kinetics.

Name _____   Section _____   Date _____

LAB 2.1   Safety of Exercise Participation: PAR-Q+

2017 PAR-Q+

The Physical Activity Readiness Questionnaire for Everyone

The health benefits of regular physical activity are clear; more people should engage in physical activity every day of the week. Participating in physical activity is very safe for MOST people. This questionnaire will tell you whether it is necessary for you to seek further advice from your doctor OR a qualified exercise professional before becoming more physically active.

GENERAL HEALTH QUESTIONS

Please read the 7 questions below carefully and answer each one honestly: check YES or NO.	YES	NO
1) Has your doctor ever said that you have a heart condition ☐ OR high blood pressure ☐?	☐	☐
2) Do you feel pain in your chest at rest, during your daily activities of living, **OR** when you do physical activity?	☐	☐
3) Do you lose balance because of dizziness **OR** have you lost consciousness in the last 12 months? Please answer **NO** if your dizziness was associated with over-breathing (including during vigorous exercise).	☐	☐
4) Have you ever been diagnosed with another chronic medical condition (other than heart disease or high blood pressure)? **PLEASE LIST CONDITION(S) HERE:** _____	☐	☐
5) Are you currently taking prescribed medications for a chronic medical condition? **PLEASE LIST CONDITION(S) AND MEDICATIONS HERE:** _____	☐	☐
6) Do you currently have (or have had within the past 12 months) a bone, joint, or soft tissue (muscle, ligament, or tendon) problem that could be made worse by becoming more physically active? Please answer **NO** if you had a problem in the past, but it *does not limit your current ability* to be physically active. **PLEASE LIST CONDITION(S) HERE:** _____	☐	☐
7) Has your doctor ever said that you should only do medically supervised physical activity?	☐	☐

☑ **If you answered NO to all of the questions above, you are cleared for physical activity.**
Go to Page 4 to sign the PARTICIPANT DECLARATION. You do not need to complete Pages 2 and 3.

▶ Start becoming much more physically active – start slowly and build up gradually.

▶ Follow International Physical Activity Guidelines for your age (www.who.int/dietphysicalactivity/en/).

▶ You may take part in a health and fitness appraisal.

▶ If you are over the age of 45 yr and **NOT** accustomed to regular vigorous to maximal effort exercise, consult a qualified exercise professional before engaging in this intensity of exercise.

▶ If you have any further questions, contact a qualified exercise professional.

⬤ **If you answered YES to one or more of the questions above, COMPLETE PAGES 2 AND 3.**

⚠ **Delay becoming more active if:**

✓ You have a temporary illness such as a cold or fever; it is best to wait until you feel better.

✓ You are pregnant - talk to your health care practitioner, your physician, a qualified exercise professional, and/or complete the ePARmed-X+ at **www.eparmedx.com** before becoming more physically active.

✓ Your health changes - answer the questions on Pages 2 and 3 of this document and/or talk to your doctor or a qualified exercise professional before continuing with any physical activity program.

✦ **OSHF** _____   Copyright © 2016 PAR-Q+ Collaboration   1 / 4
01-01-2016

LABORATORY ACTIVITIES

2017 PAR-Q+

FOLLOW-UP QUESTIONS ABOUT YOUR MEDICAL CONDITION(S)

1. Do you have **Arthritis, Osteoporosis, or Back Problems?**

If the above condition(s) is/are present, answer questions 1a-1c   If **NO** ☐ go to question 2

1a.	Do you have difficulty controlling your condition with medications or other physician-prescribed therapies? (Answer **NO** if you are not currently taking medications or other treatments)	YES ☐ NO ☐
1b.	Do you have joint problems causing pain, a recent fracture or fracture caused by osteoporosis or cancer, displaced vertebra (e.g., spondylolisthesis), and/or spondylolysis/pars defect (a crack in the bony ring on the back of the spinal column)?	YES ☐ NO ☐
1c.	Have you had steroid injections or taken steroid tablets regularly for more than 3 months?	YES ☐ NO ☐

2. Do you currently have **Cancer of any kind?**

If the above condition(s) is/are present, answer questions 2a-2b   If **NO** ☐ go to question 3

2a.	Does your cancer diagnosis include any of the following types: lung/bronchogenic, multiple myeloma (cancer of plasma cells), head, and/or neck?	YES ☐ NO ☐
2b.	Are you currently receiving cancer therapy (such as chemotherapy or radiotherapy)?	YES ☐ NO ☐

3. Do you have a **Heart or Cardiovascular Condition?** *This includes Coronary Artery Disease, Heart Failure, Diagnosed Abnormality of Heart Rhythm*

If the above condition(s) is/are present, answer questions 3a-3d   If **NO** ☐ go to question 4

3a.	Do you have difficulty controlling your condition with medications or other physician-prescribed therapies? (Answer **NO** if you are not currently taking medications or other treatments)	YES ☐ NO ☐
3b.	Do you have an irregular heart beat that requires medical management? (e.g., atrial fibrillation, premature ventricular contraction)	YES ☐ NO ☐
3c.	Do you have chronic heart failure?	YES ☐ NO ☐
3d.	Do you have diagnosed coronary artery (cardiovascular) disease and have not participated in regular physical activity in the last 2 months?	YES ☐ NO ☐

4. Do you have **High Blood Pressure?**

If the above condition(s) is/are present, answer questions 4a-4b   If **NO** ☐ go to question 5

4a.	Do you have difficulty controlling your condition with medications or other physician-prescribed therapies? (Answer **NO** if you are not currently taking medications or other treatments)	YES ☐ NO ☐
4b.	Do you have a resting blood pressure equal to or greater than 160/90 mmHg with or without medication? (Answer **YES** if you do not know your resting blood pressure)	YES ☐ NO ☐

5. Do you have any **Metabolic Conditions?** *This includes Type 1 Diabetes, Type 2 Diabetes, Pre-Diabetes*

If the above condition(s) is/are present, answer questions 5a-5e   If **NO** ☐ go to question 6

5a.	Do you often have difficulty controlling your blood sugar levels with foods, medications, or other physician-prescribed therapies?	YES ☐ NO ☐
5b.	Do you often suffer from signs and symptoms of low blood sugar (hypoglycemia) following exercise and/or during activities of daily living? Signs of hypoglycemia may include shakiness, nervousness, unusual irritability, abnormal sweating, dizziness or light-headedness, mental confusion, difficulty speaking, weakness, or sleepiness.	YES ☐ NO ☐
5c.	Do you have any signs or symptoms of diabetes complications such as heart or vascular disease and/or complications affecting your eyes, kidneys, **OR** the sensation in your toes and feet?	YES ☐ NO ☐
5d.	Do you have other metabolic conditions (such as current pregnancy-related diabetes, chronic kidney disease, or liver problems)?	YES ☐ NO ☐
5e.	Are you planning to engage in what for you is unusually high (or vigorous) intensity exercise in the near future?	YES ☐ NO ☐

 OSHF

Copyright © 2016 PAR-Q+ Collaboration   2 / 4
01-01-2016

2017 PAR-Q+

6. **Do you have any Mental Health Problems or Learning Difficulties?** *This includes Alzheimer's, Dementia, Depression, Anxiety Disorder, Eating Disorder, Psychotic Disorder, Intellectual Disability, Down Syndrome*

If the above condition(s) is/are present, answer questions 6a-6b   If **NO** ☐ go to question 7

6a.	Do you have difficulty controlling your condition with medications or other physician-prescribed therapies? (Answer **NO** if you are not currently taking medications or other treatments)	YES ☐ NO ☐
6b.	Do you have Down Syndrome **AND** back problems affecting nerves or muscles?	YES ☐ NO ☐

7. **Do you have a Respiratory Disease?** *This includes Chronic Obstructive Pulmonary Disease, Asthma, Pulmonary High Blood Pressure*

If the above condition(s) is/are present, answer questions 7a-7d   If **NO** ☐ go to question 8

7a.	Do you have difficulty controlling your condition with medications or other physician-prescribed therapies? (Answer **NO** if you are not currently taking medications or other treatments)	YES ☐ NO ☐
7b.	Has your doctor ever said your blood oxygen level is low at rest or during exercise and/or that you require supplemental oxygen therapy?	YES ☐ NO ☐
7c.	If asthmatic, do you currently have symptoms of chest tightness, wheezing, laboured breathing, consistent cough (more than 2 days/week), or have you used your rescue medication more than twice in the last week?	YES ☐ NO ☐
7d.	Has your doctor ever said you have high blood pressure in the blood vessels of your lungs?	YES ☐ NO ☐

8. **Do you have a Spinal Cord Injury?** *This includes Tetraplegia and Paraplegia*

If the above condition(s) is/are present, answer questions 8a-8c   If **NO** ☐ go to question 9

8a.	Do you have difficulty controlling your condition with medications or other physician-prescribed therapies? (Answer **NO** if you are not currently taking medications or other treatments)	YES ☐ NO ☐
8b.	Do you commonly exhibit low resting blood pressure significant enough to cause dizziness, light-headedness, and/or fainting?	YES ☐ NO ☐
8c.	Has your physician indicated that you exhibit sudden bouts of high blood pressure (known as Autonomic Dysreflexia)?	YES ☐ NO ☐

9. **Have you had a Stroke?** *This includes Transient Ischemic Attack (TIA) or Cerebrovascular Event*

If the above condition(s) is/are present, answer questions 9a-9c   If **NO** ☐ go to question 10

9a.	Do you have difficulty controlling your condition with medications or other physician-prescribed therapies? (Answer **NO** if you are not currently taking medications or other treatments)	YES ☐ NO ☐
9b.	Do you have any impairment in walking or mobility?	YES ☐ NO ☐
9c.	Have you experienced a stroke or impairment in nerves or muscles in the past 6 months?	YES ☐ NO ☐

10. **Do you have any other medical condition not listed above or do you have two or more medical conditions?**

If you have other medical conditions, answer questions 10a-10c   If **NO** ☐ read the Page 4 recommendations

10a.	Have you experienced a blackout, fainted, or lost consciousness as a result of a head injury within the last 12 months **OR** have you had a diagnosed concussion within the last 12 months?	YES ☐ NO ☐
10b.	Do you have a medical condition that is not listed (such as epilepsy, neurological conditions, kidney problems)?	YES ☐ NO ☐
10c.	Do you currently live with two or more medical conditions?	YES ☐ NO ☐

PLEASE LIST YOUR MEDICAL CONDITION(S) AND ANY RELATED MEDICATIONS HERE: _____

_____

> ## GO to Page 4 for recommendations about your current medical condition(s) and sign the PARTICIPANT DECLARATION.

OSHF

LABORATORY ACTIVITIES

2017 PAR-Q+

☑ **If you answered NO to all of the follow-up questions about your medical condition, you are ready to become more physically active - sign the PARTICIPANT DECLARATION below:**

▶ It is advised that you consult a qualified exercise professional to help you develop a safe and effective physical activity plan to meet your health needs.

▶ You are encouraged to start slowly and build up gradually - 20 to 60 minutes of low to moderate intensity exercise, 3-5 days per week including aerobic and muscle strengthening exercises.

▶ As you progress, you should aim to accumulate 150 minutes or more of moderate intensity physical activity per week.

▶ If you are over the age of 45 yr and **NOT** accustomed to regular vigorous to maximal effort exercise, consult a qualified exercise professional before engaging in this intensity of exercise.

○ **If you answered YES to one or more of the follow-up questions about your medical condition:**

You should seek further information before becoming more physically active or engaging in a fitness appraisal. You should complete the specially designed online screening and exercise recommendations program - the **ePARmed-X+ at www.eparmedx.com** and/or visit a qualified exercise professional to work through the ePARmed-X+ and for further information.

⚠ **Delay becoming more active if:**

✓ You have a temporary illness such as a cold or fever; it is best to wait until you feel better.

✓ You are pregnant - talk to your health care practitioner, your physician, a qualified exercise professional, and/or complete the ePARmed-X+ **at www.eparmedx.com** before becoming more physically active.

✓ Your health changes - talk to your doctor or qualified exercise professional before continuing with any physical activity program.

● You are encouraged to photocopy the PAR-Q+. You must use the entire questionnaire and NO changes are permitted.
● The authors, the PAR-Q+ Collaboration, partner organizations, and their agents assume no liability for persons who undertake physical activity and/or make use of the PAR-Q+ or ePARmed-X+. If in doubt after completing the questionnaire, consult your doctor prior to physical activity.

PARTICIPANT DECLARATION

● All persons who have completed the PAR-Q+ please read and sign the declaration below.

● If you are less than the legal age required for consent or require the assent of a care provider, your parent, guardian or care provider must also sign this form.

I, the undersigned, have read, understood to my full satisfaction and completed this questionnaire. I acknowledge that this physical activity clearance is valid for a maximum of 12 months from the date it is completed and becomes invalid if my condition changes. I also acknowledge that a Trustee (such as my employer, community/fitness centre, health care provider, or other designate) may retain a copy of this form for their records. In these instances, the Trustee will be required to adhere to local, national, and international guidelines regarding the storage of personal health information ensuring that the Trustee maintains the privacy of the information and does not misuse or wrongfully disclose such information.

NAME _____ DATE _____

SIGNATURE _____ WITNESS _____

SIGNATURE OF PARENT/GUARDIAN/CARE PROVIDER _____

———— For more information, please contact ————
www.eparmedx.com
Email: eparmedx@gmail.com

Citation for PAR-Q+
Warburton DER, Jamnik VK, Bredin SSD, and Gledhill N on behalf of the PAR-Q+ Collaboration. The Physical Activity Readiness Questionnaire for Everyone (PAR-Q+) and Electronic Physical Activity Readiness Medical Examination (ePARmed-X+). Health & Fitness Journal of Canada 4(2):3-23, 2011.
Key References
1. Jamnik VK, Warburton DER, Makarski J, McKenzie DC, Shephard RJ, Stone J, and Gledhill N. Enhancing the effectiveness of clearance for physical activity participation; background and overall process. APNM 36(S1):S3-S13, 2011.
2. Warburton DER, Gledhill N, Jamnik VK, Bredin SSD, McKenzie DC, Stone J, Charlesworth S, and Shephard RJ. Evidence-based risk assessment and recommendations for physical activity clearance; Consensus Document. APNM 36(S1):S266-s298, 2011.
3. Chisholm DM, Collis ML, Kulak LL, Davenport W, and Gruber N. Physical activity readiness. British Columbia Medical Journal. 1975;17:375-378.
4. Thomas S, Reading J, and Shephard RJ. Revision of the Physical Activity Readiness Questionnaire (PAR-Q). Canadian Journal of Sport Science 1992;17:4 338-345.

The PAR-Q+ was created using the evidence-based AGREE process (1) by the PAR-Q+ Collaboration chaired by Dr. Darren E. R. Warburton with Dr. Norman Gledhill, Dr. Veronica Jamnik, and Dr. Donald C. McKenzie (2). Production of this document has been made possible through financial contributions from the Public Health Agency of Canada and the BC Ministry of Health Services. The views expressed herein do not necessarily represent the views of the Public Health Agency of Canada or the BC Ministry of Health Services.

OSHF

Copyright © 2016 PAR-Q+ Collaboration 4 / 4
01-01-2016

Name _____ Section _____ Date _____

LAB 2.2 Overcoming Barriers to Being Active

Barriers to Being Active Quiz

Directions: Listed below are reasons that people give to describe why they do not get as much physical activity as they think they should. Please read each statement and circle the number that describes how likely you are to say each of the following statements.

How likely are you to say this?	Very likely	Somewhat likely	Somewhat unlikely	Very unlikely
1. My day is so busy now, I just don't think I can make the time to include physical activity in my regular schedule.	3	2	(1)	0
2. None of my family members or friends like to do anything active, so I don't have a chance to exercise.	3	2	(1)	0
3. I'm just too tired after work to get any exercise.	3	2	1	(0)
4. I've been thinking about getting more exercise, but I just can't seem to get started.	3	2	(1)	0
5. I'm getting older, so exercise can be risky.	3	2	1	(0)
6. I don't get enough exercise because I have never learned the skills for any sport.	3	2	1	(0)
7. I don't have access to jogging trails, swimming pools, bike paths, etc.	3	2	1	(0)
8. Physical activity takes too much time away from other commitments—like work, family, etc.	3	2	1	(0)
9. I'm embarrassed about how I will look when I exercise with others.	3	2	1	(0)
10. I don't get enough sleep as it is. I just couldn't get up early or stay up late to get some exercise.	3	2	1	(0)
11. It's easier for me to find excuses not to exercise than to go out and do something.	3	2	1	(0)
12. I know of too many people who have hurt themselves by overdoing it with exercise.	3	2	1	(0)
13. I really can't see learning a new sport at my age.	3	2	1	(0)
14. It's just too expensive. You have to take a class or join a club or buy the right equipment.	3	2	1	(0)
15. My free times during the day are too short to include exercise.	3	2	1	(0)
16. My usual social activities with family or friends do not include physical activity.	3	2	(1)	0
17. I'm too tired during the week, and I need the weekend to catch up on my rest.	3	2	1	(0)
18. I want to get more exercise, but I just can't seem to make myself stick to anything.	3	2	1	(0)
19. I'm afraid I might injure myself or have a heart attack.	3	2	1	(0)
20. I'm not good enough at any physical activity to make it fun.	3	2	1	(0)
21. If we had exercise facilities and showers at work, then I would be more likely to exercise.	3	(2)	(1)	0

LABORATORY ACTIVITIES

Scoring

- Enter the circled numbers in the spaces provided below, putting the number for statement 1 on line 1, statement 2 on line 2, and so on.
- Add the three scores on each line. Your barriers to physical activity fall into one or more of seven categories: lack of time, social influences, lack of energy, lack of willpower, fear of injury, lack of skill, and lack of resources. A score of 5 or above in any category shows that this is an important barrier for you to overcome.

1	+	8	+	15	= Lack of time
2	+	9	+	16	= Social influences
3	+	10	+	17	= Lack of energy
4	+	11	+	18	= Lack of willpower
5	+	12	+	19	= Fear of injury
6	+	13	+	20	= Lack of skill
7	+	14	+	21	= Lack of resources

Handwritten entries:
- Line 1: 1 + 2 + 0 = 1 (Lack of time)
- Line 2: 1 + 0 + 1 = 2 (Social influences)
- Line 3: 0 + 0 + 0 = 0 (Lack of energy)
- Line 4: 1 + 0 + 0 = 1 (Lack of willpower)
- Line 5: 0 + 0 + 0 = 0 (Fear of injury)
- Line 6: 0 + 0 + 0 = 0 (Lack of skill)
- Line 7: 0 + 0 + 2 = 2 (Lack of resources)

Using Your Results

How did you score? How many key barriers did you identify? Are they what you expected?

What should you do next? For your key barriers, try the strategies listed on the following pages and/or develop additional strategies that work for you. Check off any strategy that you try.

Suggestions for Overcoming Physical Activity Barriers

Lack of Time

_____ Identify available time slots. Monitor your daily activities for one week. Identify at least three 30-minute time slots you could use for physical activity.

_____ Add physical activity to your daily routine. For example, walk or ride your bike to work or shopping, organize social activities around physical activity, walk the dog, exercise while you watch TV, park farther from your destination, etc.

_____ Make time for physical activity. For example, walk, jog, or swim during your lunch hour, or take fitness breaks instead of coffee breaks.

_____ Select activities requiring minimal time, such as walking, jogging, or stair climbing.

_____ Other:_____

Social Influences

_____ Explain your interest in physical activity to friends and family. Ask them to support your efforts.

_____ Invite friends and family members to exercise with you. Plan social activities involving exercise.

_____ Develop new friendships with physically active people. Join a group, such as the YMCA or a hiking club.

_____ Other:_____

Lack of Energy

_____ Schedule physical activity for times in the day or week when you feel energetic.

_____ Convince yourself that if you give it a chance, exercise will increase your energy level. Then try it.

_____ Other:_____

Lack of Willpower

_____ Plan ahead. Make physical activity a regular part of your daily or weekly schedule and write it on your calendar.

_____ Invite a friend to exercise with you on a regular basis and write it on *both* your calendars.

_____ Join an exercise group or class.

_____ Other:_____

Fear of Injury

_____ Learn how to warm up and cool down to prevent injury.

_____ Learn how to exercise appropriately considering your age, fitness level, skill level, and health status.

_____ Choose activities involving minimal risk.

_____ Other:_____

Lack of Skill

_____ Select activities requiring no new skills, such as walking, jogging, or stair-climbing.

_____ Exercise with friends who are at the same skill level as you are.

_____ Find a friend who is willing to teach you some new skills.

_____ Take a class to develop new skills.

_____ Other:_____

Lack of Resources

_____ Select activities that require minimal facilities or equipment, such as walking, jogging, jumping rope, or calisthenics.

_____ Identify inexpensive, convenient resources available in your community (community education programs, park and recreation programs, worksite programs, etc.).

_____ Other:_____

LABORATORY ACTIVITIES

Are any of the following additional barriers important for you? If so, try some of the strategies listed here or invent your own.

Weather Conditions

_____ Develop a set of regular activities that are always available regardless of weather (indoor cycling, aerobic dance, indoor swimming, calisthenics, stair-climbing, rope-skipping, mall-walking, dancing, gymnasium games, etc.).

_____ Look at outdoor activities that depend on weather conditions (cross-country skiing, outdoor swimming, outdoor tennis, etc.) as "bonuses"—extra activities possible when weather and circumstances permit.

_____ Other:_____

Travel

_____ Put a jump rope in your suitcase and jump rope.

_____ Walk the halls and climb the stairs in hotels.

_____ Stay in places with swimming pools or exercise facilities.

_____ Join the YMCA or YWCA (ask about reciprocal membership agreements).

_____ Visit the local shopping mall and walk for half an hour or more.

_____ Bring a personal music player loaded with your favorite workout music.

_____ Other:_____

Family Obligations

_____ Trade babysitting time with a friend, neighbor, or family member who also has small children.

_____ Exercise *with* the kids—go for a walk together, play tag or other running games, or get an aerobic dance or exercise DVD for kids (there are several on the market) and exercise together. You can spend time together and still get your exercise.

_____ Hire a babysitter and look at the cost as a worthwhile investment in your physical and mental health.

_____ Jump rope, do calisthenics, ride a stationary bicycle, or use other home gymnasium equipment while the kids watch TV or when they are sleeping.

_____ Try to exercise when the kids are not around (e.g., during school hours or their nap time).

_____ Other:_____

Retirement Years

_____ Look on your retirement as an opportunity to become more active instead of less. Spend more time gardening, walking the dog, and playing with your grandchildren. Children with short legs and grandparents with slower gaits are often great walking partners.

_____ Learn a new skill you've always been interested in, such as ballroom dancing, square dancing, or swimming.

_____ Now that you have the time, make regular physical activity a part of every day. Go for a walk every morning or every evening before dinner. Treat yourself to an exercycle and ride every day during a favorite TV show.

_____ Other:_____

SOURCE: Adapted from CDC Division of Nutrition and Physical Activity. 2010. *Promoting Physical Activity: A Guide for Community Action,* 2nd ed. Champaign, Ill.: Human Kinetics.

Name _____ Section _____ Date _____

LAB 2.3   Using a Fitness Tracker or Smartphone Exercise App to Measure Physical Activity

How physically active are you? Would you be more motivated to increase daily physical activity if you had an easy way to monitor your level of activity? If so, consider a smartphone exercise app or fitness tracker to measure your daily physical activity. Smartphone exercise apps use sensors that accurately measure exercise time, distance, peak speed, average speed, step count, and flights of stairs climbed per day. These apps are either low cost or free.

Determine Your Baseline

Wear the fitness tracker or use your smartphone fitness app for a week to obtain a baseline average daily number of steps.

	M	T	W	Th	F	Sa	Su	Average
Steps								
Distance								
Flights of Stairs								

Set Goals

Set an appropriate goal for increasing exercise time, steps, or flights of stairs. The goal of 60 minutes of activity or 10,000 steps per day is widely recommended, but your personal goal should reflect your baseline level of steps. For example, if your current daily steps are far below 10,000, a goal of walking 2,000 additional steps each day might be appropriate. If you are already close to 10,000 steps per day, choose a higher goal. Also consider the following guidelines from health experts:

- To reduce the risk of chronic disease, aim to accumulate at least 150 minutes of moderate physical activity per week.
- To help manage body weight and prevent gradual, unhealthy weight gain, engage in 60 minutes of moderate- to vigorous-intensity activity on most days of the week.
- To sustain weight loss, engage daily in at least 60–90 minutes of moderate-intensity physical activity.

To help gauge how close you are to meeting these time-based physical activity goals, you might walk for 10–15 minutes while wearing your fitness tracker or smartphone to determine how many steps correspond with the time-based goals.

Once you have set your overall goal, break it down into several steps. For example, if your goal is to increase daily steps by 2,000, set mini-goals of increasing daily steps by 500, allowing two weeks to reach each mini-goal. Smaller goals are easier to achieve and can help keep you motivated and on track. Having several interim goals also gives you the opportunity to reward yourself more frequently. Note your goals below:

Mini-goal 1: _____   Target date: _____   Reward: _____
Mini-goal 2: _____   Target date: _____   Reward: _____
Mini-goal 3: _____   Target date: _____   Reward: _____
Overall goal: _____   Target date: _____   Reward: _____

Develop Strategies for Increasing Steps, Exercise Time, and Flights of Stairs

What can you do to become more active? The possibilities include walking when you do errands, getting off one stop from your destination on public transportation, parking an extra block or two away from your destination, and doing at least one chore every day that requires physical activity. If weather or neighborhood safety is an issue, look for alternative locations to walk. For example, find an indoor gym or shopping mall or even a long hallway. Check out locations that are near or on the way to your campus, workplace, or residence. If you think walking indoors will be dull, walk with friends or family members or wear headphones (if safe) and listen to music or audiobooks.

Are there any days of the week for which your baseline steps are particularly low and/or it will be especially difficult because of your schedule to increase your number of steps? Be sure to develop specific strategies for difficult situations.

Below, list at least five strategies for increasing daily steps, exercise time, or stair flights climbed:

_____   _____

_____   _____

_____

Track Your Progress

Based on the goals you set, fill in the goal portion of the progress chart with your target average daily steps for each week. Then carry your smartphone or fitness tracker every day and note your total daily steps, exercise time, and flights of stairs climbed. Track your progress toward each mini-goal and your final goal. Every few weeks, stop and evaluate your progress. If needed, adjust your plan and develop additional strategies for increasing steps. In addition to the chart in this worksheet, you might also want to graph your daily steps to provide a visual reminder of how you are progressing toward your goals. Make as many copies of this chart as you need.

Week	Goal	M	Tu	W	Th	F	Sa	Su	Average
1									
2									
3									
4									

Weeks 1–4 Progress Checkup

How close are you to meeting your goal? How do you feel about your program and your progress?

If needed, describe changes to your plan and additional strategies for increasing total physical activity:

Week	Goal	M	Tu	W	Th	F	Sa	Su	Average
5									
6									
7									
8									

Weeks 5–8 Progress Checkup

How close are you to meeting your goal? How do you feel about your program and your progress?

If needed, describe changes to your plan and additional strategies for increasing total physical activity:

Week	Goal	M	Tu	W	Th	F	Sa	Su	Average
9									
10									
11									
12									

Weeks 9–12 Progress Checkup

How close are you to meeting your goal? How do you feel about your program and your progress?

If needed, in the space below, describe changes to your plan and additional strategies for increasing total physical activity.

3 Cardiorespiratory Endurance

LOOKING AHEAD...

After reading this chapter, you should be able to

- Describe how the body produces the energy it needs for exercise.

- List the major effects and benefits of cardiorespiratory endurance exercise.

- Explain how cardiorespiratory endurance is measured and assessed.

- Describe how frequency, intensity, time (duration), type of exercise, volume, and progression (FITT-VP) affect the development of cardiorespiratory endurance.

- Explain the best ways to prevent and treat common exercise injuries.

TEST YOUR KNOWLEDGE

1. Compared to sedentary people, those who engage in regular moderate endurance exercise are likely to
   a. have fewer colds.
   b. be less anxious and depressed.
   c. fall asleep more quickly and sleep better.
   d. be more alert and creative.
   e. all four

2. About how much blood does the heart pump each minute during maximum-intensity aerobic exercise?
   a. 5 quarts
   b. 10 quarts
   c. 20 quarts

3. During an effective 30-minute cardiorespiratory endurance workout, you should lose 1–2 pounds. True or false?

See answers on the next page.

© Phillip Suddick/Getty Images

Cardiorespiratory endurance—the ability of the body to perform prolonged, large-muscle, dynamic exercise at moderate to high levels of intensity—is a key health-related component of fitness. As explained in Chapter 2, a healthy cardiorespiratory system is essential to high levels of fitness and wellness.

This chapter reviews the short- and long-term effects and benefits of cardiorespiratory endurance exercise. It then describes several tests commonly used to assess cardiorespiratory fitness. Finally, it provides guidelines for creating your own cardiorespiratory endurance training program—one that is geared to your current level of fitness and built around activities you enjoy.

BASIC PHYSIOLOGY OF CARDIORESPIRATORY ENDURANCE EXERCISE

A basic understanding of the body processes involved in cardiorespiratory endurance exercise can help you design a safe and effective fitness program.

The Cardiorespiratory System

The **cardiorespiratory system** consists of the heart, the blood vessels, and the respiratory system (the lungs) (Figure 3.1). The cardiorespiratory system circulates blood through the body, transporting oxygen, nutrients, and other key substances to the organs and tissues that need them. It also carries away waste products so that they can be used or expelled.

The Heart The heart is a four-chambered, fist-sized muscle located just beneath the sternum (breastbone) (Figure 3.2). It pumps oxygen-poor blood to the lungs and delivers oxygen-rich blood to the rest of the body. Blood travels through two separate circulatory systems: The right side of the heart pumps blood to the lungs through **pulmonary circulation**, and the left side pumps blood through the rest of the body in **systemic circulation**.

The path of blood flow through the heart and cardiorespiratory system is illustrated in Figure 3.2. Refer to that illustration as you trace these steps:

1. Waste-laden, oxygen-poor blood travels through large vessels, called **venae cavae**, into the heart's right upper chamber, or **atrium**.

2. After the right atrium fills, it contracts and pumps blood into the heart's right lower chamber, or **ventricle**.

3. When the right ventricle is full, it contracts and pumps blood through the pulmonary artery into the lungs.

4. In the lungs, blood picks up oxygen and discards **carbon dioxide**. Oxygen moves from the lungs to the blood and carbon dioxide moves from the blood to the lungs by a process called **diffusion**. During exercise, you breathe faster to promote diffusion of these gases.

TERMS

cardiorespiratory system   The system that circulates blood through the body; consists of the heart, blood vessels, and respiratory system.

pulmonary circulation   The part of the circulatory system that moves blood between the heart and lungs; controlled by the right side of the heart.

systemic circulation   The part of the circulatory system that moves blood between the heart and the rest of the body; controlled by the left side of the heart.

venae cavae   The large veins through which blood is returned to the right atrium of the heart.

atrium   One of the two upper chambers of the heart in which blood collects before passing to the ventricles (pl. *atria*).

ventricle   One of the two lower chambers of the heart from which blood flows through arteries to the lungs and other parts of the body.

carbon dioxide   A gas produced during the metabolism of carbohydrates, fats, protein, and acids. During exercise, the body manages increased levels of carbon dioxide by breathing faster. Plants use carbon dioxide to capture energy through photosynthesis, but high levels of carbon dioxide are toxic to the body.

diffusion   The process by which oxygen moves from the lungs to the blood and carbon dioxide moves from the blood to the lungs; faster breathing concentrates oxygen and decreases carbon dioxide in the lungs and promotes diffusion.

aorta   The body's largest artery; receives blood from the left ventricle and distributes it to the body.

tricuspid valve   The heart valve between the right atrium and the right ventricle that prevents the back flow of blood into the right atrium.

pulmonary valve   The heart valve that lies between the right ventricle and the pulmonary artery that prevents the back flow of blood into the right ventricle.

mitral valve   The heart valve that lies between the left atrium and left ventricle that prevents the back flow of blood into the left atrium.

aortic valve   The heart valve between the left ventricle and the aorta that prevents the back flow of blood into the left ventricle.

systole   Contraction of the heart.

diastole   Relaxation of the heart.

blood pressure   The force exerted by the blood on the walls of the blood vessels; created by the pumping action of the heart.

Answers (Test Your Knowledge)

1. **e. All four.** Endurance exercise has many immediate benefits that affect all the dimensions of wellness and improve overall quality of life.

2. **c.** During exercise, cardiac output increases to 20 or more quarts per minute, compared to about 5 quarts per minute at rest.

3. **False.** Any weight loss during an exercise session is due to fluid loss that needs to be replaced to prevent dehydration and enhance performance. It is best to drink enough during exercise to match fluid lost as sweat; weigh yourself before and after a workout to make sure you are drinking enough.

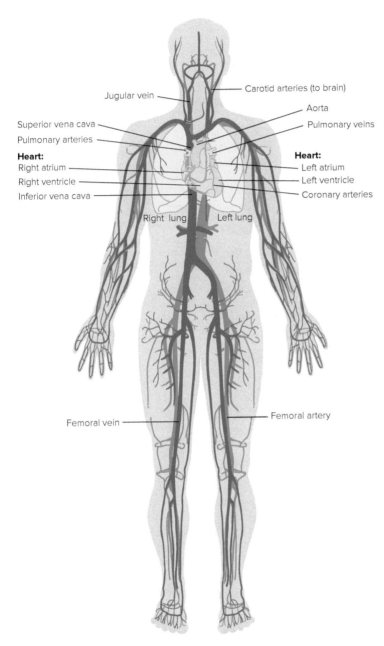

Jugular vein — Carotid arteries (to brain)

— Aorta

Superior vena cava — Pulmonary veins

Pulmonary arteries —

Heart: **Heart:**

Right atrium — Left atrium

Right ventricle — Left ventricle

Inferior vena cava — Coronary arteries

Right lung   Left lung

Femoral vein — Femoral artery

FIGURE 3.1. The cardiorespiratory system.

5. The cleaned, oxygenated blood flows from the lungs through the pulmonary veins into the heart's left atrium.

6. After the left atrium fills, it contracts and pumps blood into the left ventricle.

7. When the left ventricle is full, it pumps blood through the **aorta**—the body's largest artery—for distribution to the rest of the body's blood vessels.

The heart has four valves that prevent blood back-flow and keep blood moving in the right direction: the **tricuspid valve** opens to allow blood flow from the right atrium to right ventricle; the **pulmonary valve** allows blood flow from the right ventricle to the lungs; the **mitral valve** allows blood flow from the left atrium to the left ventricle; and the **aortic valve** allows blood flow into the aorta.

The period of the heart's contraction is called **systole**; the period of relaxation is called **diastole**. During systole, the atria contract first, pumping blood into the ventricles. A fraction of a second later, the ventricles contract, pumping blood to the lungs and the body. During diastole, blood flows into the heart.

Blood pressure, the force exerted by blood on the walls of the blood vessels, is created by the pumping action of the heart. Blood pressure is greater during systole than during diastole. A person weighing 150 pounds has about 5 quarts of blood, which are circulated about once every minute at rest. Hypertension (high blood pressure) is a major risk factor for heart and kidney disease (see Table 11.1).

The heartbeat—the split-second sequence of contractions of the heart's four chambers—is controlled by nerve impulses. These signals originate in a bundle of specialized cells in the right atrium called the *pacemaker,* or *sinoatrial (SA) node.* The heart produces nerve impulses at a steady rate—unless it is speeded up or slowed down by the brain in response to stimuli such as exercise.

The Blood Vessels Blood vessels are classified by size and function. **Veins** carry blood to the heart. **Arteries** carry it away from the heart. Veins have thin walls, but arteries have thick elastic walls that enable them to expand and relax with the volume of blood being pumped through them.

The blood vessels are lined with **endothelial cells** that secrete **nitric oxide**—a chemical messenger regulating blood flow. Inflammation, physical inactivity, poor diet, smoking, high blood pressure, or insulin resistance can promote blood vessel disease and interfere with nitric oxide secretion, which has a wide range of negative effects ranging from erectile dysfunction to heart disease. Regular physical activity helps maintain healthy blood vessels and normal nitric oxide metabolism.

After leaving the heart, the aorta branches into smaller and smaller vessels. The smallest arteries branch still further into

TERMS

veins Vessels that carry blood to the heart.

arteries Vessels that carry blood away from the heart.

endothelial cells Cells lining the blood vessels.

nitric oxide A gas released by the endothelial cells to promote blood flow. The capacity of these cells to release nitric oxide is an important marker of good health.

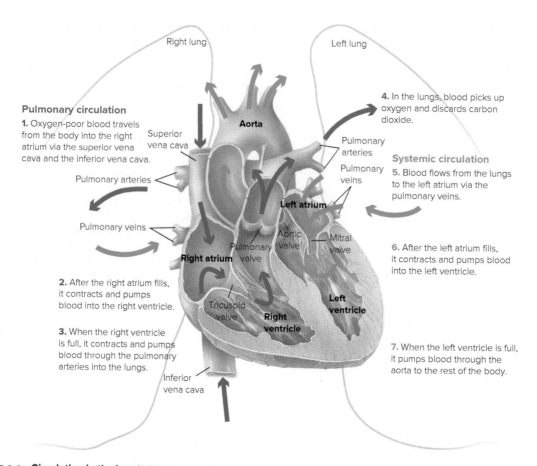

Right lung

Pulmonary circulation

1. Oxygen-poor blood travels from the body into the right atrium via the superior vena cava and the inferior vena cava.

Superior vena cava

Aorta

Pulmonary arteries

Pulmonary veins

Right atrium

Pulmonary valve

Tricuspid valve

2. After the right atrium fills, it contracts and pumps blood into the right ventricle.

3. When the right ventricle is full, it contracts and pumps blood through the pulmonary arteries into the lungs.

Inferior vena cava

Left lung

4. In the lungs, blood picks up oxygen and discards carbon dioxide.

Pulmonary arteries

Pulmonary veins

Systemic circulation

5. Blood flows from the lungs to the left atrium via the pulmonary veins.

Left atrium

Aortic valve

Mitral valve

6. After the left atrium fills, it contracts and pumps blood into the left ventricle.

Left ventricle

Right ventricle

7. When the left ventricle is full, it pumps blood through the aorta to the rest of the body.

FIGURE 3.2   Circulation in the heart. Blue arrows indicate oxygen-poor blood; red arrows indicate oxygen-rich blood.

capillaries, tiny vessels only one cell thick. The capillaries deliver oxygen and nutrient-rich blood to the tissues and pick up oxygen-poor, waste-laden blood. From the capillaries, this blood empties into small veins (*venules*) and then into larger veins that return it to the heart to repeat the cycle.

Blood pumped through the heart doesn't reach the heart's own cells, so the organ has its own network of blood vessels called the **coronary arteries**. Two large vessels, the right and left coronary arteries, branch off the aorta and supply the heart muscle with oxygenated blood. (The coronary arteries are shown in Figure 3.1). The fit-and-well lifestyle helps prevent coronary artery disease.

capillaries   Very small blood vessels that distribute blood to all parts of the body.   **TERMS**

coronary arteries   A pair of large blood vessels that branch off the aorta and supply the heart muscle with oxygenated blood.

respiratory system   The lungs, air passages, and breathing muscles; supplies oxygen to the body and removes carbon dioxide.

alveoli   Tiny air sacs in the lungs that allow the exchange of oxygen and carbon dioxide between the lungs and blood.

The Respiratory System   The **respiratory system** supplies oxygen to the body, carries off carbon dioxide—a waste product of body processes—and helps regulate acid produced during metabolism. Air passes in and out of the lungs as a result of pressure changes brought about by the contraction and relaxation of the diaphragm and rib muscles. As air is inhaled, it passes through the nasal passages, throat, larynx, trachea (windpipe), and bronchi into the lungs. The lungs consist of many branching tubes that end in tiny, thin-walled air sacs called **alveoli**.

Carbon dioxide and oxygen are exchanged between alveoli and capillaries in the lungs. Carbon dioxide passes from blood cells into the alveoli, where it is carried up and out of the lungs (exhaled). Oxygen from inhaled air is passed from the alveoli into blood cells; these oxygen-rich blood cells then return to the heart and are pumped throughout the body. Oxygen is an important component of the body's energy-producing system, so the cardiorespiratory system's ability to pick up and deliver oxygen is critical for the functioning of the body.

The Cardiorespiratory System at Rest and during Exercise   At rest and during light activity, the cardiorespiratory system functions at a fairly steady pace. Your heart beats at a rate of about 50–90 beats per minute, and you take about 12–20 breaths per minute. A typical resting blood pressure in a healthy adult, measured in millimeters of mercury, is 120 systolic and 80 diastolic (120/80 mmHg).

During exercise, the demands on the cardiorespiratory system increase. Body cells, particularly working muscles, need to obtain more oxygen and fuel and to eliminate more waste products. To meet these demands, your body makes the following changes:

- Heart rate increases, up to 170–210 beats per minute during intense exercise.

- The heart's **stroke volume** increases, meaning that the heart pumps out more blood with each beat.

- The heart pumps and circulates more blood per minute as a result of the faster heart rate and greater stroke volume. During exercise, this **cardiac output** increases to 20 or more quarts per minute, compared to about 5 quarts per minute at rest.

- Blood flow changes, so as much as 85–90% of the blood may be delivered to working muscles. At rest, about 15–20% of blood is distributed to the skeletal muscles.

- Systolic blood pressure increases, while diastolic blood pressure holds steady or declines slightly. A typical exercise blood pressure might be 175/65. Diastolic pressure is particularly important during exercise because the blood flow to the coronary arteries that supply the heart muscle is greatest during the relaxation phase of the cardiac cycle.

- To oxygenate this increased blood flow, you take deeper breaths and breathe faster, up to 40–60 breaths per minute.

All of these changes are controlled and coordinated by special centers in the brain, which use the nervous system and chemical messengers to control the process.

Energy Production

Metabolism is the sum of all the chemical processes necessary to maintain the body. Energy is required to fuel vital body functions—to build and break down tissue, contract muscles, conduct nerve impulses, regulate body temperature, and so on.

The rate at which your body uses energy—its **metabolic rate**—depends on your level of activity. At rest, you have a low metabolic rate; if you begin to walk, your metabolic rate increases. If you jog, your metabolic rate may increase more than 800% above its resting level. Olympic-caliber distance runners can increase their metabolic rate by 2,000% or more.

Energy from Food The body converts chemical energy from food into substances that cells can use as fuel. These fuels can be used immediately or stored for later use. The body's ability to store fuel is critical, because if all the energy from food were released immediately, much of it would be wasted.

The three classes of energy-containing nutrients in food are carbohydrates (sugar, wheat flour, honey), fats (meat, nuts, fried foods), and proteins (seafood, poultry, dairy food). During digestion, most carbohydrates are broken down into the simple sugar **glucose**. Some glucose circulates in the blood ("blood sugar"), where it can be used as a quick source of fuel

to produce energy. Glucose may also be converted to **glycogen** and stored mainly in the liver and muscles. If glycogen stores are full and the body's immediate need for energy is met, the remaining glucose is converted to fat and stored in the body's fatty tissues. Excess energy from fat in the diet is also stored as body fat. Protein in the diet is used primarily to build new tissue, but it can be broken down for energy or incorporated into fat stores. Glucose, glycogen, and fat are important fuels for the production of energy in the cells; protein is a significant energy source only when other fuels are lacking. (See Chapter 8 for more on the roles of carbohydrate, fat, and protein in the body.)

ATP: The Energy "Currency" of Cells The basic form of energy used by cells is **adenosine triphosphate**, or **ATP**. When a cell needs energy, it breaks down ATP, a process that releases energy in the only form the cell can use directly. Cells store a small amount of ATP; when they need more, they create it through chemical reactions that utilize the body's stored fuels—glucose, glycogen, and fat. When you exercise, your cells need to produce more energy. Consequently, your body mobilizes its stores of fuel to increase ATP production. The mitochondria of cells produce the most ATP. A high mitochondrial capacity is critical for endurance performance, health, and longevity.

Exercise and the Three Energy Systems

The muscles in your body use three energy systems to create ATP and fuel cellular activity. These systems use different fuels and chemical processes and perform different, specific functions during exercise (Table 3.1).

The Immediate Energy System The **immediate ("explosive") energy system** provides energy rapidly but for only a short period of time. It is used to fuel activities that last for about 10 or fewer seconds—such as weight lifting and shot-putting or in daily life just rising from a chair or picking up a bag of groceries. The fuels for this energy system include existing

---

stroke volume The amount of blood the heart pumps with each beat. **TERMS**

cardiac output The volume of blood pumped by the heart per minute via heart rate and stroke volume.

metabolic rate The rate at which the body uses energy.

glucose A simple sugar circulating in the blood that can be used by cells to fuel adenosine triphosphate (ATP) production.

glycogen A complex carbohydrate stored principally in the liver and skeletal muscles; the major fuel source during most forms of intense exercise. Glycogen is the storage form of glucose.

adenosine triphosphate (ATP) The energy source for cellular processes.

immediate ("explosive") energy system The system that supplies very short bursts of energy to muscle cells through the breakdown of cellular stores of ATP and creatine phosphate (CP).

Table 3.1	Characteristics of the Body's Energy Systems		
	ENERGY SYSTEM*		
	IMMEDIATE	NONOXIDATIVE	OXIDATIVE
DURATION OF ACTIVITY FOR WHICH SYSTEM PREDOMINATES	0–10 seconds	10 seconds–2 minutes	>2 minutes
INTENSITY OF ACTIVITY FOR WHICH SYSTEM PREDOMINATES	High	High	Low to moderately high
RATE OF ATP PRODUCTION	Immediate, very rapid	Rapid	Slower, but prolonged
FUEL	Adenosine triphosphate (ATP), creatine phosphate (CP)	Muscle stores of glucose and glycogen	Body stores of glycogen, glucose, fat, and protein
OXYGEN USED?	No	No	Yes
SAMPLE ACTIVITIES	Weight lifting, picking up a bag of groceries	400-meter run, running up several flights of stairs	1500-meter run, 30-minute walk, standing in line for a long time

*For most activities, all three systems contribute to energy production; the duration and intensity of the activity determine which system predominates.

SOURCE: Brooks, G. A., et al. 2005. *Exercise Physiology: Human Bioenergetics and Its Applications*, 4th ed. New York: McGraw-Hill.

cellular ATP stores and **creatine phosphate** (CP), a chemical that cells can use to make ATP. CP levels deplete rapidly during exercise, so the maximum capacity of this energy system is reached within a few seconds. Cells must then switch to the other energy systems to restore levels of ATP and CP. (Without adequate ATP, muscles will stiffen and become unusable.)

The Nonoxidative Energy System The **nonoxidative (anaerobic) energy system** is used at the start of an exercise zsession and for high-intensity activities lasting for about 10 seconds to 2 minutes, such as the 400-meter run. During daily activities, this system may be called on to help you run to

creatine phosphate A high-energy compound used to resynthesize ATP that is particularly important during high-intensity exercise.

nonoxidative (anaerobic) energy system The system that supplies energy to muscle cells for highly intense exercise of short duration by breaking down muscle stores of glucose and glycogen; called the *anaerobic system* because chemical reactions take place without oxygen and produce lactic acid.

anaerobic Occurring in the absence of oxygen.

lactic acid A metabolic acid resulting from the metabolism of glucose and glycogen. It is broken down in the body into lactate and hydrogen ions as soon as it is produced.

Lactate Lactate is lactic acid without the acid. In the body, lactic acid immediately gets rid of the acid (hydrogen ion, H+), so the body produces and uses lactate at rest and during exercise.

oxidative (aerobic) energy system The system that supplies energy to cells for long periods of activity through the breakdown of glucose, glycogen, and fats; called the *aerobic system* because its chemical reactions require oxygen.

aerobic Dependent on the presence of oxygen.

mitochondria Cell structures that convert the energy in food to a form the body can use.

TERMS

catch a bus or dash up several flights of stairs. The nonoxidative energy system creates ATP by breaking down glucose and glycogen. This system doesn't require oxygen, which is why it is sometimes referred to as the **anaerobic** system. This system's capacity to produce energy is limited, but it can generate a great deal of ATP in a short period of time. For this reason, it is the most important energy system for very intense exercise.

The nonoxidative energy system has two key limitations. First, the body's supply of glucose and glycogen is limited. If these are depleted, a person may experience fatigue, dizziness, and impaired judgment. (The brain and nervous system rely on carbohydrates as fuel.) Second, the rapid metabolism caused by this energy system increases hydrogen and potassium ions that interfere with metabolism and muscle contraction and cause fatigue. During heavy exercise, such as sprinting, large increases in hydrogen and potassium ions cause muscles to fatigue rapidly.

The anaerobic energy system also creates metabolic acids. Fortunately, exercise training increases the body's ability to cope with metabolic acids. Improved fitness allows you to exercise at higher intensities before the abrupt buildup of metabolic acids—a point that scientists call the *lactate threshold*. One metabolic acid, called **lactic acid,** is often linked to fatigue during intense exercise. Lactic acid does not last long in blood. It breaks down into **lactate** and hydrogen ions (acid) as soon as it is produced. Lactate is an important fuel at rest and during exercise. Training improves the ability to use lactate as fuel.

The Oxidative Energy System The **oxidative (aerobic) energy system** operates during any physical activity that lasts longer than about two minutes, such as distance running, swimming, hiking, or even just standing in line. The oxidative system requires oxygen to generate ATP, which is why it is considered an **aerobic** system. The oxidative system cannot produce energy as quickly as the other two systems, but it can supply energy for much longer periods of time. It is the source of our energy during most daily activities.

In the oxidative energy system, ATP production takes place in cellular structures called **mitochondria**. Because mitochondria can use carbohydrates (glucose and glycogen) or fats to produce ATP, the body's stores of fuel for this system are much greater than those for the other two energy systems. The actual fuel used depends on the intensity and duration of exercise and on the fitness status of the individual. Carbohydrates are favored during more intense exercise (more than 65% of maximum capacity); fats are used for mild, low-intensity activities. During a prolonged exercise session, carbohydrates are the predominant fuel at the start of the workout, but fat utilization increases over time. Fit individuals use a greater proportion of fat as fuel because increased fitness allows people to do activities at lower intensities. This is an important adaptation because glycogen depletion is one of the limiting factors for the oxidative energy system. By being able to use more fat as fuel, a fit individual can exercise for a longer time before glycogen is depleted and muscles become fatigued. Aerobic exercise and high-intensity interval training increase the number and capacity of mitochondria. Increased mitochondrial capacity is the most important benefit of exercise. Mitochondrial health and fitness are linked to a reduced risk of disease and increased longevity.

Oxygen is another factor limiting exercise capacity. The oxygen requirement of this energy system is proportional to the intensity of exercise. As intensity increases, so does oxygen consumption. The body's ability to increase oxygen use is limited; this limit, known as **maximal oxygen consumption**, or $\dot{V}O_{2max}$, refers to the highest rate of oxygen consumption an individual is capable of during maximum physical effort. It is expressed in milliliters of oxygen per kilogram of body weight per minute or as liters per minute. In the symbol, the V stands for volume, the dot over the V means per minute, the O_2 stands for oxygen, and the max means maximum. $\dot{V}O_{2max}$ determines how intensely a person can perform endurance exercise and for how long, and it is considered the best overall measure of the capacity of the cardiorespiratory system. (The assessment tests described later in the chapter are designed to help you evaluate your $\dot{V}O_{2max}$.)

The Energy Systems in Combination Your body typically uses all three energy systems when you exercise. The intensity and duration of the activity determine which system predominates. For example, when you play tennis, you use the immediate energy system when hitting the ball, but you replenish cellular energy stores by using the nonoxidative and oxidative systems. When cycling, the oxidative system predominates. However, if you must suddenly exercise intensely—by riding up a steep hill, for example—the other systems become important because the oxidative system is unable to supply ATP fast enough to sustain high-intensity effort.

Physical Fitness and Energy Production Physically fit people can increase their metabolic rate substantially, generating the energy needed for powerful or sustained exercise. People who are not fit cannot respond to exercise in the same way. Their bodies are less capable of delivering oxygen and fuel to exercising muscles, they can't burn as many calories during or after exercise, and they are less able to cope with lactate and other substances produced during intense physical activity that contribute to fatigue. Because of this, they become fatigued more rapidly; their legs hurt and they breathe heavily walking up a flight of stairs, for example. Regular physical training can substantially improve the body's ability to produce energy and meet the challenges of increased physical activity.

In designing an exercise program, focus on the energy system most important to your goals. Because improving the functioning of the cardiorespiratory system is critical to overall wellness, endurance exercise that utilizes the oxidative energy system—activities performed at moderate to high intensities for a prolonged duration—is a key component of any health-related fitness program.

BENEFITS OF CARDIORESPIRATORY ENDURANCE EXERCISE

Cardiorespiratory endurance exercise helps the body become more efficient and better able to cope with physical challenges. It also lowers risk for many chronic diseases.

Improved Cardiorespiratory Functioning

Earlier, this chapter described some of the major changes that occur in the cardiorespiratory system when you exercise, such as increases in cardiac output and blood pressure, breathing rate, and blood flow to the skeletal muscles. In the short term, all these changes help the body respond to the challenge of exercise. When performed regularly, endurance exercise also leads to permanent adaptation in the cardiorespiratory system (Figure 3.3). This improvement reduces the effort required to perform everyday tasks and enables the body to respond to physical challenges. This, in a nutshell, is what it means to be physically fit.

Endurance exercise enhances the heart's health by doing the following:

- Maintaining or increasing the heart's own blood and oxygen supply.
- Improving the heart muscle's function, enabling the heart to pump more blood per beat. This improved function keeps

---

Ask Yourself

QUESTIONS FOR CRITICAL THINKING AND REFLECTION

When you think about the types of physical activity you engage in during your typical day or week, which ones use the immediate energy system? The nonoxidative energy system? The oxidative energy system? How can you increase activities that use the oxidative energy system?

---

maximal oxygen consumption ($\dot{V}O_{2max}$) The **TERMS** highest rate of oxygen consumption an individual is capable of during maximum physical effort, reflecting the body's ability to transport and use oxygen; measured in milliliters of oxygen used per kilogram of body weight per minute.

the heart rate lower both at rest and during exercise. The resting heart rate of a fit person is often 10–20 beats per minute lower than that of an unfit person. This translates into as many as 10 million fewer beats in the course of a year.

- Strengthening the heart's contractions.
- Increasing the heart's cavity size (in young adults).
- Increasing blood volume, enabling the heart to push more blood into the circulatory system during each contraction (larger stroke volume). Increased blood volume also improves temperature regulation, which reduces the load on the heart.
- Reducing blood pressure.

- Reducing blood cholesterol and triglycerides and increasing HDL (good cholesterol), all of which reduce the risk of coronary artery disease.
- Stabilizing the electrical activity of the heart, which protects against **cardiac arrest**.

Improved Cellular Metabolism

Regular endurance exercise improves the body's metabolism, down to the cellular level, enhancing your ability to produce and use energy efficiently. Cardiorespiratory training improves metabolism by doing the following (see Figure 3.3):

Immediate effects

Increases levels of neurotransmitters; constant or slightly increased blood flow to the brain.

Increases heart rate and stroke volume (amount of blood pumped per beat).

Increases pulmonary ventilation (amount of air breathed into the body per minute). More air is taken into the lungs with each breath and breathing rate increases.

Reduced blood flow to the stomach, intestines, liver, and kidneys, resulting in less activity in the digestive tract and less urine output.

Increases energy (ATP) production.

Increases cell pump activity, normalizing cell function during excercise and preventing heart rhythm problems.

Increases blood flow to the skin and increased sweating to help maintain a safe body temperature.

Increases systolic blood pressure; increased blood flow and oxygen transport to working skeletal muscles and the heart; increased oxygen consumption. As exercise intensity increases, blood levels of lactate.

Long-term effects

Improved self-image, cognitive functioning, and ability to manage stress; enhanced learning, memory, energy level, and sleep; decreased depression, anxiety, and risk for stroke.

Increased heart size and resting stroke volume; lower resting heart rate. Risk of heart disease and heart attack reduced significantly.

Improved ability to extract oxygen from air during exercise. Reduced risk of colds and upper respiratory tract infections.

Increased sweat rate and earlier onset of sweating, helping to cool the body.

Decreased body fat.

Reduced risk of colon cancer and certain other forms of cancer.

Increased number and size of mitochondria in muscle cells; increased amount of stored glycogen; improved ability to use lactate and fats as fuel. All of these changes allow for greater energy production and power output. Insulin sensitivity remains constant or improves, helping to prevent type 2 diabetes. Fat-free mass may also increase somewhat.

Increased density and breaking strength of bones, ligaments, and tendons; reduced risk for low-back pain, injuries, and osteoporosis.

Increased blood volume and capillary density; higher levels of high-density lipoproteins (HDL) and lower levels of triglycerides; lower resting blood pressure; increased ability of blood vessels to secrete nitric oxide; and reduced platelet stickiness (a factor in coronary artery disease).

FIGURE 3.3   Immediate and long-term effects of regular cardiorespiratory endurance exercise. When endurance exercise is performed regularly, short-term changes in the body develop into more permanent adaptations; these include improved ability to exercise, reduced risk of many chronic diseases, and improved psychological and emotional well-being.

- Increasing the number of capillaries in the muscles. Additional capillaries supply the muscles with more fuel and oxygen and more quickly eliminate waste products. Greater capillary density also helps heal injuries and reduce muscle aches.
- Training muscles to make the most of oxygen and fuel so that they work more efficiently.
- Increasing the size and number of mitochondria in muscle and brain cells, thereby increasing the cells' energy capacity.
- Preventing glycogen depletion and increasing the muscles' ability to use lactate and fat as fuels.
- Increasing the activity of cell pumps for sodium, potassium, and calcium, which normalizes cell function and prevents fatigue and abnormal heart rhythms.

Regular exercise may also help protect cells from chemical damage caused by agents called *free radicals.* (See Chapter 8 for details on free radicals and the special enzymes the body uses to fight them.)

Fitness programs that best develop metabolic efficiency include both long-duration, moderately intense endurance exercise and brief periods of more intense effort. For example, climbing a small hill while jogging or cycling introduces the kind of intense exercise that leads to more efficient use of lactate and fats.

Reduced Risk of Chronic Disease

Regular endurance exercise lowers your risk of many chronic, disabling diseases. It can also help people with those diseases improve their health (see the box "Benefits of Exercise for Older Adults"). The most significant health benefits occur when someone who is sedentary becomes moderately active.

Cardiovascular Diseases Sedentary living is a key contributor to cardiovascular disease (CVD). CVD is a general category that encompasses several diseases of the heart and blood vessels, including coronary heart disease (which can cause heart attacks), stroke, and high blood pressure (see the box "Combine Aerobic Exercise with Strength Training"). Sedentary people are significantly more likely to die of CVD than are fit individuals.

Cardiorespiratory endurance exercise lowers your risk of CVD by doing the following:

- Promoting a healthy balance of fats in the blood. High concentrations of blood fats such as cholesterol and triglycerides are linked to CVD. Exercise raises levels of "good cholesterol" (high-density lipoproteins, or HDL) and may lower levels of "bad cholesterol" (low-density lipoproteins, or LDL).
- Reducing high blood pressure, which is a contributing factor to several kinds of CVD.
- Boosting **cell pump** activity (sodium-potassium and calcium pumps) that help maintain internal cellular health.
- Enhancing the capacity of cell mitochondria.

- Enhancing the function of the cells that line the arteries (endothelial cells).
- Reducing chronic inflammation.
- Preventing obesity and type 2 diabetes, both of which contribute to CVD.

Details on various types of CVD, their associated risk factors, and a lifestyle that can reduce your risk for developing CVD are discussed in Chapter 11.

Cancer Although the findings are not conclusive, some studies have shown a relationship between increased physical activity and a reduction in a person's risk of cancer. Exercise reduces the risk of colon cancer, and it may reduce the risk of cancers of the breast and reproductive organs. Physical activity during the high school and college years may be particularly important for preventing breast cancer later in life. Exercise may also reduce the risk of lung cancer, endometrial cancer, pancreatic cancer, and prostate cancer. (See Chapter 12 for more information on various types of cancer.)

Type 2 Diabetes Regular exercise helps prevent the development of type 2 diabetes, the most common form of diabetes. Physical activity is also an important part of treating the disease. Obesity is a key risk factor for diabetes, and exercise helps keep body fat at healthy levels. But even without fat loss, exercise improves control of blood sugar levels in many people with diabetes. Exercise metabolizes (burns) excess sugar and makes cells more sensitive to the hormone insulin, which helps regulate blood sugar levels. (See Chapter 11 for more on diabetes and insulin resistance.)

Osteoporosis A special benefit of exercise, especially for women, is protection against osteoporosis, a disease that results in loss of bone density and strength. Weight-bearing exercise—particularly weight training—helps build bone during the teens and 20s. People with denser bones can better endure the bone loss that occurs with aging. With stronger bones and muscles and better balance, fit people are less likely to experience debilitating falls and bone fractures. (See Chapter 8 for more on osteoporosis.)

Inflammation **Inflammation** is the body's response to tissue and cell damage (from injury, high blood pressure, or intense exercise), environmental poisons (e.g., cigarette smoke), or poor metabolic health (high blood fats, poor blood

---

cardiac arrest Malfunctioning of the heart, in which it suddenly stops beating due to "electrical" problems in the heart cells. **TERMS**

cell pump Structures in cell walls that work to maintain normal cell levels of sodium, potassium, and calcium. Exercise training increases the activity of these pumps, which helps prevent fatigue.

inflammation The body's response to tissue and cell damage, environmental poisons, or poor metabolic health.

DIVERSITY MATTERS
Benefits of Exercise for Older Adults

Research has shown that most aspects of physiological functioning peak when people are about 30 years old, then decline at a rate of about 0.5–1.0% per year. This decline in physical capacity shows up in decreases in maximal oxygen consumption, cardiac output, muscular strength, fat-free mass, joint mobility, and other factors. However, regular exercise can substantially alter the rate of decline and promote both longevity and improved quality of life.

Regular endurance exercise can improve maximal oxygen consumption in older adults by up to 15–30%—the same degree of improvement seen in younger adults. In fact, studies have shown that masters athletes in their 70s have $\dot{V}O_{2max}$ values equivalent to those of sedentary 20 year olds.

At any age, endurance training can improve cardiorespiratory functioning, cellular metabolism, body composition, and psychological and emotional well-being. Older adults who exercise regularly have better balance and greater bone density and are less likely than their sedentary peers to suffer injuries as a result of falls. Endurance and interval training also increase the cell mitochondria (powerhouses of the cell), a factor linked to increased longevity. Moreover, regular endurance training substantially reduces the risk of many chronic and disabling diseases, including heart disease, cancer, diabetes, osteoporosis, and dementia.

Other forms of exercise training are also beneficial for older adults. Resistance training, a safe and effective way to build strength and fat-free mass, helps people remain independent as they age. Lifting weights also benefits older people; improvements in strength appear quickly and are easily applied to everyday tasks such as climbing stairs and carrying groceries. Flexibility exercises can improve the ranges of motion in joints, another aid in helping people maintain functional independence as they age.

It's never too late to start exercising. Even those over 80 can see improved physical functioning and quality of life after beginning an exercise program. In 2017, 105-year-old French cyclist Robert Marchand set a masters world record by riding 22.5 kilometers (14 miles) in one hour. He didn't start competitive cycling until he was 68. Most older adults can participate in moderate walking and strengthening and stretching exercises, and modified programs can be created for people with chronic conditions and other special health concerns. The wellness benefits of exercise are available to people of all ages and levels of ability.

105-year-old cyclist Robert Marchand
© Nolwenn Le Gouic/Icon Sport/Getty Images
Box icon: © Rawpixel Ltd/Getty Images RF

sugar control). Acute inflammation is a short-term response to exercise and is an important way that the body improves physical fitness. For example, short-term inflammation triggers increased muscle protein synthesis, which promotes muscle fitness and recovery from exercise. Chronic inflammation, by contrast, is a prolonged, abnormal process that causes tissue breakdown and diseases such as atherosclerosis, cancer, and rheumatoid arthritis.

Although exercise increases acute inflammation during and shortly after a workout, it reduces chronic levels of inflammation—if the training program is not too severe. For example, practicing endurance training three to five days a week will reduce inflammation, particularly when accompanied by weight and fat loss. Training excessively, such as running a marathon several times a month or doing severe cross-training workouts five to seven days per week, will cause overtraining and chronic inflammation. We could call this the Goldilocks effect: The training program should not be too much or too little; it should be just right.

Deaths from All Causes Physically active people have a reduced risk of dying prematurely from all causes, with the greatest benefits found for people with the highest levels of physical activity and fitness (Figure 3.4). Physical inactivity is a predictor of premature death and is as important a risk factor as smoking, high blood pressure, obesity, and diabetes.

Better Control of Body Fat

Too much body fat is linked to a variety of health problems, including cardiovascular disease, cancer, and type 2 diabetes. Healthy body composition can be difficult to achieve and maintain—especially for someone who is sedentary—because a diet that contains all essential nutrients can be relatively high in calories. Excess calories are stored in the body as fat. Regular exercise increases daily calorie expenditure, which means that a healthy diet is less likely to lead to weight gain. Endurance exercise burns calories directly and, if intense enough, continues to do so by raising resting metabolic rate for several hours following an exercise session. A higher metabolic rate makes it easier for a person to maintain a healthy weight or to lose weight. However, exercise alone cannot ensure a healthy body composition. As described in Chapters 6 and 9, you will lose more weight more rapidly and keep it off longer if you decrease your calorie intake and boost your calorie expenditure through exercise.

THE EVIDENCE FOR EXERCISE
Combine Aerobic Exercise with Strength Training

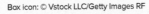

Emphasizing one aspect of fitness at the expense of others may be a special concern for those exercising with weights who don't do enough cardiorespiratory conditioning. Although exercise experts universally agree that resistance training is beneficial for a variety of reasons (as detailed in Chapter 4), it also has a downside.

A number of global studies have tracked the impact of weight training exercises on the cardiovascular system to find out if such training helps or harms the heart and blood vessels. These studies have shown that intense strength training poses short- and long-term risks to cardiovascular health and especially to arterial health. Aside from the risk of injury, lifting weights has been shown to have the following adverse effects on the cardiovascular system:

- Weight training promotes short-term stiffness of the blood vessels, which could promote hypertension (high blood pressure) over time and increase the load on the heart.

- Lifting weights (especially heavy weights) causes extreme short-term boosts in blood pressure; a Canadian study revealed that blood pressure can reach 480/350 mmHg during heavy lifting. Over the long term, sharp elevations in blood pressure can damage arteries, even if each pressure increase lasts only a few seconds.

- Weight training places stress on the endothelial cells that line blood vessels. Because these cells secrete nitric oxide (a chemical messenger involved in a variety of bodily functions), this stress can contribute to a wide range of negative effects, from erectile dysfunction to heart disease.

A variety of studies have shown that the best way to offset cardiovascular stress caused by strength training is to do cardiorespiratory endurance exercise (such as brisk walking or using an elliptical machine) immediately after a weight training session. Groundbreaking Japanese research showed that following resistance training with aerobic exercise prevents the stiffening of blood vessels and its associated damage. In this eight-week

study, participants did aerobics before lifting weights, after lifting weights, or not at all. The group that did aerobics *after* weight training saw the greatest positive impact on arterial health; participants who did aerobics before lifting weights did not see any improvement in the health of their blood vessels.

Strength training promotes endurance fitness by improving nervous control of the muscles, increasing type IIa motor units (muscle fibers that have a blend of strength and endurance capacity), and increasing tendon strength. These changes increase muscle strength and the rate of force development, enhance the economy of movement, and increase the speed with which blood cells travel through the muscles.

The bottom line of all this research? Both resistance training and cardiorespiratory exercise are good for you, if you do them in the right order. So, when you plan your workouts, be sure to do 15–60 minutes of aerobic exercise after each weight training session.

SOURCES: Kingsley, J. D., et al. 2016. "Arterial stiffness and autonomic modulation after free-weight resistance exercise in resistance trained individuals," *Journal of Strength Conditioning Research* 30(12), 3373–3380; Ashor, A. W., et al. 2014. "Effects of exercise modalities on arterial stiffness and wave reflection: A systematic review and meta-analysis of randomized controlled trials," *PLoS ONE* 9(10), e110034; Okamoto, T. M., et al. 2007. "Combined aerobic and resistance training and vascular function: Effect of aerobic exercise before and after resistance training," *Journal of Applied Physiology* 103(5), 1655–1661.

Box icon: © Vstock LLC/Getty Images RF

© Paul Burns/Digital Vision/Getty Images RF

Improved Immune Function

Exercise can have either positive or negative effects on the **immune system**, the physiological processes that protect us from diseases such as colds, bacterial infections, and even cancer. Moderate endurance exercise boosts immune function, whereas overtraining (excessive training) depresses it, at least temporarily. Physically fit people get fewer colds and upper respiratory tract infections than people who are not fit.

Exercise affects immune function by influencing levels of specialized cells and chemicals involved in the immune response. As discussed in Chapter 2, physically active people also have healthier, more resilient genes, which promotes immunity. Exercise preserves the telomeres, which form the ends of the DNA strands and holds them together. Without exercise, the telomeres shorten over time, eventually reducing the effectiveness of the immune system. In addition to getting regular

moderate exercise, you can further strengthen your immune system by eating a well-balanced diet, managing stress, and getting seven to eight hours of sleep every night.

Improved Psychological and Emotional Well-Being

Most people who participate in regular endurance exercise experience social, psychological, and emotional benefits. Skill mastery and self-control enhance one's self-image. Recreational sports provide an opportunity to socialize, have fun, and strive

> **immune system** The physiological processes that protect us from diseases such as colds, bacterial infections, and even cancer.
>
> TERMS

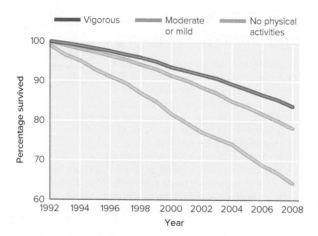

FIGURE 3.4   Survival rates for older adults doing vigorous, moderate, or no exercise, 1992–2008. The Health and Retirement Study—a long-term study of older adults—found that people who exercised vigorously over a 16-year period (1992–2008) had a lower death rate than those who exercised at moderate intensities or did no physical activity. After 16 years, the survival rate was 84% for those doing vigorous exercise, 78% for those doing moderate-intensity physical activity, and only 65% for those doing no physical activity. Exercising longer or more intensely reduces the risk of dying prematurely from a variety of causes.

SOURCE: Wen, M., et al. 2014. "Physical activity and mortality among middle-aged and older adults in the United States," *Journal Physical Activity & Health* 11(2), 303–312.

to excel. Endurance exercise lessens anxiety, depression, stress, anger, and hostility, thereby improving mood while boosting cardiovascular health. Regular exercise also improves sleep.

ASSESSING CARDIORESPIRATORY FITNESS

The body's ability to maintain a level of exertion (exercise) for an extended time is a direct reflection of cardiorespiratory fitness. One's level of fitness is determined by the body's ability to take up, distribute, and use oxygen during physical activity. As explained earlier, the best quantitative measure of cardiorespiratory endurance is maximal oxygen consumption, expressed as $\dot{V}O_{2max}$, the amount of oxygen the body uses when a person reaches his or her maximum ability to supply oxygen during exercise. Maximal oxygen consumption can be measured precisely in an exercise physiology laboratory through analysis of the air a person inhales and exhales when exercising to a level of exhaustion (maximum intensity). This procedure can be expensive and time-consuming, however, making it impractical for the average person.

Choosing an Assessment Test

Fortunately, several simple assessment tests provide reasonably good estimates of maximal oxygen consumption (within 10–15% of the results of a laboratory test). Four commonly used assessments are the following:

- *The 1-Mile Walk Test.* This test measures the amount of time it takes you to complete 1 mile of brisk walking and your

heart rate at the end of your walk. A fast time and a low heart rate indicate a high level of cardiorespiratory endurance.

- *The 3-Minute Step Test.* In the step test, you step continually at a steady rate for 3 minutes and then monitor your heart rate during recovery. The rate at which the pulse returns to normal is a good measure of cardiorespiratory capacity; heart rate remains lower and recovers faster in people who are more physically fit.

- *The 1.5-Mile Run-Walk Test.* Oxygen consumption increases with speed in distance running, so a fast time on this test indicates high maximal oxygen consumption.

- *The Beep Test.* This test predicting maximal oxygen consumption is excellent for people who are physically fit and wish to measure their capacity for high-intensity exercise, such as sprints. A prerecorded series of "beeps" (tones) sound off at faster and faster intervals. Your task is to keep up with the beeps during the exercise.

Lab 3.1 provides detailed instructions for each of these tests. An additional assessment, the 12-Minute Swim Test, is also provided. To assess yourself, choose one of these methods based on your access to equipment, your current physical condition, and your own preference.

Don't take any of these tests without checking with your physician if you are ill or have any of the risk factors for exercise discussed in Chapter 2 and Lab 2.1.

Monitoring Your Heart Rate

Each time your heart contracts, it pumps blood into your arteries. You can measure your heart rate—the number of heart contractions per minute—by using a heart rate monitor or counting your pulse beats. Modern heart rate monitors are inexpensive and fairly accurate. Several companies make heart rate monitor apps that are used with smartphones to measure heart rate, distances, route maps, running or cycling speed, calories burned, and even the electrical activity of the heart as it beats, which is what an electrocardiogram (ECG, or EKG) does. Counting your pulse is the traditional method of measuring heart rate. Each contraction of the heart produces a surge of blood that causes a pulse you can feel by holding your fingers against an artery. Heart rate is a good way to monitor exercise intensity during a workout. (Intensity is described in more detail in the next section.)

The radial artery in the wrist is the most common site to measure pulse rate (Figure 3.5). To take your pulse, press your index and middle fingers gently on the correct site. You may have to shift position several times to find the best place to feel your pulse. A good technique is to bend your fingers slightly and take your pulse with the tops of your fingers where you have many nerve endings. Don't use your thumb to check your pulse; it has a pulse of its own that can confuse your count.

Heart rates are usually assessed in beats per minute (bpm). But counting your pulse for an entire minute isn't practical when you're exercising. And because heart rate slows rapidly when you stop exercising, a full minute's worth of counting can give inaccurate results. It's best to do a shorter count—15

WELLNESS IN THE DIGITAL AGE
Fitness Trackers, Heart Rate Monitors, and GPS Devices

Technology has transformed the market for trackers and monitors. It is difficult to keep up with the latest exercise monitors designed as stand-alone units, smartphone apps, and GPS accessories. A heart rate monitor is an electronic device that checks the user's pulse, either continuously or on demand. These devices make it easy to monitor your heart rate before, during, and after exercise. Some include global positioning system (GPS) receivers that help you track the distance you walk, run, or bike. Wearable fitness trackers, made by Fitbit, Polar, Timex, Mio, and Garmin, among others, measure distance and steps covered, calories burned, and exercise intensity. Most studies show that the heart rate monitors are highly accurate, but the calorie counters are less so. However, the activity trackers are excellent motivators and provide a relative benchmark from one workout to the next.

Fitness Trackers

High-tech monitors and phone apps such as the Nike + Fuel-Band, Cyclemeter, Nike + Sensor, and Adidas miCoach track daily activities including running and walking and sports like basketball. They track steps taken, distance covered, and calories burned. Fitness trackers allow you to keep track of your progress, compete against other people, and meet challenges.

Wearable Heart Rate Monitors

Heart rate monitors use either a chest strap that measures the electrical activity of the heart or an optical sensor worn on the wrist that measures heart rate by detecting changes in wrist blood flow. Chest-strap monitors are more accurate, but wrist monitors are more convenient. A wide variety of monitors are available, many at modest cost.

Monitors in Gym Equipment

Many pieces of workout equipment—including newer-model treadmills, stationary bikes, and elliptical trainers—feature built-in heart rate monitors. The monitor is usually mounted into the device's handles. To check your heart rate at any time while working out, simply grip the handles in the appropriate place; within a few seconds, your current heart rate will appear on the device's console.

Other Features

Heart rate monitors can do more than just check your pulse. Most can also tell you the following:

- Highest and lowest heart rate during a session
- Average heart rate

- Target heart rate range, based on your age, weight, and other factors
- Time spent within the target range
- Number of calories burned during a session

Some monitors can upload their data to a computer so that information can be stored and analyzed. The analytical software can help you track your progress over a period of time or a number of workouts. AliveCor is a phone app that can produce a medical-quality ECG and store it or send it to a physician by e-mail. Monitors with GPS provide an accurate estimate of distance traveled during a workout or over an entire day.

Choosing and Using Monitors

Heart rate monitors are useful if close tracking of heart rate is important in your program. They offer several advantages:

- They are fairly accurate, and they reduce the risk of mistakes when checking your own pulse. (*Note:* Chest-strap monitors are considered more accurate than strapless models. If you use a monitor built in to gym equipment, its accuracy will depend on how well the device is maintained.)

- They are easy to use, although a sophisticated, multifunction monitor may take some time to master.

- They do the monitoring for you, so you don't have to worry about checking your own pulse.

When shopping for a heart rate, fitness tracker, phone app, or exercise GPS monitor, do your homework. Quality, reliability, and warranties vary. Ask personal trainers in your area for their recommendations, and look for independent product reviews and comparison accuracy tests in consumer magazines or online. Remember that the vast majority of devices on the market are for general, and not medical, use; only a few have been formally evaluated and approved by the U.S. Food and Drug Administration (FDA) as accurate enough for medical purposes

© Sasils/Shutterstock.com RF

Box icon: © Hong Li/Getty Images RF

---

seconds—and then multiply the result by 4 to get your heart rate in beats per minute. (You can also use a heart rate monitor to check your pulse. See the box "Fitness Trackers, Heart Rate Monitors, and GPS Devices" for more information.)

Interpreting Your Score

After you've completed one or more of the assessment tests, use the table under "Rating Your Cardiovascular Fitness" in

Lab 3.1 to determine your current level of cardiorespiratory fitness. As you interpret your score, remember that field tests of cardiorespiratory fitness are not precise scientific measurements and have up to a 10–15% margin of error.

You can use the assessment tests to monitor the progress of your fitness program by retesting yourself from time to time. Always compare scores for the *same* test: Your scores on different tests may vary considerably because of differences in skill and motivation and quirks in the tests themselves.

The radial pulse is felt on the wrist just under the thumb.

FIGURE 3.5 **Checking your pulse.** Take your pulse at the radial artery in the wrist.

Courtesy Robin Mouat

DEVELOPING A CARDIORESPIRATORY ENDURANCE PROGRAM

Cardiorespiratory endurance exercises are best for developing the type of fitness associated with good health, so they should serve as the focus of your exercise program. To create a successful endurance exercise program, follow these guidelines:

- Set realistic goals.
- Set your starting frequency, intensity, and duration of exercise at appropriate levels.
- Choose suitable activities.
- Warm up and cool down.
- Adjust your program as your fitness improves.

Setting Goals

You can use the results of cardiorespiratory fitness assessment tests to set a specific oxygen consumption goal for your cardiorespiratory endurance program. Your goal should be high enough to ensure a healthy cardiorespiratory system, but not so high that it will be impossible to achieve. Scores in the fair and good ranges for maximal oxygen consumption suggest good fitness; scores in the excellent and superior ranges indicate a high standard of physical performance.

Through endurance training, an individual may be able to improve maximal oxygen consumption $\dot{V}O_{2max}$ by about 10–30%. The amount of improvement possible depends on genetics, age, health status, and initial fitness level. People who start at a very low fitness level can improve by a greater percentage than elite athletes because the latter are already at a much higher fitness level, one that may approach their genetic physical limits. If you are tracking $\dot{V}O_{2max}$ by using the field tests described in this chapter, you may be able to increase your score by more than 30% due to improvements in other physical

factors, such as muscle power, which can affect your performance on the tests.

Other physical factors you can track to monitor progress are resting heart rate—your heart rate at complete rest—and blood pressure, measured in the morning before you get out of bed and move around. Resting heart rate may decrease by as much as 10–15 beats per minute and resting systolic and diastolic blood pressure by 5 mmHg in response to endurance training. These changes may be noticeable after only about four to six weeks of training.

You may want to set other types of goals for your fitness program. For example, if you walk, jog, or cycle as part of your fitness program, you may want to set a time or distance goal—working up to walking 5 miles in one session, completing a 4-mile run in 28 minutes, or cycling a total of 35 miles per week. A more modest goal might be to achieve the recommendation of the U.S. Department of Health and Human Services and American College of Sports Medicine (ACSM) of 150 minutes per week of moderate-intensity physical activity. Although it's best to base your program on "SMART" goals (those that are **s**pecific, **m**easurable, **a**ttainable, **r**ealistic, and **t**ime frame–specific), you may also want to set more qualitative goals, such as becoming more energetic, sleeping better, and improving the fit of your clothes.

Applying the FITT-VP Principle

As described in Chapter 2, you can use the acronym FITT-VP to set key parameters of your fitness program: **F**requency, **I**ntensity, **T**ime (duration), **T**ype of activity, **V**olume, and **P**rogression.

Frequency of Training Accumulatizng at least 150 minutes per week of moderate-intensity physical activity (or at least 75 minutes per week of vigorous physical activity) is enough to promote health. Most experts recommend that people exercise three to five days per week to build cardiorespiratory endurance. Training more than five days per week can lead to injury and isn't necessary for the typical person on an exercise program designed to promote wellness. It is safe to do moderate-intensity activity such as walking and gardening every day. Training fewer than three days per week makes it difficult to improve your fitness (unless exercise intensity is very high) or to lose weight through exercise. Remember, however, that some exercise is better than none.

Intensity of Training Intensity is the most important factor for increasing aerobic fitness. You must exercise intensely enough to stress your body so that fitness improves. Four methods of monitoring exercise intensity are described in the following sections; choose the method that works best for you. Be sure to make adjustments in your intensity levels for environmental or individual factors. For example, on a hot and humid day or on your first day back to your program after an illness, you should decrease your intensity level.

TARGET HEART RATE ZONE One of the best ways to monitor the intensity of cardiorespiratory endurance exercise is to measure your heart rate (calculated in beats per minute). It isn't

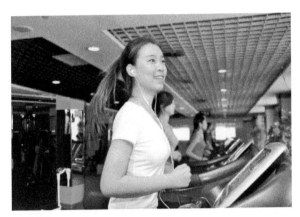

Fitness Tip Listen to fast-paced music for a better workout! In a recent study, students rode a stationary bike while listening to music at different tempos. The subjects rode harder when listening to faster music and performed less exercise in response to slower music.

© Yaping/Shutterstock.com RF

necessary to exercise at your maximum heart rate to improve maximal oxygen consumption. Fitness adaptations occur at lower heart rates with a much lower risk of injury.

According to the ACSM, your **target heart rate zone**—the range of rates at which you should exercise to experience cardiorespiratory benefits—is between 65% and 90% of your maximum heart rate. To calculate your target heart rate zone, follow these steps:

1. Estimate your maximum heart rate (MHR) by subtracting your age from 220, or have it measured precisely by undergoing an exercise stress test in a doctor's office, hospital, or sports medicine lab. (*Note:* The formula to estimate MHR carries an error of about ±10–15 bpm and can be very inaccurate for some people, particularly older adults and young children. If your exercise heart rate seems inaccurate—that is, exercise within your target zone seems either too easy or too difficult—then use the perceived exertion method described in the next section, or have your MHR measured precisely.) You can get a reasonable estimate of maximal heart rate by exercising at maximal intensities on a stationary bike, treadmill, or elliptical trainer that has a built-in heart rate monitor. This method is not recommended unless you are physically fit and accustomed to intense exercise.

2. Multiply your MHR by 65% and 90% to calculate your target heart rate zone. Very unfit people should use 55% of MHR for their training threshold. For example, a 19 year old would calculate her target heart rate zone as follows:

$$\text{MHR} = 220 - 19 = 201 \text{ bpm}$$

$$65\% \text{ training intensity} = 0.65 \times 201 = 131 \text{ bpm}$$

$$90\% \text{ training intensity} = 0.90 \times 201 = 181 \text{ bpm}$$

To gain fitness benefits, the young woman in our example would have to exercise at an intensity that raises her heart rate to between 131 and 181 bpm.

An alternative method for calculating target heart rate zone uses **heart rate reserve**, the difference between maximum heart rate and resting heart rate. Using this method, target heart rate is equal to resting heart rate plus between 50% (40% for very unfit people) and 85% of heart rate reserve. Although some people (particularly those with very low levels of fitness) will obtain more accurate results using this more complex method, both methods provide reasonable estimates of an appropriate target heart rate zone. Lab 3.2 gives formulas for both methods of calculating target heart rate.

If you have been sedentary, start by exercising at the lower end of your target heart rate zone (65% of maximum heart rate or 50% of heart rate reserve) for at least four to six weeks. Exercising closer to the top of the range can cause fast and significant gains in maximal oxygen consumption, but you may increase your risk of injury and overtraining. You *can* achieve significant health benefits by exercising at the bottom of your target zone, so don't feel pressure to exercise at an unnecessarily intense level. If you exercise at a lower intensity, you can increase the duration or frequency of training to obtain as much benefit to your health, as long as you are above the 65% training threshold. For people with a very low initial level of fitness, a lower training intensity of 55–64% of maximum heart rate or 40–49% of heart rate reserve may be sufficient to achieve improvements in maximal oxygen consumption, especially at the start of an exercise program. Intensities of 70–85% of maximum heart rate are appropriate for individuals with an average level of fitness.

By monitoring your heart rate, you will always know if you are working hard enough to improve, not hard enough, or too hard. As your program progresses and your fitness improves, you will need to jog, cycle, or walk faster to reach your target heart rate zone. To monitor your heart rate during exercise, use a heart rate monitor or count your pulse while you're still moving or immediately after you stop exercising. Count beats for 15 seconds, then multiply that number by 4 to see if your heart rate is in your target zone. Table 3.2 shows target heart rate ranges and 15-second counts based on the maximum heart rate formula.

METS One way scientists describe fitness is in terms of the capacity to increase metabolism (energy usage level) above rest. Scientists use METs to measure the metabolic cost of an exercise. One **MET** represents the body's resting metabolic rate—that is, the energy or calorie requirement of the body at rest. Exercise intensity is expressed in multiples of resting

Table 3.2	Target Heart Rate Zone and 15-Second Counts	
AGE (years)	TARGET HEART RATE ZONE (bpm)*	15-SECOND COUNT (beats)
20–24	127–180	32–45
25–29	124–176	31–44
30–34	121–171	30–43
35–39	118–167	30–42
40–44	114–162	29–41
45–49	111–158	28–40
50–54	108–153	27–38
55–59	105–149	26–37
60–64	101–144	25–36
65+	97–140	24–35

*Target heart rates lower than those shown here are appropriate for individuals with a very low initial level of fitness. Ranges are based on the following formula: target heart rate = 0.65 to 0.90 of maximum heart rate, assuming maximum heart rate = 220 − age.

Table 3.3	Approximate MET and Energy Costs of Selected Activities for a 154-Pound Person	
ACTIVITY	METs	ENERGY COST (CALORIES PER MINUTE)
Rest	1	1.2
Light housework	2–4	2.4–4.8
Bowling	2–4	2.5–5
Walking	2–7	2.5–8.5
Archery	3–4	3.7–5
Dancing	3–7	3.7–8.5
Activity-promoting video game	3–7	3.7–8.5
Hiking	3–7	3.7–8.5
Horseback riding	3–8	3.7–10
Fishing (fly, stream)	4–6	5–7.5
Circuit training	4–8	5–10
Basketball (recreational)	4–9	5–11
Cycling	4–10	5–12
In-line skating	5–8	6–10
Skiing (downhill)	5–8	6–10
Swimming	5–9	6–11
Tennis	5–9	6–11
Rock climbing	5–10	6–12
Scuba diving	5–10	6–12
Rowing machine	5–12	6–15
Skiing (cross-country)	6–12	7.5–15
Jogging	8–12	10–15

NOTE: Intensity varies greatly with effort, skill, and motivation.

SOURCE: American College of Sports Medicine. 2018. *ACSM's Guidelines for Exercise Testing and Prescription*, 10th ed. Philadelphia: Wolters Kluwer/Lippincott Williams & Wilkins Health; Ainsworth B.E., et al. 2011. *The Compendium of Physical Activities Tracking Guide*. (https://sites.google.com/site/compendiumofphysicalactivities/home)

metabolic rate. For example, an exercise intensity of 2 METs is twice the resting metabolic rate.

METs are used to describe exercise intensities for occupational activities and exercise programs. Exercise intensities of less than 3–4 METs are considered low. Household chores and most industrial jobs fall into this category. Exercise at these intensities does not improve fitness for most people, but it will improve fitness for people with low physical capacities. Activities that increase metabolism by 3–7 METs are classified as moderate-intensity exercises and are suitable for most people beginning an exercise program. Vigorous exercise increases metabolic rate by 8 to 12 METs. Fast running or cycling, as well as intense play in sports like racquetball, can place people in this category. Table 3.3 lists the MET ratings for various activities.

METs are intended to be only an approximation of exercise intensity. Skill, body weight, body fat, and environment affect the accuracy of METs. As a practical matter, however, we can disregard these limitations. METs are a good way to express exercise intensity because this system is easy for people to remember and apply.

RATINGS OF PERCEIVED EXERTION   Another way to monitor intensity is to monitor your perceived level of exertion. Repeated pulse counting during exercise can become a nuisance if it interferes with the activity. As your exercise program progresses, you will probably become familiar with the amount of exertion required to raise your heart rate to target levels. In other words, you will know how you feel when you have exercised intensely enough. If this is the case, you can use the scale of **ratings of perceived exertion (RPE)** shown in Figure 3.6 to monitor the intensity of your exercise session without checking your pulse.

ratings of perceived exertion (RPE)   A system   TERMS
of monitoring exercise intensity by assigning a number
to the subjective perception of target intensity.

To use the RPE scale, select a rating that corresponds to your subjective perception of how hard you are exercising when you are training in your target heart rate zone. If your target zone is about 135–155 bpm, exercise intensely enough to raise your heart rate to that level, and then associate a rating—for example, "somewhat hard" or "hard" (4 or 5)—with how hard you feel you are working. To reach and maintain a similar intensity in future workouts, exercise hard enough to reach what you feel is the same level of exertion. You should periodically check your RPE against your target heart rate zone to make sure it's correct. RPE is an accurate means of monitoring exercise intensity, and you may find it easier and more convenient than pulse counting.

TALK TEST   Another easy method of monitoring exercise exertion—in particular, to prevent overly intense exercise—is the talk test. Although your breathing rate will increase during moderate-intensity cardiorespiratory endurance exercise, you should not work out so intensely that you cannot communicate. Speech is limited to short phrases during vigorous-intensity exercise. The talk test is an effective gauge of intensity for many types of activities.

RATING	DEFINITION
0	Nothing at all
0.5	Very, very easy
1	Very easy
2	Easy
3	Moderate
4	Somewhat hard
5	Hard
6	
7	Very hard
8	
9	Very, very hard
10	Impossible

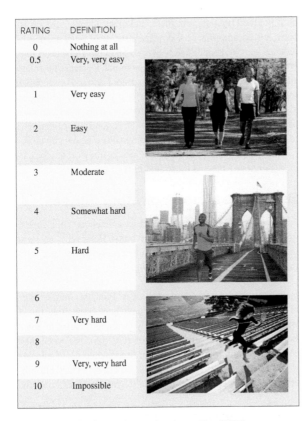

FIGURE 3.6 **Ratings of perceived exertion (RPE).**
Experienced exercisers may use this subjective scale to estimate how near they are to their target heart rate zone.

SOURCE: Borg, G. 1990. "Psychophysical scaling with applications in physical work and the perception of exertion," *Scandinavian Journal of Work and Environmental Health* 16(suppl 1), 55-58.

Photo credits, top to bottom: © leaf/Getty Images RF; © Diane Collins and Jordan Hollender/Getty Images RF; © Peathegee Inc/Getty Images RF

Table 3.4	Estimating Exercise Intensity	
METHOD	MODERATE INTENSITY	VIGOROUS INTENSITY
Target heart rate (maximum heart rate method)	55–69%	70–90%
Target heart rate (heart rate reserve method)	40–59%	60–85%
METs	3-7 METs	8-12 METs
Ratings of perceived exertion	4–5 (somewhat hard)	5–8 (hard to very hard)
Talk test	Speech with some difficulty	Speech limited to short phrases

Type of Activity Cardiorespiratory endurance exercises include activities that involve the rhythmic use of large-muscle groups for an extended period of time, such as jogging, walking, cycling, aerobic dancing and other forms of group exercise, cross-country skiing, and swimming. Start-and-stop sports, such as tennis and racquetball, also qualify if you have enough skill to play continuously and intensely enough to raise your heart rate to target levels. Other important considerations are access to facilities, expense, equipment, and the time required to achieve an adequate skill level and workout.

Volume of Activity Training volume is the product of frequency, intensity, and time. Increasing volume is the best way to improve fitness. Excessive volume, however, can lead to injury and overtraining. Activity trackers can help you gauge and monitor your progress. They can also help quantify your program in total energy expenditure in terms of calories (**calories per session**, week, month, and/or year) and **MET-minutes** (exercise intensity in METs times minutes of exercise). Exercise volume for cardiorespiratory endurance can be estimated using several different measures; each of the following is approximately equivalent:

- 150 minutes per week of moderate intensity activity
- Calories: 1,000 calories per week in moderate intensity exercise
- MET-minutes: 500 to 1,000 MET-mins per week
- Steps: 5,400 to 7,900 steps or more per day; for accuracy, combine step counts with recommend time (duration) of exercise

Table 3.4 provides a quick reference to each of the methods of estimating exercise intensity discussed here.

Time (Duration) of Training A total duration of 20–60 minutes per day is recommended; exercise can take place in a single session or in multiple sessions lasting 10 or more minutes. The total duration of exercise depends on its intensity. To improve cardiorespiratory endurance during a low- to moderate-intensity activity such as walking or slow swimming, you should exercise for 30–60 minutes. For high-intensity exercise performed at the top of your target heart rate zone, a duration of 20 minutes is sufficient.

Some studies have shown that 5–10 minutes of extremely intense exercise (greater than 90% of maximal oxygen consumption) improves cardiorespiratory endurance. However, training at high intensity, particularly during high-impact activities, increases the risk of injury. Also, if you experience discomfort in high-intensity exercise, you are more likely to discontinue your exercise program. Longer-duration, low- to moderate-intensity activities generally result in more gradual gains in maximal oxygen consumption. In planning your program, start with less vigorous activities and gradually increase intensity.

calories per session   The energy expenditure of an exercise session expressed in calories; as described earlier, in common usage *calories* represents the larger energy unit *kilocalories*.

MET-minute   A measure of training volume equal to exercise intensity expressed in METs times the total exercise time (METs × time).

TERMS

Progression The rate of progression depends on your goals, fitness, health, age, and adaptation to training. For general health, most benefits occur at moderate training intensities for about 150 minutes per week. Higher levels of fitness require more intense training programs. Increasing intensity is most important for increasing fitness, while increasing time and frequency can promote a healthy body composition by increasing overall energy expenditure with moderate-intensity activity.

Motivation determines your adherence to an exercise program. Highly motivated people are willing to put up with the high levels of discomfort that accompany intense training programs. Less motivated people often stop exercising if the program is too intense or uncomfortable.

Fitness determines your capacity to improve. Untrained people make rapid gains, whereas highly fit people improve more slowly. Genetics also determine how fast you will improve. People vary in their response to identical training programs. Finally, health and age influence your adaptability and capacity for training progression.

Warming Up and Cooling Down

As we saw in Chapter 2, it's important to warm up before every session of cardiorespiratory endurance exercise and to cool down afterward. Because the body's muscles work better when their temperature is slightly above resting level, warming up enhances performance and decreases the chance of injury. It gives the body time to redirect blood to active muscles and the heart time to adapt to increased demands. Warming up also helps spread protective fluid throughout the joints, preventing injury to their surfaces.

A warm-up session should include low-intensity, whole-body movements similar to those in the activity that will follow, such as walking slowly before beginning a brisk walk. An active warm-up of 5–10 minutes is adequate for most types of exercise. However, warm-up time will depend on your level of fitness, experience, and individual preferences.

What about stretching as part of a warm-up? Performing *static* stretches—those in which you move a joint to the end of the range of motion and hold the position—as part of your pre-exercise warm-up has not been found to prevent injury and has little or no effect on post-exercise muscle soreness. Static stretching before exercise may also adversely affect strength, power, balance, reaction time, and movement time. (Stretching may interfere with muscle and joint receptors that are used in the performance of sport and movement skills.) For these reasons, it is often recommended that static stretches be performed at the end of your workout, after your cool-down but while your muscles are still warm and your joints are lubricated. On the flip side, *dynamic* stretches—those involving continuous movement of joints through a range of motion—can be an appropriate part of a warm-up. Slow and controlled movements such as walking lunges, heel kicks, and arm circles can raise muscle temperature while moving joints through their range of motion. (See Chapter 5 for a detailed discussion of stretching and flexibility exercises.)

Cooling down after exercise is important for returning the body to a nonexercising state. A cool-down helps maintain blood flow to the heart and brain and redirects blood from working muscles to other areas of the body. This helps prevent a large drop in blood pressure, dizziness, and other potential cardiovascular complications. A cool-down, consisting of 5–10 minutes of reduced activity, should follow every workout to allow heart rate, breathing, and circulation to return to normal. Decrease the intensity of exercise gradually during your cool-down. For example, following a running workout, begin your cool-down by jogging at half speed for 30 seconds to a minute; then do several minutes of walking, reducing your speed slowly. A good rule of thumb is to cool down at least until your heart rate drops below 100 bpm.

The general pattern of a safe and successful workout for cardiorespiratory fitness is illustrated in Figure 3.7.

Building Cardiorespiratory Fitness

Building fitness is as much an art as a science. Your fitness improves when you overload your body. However, you must increase the frequency, intensity, and duration of exercise carefully to avoid injury and overtraining.

General Program Progression For the initial stage of your program, which may last anywhere from three to six weeks, exercise at the low end of your target heart rate zone. Begin with a frequency of three or four days per week, and choose a duration appropriate for your fitness level: 12–15 minutes if you are very unfit, 20 minutes if you are sedentary but otherwise healthy, and 30–40 minutes if you are an experienced

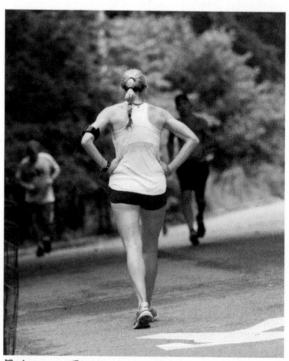

Fitness Tip Make warming up and cooling down a part of your exercise routine. Starting an exercise activity with a low-intensity version and slowing down gradually at the end helps your body adapt to being more active, protects you from certain injuries, and may make the health benefits of exercise last longer.

© keepics/Alamy Stock photo

Frequency: 3–5 days per week

Intensity: 55/65–90% of maximum heart rate, 40/50–85% of heart rate reserve plus resting heart rate, or an RPE rating of about 4–8 (lower intensities—55–64% of maximum heart rate and 40–49% of heart rate reserve—are applicable to people who are quite unfit; for average individuals, intensities of 70–85% of maximum heart rate are appropriate)

Time (duration): 20–60 minutes (one session or multiple sessions lasting 10 or more minutes)

Type of activity: Cardiorespiratory endurance exercises, such as walking, jogging, biking, swimming, cross-country skiing, and rope skipping

Volume of activity: Equivalent to 150 minutes or 1,000 or more calories per week of moderate-intensity activity, consistent with individual fitness status and goals.

Progression: Gradually increase volume (frequency, intensity, and/or time) over time, as appropriate for goals, fitness status, age, and adaptability

FIGURE 3.7 The FITT-VP principle for a cardiorespiratory endurance program. Longer-duration exercise at lower intensities can often be as beneficial for promoting health as shorter-duration, high-intensity exercise.

Table 3.5 Sample Progression for an Endurance Program

STAGE/WEEK	FREQUENCY (days/week)	INTENSITY* (beats/minute)	TIME (duration in minutes)
Initial stage			
1	3	120–130	15–20
2	3	120–130	20–25
3	4	130–145	20–25
4	4	130–145	25–30
Improvement stage			
5–7	3–4	145–160	25–30
8–10	3–4	145–160	30–35
11–13	3–4	150–165	30–35
14–16	4–5	150–165	30–35
17–20	4–5	160–180	35–40
21–24	4–5	160–180	35–40
Maintenance stage			
25+	3–5	160–180	20–60

*The target heart rates shown here are based on calculations for a healthy 20 year old with a resting heart rate of 60 bpm; the program progresses from an initial target heart rate of 50% to a maintenance range of 70–85% of heart rate reserve.

SOURCE: American College of Sports Medicine. 2018. *ACSM's Guidelines for Exercise Testing and Prescription,* 10th ed. Philadelphia: Wolters Kluwer/Lippincott Williams & Wilkins Health.

exerciser. Use this stage of your program to allow both your body and your schedule to adjust to your new exercise routine. When you can exercise at the upper levels of frequency (four or five days per week) and duration (30–40 minutes) without excessive fatigue or muscle soreness, you are ready to progress.

The next phase of your program is the improvement stage, lasting from four to six months. During this phase, slowly and gradually increase the amount of overload until you reach your target level of fitness (see the sample training progression in Table 3.5). Take care not to increase overload too quickly. It is usually best to avoid increasing both intensity and duration during the same session or increasing all three training variables (frequency, intensity, and duration) in one week. Increasing duration in increments of 5–10 minutes every two or three weeks is usually appropriate. Signs that you are increasing overload too quickly include muscle aches and pains, lack of usual interest in exercise, extreme fatigue, and inability to complete a workout. Keep an exercise log or training diary to monitor your workouts and progress; use a tracking app, spreadsheet, or paper journal—whatever works best for you.

Interval Training You will not improve your fitness indefinitely. The more fit you become, the harder you must work to improve. Few exercise techniques are more effective at improving fitness rapidly than *high-intensity interval training (HIIT)*—a series of very brief, high-intensity exercise sessions interspersed with short rest periods. The four components of interval training are distance, repetition, intensity, and rest, defined as follows:

- *Distance* refers to either the distance or the time of the exercise interval.
- *Repetition* is the number of times the exercise is repeated.
- *Intensity* is the speed at which the exercise is performed.
- *Rest* is the time spent recovering between exercises.

You can use interval training in your favorite aerobic exercises. In fact, the type of exercise you select is not important as long as you exercise at a high intensity and rest 3–5 minutes between repetitions. HIIT training can even be used to help develop sports skills. For example, a runner might do 4–8 repetitions of 200-meter sprints at near-maximum effort. A tennis player might practice volleys against a wall as fast as possible for 4–8 repetitions lasting 30 seconds each. A swimmer might swim 4–8 repetitions of 50 meters at 100% effort.

If you add HIIT to your exercise program, do not practice interval training more than three days per week. Intervals are exhausting and easily lead to injury. Let your body tell you how many days you can tolerate. If you become overly tired after doing interval training three days per week, cut back to two days.

If you feel good, try increasing the intensity or number of intervals (but not the number of days per week) and see what happens. As with any kind of exercise program, begin HIIT training slowly and progress conservatively. Although HIIT training produces substantial fitness improvements, it is best to integrate it into your total exercise program.

PROS   Canadian researchers found that practicing HIIT for 3 minutes per week (exercise, not counting rest, warm-up, and cool-down) for 12 weeks produced the same changes in cardiorespiratory fitness, blood sugar regulation, and skeletal muscle mitochondria as training continuously for 150 minutes per week at a moderate intensity. Each workout consisted of three 20-second maximum sprints on a stationary bike, interspersed with 2 minutes of extremely light exercise. Continuous exercise involved 50 minutes of moderate-intensity exercise (70% of maximal heart rate) for 50 minutes, three times per week. Both programs involved a 2-minute warm-up and 3-minute cool-down. This study (and more than 50 others) showed the value of HIIT for building aerobic capacity and endurance.

CONS   High-intensity interval training appears to be safe and effective in the short term, but there are concerns about the long-term safety and effectiveness of this type of training, so consider the following issues:

- High-intensity training could be dangerous for some people. A physician might be reluctant to give certain patients the green light for this type of exercise.

- Always warm up with several minutes of low-intensity exercise before practicing HIIT. High-intensity exercise without a warm-up can cause cardiac arrhythmias (abnormal heart rhythms), even in healthy people.

- HIIT might trigger overuse injuries in unfit people. For this reason, it is essential to start gradually, especially for someone at a low level of fitness. Exercise at submaximal intensities for at least four to six weeks before starting HIIT. Cut back on interval training or rest if you feel overly fatigued or develop overly sore joints or muscles.

Other types of high-intensity training may combine intervals with other types of exercises and training techniques; see the box "High-Intensity Conditioning Programs."

Maintaining Cardiorespiratory Fitness

There are limits to the level of fitness you can achieve, and if you increase intensity and duration indefinitely, you are likely to become injured or overtrained. After an improvement stage of four to six months, you may reach your goal of an acceptable level of fitness. You can then maintain fitness by continuing to exercise at the same intensity at least three nonconsecutive days every week. If you stop exercising, you lose your gains in fitness fairly rapidly.

Fitness Tip High-intensity interval training can be an effective technique for boosting fitness. For a runner, HIIT might be half a dozen 200-meter sprints one to three times a week. If you decide to try HIIT, be sure to start slowly, progress gradually, and listen to your body to avoid injury

© Cultura RM/Edwin Jimenez/Getty Images

If you take time off for any reason, start your program again at a lower level and rebuild your fitness in a slow and systematic way.

When you reach the maintenance stage, you may want to set new goals for your program and make some adjustments to maintain your motivation. For example, you might set a new goal of participating in a local 5K race. Or you might add new buddies to your program, or mix up your exercise sessions by working out in a new setting. Adding variety to your program can be a helpful strategy. Engaging in multiple types of endurance activities, an approach known as **cross-training**, can help boost enjoyment and prevent some types of injuries. For example, someone who has been jogging five days a week may change her program so that she jogs three days a week, plays tennis one day a week, and goes for a bike ride one day a week.

Although all these activities build endurance, alternating between them reduces the strain on specific joints and muscles. Varying your activities also offers new physical and mental challenges that can keep your fitness program fresh and fun.

EXERCISE SAFETY AND INJURY PREVENTION

Exercising safely and preventing injuries are two important challenges for people who engage in cardiorespiratory endurance exercise. This section provides basic safety guidelines that can be applied to a variety of fitness activities. Chapters 4 and 5 include additional advice specific to strength training and flexibility training.

Hot Weather and Heat Stress

Human beings require a relatively constant body temperature to survive. A change of just a few degrees can quickly lead to distress and even death. If you lose too much water or if your body

cross-training   Training in two or more sports or types of exercises in order to produce more diverse fitness.   TERMS

TAKE CHARGE
High-Intensity Conditioning Programs

In recent years, high-intensity power-based "extreme" conditioning programs, such as CrossFit, Gym Jones, and Insanity, have grown in popularity. The programs typically incorporate a range of activity types and may include high-intensity aerobic exercise, interval training, free-weight exercises, and gymnastics moves. The programs may be geared toward developing whole-body fitness, limiting workout time by utilizing short but high-intensity sessions, and/or adding a competitive aspect to fitness training.

CrossFit is a popular example of a high-intensity program that emphasizes use of broad and constantly changing training stimuli. It includes activities designed to develop not only cardiorespiratory endurance but also strength, power, speed, coordination, ability, balance, and accuracy. Workouts are short and intense but should be tailored to an individual's current fitness level and age. They may include aerobic activities such as running and rope-skipping, plus whole-body strength training activities such as power lifts, plyometrics, sled pulls, and kettlebell exercises. Do not attempt these rigorous training programs without thorough instruction in technical weight lifting and gymnastic exercises, and always use good technique.

These sample workouts provide a flavor of this type of high-intensity training.

Sample Workouts

Complete three circuits (series) of the activities, but do not exceed 20—30 minutes for the workout. Break the exercises into sets if you cannot complete all the repetitions (e.g., 20 pull-ups). Record your time. Train as hard and as fast as you can while maintaining good technique. Select a weight that allows you to complete the reps in the sets. (Principles of resistance exercise are described in Chapter 4.) Change the exercises with every workout.

Workout 1

40 push-ups

10 standing long jumps

40 squats with hands on your hips

20 dumbbell or kettlebell swings

Skip rope rapidly for 3 minutes

Rest 3 minutes; repeat circuit 2 more times

Workout 2

20 pull-ups

20 dumbbell thrusters (front squat with barbell or dumbbells, then immediately perform an overhead press)

20 overhead squats

10 kettlebell snatches (10 for each arm)

2 minutes spinning on bike while standing, maximum intensity

Rest 3 minutes; repeat circuit 2 more times

Cautions and Guidelines

High-intensity training programs have their critics, who point to the increased risk of severe injury and lack of concern for the principle of specificity (training the way you want your body to adapt) with this type of training. Good technique is essential: The emphasis on speed and intensity can make it difficult to achieve good technique, but performing high-speed free-weight exercises such as cleans and squats improperly can lead to severe injury.

Performing high-speed, high-repetition sit-ups or squats often pushes muscles and joints to failure, causing severe knee or back injury or muscle destruction (rhabdomyolysis or "rhabdo"). Until recently, physicians encountered rhabdo only after extreme trauma from automobile accidents. These days, rhabdo may become more common because of the popularity of "feel the burn" high-intensity training programs. Biomechanical studies suggest that high-speed sit-ups and squats can damage the spine. The benefits of high levels of fitness are counterbalanced by the risk of injury.

In spite of the potential risks of high-intensity training, it can be a suitable option for fit individuals who enjoy and are motivated by varied, high-intensity workouts that require little time or equipment. If you are considering this type of training, note the following:

• Follow general guidelines for medical clearance for exercise (see Chapter 2).

• Use good form and appropriate safety equipment for all exercises and activities; do not sacrifice form for speed, number of repetitions, or any other goal.

• Drink plenty of water and avoid exercise in hot and humid environments.

• Don't push yourself beyond the limits of your strength or conditioning level. Monitor yourself for signs of overtraining (unusual fatigue or muscle soreness), injuries, and rhabdomyolysis (severe muscle pain or weakness; dark red or cola-colored urine).

• Get advice from a qualified professional; when choosing a class, fitness facility, or trainer, follow the guidelines presented in Chapter 2.

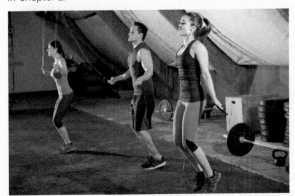

© Tetra Images/Alamy Stock photo RF

SOURCES: Aune, K. T., and J. M. Powers. 2017. "Injuries in an extreme conditioning program," *Sports Health* 9(1), 52–58; Smith, M. M., A. J. Sommer, B. E. Starkoff, and S. T. Devor. 2013. "CrossFit-based high intensity power training improves maximal aerobic fitness and body composition," *Journal of Strength Conditioning Research* 27(11), 3159–3172; Heinrich, K. M. 2014. "High-intensity compared to moderate-intensity training for exercise initiation, enjoyment, adherence, and intentions: An intervention study," *BMC Public Health* 14, 789.

Box Icon: © VisualCommunications/Getty Images RF

temperature gets too high, you may suffer from heat stress. Problems associated with heat stress include dehydration, heat cramps, heat exhaustion, and heatstroke.

When it is hot, exercise safety depends on the body's ability to dissipate heat and maintain blood flow to active muscles. The body releases heat from exercise through the evaporation of sweat. This process cools the skin and the blood circulating near the body's surface. Sweating is an efficient process as long as the air is relatively dry. As humidity increases, however, the sweating mechanism becomes less efficient because extra moisture in the air inhibits the evaporation of sweat from the skin. This is why it takes longer to cool down in humid weather than in dry weather.

You can avoid significant heat stress by staying fit, avoiding overly intense or prolonged exercise for which you are not prepared, drinking adequate fluids before and during exercise, and wearing clothes that allow heat to dissipate.

Dehydration Your body needs water to carry out many chemical reactions and to regulate body temperature. Sweating during exercise depletes your body's water supply and can lead to **dehydration**, excessive loss of body fluids, if fluids aren't replaced. Although dehydration is most common in hot weather, it can occur even in comfortable temperatures if fluid intake is insufficient.

Dehydration increases body temperature and decreases sweat rate, plasma volume, cardiac output, maximal oxygen consumption, exercise capacity, muscular strength, and stores of liver glycogen. You may begin to feel thirsty when you have a fluid deficit greater than about 1% of total body weight.

Drinking fluids before and during exercise is important to prevent dehydration and enhance performance. As a general rule, drink 16–20 ounces (about 2 cups) of fluid four hours before exercise, and 8–12 ounces 15 minutes immediately before exercise. During exercise lasting less than 60 minutes, drink 3–8 ounces of water every 15–20 minutes. Consume a sports drink with electrolytes every 15–20 minutes when exercising longer than 60 minutes.

Don't drink more than one quart of water per hour. Very rarely, active people consume too much water and develop *hyponatremia (water intoxication),* a condition that can cause lung congestion, muscle weakness, nervous system problems, and even death. Following the guidelines presented here can help prevent this condition.

To determine if you're drinking enough fluid, weigh yourself before and after an exercise session; any weight loss is due to fluid loss that needs to be replaced. Urine color is a good marker of hydration (see Figure 3.8). A dark color means that you might be dehydrated. Diet and supplements can affect urine color, which affects the accuracy of the test.

Bring a water bottle when you exercise so that you can replace your fluids while they're being depleted. For exercise sessions lasting less than 60 minutes, cool water is an excellent fluid replacement. For longer workouts, choose sports drinks containing water and small amounts of electrolytes (sodium, potassium, and magnesium) and simple carbohydrates ("sugar," usually in the form of sucrose, glucose, lactate, or glucose polymers). Electrolytes, which are lost from the body in sweat, are important because they help regulate the balance of fluids in body cells and the bloodstream. The carbohydrates in typical sports drinks are rapidly digestible, which enables them to help maintain blood glucose levels. Choose a beverage with no more than eight grams of simple carbohydrate per 100 milliliters of fluid. Nonfat milk and chocolate milk, for those who can tolerate dairy products, are excellent fluid replacement beverages because they promote long-term hydration. See Chapter 8 for more on diet and fluid recommendations for active people.

Heat Cramps Involuntary cramping and spasms in the muscle groups used during exercise are sometimes called **heat cramps**. Although depletion of sodium and potassium from the muscles is involved with the problem, the primary cause of cramps is muscle fatigue. Children are particularly susceptible to heat cramps, but the condition can also occur in adults, even those who are fit. The best treatment for heat cramps is a combination of gentle stretching, replacement of fluid and electrolytes, and rest.

Heat Exhaustion Symptoms of **heat exhaustion** include the following:

- Rapid, weak pulse
- Low blood pressure
- Headache
- Faintness, weakness, dizziness
- Profuse sweating
- Pale face

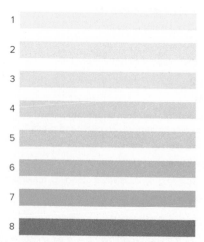

FIGURE 3.8 Urine chart to assess hydration. A large amount of light-colored urine means you are well hydrated. The darker the color, the more dehydrated you are. Vitamins and some foods can make urine darker.

SOURCE: American College of Sports Medicine. 2011. *Selecting and Effectively Using Hydration for Fitness.* Indianapolis, IN: American College of Sports Medicine.

---

dehydration Excessive loss of body fluids.

TERMS

heat cramps Sudden muscle spasms and pain associated with intense exercise in hot weather.

heat exhaustion Heat illness resulting from exertion in hot weather.

- Psychological disorientation (in some cases)
- Normal or slightly elevated core body temperature

Heat exhaustion occurs when an insufficient amount of blood returns to the heart because so much of the body's blood volume is being directed to working muscles (for exercise) and to the skin (for cooling). Treatment for heat exhaustion includes resting in a cool area, removing excess clothing, applying cool or damp towels to the body, and drinking fluids. An affected individual should rest for the remainder of the day and drink plenty of fluids for the next 24 hours.

Heatstroke Heatstroke is a major medical emergency resulting from the failure of the brain's temperature regulatory center. The body does not sweat enough, and body temperature rises dramatically to extremely dangerous levels. In addition to high body temperature, symptoms can include the following:

- Hot, flushed skin (dry or sweaty), red face
- Chills, shivering
- Very high or very low blood pressure
- Confusion, erratic behavior
- Convulsions, loss of consciousness

A heatstroke victim should be cooled as rapidly as possible and immediately transported to a hospital. To lower body temperature, get out of the heat, remove excess clothing, drink cold fluids, and apply cool or damp towels to the body or immerse the body in cold water. People experiencing heatstroke during exercise may still be sweating.

Cold Weather

In extremely cold conditions, problems can occur if a person's body temperature drops or if particular parts of the body are exposed. If the body's ability to warm itself through shivering or exercise can't keep pace with heat loss, the core body temperature begins to drop. This condition, known as **hypothermia**, depresses the central nervous system, resulting in sleepiness and a lower metabolic rate. As metabolic rate drops, body temperature declines even further, and coma and death can result. The risk of hypothermia is particularly severe in cold water.

Frostbite—the freezing of body tissues—is another potential danger of exercise in extremely cold conditions. Frostbite most commonly occurs in exposed body parts like earlobes, fingers, and the nose. It can cause permanent circulatory damage; its symptoms are numbness, pale color, and lack of sensation to cold in the affected areas. Both hypothermia and frostbite require immediate medical treatment.

To exercise safely in cold conditions, don't stay out in very cold temperatures for too long. Take both the temperature and the wind into account when planning your exercise session. Frostbite is possible within 30 minutes in calm conditions when the temperature is colder than −5°F, or in windy conditions (30 mph or more) if the temperature is below 10°F. **Wind chill** values that reflect a combination of the temperature and the wind speed are available as part of a local weather forecast and from the National Weather Service (http://www.weather.gov).

Appropriate clothing provides insulation and helps trap warm air next to the skin. Dress in layers so that you can remove them as you warm up and can put them back on if you get cold. A substantial amount of heat loss comes from the head and neck, so keep these areas covered. In subfreezing temperatures, protect the areas of your body most susceptible to frostbite— fingers, toes, ears, nose, and cheeks—with warm socks, mittens or gloves, and a cap, hood, or ski mask. Wear clothing that breathes and will wick moisture away from your skin to avoid being cooled or overheated by trapped perspiration. Many types of comfortable, lightweight clothing that provide good insulation are available. It's also important in cold conditions to warm up thoroughly and to drink plenty of fluids.

Poor Air Quality

Air pollution can decrease exercise performance and negatively affect health, particularly if you smoke or have respiratory problems such as asthma, bronchitis, or emphysema. The effects of smog are worse during exercise than at rest because air enters the lungs faster. Polluted air may also contain carbon monoxide, which displaces oxygen in the blood and reduces the amount of oxygen available to working muscles. One study found that exercise in polluted air could decrease lung function to the same extent as heavy smoking. Another study found that training in a polluted environment counteracted the normally beneficial effects of exercise on the brain. Symptoms of exercising in poor air quality include eye and throat irritations, difficulty breathing, and possibly headache and malaise.

Do not exercise outdoors during a smog alert or if air quality is very poor. If you have any type of cardiorespiratory difficulty, you should take particular care to avoid exertion outdoors in poor air quality. You can avoid some smog and air pollution by exercising in indoor facilities, in parks, near water (riverbanks, lakeshores, and ocean beaches), or in residential areas with less traffic. Air quality is also usually better in the early morning and late evening, before and after the commute hours.

Exercise Injuries

Most injuries are annoying rather than serious or permanent. However, an injury that isn't cared for properly can escalate into a chronic problem, sometimes serious enough to permanently curtail the activity. It's important to learn how to deal with injuries so that they don't derail your fitness program. Strategies for the care of common exercise injuries and discomforts appear in Table 3.6; some general guidelines are given in the following sections.

TERMS

heatstroke A severe and often fatal heat illness characterized by significantly elevated core body temperature.

hypothermia Low body temperature due to exposure to cold conditions.

frostbite Freezing of body tissues characterized by pallor, numbness, and a loss of cold sensation.

wind chill A measure of how cold it feels based on the rate of heat loss from exposed skin caused by cold and wind.

When to Call a Physician Some injuries require medical attention. Consult a physician for the following:

- Head and eye injuries
- Possible ligament injuries
- Broken bones
- Internal disorders: chest pain, fainting, elevated body temperature, intolerance to hot weather

Also seek medical attention for ostensibly minor injuries that do not get better within a reasonable amount of time. You may need to modify your exercise program for a few weeks to allow an injury to heal.

Managing Minor Exercise Injuries For minor cuts and scrapes, stop the bleeding and clean the wound. Treat injuries to soft tissue (muscles and joints) with the R-I-C-E principle: rest, ice, compression, and elevation.

- *Rest:* Stop using the injured area as soon as you experience pain. Avoid any activity that causes pain.
- *Ice:* Apply ice to the injured area to reduce swelling and alleviate pain. Apply ice immediately for 10–20 minutes, and repeat every few hours as needed for pain. Let the injured part return to normal temperature between icings, and do not apply ice to one area for more than 20 minutes. An easy method for applying ice is to freeze water in a paper cup, peel some of the paper away, and rub the exposed ice on the injured area. If the injured area is large, you can surround it with several bags of crushed ice or ice cubes, or bags of frozen vegetables. Place a thin towel between the bag and your skin. If you use a cold gel pack, limit application time to 10 minutes. Some experts recommend regular icing for up to about 6 hours after an injury, while others suggest continuing as long as swelling persists.

- *Compression:* Wrap the injured area firmly with an elastic or compression bandage between icings. If the area starts throbbing or begins to change color, the bandage may be wrapped too tightly. Do not sleep with the wrap on.
- *Elevation:* Raise the injured area above heart level to decrease the blood supply and reduce swelling. When lying down, use pillows, books, or a low chair or stool to raise the injured area.

Some experts recommend also taking an over-the-counter medication, such as aspirin, ibuprofen, or naproxen, the day after the injury, to decrease inflammation. To rehabilitate your body, follow the steps listed in the box "Rehabilitation Following a Minor Athletic Injury."

Preventing Injuries The best method for dealing with exercise injuries is to prevent them. If you choose activities

---

Table 3.6	Care of Common Exercise Injuries and Discomforts	
INJURY	**SYMPTOMS**	**TREATMENT**
Blister	Accumulation of fluid in one spot under the skin	Don't pop or drain it unless it interferes too much with your daily activities. If it does pop, clean the area with antiseptic and cover with a bandage. Do not remove the skin covering the blister.
Bruise (contusion)	Pain, swelling, and discoloration	R-I-C-E: rest, ice, compression, elevation.
Fracture and/or dislocation	Pain, swelling, tenderness, loss of function, and deformity	Seek medical attention, immobilize the affected area, and apply cold.
Joint sprain	Pain, tenderness, swelling, discoloration, and loss of function	R-I-C-E; apply heat when swelling has disappeared. Stretch and strengthen affected area.
Muscle cramp	Painful, spasmodic muscle contractions	Gently stretch for 15–30 seconds at a time and/or massage the cramped area. Drink fluids and increase dietary salt intake if exercising in hot weather.
Muscle soreness or stiffness	Pain and tenderness in the affected muscle	Stretch the affected muscle gently; exercise at a low intensity; apply heat. Nonsteroidal anti-inflammatory drugs, such as ibuprofen, help some people.
Muscle strain	Pain, tenderness, swelling, and loss of strength in the affected muscle	R-I-C-E; apply heat when swelling has disappeared. Stretch and strengthen the affected area.
Plantar fasciitis	Pain and tenderness in the connective tissue on the bottom of the foot	Apply ice, take nonsteroidal anti-inflammatory drugs, and stretch. Wear night splints when sleeping.
Shin splint	Pain and tenderness on the front of the lower leg; sometimes also pain in the calf muscle	Rest; apply ice to the affected area several times a day and before exercise; wrap with tape for support. Stretch and strengthen muscles in the lower legs. Purchase good-quality footwear and run on soft surfaces.
Side stitch	Pain on the side of the abdomen	Stretch the arm on the affected side as high as possible; if that doesn't help, try bending forward while tightening the abdominal muscles.
Tendinitis	Pain, swelling, and tenderness of the affected area	R-I-C-E; apply heat when swelling has disappeared. Stretch and strengthen the affected area.

TAKE CHARGE
Rehabilitation Following a Minor Athletic Injury

- Reduce the initial inflammation using the R-I-C-E principle (see text).

- After 36–48 hours, apply heat *if the swelling has disappeared completely.* Immerse the affected area in warm water or apply warm compresses, a hot water bottle, or a heating pad. As soon as you feel comfortable, begin moving the affected joints slowly. If you feel pain, or if the injured area begins to swell again, reduce the amount of movement. Continue gently stretching and moving the affected area until you have regained normal range of motion.

- Gradually begin exercising the injured area to build strength and endurance. Depending on the type of injury, weight training, walking, and resistance training can all be effective.

- Gradually reintroduce the stress of an activity until you can return to full intensity. Don't progress too rapidly or you'll re-injure yourself. Before returning to full exercise participation, you should have a full range of motion in your joints, normal strength and balance among your muscles, normal coordinated patterns of movement (with no injury compensation movements, such as limping), and little or no pain.

for your program carefully and follow the training guidelines described here and in Chapter 2, you should be able to avoid most types of injuries. Important guidelines for preventing athletic injuries include the following:

- Train regularly and stay in condition.
- Gradually increase the frequency, intensity, or duration of your workouts.
- Avoid or minimize high-impact activities such as running; alternate them with low-impact activities such as swimming or cycling.
- Get proper rest between exercise sessions.
- Drink plenty of fluids.
- Warm up thoroughly before you exercise and cool down afterward.
- Achieve and maintain a normal range of motion in your joints.
- Use proper body mechanics when lifting objects or executing sports skills.
- Don't exercise when you are ill or overtrained.
- Use proper equipment, particularly shoes, and choose an appropriate exercise surface. If you exercise on a grass field, soft track, or wooden floor, you are less likely to be injured than on concrete or a hard track. (For information on athletic shoes, see the box "Choosing Exercise Footwear.")

- Don't return to your normal exercise program until any athletic injuries have healed. Restart your program at a lower intensity and gradually increase the amount of overload.

TIPS FOR TODAY AND THE FUTURE

Regular, moderate exercise, even in short bouts spread through the day, can improve cardiorespiratory fitness.

RIGHT NOW YOU CAN

- Assess your cardiorespiratory fitness by using one of the methods discussed in this chapter and in Lab 3.1.
- Do a short bout of endurance exercise, such as 10–15 minutes of walking, jogging, or cycling.
- If you have physical activity planned for later in the day, drink some fluids now to make sure you are fully hydrated for your workout.
- Consider the exercise equipment, including shoes, you currently have on hand. If you need new equipment, start researching your options to get the best equipment you can afford.

IN THE FUTURE YOU CAN

- Graduate to a different, more challenging fitness assessment as your cardiorespiratory fitness improves.
- Vary the exercises in your cardiorespiratory endurance training to keep yourself challenged and motivated.

SUMMARY

- The cardiorespiratory system consists of the heart, blood vessels, and respiratory system; it picks up and transports oxygen, nutrients, and waste products.

- The body takes chemical energy from food and uses it to produce ATP and fuel cellular activities. ATP is stored in the body's cells as the basic form of energy.

- During exercise, the body supplies ATP and fuels cellular activities by combining three energy systems: immediate, for short periods of activity; nonoxidative (anaerobic), for intense activity; and oxidative (aerobic), for prolonged activity. Which energy system predominates depends on the duration and intensity of the activity.

- Cardiorespiratory endurance exercise improves cardiorespiratory functioning and cellular metabolism; it reduces the risk of chronic diseases such as heart disease, cancer, type 2 diabetes, obesity, and

CRITICAL CONSUMER
Choosing Exercise Footwear

Footwear is perhaps the most important item of equipment for almost any activity. Shoes protect and support your feet and improve your traction. When you jump or run, you place as much as six times more force on your feet than when you stand still. Shoes can help cushion against the stress that this additional force places on your lower legs, thereby preventing injuries. Some athletic shoes are also designed to help prevent ankle rollover, another common source of injury.

©chictype/Getty Images RF

General Guidelines

When choosing athletic shoes, first consider the activity you've chosen for your exercise program. Shoes appropriate for different activities have very different characteristics. Foot type is another important consideration. If your feet tend to roll inward excessively, you may need shoes with additional stability features on the inner side of the shoe to counteract this movement. If your feet tend to roll outward excessively, you may need highly flexible and cushioned shoes that promote foot motion. Most women will get a better fit if they choose shoes specifically designed for women's feet rather than downsized versions of men's shoes.

Successful Shopping

For successful shoe shopping, keep the following strategies in mind:

- Shop late in the day or, ideally, following a workout. Your foot size increases over the course of the day and after exercise.

- Wear socks like those you plan to wear during exercise.

- Try on both shoes and wear them for 10 or more minutes. Try walking on a noncarpeted surface. Approximate the movements of your activity: walk, jog, run, jump, and so on.

- Check the fit and style carefully:

  - Is the toe box roomy enough? Your toes will spread out when your foot hits the ground or when you push off. There should be at least one thumb's width of space from the longest toe to the end of the toe box.

  - Do the shoes have enough cushioning? Do your feet feel supported when you bounce up and down? Try bouncing on your toes and on your heels.

- Do your heels fit snugly into the shoe? Do they stay put when you walk, or do they slide up?

- Are the arches of your feet right on top of the shoes' arch supports?

- Do the shoes feel stable when you twist and turn on the balls of your feet? Try twisting from side to side while standing on one foot.

- Do you feel any pressure points?

- If you exercise at dawn or dusk, choose shoes with reflective sections for added visibility and safety.

- Replace athletic shoes about every three months or 300–500 miles of jogging or walking.

Barefoot Shoes or Minimalist Footwear

Two-thirds of runners experience an injury every year. Humans have evolved to run, so some scientists blame running shoes for the high injury rate. Most runners strike heel first when using heavily padded running shoes. Barefoot runners strike the ground with their forefoot (at least they're supposed to), which better uses the shock absorbing capacity of the skeleton. Some researchers speculate that using "minimalist" footwear allows people to run more naturally, which should cut down on the injury rate. Other research suggests that traditional running shoes provide a physiological advantage that makes running easier. We need more research to determine whether barefoot running is safe and viable or just the latest running fad.

Box icon: © sam74100/Getty Images RF

---

osteoporosis; and it improves immune function and psychological and emotional well-being.

- Cardiorespiratory fitness is measured by determining how well the cardiorespiratory system transports and uses oxygen. The upper limit of this measure, called maximal oxygen consumption, or $\dot{V}O_{2max}$, can be measured precisely in a laboratory, or it can be estimated reasonably well through self-assessment tests.

- To create a successful exercise program, set realistic goals, choose suitable activities, begin slowly, and always warm up and cool down. As fitness improves, exercise more often, harder, and/or longer.

Program design should consider the FITT-VP principle: **F**requency, **I**ntensity, **T**ime, **T**ype, **V**olume, and **P**rogression.

- Intensity of training can be measured through target heart rate zone, ratings of perceived exertion, METs, or the talk test.

- With careful attention to fluid intake, clothing, duration of exercise, and exercise intensity, endurance training can be safe in hot and cold weather conditions.

- Serious injuries require medical attention. Application of the R-I-C-E principle (rest, ice, compression, elevation) is appropriate for treating many types of muscle or joint injuries.

COMMON QUESTIONS ANSWERED

Q Do I need a special diet for my endurance exercise program?

A No. For most people, a nutritionally balanced diet contains all the energy and nutrients needed to sustain an exercise program. Don't waste your money on unnecessary supplements. (Chapter 8 provides detailed information about putting together a healthy diet.)

Q How can I measure how far I walk or run?

A The simplest way to measure distance is with a GPS-based phone app, which measures your distance, speed, and change in elevation. You can also use a pedometer, which counts your steps. Although stride length varies among individuals, 2,000 steps typically equals about one mile, and 10,000 steps equals about five miles. To track your distance and your progress using a phone app or pedometer, follow the guidelines in Lab 2.3.

Q How can I avoid being so sore when I start an exercise program?

A Post-exercise muscle soreness is caused by muscle injury followed by muscle inflammation. Muscles get stronger and larger in response to muscle tension and injury. However, excessive injury can delay progress. The best approach is to begin conservatively with low-volume, low-intensity workouts, and gradually increase the intensity of the exercise sessions. If you are currently sedentary, begin with 5–10 minutes of exercise and gradually increase the distance and speed you walk, run, cycle, or swim.

Q Is it OK to do cardiorespiratory endurance exercise while menstruating?

A Yes. There is no evidence that exercise during menstruation is unhealthy or that it has negative effects on performance. If you have headaches, backaches, and abdominal pain during menstruation, you may not feel like exercising. For some women, exercise helps relieve these symptoms. Listen to your body and exercise at whatever intensity is comfortable for you.

Q Will high altitude affect my ability to exercise?

A At high altitude (above 1,500 meters, or about 4,900 feet), there is less oxygen available in the air than at lower altitude. High altitude doesn't affect anaerobic exercise, such as stretching and weight lifting, but it does affect aerobic activities—that is, any type of cardiovascular endurance exercise—because the heart and lungs have to work harder, even when the body is at rest, to deliver enough oxygen to body cells. The increased cardiovascular strain of exercise at high altitude reduces endurance. To play it safe when at high altitude, avoid heavy exercise—at least for the first few days—and drink plenty of water. And don't expect to reach your normal lower-altitude exercise capacity.

FOR FURTHER EXPLORATION

American Academy of Orthopaedic Surgeons: Sports Injuries & Prevention. Provides fact sheets on many fitness and sports topics, including how to begin a program, how to choose equipment, and how to prevent and treat many types of injuries.
http://orthoinfo.aaos.org/menus/sports.cfm

American Cancer Society: Eat Healthy and Get Active. Provides tools for managing an exercise program and discusses the links between cancer and lifestyle, including the importance of physical activity in preventing some cancers.
http://www.cancer.org/healthy/eathealthygetactive/

American Heart Association: Exercise and Fitness. Provides information on cardiovascular health and disease, including the role of exercise in maintaining heart health and exercise tips for people of all ages.
http://www.heart.org/HEARTORG/GettingHealthy/PhysicalActivity/Physical-Activity_UCM_001080_SubHomePage.jsp

Centers for Disease Control and Prevention: Physical Activity for Everyone. Explains the latest government recommendations on exercise and physical activity and provides strategies for getting the appropriate type and amount of exercise.
http://www.cdc.gov/physicalactivity/

CrossFit Journal. A fitness, health, and lifestyle publication dedicated to the improvement of athletic performance, with new articles published daily and an archive of articles, videos, and audio files covering exercise technique, nutrition, injuries and rehab, equipment, coaching, and more.
http://journal.crossfit.com/

Exercise Is Medicine. A global health initiative managed by the American College of Sports Medicine that promotes physical activity for the treatment and prevention of many diseases.
http://www.exerciseismedicine.org/

Runner's World Online. Contains a wide variety of information about running, including tips for beginning runners, advice about training, and a shoe buyer's guide.
http://www.runnersworld.com

Weight-control Information Network: Walking. An online fact sheet that explains the benefits of walking for exercise, tips for starting a walking program, and techniques for getting the most from walking workouts.
http://win.niddk.nih.gov

Women's Sports Foundation. Provides information and links about training and about many specific sports activities.
http://www.womenssportsfoundation.org

SELECTED BIBLIOGRAPHY

American College of Sports Medicine. 2009. *ACSM's Resource Manual for Guidelines for Exercise Testing and Prescription,* 6th ed. Philadelphia: Lippincott Williams and Wilkins.

American College of Sports Medicine. 2012. *ACSM's Health/Fitness Facility Standards and Guidelines,* 4th ed. Champaign, Ill: Human Kinetics.

American College of Sports Medicine. 2018. *ACSM's Guidelines for Exercise Testing and Prescription,* 10th ed. Philadelphia: Wolters Kluwer.

Arem, H., et al. 2015. Leisure time physical activity and mortality: A detailed pooled analysis of the dose-response relationship. *Journal of the American Medical Association Internal Medicine* 175(6): 959–967.

Brooks, G. A., et al. 2005. *Exercise Physiology: Human Bioenergetics and Its Applications,* 4th ed. New York: McGraw-Hill.

Centers for Disease Control and Prevention. 2010. *Promoting Physical Activity: A Guide for Community Action,* 2nd ed. Champaign, Ill.: Human Kinetics.

Denis, G. V., and M. S. Obin. 2013. Metabolically healthy obesity: origins and implications. *Molecular Aspects of Medicine* 34(1): 59–70.

Dimitrov, S., Hulteng, E., and S. Hong. 2017. Inflammation and exercise: Inhibition of monocytic intracellular TNF production by acute exercise via β2-adrenergic activation. *Brain, Behavior, and Immunity* 61: 60–68.

Doral, M. N., and J. Karlsson. 2015. *Sports Injuries: Prevention, Diagnosis, Treatment and Rehabilitation.* New York: Springer.

Falcone, P. H., et al. 2015. Caloric expenditure of aerobic, resistance, or combined high-intensity interval training using a hydraulic resistance system in healthy men. *Journal of Strength and Conditioning Research* 29(3): 779–785.

Fenesi, B., et al. 2017. Physical exercise moderates the relationship of apolipoprotein E (APOE) genotype and dementia risk: A population-based study. *Journal of Alzheimer's Disease* 56(1): 297-303.

Garber, C. E., et al. 2011. Quantity and quality of exercise for developing and maintaining cardiorespiratory, musculoskeletal, and neuromotor fitness in apparently healthy adults: Guidance for prescribing exercise. *Medicine and Science in Sport and Exercise* 43(7):1334–1359.

Gebel, K., et al. 2015. Effect of moderate to vigorous physical activity on all-cause mortality in middle-aged and older Australians. *Journal of the American Medical Association Internal Medicine* 175(6): 970–977.

Gillen, J. B. 2016. Twelve Weeks of Sprint Interval Training Improves Indices of Cardiometabolic Health Similar to Traditional Endurance Training despite a Five-Fold Lower Exercise Volume and Time Commitment. *PlosOne* 11(4):e0154075.

Gonzales, M. M., et al. 2013. Aerobic fitness and the brain: Increased N-acetyl aspartate and choline concentrations in endurance-trained middle-aged adults. *Brain Topography* 26(1): 126–134.

Hanssen, H., et al. 2015. Acute effects of interval versus continuous endurance training on pulse wave reflection in healthy young men. *Atherosclerosis* 238(2): 399–406.

Hardee, J. P., et al. 2014. The effect of resistance exercise on all-cause mortality in cancer survivors. *Mayo Clinic Proceedings* 89(8): 1108–1115.

He, F. 2016. Redox mechanism of reactive oxygen species in exercise. *Frontiers of Physiology* 7: 486.

Howley, E., and D. Thompson. 2012. *Fitness Professional's Handbook,* 6th ed. Champaign, Ill.: Human Kinetics.

Kingsley, J. D., et al. 2016. Arterial stiffness and autonomic modulation after free-weight resistance exercise in resistance trained individuals. *Journal of Strength and Conditioning Research* 30(12): 3373–3380.

Larsen, S., et al. 2015. The effect of high-intensity training on mitochondrial fat oxidation in skeletal muscle and subcutaneous adipose tissue. *Scandinavian Journal of Medicine and Science in Sports* 25(1): e59–69.

Lucas, S. J., et al. 2015. High-intensity interval exercise and cerebrovascular health: Curiosity, cause, and consequence. *Journal of Cerebral Blood Flow and Metabolism* 35(6): 902–911.

MacIntosh, B. J., et al. 2014. Impact of a single bout of aerobic exercise on regional brain perfusion and activation responses in healthy young adults. *PLoS One* 9(1): e85163.

Meeusen, R. 2014. Exercise, nutrition and the brain. *Sports Medicine* 44 (Suppl 1): S47–56.

Metzl, J., and C. Kowalchik. 2015. *Dr. Jordan Metzl's Running Strong: The Sports Doctor's Complete Guide to Staying Healthy and Injury-Free for Life.* New York: Rodale.

Mozaffarian, D., et al. 2016. *Heart Disease and Stroke Statistics—2016 Update. Circulation* 133 (4): e38–360.

Muller, J., et al. 2015. Acute effects of submaximal endurance training on arterial stiffness in healthy middle- and long-distance runners. *Journal of Clinical Hypertension* 17(5): 371–374.

Nagamatsu, L. S., et al. 2014. Exercise is medicine, for the body and the brain. *British Journal of Sports Medicine* 48(12): 943–944.

Nieman, D. C. 2010. *Exercise Testing and Prescription: A Health-Related Approach,* 7th ed. New York: McGraw-Hill.

Physical Activity Guidelines Advisory Committee. 2008. *Physical Activity Guidelines Advisory Committee Report, 2008.* Washington, DC: U.S. Department of Health and Human Services.

Puterman, E., et al. 2015. Determinants of telomere attrition over 1 year in healthy older women: stress and health behaviors matter. *Molecular Psychiatry* 20(4): 529–535.

Ramos, J. S., et al. 2015. The impact of high-intensity interval training versus moderate-intensity continuous training on vascular function: A systematic review and meta-analysis. *Sports Medicine* 45(5): 679–692.

Schnohr, P., et al. 2015. Dose of jogging and long-term mortality: The Copenhagen City Heart Study. *Journal of the American College of Cardiology* 65(5): 411–419.

U.S. Department of Health and Human Services. 2008. *Physical Activity Guidelines for Americans.* Washington, DC: U.S. Department of Health and Human Services.

Vardar Yagli, N., et al. 2015. Do yoga and aerobic exercise training have impact on functional capacity, fatigue, peripheral muscle strength, and quality of life in breast cancer survivors? *Integrative Cancer Therapies* 14(2): 125–132.

Vincent, G., et al. 2015. Changes in mitochondrial function and mitochondria associated protein expression in response to 2 weeks of high intensity interval training. *Frontiers in Physiology* 6: 51.

Watson, R. R. 2017. *Exercise and the Aging Brain: Effects of Exercise on Neurological Function.* London: Academic Press.

Weston, M., et al. 2014. Effects of low-volume high-intensity interval training (HIIT) on fitness in adults: A meta-analysis of controlled and non-controlled trials. *Sports Medicine* 44(7): 1005–1017.

Wilson, M., et al. 2017. *IOC Manual of Sports Cardiology.* New York: Wiley.

Xiang, L., and R. L. Hester. 2017. *Cardiovascular Responses to Exercise,* 2nd ed. Williston, VT:Morgan & Claypool.

Zwetsloot, K. A., et al. 2014. High-intensity interval training induces a modest systemic inflammatory response in active, young men. *Journal of Inflammation Research* 7: 9–17.

LABORATORY ACTIVITIES

Name _____ Section _____ Date _____

LAB 3.1 Assessing Your Current Level of Cardiorespiratory Endurance

The conditions for exercise safety given in Chapter 2 apply to all fitness assessment tests. Talk to a physician if needed, and if you experience any unusual symptoms while taking a test, stop exercising and discuss your condition with your instructor. Additional cautions and prerequisites for the five test options presented in this lab are described below.

1-Mile Walk Test	Recommended for anyone who meets the criteria for safe exercise. This test can be used by people who cannot perform other tests because of low fitness level or injury.
3-Minute Step Test	If you suffer from joint problems in your ankles, knees, or hips or are significantly overweight, check with your physician before taking this test. People with balance problems or for whom a fall would be particularly dangerous, including older adults and pregnant women, should use special caution or avoid this test.
1.5-Mile Run-Walk Test	Recommended for people who are healthy and at least moderately active. If you have been sedentary, you should participate in a 4- to 8-week walk-run program before taking the test. Don't take this test in extremely hot or cold weather or if you aren't used to exercising under those conditions.
Beep Test	Recommended for fit individuals; the test is highly strenuous and requires the ability to jog, run, and sprint. Don't take this test unless you can complete at least 10 sets of 50-meter sprints.
12-Minute Swim Test	Recommended for relatively strong swimmers who are confident in the water; if needed, ask a qualified swimming instructor to evaluate your swimming ability before attempting this test.

Choose one of the tests based on your fitness level and available facilities. For best results, don't exercise strenuously or consume caffeine the day of the test, and don't smoke or eat a heavy meal within about three hours of the test.

The 1-Mile Walk Test

Equipment

1. A track or course that provides a measurement of 1 mile
2. A stopwatch, clock, or watch with a second hand
3. A weight scale

Preparation

Measure your body weight (in pounds) before taking the test.
Body weight: _____ lbs

Instructions

1. Warm up before taking the test. Do some walking, easy jogging, or calisthenics.
2. Cover the 1-mile course as quickly as possible. Walk at a pace that is brisk but comfortable. You must raise your heart rate above 120 beats per minute (bpm).
3. As soon as you complete the distance, note your time and take your pulse for 15 seconds.

    Walking time: _____ min _____ sec
    15-second pulse count: _____ beats
4. Cool down after the test by walking slowly for several minutes.

Determining Maximal Oxygen Consumption

1. Convert your 15-second pulse count into a value for exercise heart rate by multiplying it by 4.

    Exercise heart rate: _____ × 4 = _____ bpm
2. Convert your walking time from minutes and seconds to a decimal figure. For example, a time of 14 minutes and 45 seconds would be 14 + (45/60), or 14.75 minutes.

    Walking time: _____ min + (_____ sec ÷ 60 sec/min) = _____ min
3. Insert values for your age, gender, weight, walking time, and exercise heart rate in the following equation, where

    W = your weight (in pounds)
    A = your age (in years)

LABORATORY ACTIVITIES

G = your gender (male = 1; female = 0)

T = your time to complete the 1-mile course (in minutes)

H = your exercise heart rate (in beats per minute)

$\dot{V}O_{2max} = 132.853 - (0.0769 \times W) - (0.3877 \times A) + (6.315 \times G) - (3.2649\, T) - (0.1565 \times H)$ = ml/kg/min (maximum oxygen consumption measured in milliliters of oxygen used per kilogram of body weight per minute)

For example, a 20-year-old, 190-pound male with a time of 14.75 minutes and an exercise heart rate of 152 bpm would calculate maximal oxygen consumption as follows:

$\dot{V}O_{2max} = 132.853 - (0.0769 \times 190) - (0.3877 \times 20) + (6.315 \times 1) - (3.2649 \times 14.75) - (0.1565 \times 152) = 45$ *ml/kg/min*

$\dot{V}O_{2max} = \mathbf{132.853 - (0.0769 \times}$ _____ **)** $\mathbf{- (0.3877 \times}$ _____ **)** $\mathbf{+ (6.315 \times}$ _____ **)**
                          weight (lb)   age (years)   gender

$\mathbf{- (3.2649 \times}$ _____ **)** $\mathbf{- (0.1565 \times}$ _____ **)** = _____ **ml/kg/min**
                walking time (min)   exercise heart rate (bpm)

4. Copy this value for $\dot{V}O_{2max}$ into the appropriate place in the chart in the "Rating Your Cardsiovascular Fitness" section.

The 3-Minute Step Test

Equipment

1. A step, bench, or bleacher step that is 16.25 inches from ground level

2. A stopwatch, clock, or watch with a second hand

3. A metronome

Preparation

Practice stepping up onto and down from the step before you begin the test. Each step has four beats: up-up-down-down. Males should perform the test with the metronome set for a rate of 96 beats per minute, or 24 steps per minute. Females should set the metronome at 88 beats per minute, or 22 steps per minute.

Instructions

1. Warm up before taking the test. Do some walking or easy jogging.

2. Set the metronome at the proper rate. Your instructor or a partner can call out starting and stopping times; otherwise, have a clock or watch within easy viewing during the test.

3. Begin the test and continue to step at the correct pace for three minutes.

4. Stop after three minutes. Remain standing and count your pulse for the 15-second period from 5 to 20 seconds into recovery.
   15-second pulse count: _____ beats

5. Cool down after the test by walking slowly for several minutes.

Determining Maximal Oxygen Consumption

1. Convert your 15-second pulse count to a value for recovery heart rate by multiplying by 4.
   Recovery heart rate: _____ × 4 = _____ **bpm**
                        15-sec pulse count

2. Insert your recovery heart rate in the equation below, where
   H = recovery heart rate (in beats per minute)
   Males: $\dot{V}O_{2max} = 111.33 - (0.42 \times H)$
   Females: $\dot{V}O_{2max} = 65.81 - (0.18470 \times H)$
   For example, a man with a recovery heart rate of 162 bpm would calculate maximal oxygen consumption as follows:
   $\dot{V}O_{2max} = 111.33 - (0.42 \times 162) = 43$ *ml/kg/min*
   Males: $\dot{V}O_{2max} = 111.33 - (0.42 \times$ _____ **)** = _____ **ml/kg/min**
                                      recovery heart rate (bpm)

   Females: $\dot{V}O_{2max} = 65.81 - (0.1847 \times$ _____ **)** = _____ **ml/kg/min**
                                        recovery heart rate (bpm)

3. Copy this value for $\dot{V}O_{2max}$ into the appropriate place in the chart in the "Rating Your Cardiovascular Fitness" section.

The 1.5-Mile Run-Walk Test

Equipment

1. A running track or course that is flat and provides exact measurements of up to 1.5 miles

2. A stopwatch, clock, or watch with a second hand

Preparation

You may want to practice pacing yourself prior to taking the test to avoid going too fast at the start and becoming prematurely fatigued. Allow yourself a day or two to recover from your practice run before taking the test.

Instructions

1. Warm up before taking the test. Do some walking or easy jogging.

2. Try to cover the distance as fast as possible without overexerting yourself. If possible, monitor your own time, or have someone call out your time at various intervals of the test to determine whether your pace is correct.

3. Record the amount of time, in minutes and seconds, it takes you to complete the 1.5-mile distance.
   Running-walking time: _____ min _____ sec

4. Cool down after the test by walking or jogging slowly for about five minutes.

Determining Maximal Oxygen Consumption

1. Convert your running time from minutes and seconds to a decimal figure. For example, a time of 14 minutes and 25 seconds would be 14 + (25/60), or 14.4 minutes.
   Running-walking time: __11__ min + (__31__ sec ÷ 60 sec/min) = __11.51__ min

2. Insert your running time into the equation below, where

   T = running time (in minutes)

   $\dot{V}O_{2max} = (483 \div T) + 3.5$

   For example, a person who completes 1.5 miles in 14.4 minutes would calculate maximal oxygen consumption as follows:

   $\dot{V}O_{2max} = (483 \div 14.4) + 3.5 = 37$ *ml/kg/min*

   $\dot{V}O_{2max} = (483 \div \underset{\text{run-walk time (min)}}{\underline{11.51}}) + 3.5 = \underline{45.46}$ ml/kg/min

3. Copy this value for $\dot{V}O_{2max}$ into the appropriate place in the chart in the "Rating Your Cardiovascular Fitness" section.

The Beep Test

This is also called the Multi-Stage Fitness Test, Pacer Test, Yo Yo test, or 20-Meter Shuttle Run Test.

Description

The Beep Test involves running a series of 20-meter shuttles at a specified pace. The pace gets faster each minute as you go to another level. For example, the series begins at a speed of 8.5 kilometers per hour and then increases by 0.5 kilometers per hour with each advancing level. The MP3 audio recording or phone app signals the end of a shuttle with a single beep and the start of the next level with three beeps. The object of the test is to keep up with the beeps as long as possible.

Facilities and Equipment

1. Running track, open field, or gymnasium

2. Two cones or field markers set 20 meters (21 yards, 32 inches) apart (use four cones if testing a large group)

3. Beep Test app or MP3 recording of beeps (widely available free on the Internet—e.g., http://www.beeptestacademy.com; free Beep Test apps are also available for the iPhone and Android smartphones)

4. Method of playing Beep Test: MP3 player with speaker, smartphone with speaker, iPad with speaker. You could run this test by yourself if you have an MP3 player with earphones.

Preparation

Don't take this test until you are prepared. A good technique is to run intervals on a track or playing field. For example, run 50 meters, rest 30 seconds, repeat. Gradually, increase the speed and number of repetitions until you can complete at least 10 sets of 50-meter sprints.

Instructions

The Beep Test is a popular assessment of cardiovascular endurance levels and maximal oxygen consumption.

1. Set up the audio alert system for the test (MP3 player with speaker, or personal MP3 player, or smartphone with headphones).

2. Run back and forth between two cones or field markers placed 20 meters apart, keeping pace with an audio beep that plays during the test. The test is arranged in levels. The beeps get faster with each increasing stage. A single beep will sound at the end of the time for each shuttle. A triple beep sounds at the end of each level. The triple beep is a signal that the pace will get faster. Do not stop when you hear the triple beat; continue running toward the other field marker or cone.

LABORATORY ACTIVITIES

3. The test ends when you can't keep pace with the beeps for two consecutive shuttles.

4. Note your level and the total number of shuttles you completed. Record your maximal oxygen consumption and enter it on the chart labeled "Rating Your Cardiovascular Fitness."

Videos of the test are widely available on the Internet.

Level	Speed (miles per hour)	Minutes per Mile	Total Shuttles	Predicted $\dot{V}O_{2max}$ (milliliters oxygen per kilogram body weight)
1	5.3	11.4	2	16.6
1	5.3	11.4	4	17.5
1	5.3	11.4	6	18.5
2	5.6	10.7	8	20.0
2	5.6	10.7	10	20.9
2	5.6	10.7	12	21.8
2	5.6	10.7	14	22.6
3	5.9	10.2	16	23.4
3	5.9	10.2	18	24.3
3	5.9	10.2	20	25.1
3	5.9	10.2	22	26.0
4	6.2	9.7	24	26.8
4	6.2	9.7	26	27.6
4	6.2	9.7	28	28.3
4	6.2	9.7	31	29.5
5	6.5	9.2	33	30.2
5	6.5	9.2	35	31.0
5	6.5	9.2	37	31.8
5	6.5	9.2	40	32.9
6	6.8	8.8	42	33.6
6	6.8	8.8	44	34.3
6	6.8	8.8	46	35.0
6	6.8	8.8	48	35.7
6	6.8	8.8	50	36.4
7	7.2	8.4	52	37.1
7	7.2	8.4	54	37.8
7	7.2	8.4	56	38.5
7	7.2	8.4	58	39.2
7	7.2	8.4	60	39.9
8	7.5	8.0	62	40.5
8	7.5	8.0	64	41.1
8	7.5	8.0	66	41.8
8	7.5	8.0	68	42.4
8	7.5	8.0	71	43.3
9	7.8	7.7	73	43.9
9	7.8	7.7	75	44.5
9	7.8	7.7	76	45.2 ⟩ 45.46
9	7.8	7.7	78	45.8
9	7.8	7.7	81	46.8
10	8.1	7.4	83	47.4
10	8.1	7.4	85	48.0
10	8.1	7.4	87	48.7
10	8.1	7.4	89	49.3
10	8.1	7.4	92	50.2

Level	Speed (miles per hour)	Minutes per Mile	Total Shuttles	Predicted $\dot{V}O_{2max}$ (milliliters oxygen per kilogram body weight)
11	8.4	7.2	94	50.8
11	8.4	7.2	96	51.4
11	8.4	7.2	98	51.9
11	8.4	7.2	100	52.5
11	8.4	7.2	102	53.1
11	8.4	7.2	104	53.7
12	8.7	6.9	106	54.3
12	8.7	6.9	108	54.8
12	8.7	6.9	110	55.4
12	8.7	6.9	112	56.0
12	8.7	6.9	114	56.5
12	8.7	6.9	116	57.1
13	9.0	6.7	118	57.6
13	9.0	6.7	120	58.2
13	9.0	6.7	122	58.7
13	9.0	6.7	124	59.3
13	9.0	6.7	126	59.8
13	9.0	6.7	129	60.6
14	9.3	6.4	131	61.1
14	9.3	6.4	133	61.7
14	9.3	6.4	135	62.2
14	9.3	6.4	137	62.7
14	9.3	6.4	139	63.2
14	9.3	6.4	142	64.0
15	9.6	6.2	144	64.6
15	9.6	6.2	146	65.1
15	9.6	6.2	148	65.6
15	9.6	6.2	150	66.2
15	9.6	6.2	152	66.7
15	9.6	6.2	154	67.5
16	9.9	6.0	156	68.0
16	9.9	6.0	158	68.5
16	9.9	6.0	160	69.0
16	9.9	6.0	162	69.5
16	9.9	6.0	164	69.9
16	9.9	6.0	166	70.5
16	9.9	6.0	168	70.9
17	10.3	5.9	170	71.4
17	10.3	5.9	172	71.9
17	10.3	5.9	174	72.4
17	10.3	5.9	176	72.9
17	10.3	5.9	178	73.4
17	10.3	5.9	180	73.9
17	10.3	5.9	182	74.4
18	10.6	5.7	184	74.8
18	10.6	5.7	186	75.3
18	10.6	5.7	188	75.8
18	10.6	5.7	190	76.2
18	10.6	5.7	192	76.7
18	10.6	5.7	194	77.2
18	10.6	5.7	197	77.9

LABORATORY ACTIVITIES

Level	Speed (miles per hour)	Minutes per Mile	Total Shuttles	Predicted $\dot{V}O_{2max}$ (milliliters oxygen per kilogram body weight)
19	10.9	5.5	199	78.3
19	10.9	5.5	201	78.8
19	10.9	5.5	203	79.2
19	10.9	5.5	205	79.7
19	10.9	5.5	207	80.2
19	10.9	5.5	209	80.6
19	10.9	5.5	212	81.3
20	11.2	5.4	214	81.8
20	11.2	5.4	216	82.2
20	11.2	5.4	218	82.6
20	11.2	5.4	220	83.0
20	11.2	5.4	222	83.5
20	11.2	5.4	224	83.9
20	11.2	5.4	226	84.8

SOURCE: Ramsbottom, R., J. Brewer, and C. Williams, "A progressive shuttle run test to estimate maximal oxygen uptake," *British Journal of Sports Medicine* 22(4), 1988, 141–144.

Record your score. Copy this value for $\dot{V}O_{2max}$ into the appropriate place in the chart below:

Highest level: _____

Total shuttles run: _____

Predicted $\dot{V}O_{2max}$: _____

SOURCE: Adapted from Ramsbottom, R., J. Brewer, and C. Williams. 1988. A progressive shuttle run test to estimate maximal oxygen uptake. *British Journal of Sports Medicine* 22(4): 141–144.

Rating Your Cardiovascular Fitness

Record your $\dot{V}O_{2max}$ score(s) and the corresponding fitness rating from the table below.

Women	Very Poor	Poor	Fair	Good	Excellent	Superior
Age: 18–29	Below 31.6	31.6–35.4	35.5–39.4	39.5–43.9	44.0–50.1	Above 50.1
30–39	Below 29.9	29.9–33.7	33.8–36.7	36.8–40.9	41.0–46.8	Above 46.8
40–49	Below 28.0	28.0–31.5	31.6–35.0	35.1–38.8	38.9–45.1	Above 45.1
50–59	Below 25.5	25.5–28.6	28.7–31.3	31.4–35.1	35.2–39.8	Above 39.8
60–69	Below 23.7	23.7–26.5	26.6–29.0	29.1–32.2	32.3–36.8	Above 36.8
Men						
Age: 18–29	Below 38.1	38.1–42.1	42.2–45.6	45.7–51.0	51.1–56.1	Above 56.1
30–39	Below 36.7	36.7–40.9	41.0–44.3	44.4–48.8	48.9–54.2	Above 54.2
40–49	Below 34.6	34.6–38.3	38.4–42.3	42.4–46.7	46.8–52.8	Above 52.8
50–59	Below 31.1	31.1–35.1	35.2–38.2	38.3–43.2	43.3–49.6	Above 49.6
60–69	Below 27.4	27.4–31.3	31.4–34.9	35.0–39.4	39.5–46.0	Above 46.0

SOURCE: Ratings based on norms from *The Physical Fitness Specialist Manual*, The Cooper Institute of Aerobic Research, Dallas, Tex.; Revised 2002.

	$\dot{V}O_{2max}$	Cardiovascular Fitness Rating
1-Mile Walk Test		
3-Minute Step Test		
1.5-M Run-Walk Test		
Beep Test		

The 12-Minute Swim Test

If you enjoy swimming and prefer to build a cardiorespiratory training program around this type of exercise, you can assess your cardiorespiratory endurance by taking the 12-Minute Swim Test. You will receive a rating based on the distance you can swim in 12 minutes. A complete fitness program based on swimming is presented in Chapter 7.

Note, however, that this test is appropriate only for relatively strong swimmers who are confident in the water. If you are unsure about your swimming ability, this test may not be appropriate for you. If necessary, ask your school's swim coach or a qualified swimming instructor to evaluate your ability in the water before attempting this test.

Equipment

1. A swimming pool that provides measurements in yards
2. A wall clock that is clearly visible from the pool, or someone with a watch who can time you

Preparation

You may want to practice pacing yourself before taking the test to avoid going too fast at the start and becoming prematurely fatigued. Allow yourself a day or two to recover from your practice swim before taking the test.

Instructions

1. Warm up before taking the test. Do some walking or light jogging before getting in the pool. Once in the water, swim a lap or two at an easy pace to make sure your muscles are warm and you are comfortable.
2. Try to cover the distance as fast as possible without overexerting yourself. If possible, monitor your own time, or have someone call out your time at various intervals of the test to determine whether your pace is correct.
3. Record the distance, in yards, that you were able to cover during the 12-minute period.
4. Cool down after the test by swimming a lap or two at an easy pace.
5. Use the following chart to gauge your level of cardiorespiratory fitness.

	DISTANCE IN YARDS				
Men	*Needs Work*	*Better*	*Fair*	*Good*	*Excellent*
Age: 13–19	Below 500	500–599	600–699	700–799	Above 800
20–29	Below 400	400–499	500–599	600–699	Above 700
30–39	Below 350	350–449	450–549	550–649	Above 650
40–49	Below 300	300–399	400–499	500–599	Above 600
50–59	Below 250	250–349	350–449	450–549	Above 550
60 and over	Below 250	250–299	300–399	400–499	Above 500
Women					
Age: 13–19	Below 400	400–499	500–599	600–699	Above 700
20–29	Below 300	300–399	400–499	500–599	Above 600
30–39	Below 250	250–349	350–449	450–549	Above 550
40–49	Below 200	200–299	300–399	400–499	Above 500
50–59	Below 150	150–249	250–349	350–449	Above 450
60 and over	Below 150	150–199	200–299	300–399	Above 400

100 yards = 91 meters

SOURCE: Cooper, K. H., *The Aerobics Program for Total Well-Being*. New York: Bantam Books, 1982.

Record your fitness rating:

	Cardiovascular Fitness Rating
12-Minute Swim Test	

LABORATORY ACTIVITIES

Using Your Results

How did you score? Does your rating for cardiovascular fitness surprise you? Are you satisfied with your current rating?

If you're not satisfied, set a realistic goal for improvement: _____

_____

Are you satisfied with your current level of cardiovascular fitness as evidenced in your daily life—your ability to walk, run, bicycle, climb stairs, do yard work, or engage in recreational activities?

If you're not satisfied, set some realistic goals for improvement, such as completing a 5K run or 25-mile bike ride: _____

_____

What should you do next? Enter the results of this lab in the Preprogram Assessment column in Appendix B. If you've set goals for improvement, begin planning your cardiorespiratory endurance exercise program by completing the plan in Lab 3.2. After several weeks of your program, complete this lab again, and enter the results in the Postprogram Assessment column of Appendix B. How do the results compare? (Remember, it's best to compare $\dot{V}O_{2max}$ scores for the same test.)

SOURCES: Brooks, G. A., T. D. Fahey, and K. Baldwin. 2005. *Exercise Physiology: Human Bioenergetics and its Applications.* New York: McGraw Hill; Kline, G. M., et al. 1987. "Estimation of $\dot{V}O_{2max}$ from a one-mile track walk, gender, age, and body weight," *Medicine and Science in Sports and Exercise* 19(3), 253–259; McArdle, W. D., F. I. Katch, and V. L. Katch. 2017. *Exercise Physiology: Nutrition, Energy, and Human Performance,* 8th ed. Philadelphia: Lea and Febiger.

LABORATORY ACTIVITIES

Name _____   Section _____   Date _____

LAB 3.2   Developing an Exercise Program for Cardiorespiratory Endurance

1. *Goals.* List goals for your cardiorespiratory endurance exercise program. Your goals can be specific or general, short or long term. In the first section, include specific, measurable goals that you can use to track the progress of your fitness program. These goals might be things like raising your cardiorespiratory fitness rating from fair to good or swimming laps for 30 minutes without resting. In the second section, include long-term and more qualitative goals, such as improving self-confidence and reducing your risk for chronic disease.

   Specific Goals: Current Status   Final Goals

   _____   _____
   _____   _____
   _____   _____

   Other goals: _____
   _____

2. *Type of Activities.* Choose one or more endurance activities for your program. These can include any activity that uses large-muscle groups, can be maintained continuously, and is rhythmic and aerobic in nature. Examples include walking, jogging, cycling, ebike cycling, group exercise such as aerobic dance, rowing, rope-skipping, stair-climbing, cross-country skiing, swimming, skating, and endurance game activities such as soccer and tennis. Choose activities that are both convenient and enjoyable. Fill in the activity names on the program plan.

3. *Frequency.* On the program plan, fill in how often you plan to participate in each activity; the ACSM recommends participating in cardiorespiratory endurance exercise three to five days per week.

Program Plan

Type of Activity	Frequency (check ✓)							Intensity (bpm or RPE)	Time (min)
	M	T	W	TH	F	SA	SU		

4. *Intensity.* Determine your exercise intensity using one of the following methods, and enter it on the program plan. Begin your program at a lower intensity and slowly increase intensity as your fitness improves, so select a range of intensities for your program.

   a. *Target heart rate zone:* Calculate target heart rate zone in beats per minute and then calculate the corresponding 15-second exercise count by dividing the total count by 4. For example, the 15-second exercise counts corresponding to a target heart rate zone of 122–180 bpm would be 31–45 beats.

   Maximum heart rate: 220 − _____ = _____ bpm
   age (years)

   #### Maximum Heart Rate Method

   65% training intensity = _____ bpm × 0.65 = _____ bpm
   maximum heart rate

   90% training intensity = _____ bpm × 0.90 = _____ bpm
   maximum heart rate

   Target heart rate zone = _____ to _____ bpm   **15-second count** = _____ to _____

LABORATORY ACTIVITIES

Heart Rate Reserve Method

Resting heart rate: _____ bpm (taken after 10 minutes of complete rest)

Heart rate reserve = _____ bpm − _____ bpm = _____ bpm
　　　　　　　　　　　maximum heart rate　　　　　resting heart rate

50% training intensity = (_____ bpm × 0.50) + _____ bpm = _____ bpm
　　　　　　　　　　　　　heart rate reserve　　　　　　　resting heart rate

85% training intensity = (_____ bpm × 0.85) + _____ bpm = _____ bpm
　　　　　　　　　　　　　heart rate reserve　　　　　　　resting heart rate

Target heart rate zone = _____ to _____ bpm　　　15-second count = _____ to _____

　　b. *Ratings of perceived exertion (RPE):* If you prefer, determine an RPE value that corresponds to your target heart rate range (see Figure 3.6).

5. *Time (Duration).* A total time of 20–60 minutes per exercise session is recommended; your duration of exercise will vary with intensity. For developing cardiorespiratory endurance, higher-intensity activities can be performed for a shorter duration; lower-intensity activities require a longer duration. Enter a duration (or a range of duration) on the program plan.

6. *Volume.* Volume is the product of frequency, intensity, and time. Vary each factor for variety. Sometimes use high-intensity interval training (HIIT) to boost fitness quickly. Other times, exercise longer but at a lower intensity.

7. *Monitoring Your Program.* Complete a log like the one below to monitor your program and track your progress. Note the date on top, and fill in the intensity and time (duration) for each workout. If you prefer, you can also track other variables such as distance. For example, if your cardiorespiratory endurance program includes walking and swimming, you may want to track miles walked and yards swum in addition to the duration of each exercise session.

Activity/Date												
1	Intensity											
	Time											
	Distance											
2	Intensity											
	Time											
	Distance											
3	Intensity											
	Time											
	Distance											
4	Intensity											
	Time											
	Distance											

8. *Progression and Making Progress.* Follow the guidelines in the chapter and in Table 3.5 and Figure 3.7 to slowly increase the amount of overload in your program. Continue keeping a log, and periodically evaluate your progress.

Progress Checkup: Week _____ of program

Goals: Original Status　　　　　　　　　　　　　　　　Current Status

_____　　　　_____

_____　　　　_____

_____　　　　_____

　　List each activity in your program and describe how satisfied you are with the activity and with your overall progress. List any problems you've encountered or any unexpected costs or benefits of your fitness program so far.

4 Muscular Strength and Endurance

LOOKING AHEAD...

After reading this chapter, you should be able to

- Describe the basic physiology of muscles and explain how strength training affects muscles.

- Define muscular strength and endurance, and describe how they relate to wellness.

- Assess muscular strength and endurance.

- Apply the FITT-VP principle to create a safe and successful strength-training program.

- Describe the effects of supplements and drugs that are marketed to active people and athletes.

- Explain how to safely perform common strength-training exercises using body weight, free weights, and weight machines.

TEST YOUR KNOWLEDGE

1. For women, weight training typically results in which of the following?
   a. bulky muscles
   b. significant increases in body weight
   c. improved body image

2. To maximize strength gains, it is a good idea to hold your breath as you lift a weight. True or false?

3. Regular strength training is associated with which of the following benefits?
   a. denser bones
   b. reduced risk of heart disease
   c. improved body composition
   d. fewer injuries
   e. improved metabolic health
   f. increased longevity
   g. All six

See answers on the next page.

©SG Hirst/Image Source/Getty Images RF

M uscles make up more than 40% of your body mass. You depend on them for movement, and, because of their mass, they are the sites of a large portion of the energy reactions (metabolism) that take place in your body. Strong, well-developed muscles help you perform daily activities with greater ease, protect you from injury, and enhance your well-being in other ways.

As described in Chapter 2, muscular strength is the amount of force a muscle can produce with a single maximum effort, and muscular endurance is the ability to hold or repeat a muscular contraction for a long time. This chapter explains the benefits of *strength training* (also called *resistance training* or *weight training*) and describes methods of assessing muscular strength and endurance. It then explains the basics of strength training and provides guidelines for setting up your own training program.

BASIC MUSCLE PHYSIOLOGY AND THE EFFECTS OF STRENGTH TRAINING

Muscles move the body and enable it to exert force. When a muscle contracts (shortens), it moves a bone by pulling on the **tendon** that attaches the muscle to the bone.

Answers (Test Your Knowledge)

1. **c.** Because the vast majority of women have low levels of testosterone, they do not develop large muscles or gain significant amounts of weight in response to a moderate-intensity weight training program. Men have higher levels of testosterone, so they can build large muscles more easily.

2. **False.** Holding one's breath while lifting weights can significantly elevate blood pressure; it also reduces blood flow to the heart and may cause faintness. You should breathe smoothly and normally while weight training. Some experts recommend that you exhale during the most difficult part of each exercise.

3. **g, all six.** Regular strength training has many benefits for both men and women.

Muscle Fibers

Muscles consist of individual muscle cells, or **muscle fibers**, connected in bundles called fascicles (Figure 4.1). A single muscle is made up of many bundles of muscle fibers and is covered by layers of connective tissue that hold the fibers together. Muscle fibers, in turn, are made up of smaller protein structures called **myofibrils**. Myofibrils consist of a series of contractile units called *sarcomeres,* which are composed largely of actin and myosin molecules. Muscle cells contract when the myosin molecules glide across the actin molecules in a ratchet-like movement. Each muscle cell has many **nuclei** containing genes that control cell function and direct the production of enzymes and structural proteins required for muscle contraction. Strength training activates structures called **satellite cells** that provide additional muscle cell nuclei, which in turn enhances muscle repair and muscle protein synthesis. These cells improve muscle function, and they persist even if you stop training intensely.

In response to strength training, myofibrils increase in size (thicken) and in number, resulting in larger individual muscle fibers. Larger muscle fibers mean a larger and stronger muscle. The development of large muscle fibers is called **hypertrophy** (Figure 4.2). The process of hypertrophy begins after about six to eight weeks of strength training. In some species, muscles can increase in size through a separate process called **hyperplasia**, which involves an increase in the *number* of muscle fibers rather than the *size* of muscle fibers. In humans, hyperplasia is not thought to play a significant role in determining muscle size. Consistent with the fitness principle of reversability, inactivity causes a decrease in muscle fiber size, known as **atrophy**, the reversal of this process.

Muscle fibers are classified as slow-twitch or fast-twitch fibers according to their strength, speed of contraction, and energy source. (See Chapter 3 for more on energy systems.)

- **Slow-twitch muscle fibers** are relatively fatigue resistant, but they don't contract as rapidly or strongly as fast-twitch

FIGURE 4.1 Components of skeletal muscle tissue.

FIGURE 4.2 **Process of muscle hypertrophy.** Strength training leads to muscle hypertrophy, an increase in muscle mass and size. The increase occurs as a result of cellular enlargement—and increase in the size of individual muscle fibers—which in turn is due to an increase in the size and number of myofibrils. In this way, muscle fibers increase in size and in their capacity for generating force.

fibers. The principal energy system that fuels slow-twitch fibers is aerobic (oxidative). Slow-twitch muscle fibers are typically reddish in color.

- **Fast-twitch muscle fibers** contract more rapidly and forcefully than slow-twitch fibers but fatigue more quickly. Although oxygen is important in the energy system that fuels fast-twitch fibers, they rely more on anaerobic (nonoxidative) metabolism than do slow-twitch fibers. Fast-twitch muscle fibers are typically whitish in color (e.g., white meat versus dark meat in a turkey).

Most muscles contain both slow-twitch and fast-twitch fibers. The proportion of the types of fibers varies significantly among different muscles and different individuals, and that proportion is largely fixed at birth, although fibers can contract faster or slower following a period of training or a period of inactivity. The type of fiber that acts during a particular activity depends on the type of work required. Endurance activities like jogging tend to use slow-twitch fibers, whereas strength and **power** activities like sprinting, use fast-twitch fibers. Strength training can increase the size and strength of both fast-twitch and slow-twitch fibers, although fast-twitch fibers are preferentially increased.

Motor Units

To exert force, a muscle recruits one or more motor units to contract. A **motor unit** is made up of a nerve connected to a number of muscle fibers. The number of muscle fibers in a motor unit varies from two to hundreds. Small motor units contain slow-twitch fibers, whereas large motor units contain fast-twitch fibers. When a motor unit calls on its fibers to contract, all fibers contract to their full capacity. The number of motor units recruited depends on the amount of strength required: When you pick up a small weight, you use fewer and smaller motor units than when picking up a large weight.

The nervous system controls motor unit activation. Nerve cell components called **axons** are often covered in a special

tissue called **myelin**, which speeds the rate of nerve conduction. Practicing a skill causes the nervous system to lay down more myelin, which increases the speed, efficiency,

TERMS

tendon A tough band of fibrous tissue that connects a muscle to a bone or other body part and transmits the force exerted by the muscle.

muscle fiber A single muscle cell, usually classified according to strength, speed of contraction, and energy source.

myofibrils Protein structures that make up muscle fibers.

nucleus A cell structure containing DNA and genes that direct the production of proteins; plural, *nuclei.*

satellite cells Cells that provide additional cell nuclei in skeletal muscle, which enhances muscle protein synthesis and cell repair.

hypertrophy An increase in the size of muscle fibers, usually stimulated by muscular overload, as occurs during strength training.

hyperplasia An increase in the number of muscle fibers.

atrophy A decrease in the size of muscle fibers, usually attributable to inactivity.

slow-twitch muscle fibers Red muscle fibers that are fatigue resistant but have a slow contraction speed and a lower capacity for tension; usually recruited for endurance activities.

fast-twitch muscle fibers White muscle fibers that contract rapidly and forcefully but fatigue quickly; usually recruited for actions requiring strength, power, or speed.

power The ability to exert force rapidly.

motor unit A motor nerve (one that initiates movement) connected to one or more muscle fibers.

axon A long, slender part of the nerve cell that conducts the nerve impulse away from the nerve cell body.

Table 4.1 Physiological Changes and Benefits from Strength Training

CHANGE	BENEFITS
Increased muscle mass* and strength	Increased muscular strength
	Improved body composition
	Higher rate of metabolism
	Improved capacity to regulate fuel use with aging
	Toned, healthy-looking muscles
	Increased longevity
	Improved quality of life
Increased utilization of motor units during muscle contractions	Increased muscular strength and power
Improved coordination of motor units	Increased muscular strength and power
Increased strength of tendons, ligaments, and bones	Lower risk of injury to these tissues
Increased storage of fuel in muscles	Increased resistance to muscle fatigue
Increased size of fast-twitch muscle fibers (from a high-resistance program)	Increased muscular strength and power
Increased size of slow-twitch muscle fibers (from a high-repetition program)	Increased muscular endurance
Increased blood supply to muscles (from a high-repetition program) and improved blood vessel health	Increased delivery of oxygen and nutrients Faster elimination of wastes
Biochemical improvements (e.g., increased sensitivity to insulin)	Enhanced metabolic health and, possibly, increased life span
Improved blood fat levels	Reduced risk of heart disease
Increased muscle endurance	Enhanced ability to exercise for long periods and maintain good body posture

*Due to genetic and hormonal differences, men will build more muscle mass than women, but both men and women make about the same percentage gains in strength through a good program.

and coordination of the movement. In this way, basic movement skills become almost reflexive. The old adage that practice makes perfect should be changed to "practice makes myelin." The nervous system contains more than one billion nerve cells, an indicator of how complex it is to control movement.

Strength training improves the body's ability to recruit motor units—a phenomenon called **muscle learning**—which increases strength even before muscle size increases. The physiological changes and benefits that result from strength training are summarized in Table 4.1; see the box "Gender Differences in Muscular Strength" for additional information on hormonal and nervous system influences on muscle tissue.

As a person ages, motor nerves can become disconnected from the portion of muscle they control. By age 70, 15% of the motor nerves in most people are no longer connected to muscle tissue. Aging and inactivity also cause muscles to become slower and therefore less able to perform quick, powerful movements. Strength training helps maintain motor nerve connections and the quickness of muscles, particularly when engaged in **purposeful strength training**.

Osteoporosis (bone loss) is common in people over age 55, particularly postmenopausal women. Osteoporosis leads to fractures that can be life threatening. Hormonal changes from aging account for much of the bone loss that occurs, but lack of bone mass due to inactivity and a poor diet are contributing factors. Strength training can lessen bone loss even if it is taken up later in life; if practiced regularly, strength training may even build bone mass in postmenopausal women and older men. Strength training can also help prevent falls, which are a major cause of injury in people with osteoporosis (see the box "Benefits of Muscular Strength and Endurance").

Metabolic and Heart Health

Strength training helps prevent and manage both cardiovascular disease and diabetes by doing the following:

- Improving glucose metabolism
- Increasing maximal oxygen consumption
- Reducing blood pressure
- Increasing HDL cholesterol and reducing LDL cholesterol (in some people)
- Improving blood vessel health

myelin   A fatty material covering the nerve cell that insulates the axon. Practicing a motor skill lays down more myelin on the axon, which speeds neural conduction and improves skills such as hitting a tennis ball or baseball or skiing down a hill.

muscle learning   The improvement in the body's ability to recruit motor units, brought about through strength training.

purposeful strength training   Activating muscle contractions explosively, regardless of weight used. Also called compensatory acceleration training.

TERMS

DIVERSITY MATTERS
Gender Differences in Muscular Strength

Men are generally stronger than women because they typically have larger bodies and a larger proportion of their total body mass is made up of muscle. But when strength is expressed per unit of cross-sectional area of muscle tissue (i.e., relative strength), men are only 1–2% stronger than women in the upper body and about equal to women in the lower body. However, because of the larger proportion of muscle tissue in the upper male body, men can more easily build upper-body strength than women can. Individual muscle fibers are larger in men, but the metabolism of cells within those fibers is the same in both sexes.

Two factors that help explain these disparities are **testosterone** levels and the speed of nervous control of muscle. Testosterone promotes the growth of muscle tissue in both males and females, but testosterone levels are 5—10 times higher in men than in women, allowing men to have larger muscles. Also, because the male nervous system can activate muscles faster, men tend to have more power.

Women are often concerned that they will develop large muscles from strength training. Because of hormonal differences, however, most women do not develop big muscles unless they train intensely over many years or take anabolic steroids. Women do gain muscle and improve body composition through strength training, but they don't develop bulky muscles or gain significant amounts of weight. A study of average women who weight trained two or three days per week for eight weeks found that they gained about 1.75 pounds of muscle and lost about 3.5 pounds of fat. Losing muscle over time is a much greater health concern for women than small gains in muscle weight, especially because any gains in muscle weight are typically more than offset by loss of fat weight. Both men and women lose muscle mass and power as they age, but because men start out with more muscle and don't lose power as quickly, older

women tend to have greater impairment of muscle function than older men. This may partially account for the higher incidence of life-threatening falls in older women.

The bottom line is that both men and women can increase strength through strength training. Women may not be able to lift as much weight as men, but pound for pound of muscle, they have nearly the same capacity to gain strength as men.

Box icon: ©Rawpixel Ltd/Getty Images RF

©JGI/Tom Grill/Getty Images RF

Stronger muscles reduce the demand on the heart during ordinary daily activities such as lifting and carrying objects. The benefits of resistance exercise to the heart are so great that the American Heart Association recommends strength training two or three days per week for healthy adults and many low-risk cardiac patients. Resistance training may not be appropriate for people with some types of heart disease.

ASSESSING MUSCULAR STRENGTH AND ENDURANCE

Muscular strength is usually assessed by measuring the maximum amount of weight a person can lift in a single effort. This single maximum effort is called a **repetition maximum (RM)**. You can assess the strength of your major muscle groups by taking the one–repetition maximum (1-RM) test for the bench press and by taking functional leg strength tests. You can measure 1 RM directly or estimate it by doing multiple repetitions with a submaximal (lighter) weight. It is best to learn proper lifting techniques and to train for several weeks before attempting

a direct 1-RM test; after you have a baseline value, you can retest after 6–12 weeks to check your progress. See Lab 4.1 for guidelines on taking these tests. For more accurate results, avoid strenuous weight training for 48 hours beforehand.

TERMS

testosterone   The principal male hormone, responsible for the development of secondary sex characteristics and important in increasing muscle size.

repetition maximum (RM)   The maximum amount of resistance that can be moved a specified number of times. 1-RM is the maximum amount of weight that can be lifted one time; 5-RM is the maximum amount of weight that can be lifted five times.

core muscles   The trunk muscles extending from the hips to the upper back.

ligament   A tough band of tissue that connects the ends of bones to other bones or supports organs in place.

cartilage   Tough, resilient tissue that acts as a cushion between the bones in a joint.

THE EVIDENCE FOR EXERCISE
Benefits of Muscular Strength and Endurance

Enhanced muscular strength and endurance can lead to improvements in the areas of performance, injury prevention, body composition, self-image, lifetime muscle and bone health, and metabolic health. Most important, greater muscular strength and endurance reduce the risk of premature death. Stronger people—particularly men—have a lower death rate due to all causes, including cardiovascular disease (CVD) and cancer. The link between strength and death rate is independent of age, physical activity, smoking, alcohol intake, body composition, and family history of CVD.

Improved Performance of Physical Activities

A person with a moderate to high level of muscular strength and endurance can perform everyday tasks—such as climbing stairs and carrying groceries—with ease. Increased strength can enhance enjoyment of recreational sports by making it possible to achieve high levels of performance and to handle advanced techniques. Strength training also results in modest improvements in maximal oxygen consumption. People with poor muscle strength tire more easily and are less effective in both everyday and recreational activities.

Injury Prevention

Increased muscular strength and endurance help protect you from injury in two key ways:

• By enabling you to maintain good posture. Good muscle strength and endurance help stabilize the spine and stiffen the **core**, which protects against back and neck injuries.

• By encouraging proper body mechanics during everyday activities such as walking and lifting.

Good muscle strength and, particularly, endurance in the abdomen, hips, lower back, and legs maintain the spine in proper alignment and help prevent low-back pain, which afflicts more than 85% of Americans at some time in their lives. (Prevention of low-back pain is discussed in Chapter 5.)

Training for muscular strength and endurance also makes the tendons, **ligaments**, and **cartilage** cells stronger and less susceptible to injury and improves bone marrow metabolism. Resistance exercise prevents injuries best when the training program is gradual and progressive and builds all the major muscle groups.

Improved Body Composition

Healthy body composition means that the body has a high proportion of fat-free mass and a relatively small proportion of fat. Strength training improves body composition by increasing muscle mass, thereby tipping the body composition ratio toward fat-free mass and away from fat.

Building muscle mass through strength training also helps with losing fat because metabolic rate is related to muscle mass: The greater your muscle mass, the higher your metabolic rate. A high metabolic rate means that a nutritionally sound diet coupled with regular exercise will not lead to an increase in body fat. Strength training can boost resting metabolic rate by up to 15%, depending on how hard you train. Resistance exercise also increases muscle temperature, which in turn slightly increases the rate at which you burn calories over the hours following a weight-training session.

Enhanced Self-Image and Quality of Life

Strength training leads to an enhanced self-image in both men and women by providing stronger, firmer muscles and a toned, healthy-looking body. Women tend to lose inches, increase strength, and develop greater muscle definition. Men tend to build larger, stronger muscles and improve muscle tone. The larger muscles in men combine with high levels of the hormone testosterone for a strong tissue-building effect; see the box "Gender Differences in Muscular Strength."

Because strength training involves measurable objectives (pounds lifted, repetitions accomplished), a person can easily recognize improved performance, leading to greater self-confidence and self-esteem. Strength training also improves quality of life by increasing energy, preventing injuries, and making daily activities easier and more enjoyable.

Improved Muscle and Bone Health with Aging

Research has shown that good muscular strength helps people live healthier lives. A lifelong program of regular strength training prevents muscle and nerve degeneration that can compromise the quality of life and increase the risk of hip fractures and other potentially life-threatening injuries.

In the general population, people begin to lose muscle mass after age 30, a condition called *sarcopenia*. At first they may notice that they cannot play sports as well as they could in high school. After more years of inactivity and strength loss, people may have trouble performing even the simple movements of daily life, such as walking up a flight of stairs or doing yard work. By age 75, strength decreases by 30% and power by 40%. Although aging contributes to decreased strength, inactivity causes most of the loss. Poor strength and power make it much more likely that a person will be injured during everyday activities.

Increased Longevity

Strength training helps you live longer. Greater muscular strength is linked to lower rates of death from all causes, including cancer and CVD. A study of more than 9,000 men showed that compared to men with the lowest levels of muscular strength, stronger men were 1.5 times less likely to die from all causes; 1.6 times less likely to die from CVD; and 1.25 times less likely to die from cancer. The results were particularly striking in men age 60 and older with low levels of muscular strength, who were more than four times more likely to die from cancer than similar-age men with greater muscular strength.

Box Icon: ©Vstock LLC/Getty Images RF

Muscular endurance is usually assessed by counting the maximum number of **repetitions** of an exercise a person can do (such as in push-ups or kettlebell snatches) or the maximum amount of time a person can hold a muscular contraction (such as in the flexed-arm hang). You can test the muscular endurance of major muscle groups in your body by taking the curl-up test, the push-up test, and the squat endurance test. See Lab 4.2 for complete instructions on taking these assessment tests. Additional tests for low-back muscle endurance are found in Chapter 5.

CREATING A SUCCESSFUL STRENGTH TRAINING PROGRAM

When the muscles are stressed by a greater load than they are used to, they adapt and improve their function. The type of adaptation that occurs depends on the type of stress applied.

Static versus Dynamic Strength Training Exercises

Strength training exercises are generally classified as static or dynamic. Each involves a different way of using and strengthening muscles.

Static Exercise Also called **isometric** exercise, **static exercise** causes a muscle contraction without changing the length of the muscle or the angle in the joint on which the muscle acts (Figure 4.3A). In isometrics, the muscle contracts, but there is no movement. To perform an isometric exercise, a person can use an immovable object like a wall to provide resistance, or simply tighten a muscle while remaining still (e.g., tightening the abdominal muscles while sitting at a desk). The spine extension and the side bridge, shown in Exercises 5 and 6 (later in the chapter), are both isometric exercises.

Static exercises are particularly important for developing stiff core or torso muscles that support the spine and provide a firm foundation for whole body motions. During almost all movements some muscles contract statically to support the skeleton so other muscles can contract dynamically. For example, when you throw something, hit a ball, or ski, the core muscles in the abdomen and back stabilize the spine. This stability allows more powerful contractions in the lower- and upper-body muscles. The core muscles also contract statically during dynamic exercises, such as squats, lunges, and overhead presses.

Static exercises are useful in strengthening muscles after an injury or surgery, when movement of the affected joint could delay healing. Isometrics are also used to overcome weak points in an individual's range of motion. Statically strengthening a muscle at its weakest point will allow more weight to be lifted with that muscle during dynamic exercise. Certain types of calisthenics and Pilates exercises (described in more detail later in the chapter) also involve static contractions. For maximum strength gains, hold the isometric contraction maximally for six seconds; do 2–10 repetitions.

Dynamic Exercise Also called **isotonic** exercise, **dynamic exercise** causes a muscle contraction and a change in the length

FIGURE 4.3 Static versus dynamic exercise. A static (isometric) exercise such as a plank (A) involves muscle contraction without movement; the position is held. A dynamic exercise such as a biceps curl involves muscle contraction with a change in the length of the muscle and angle of the joint. Dynamic muscle contractions can be concentric (B), in which the muscle shortens as it contracts, or eccentric (C), in which the muscle lengthens as it contracts.

(a): ©Taylor Robertson Photography; (b-c): Courtesy Neil A. Tanner

of the muscle and the angle of the joint (Figure 4.3 B, C). Dynamic exercises are the most popular type of exercises for increasing muscle strength and seem to be most valuable for developing strength that can be transferred to other forms of

---

repetitions The number of times an exercise is performed during one set. **TERMS**

isometric (static) exercise Exercise causing a muscle contraction without a change in the muscle's length or a joint's angle.

isotonic (dynamic) exercise Exercise causing a muscle contraction and a change in the muscle's length.

physical activity. They can be performed with weight machines, free weights, or a person's own body weight (as in pull-ups or push-ups).

There are two kinds of dynamic muscle contractions:

- A **concentric muscle contraction** (also called a *miometric contraction*) occurs when the muscle applies enough force to overcome resistance and shortens as it contracts.

- An **eccentric muscle contraction** (also called *a pliometric contraction*) occurs when the resistance is greater than the force applied by the muscle and the muscle lengthens as it contracts.

For example, in an arm curl, the biceps muscle works concentrically as the weight is raised toward the shoulder and eccentrically as the weight is lowered.

CONSTANT AND VARIABLE RESISTANCE   Two of the most common dynamic exercise techniques are constant resistance exercise and variable resistance exercise. Both exercises are extremely effective for building muscular strength and endurance.

- **Constant resistance exercise** uses a constant load (weight) throughout a joint's full range of motion. Training with free weights is a form of constant resistance exercise; the amount of weight you move is the same during the entire exercise. A problem with this technique is that, because of differences in leverage, there are points in a joint's range of motion where the muscle controlling the movement is stronger and points where it is weaker. The weakest point in the range limits the amount of weight a person can lift.

TERMS

concentric muscle contraction   A dynamic contraction in which the muscle gets shorter as it contracts; also called a *miometric contraction*.

eccentric muscle contraction   A dynamic contraction in which the muscle lengthens as it contracts; also called a *pliometric contraction*.

constant resistance exercise   A type of dynamic exercise that uses a constant load throughout a joint's full range of motion.

variable resistance exercise   A type of dynamic exercise that uses a changing load, providing a maximum load at the strongest point in the affected joint's range of motion.

eccentric (pliometric) loading   Loading the muscle while it is lengthening; sometimes called *negatives*.

plyometrics   Rapid stretching of a muscle group that is undergoing eccentric stress (that is, the muscle is exerting force while it lengthens), followed by a rapid concentric contraction.

speed loading   Moving a load as rapidly as possible.

kettlebell   A large iron weight with a connected handle; used for ballistic weight-training exercises such as swings and one-arm snatches.

isokinetic exercise   A type of dynamic exercise that provides variable resistance to a movement, so that the movement occurs at a constant speed no matter how much effort is exerted.

- In **variable resistance exercise**, the load is changed to provide maximum load throughout the entire range of motion. This form of exercise uses machines that place more stress on muscles at the end of the range of motion, where a person has better leverage and can exert more force. Use elastic bands and chains with free weights to add variable resistance to the exercises.

OTHER DYNAMIC EXERCISE TECHNIQUES   Athletes use four other kinds of isotonic techniques, primarily for training and rehabilitation.

- **Eccentric (pliometric) loading** places a load on a muscle as it lengthens. The muscle contracts eccentrically to control the weight. Eccentric loading is practiced during most types of resistance training, such as when you lower the weight to your chest during a bench press in preparation for the active movement. You can also perform exercises designed specifically to overload a muscle eccentrically, a technique called *negatives*.

- **Plyometrics** is the sudden eccentric loading and stretching of muscles followed by a forceful concentric contraction—a movement that scientists call the stretch-shortening cycle. An example would be the action of the lower-body muscles when jumping from a bench to the ground and then jumping back onto the bench. This type of exercise helps develop explosive strength; it also helps build and maintain bone density.

- In **speed loading** you move a weight as rapidly as possible in an attempt to approach the speeds used in movements like throwing a softball or sprinting. In the bench press, for example, speed loading might involve doing 5 repetitions as fast as possible using a weight that is half the maximum load you can lift. You can gauge your progress by timing how fast you can perform the repetitions. Purposeful strength training—performing exercises explosively, regardless of weight—is a type of speed loading that builds neuromuscular power and is useful in high-intensity power sports such as basketball, tennis, skiing, and volleyball.

  Training with a **kettlebell**—an iron ball with a handle—is another type of speed loading. Kettlebell training is highly ballistic, meaning that many exercises involve fast, pendulum-type motions, extreme decelerations, and high-speed eccentric muscle contractions. Kettlebell swings require dynamic concentric muscle contractions during the upward phase of the exercise followed by high-speed eccentric contractions to control the movement when returning to the starting position.

- **Isokinetic exercise** involves exerting force at a constant speed against an equal force exerted by a special strength-training machine. The isokinetic machine provides variable resistance at different points in the joint's range of motion, matching the effort applied by the individual while keeping the speed of the movement constant. Isokinetic exercises are excellent for building strength and endurance.

Comparing Static and Dynamic Exercise Static exercises require no equipment, so they can be done virtually anywhere. They build strength rapidly and are useful for rehabilitation of joints after injury or surgery and for stabilizing joints in the shoulder and spine. On the other hand, they have to be performed at several different angles for each joint to improve strength throughout its entire range of motion. Dynamic exercises can be performed without equipment (calisthenics) or with equipment (weight training). Not only are they excellent for building muscular strength and endurance, but they also tend to build strength through a joint's full range of motion. Most people develop muscular strength and endurance using dynamic exercises. Ultimately, however, the type of exercise a person chooses depends on individual goals, preferences, and access to equipment.

Weight Machines, Free Weights, and Body Weight Exercises

Muscles get stronger when made to work against resistance. Resistance can be provided by free weights, body weight, or exercise machines. Many people prefer machines because they are safe, convenient, and easy to use. You just set the resistance, sit down at the machine, and start working. Machines make it easy to isolate and work specific muscles. You don't need a **spotter**—someone who stands by to assist when free weights are used—and you don't have to worry about dropping a weight on yourself. Many machines provide support for the back.

Free weights, such as barbells and kettlebells, require more care, balance, and coordination to use than machines, but they strengthen your body in ways that are more adaptable to real life. They are also more popular with athletes for developing functional strength for sports, especially sports that require a great deal of strength. Free weights are widely available, inexpensive, and convenient for home use.

Exercises that use body weight, elastic bands, rocks, or soup cans as resistance enable you to do workouts at home. You can purchase elastic bands at sporting good stores or any home improvement or hardware store. A basic principle of resistance exercise is to "train movements and not muscles." This means that you can overload the body in everyday movements like sitting and standing from a chair, climbing a fence, getting out of a swimming pool without a ladder, and standing after lying on the ground.

Other Training Methods and Types of Equipment

You don't need a fitness center or expensive equipment to strength train. If you prefer to train at home or like low-cost alternatives, consider the following options.

Resistance Bands Resistance or exercise bands are elastic strips or tubes of rubber material that are inexpensive, lightweight, and portable. They are available in a variety of styles and levels of resistance. Some are sold with instructional guides or online videos, and classes may be offered at fitness centers.

Many free-weight exercises can be adapted for resistance bands. For example, you can do biceps curls by standing on the center of the band and holding one end of the band in each hand; the band provides resistance when you stretch it to perform the curl.

Exercise (Stability) Balls The exercise or stability ball is an extra-large inflatable ball. It was originally developed for use in physical therapy but has become a popular piece of exercise equipment for use in the home or gym. It can be used to work the entire body, but it is particularly effective for working the core stabilizing muscles in the abdomen, chest, and back—muscles that are important for preventing back problems. The ball's instability forces the exerciser to use the stability muscles to balance the body, even when just sitting on the ball. The "stir-the-pot" exercise—a plank position with elbows resting on the ball, which is then moved in small circles—is an example of a core-building exercise that uses the stability ball.

You can incorporate a stability ball into a typical workout in many ways. For example, you can perform curl-ups while lying on a ball instead of on the floor. Lying facedown across a ball provides different leverage points for push-ups. A variety of resistance training exercises can be performed on a stability ball, but experts recommend using dumbbells rather than barbells when lifting weights on a ball.

When selecting a ball, make sure your thighs are parallel to the ground when you sit on it; if you are a beginner or have back problems, choose a larger ball so that your thighs are at an angle, with hips higher than knees. Beginners should use caution until they feel comfortable with the movements and take care to avoid poor form due to fatigue (Table 4.2).

Vibration Training Vibration training consists of doing basic exercises, such as squats, push-ups, lunges, and modified pull-ups, on a vibrating platform. Vibration is transferred to whichever part of the body is in contact with the vibrating plate

Fitness Tip Many options are available for resistance training, and many are low cost. Try different types of exercises to see what you enjoy and to add variety to your program. Shown here are exercises using an elastic band (left), stability ball (center), and medicine ball (right)
©McGraw-Hill Education/David Scott, photographer: ©Wavebreakmedia/Getty Images RF: ©Taylor Robertson Photography

spotter A person who assists with a weight-training exercise done with free weights. **TERMS**

Table 4.2	The Pros and Cons of Stability Balls

PROS	CONS
Stability balls activate muscle and nerve groups that might not otherwise get involved in a particular exercise.	Muscle activation when training on unstable surfaces is less effective than traditional training for building strength in muscle groups responsible for a movement or in trunk-stabilizing muscle groups.
Some exercises, such as the stir-the-pot exercise, can enhance the stability of supporting joints throughout the body.	Some exercises (such as curl-ups) can be more stressful to certain joints and muscles and promote back or shoulder pain in susceptible people.
Stability balls can be useful for some older adults because they require balance and can enhance overall stability.	Falling off an unstable surface, especially while holding weights, can cause serious injury.
Stability balls add variety and challenge to a workout.	

or handlebars. Vibration activates stretch receptors in the muscles, which triggers thousands of small reflex muscle contractions. Most studies have found that vibration training caused little or no additional effects above weight training alone.

Pilates Pilates (*pil LAH teez*) was developed by German gymnast and boxer Joseph Pilates early in the 20th century. Pilates focuses on strengthening and stretching the core muscles in the back, abdomen, and buttocks to create a solid base of support for whole-body movement; the emphasis is on concentration, control, movement flow, and breathing. Pilates often makes use of specially designed resistance training devices, although some classes feature just mat or floor work. Mat exercises can be done at home, but because there are hundreds of Pilates exercises, some of them strenuous, it is best to begin with some qualified instruction.

Medicine Balls, Suspension Training, Stones, and Carrying Exercises Almost anything that provides resistance to movement will develop strength. Rubber medicine balls weighing up to 50 pounds can be used for a variety of functional movements, such as squats and overhead throws. Suspension training (e.g., TRX system) uses body weight as the resistance in exercises using ropes or cords attached to a hook, bar, door jam, or sturdy tree branch. You can train with a stone found in your backyard or local riverbank in performing exercises such as squats, presses, and carries. Walking while carrying dumbbells, farmer's bars, or heavy stones is an easy and effective way to develop whole-body strength. Carrying exercises are particularly useful for building core muscle fitness.

Power-Based Conditioning Programs This type of training combines aerobics, weight training, gymnastics, and high-intensity interval training. Programs such as CrossFit and Gym Jones employ different exercises every day. More traditional circuit training methods often use the same exercises set up in series. (See the box "High-Intensity Conditioning Programs" in Chapter 3.)

blood flow restriction training Exercising with restricted blood flow to working muscles. Also called Kaatsu training.   TERMS

Blood Flow Restriction Resistance Training **Blood flow restriction training** involves exercising with restricted blood flow to the working muscles. Blood flow restriction during low-intensity weight training promotes muscle hypertrophy because it creates severe metabolic stress that stimulates muscle protein synthesis and hypertrophy. Although blood flow restriction might be effective for injury rehabilitation, it is less effective than traditional training and may cause severe muscle injury in some people.

Applying the FITT-VP Principle: Selecting Exercises and Putting Together a Program

A complete weight training program works all the major muscle groups. It usually takes about 8–10 different exercises to get a complete full-body workout. Use the FITT-VP principle—frequency, intensity, time, type, volume, and progression—to set the parameters of your program.

Frequency of Exercise For general fitness, the American College of Sports Medicine (ACSM) recommends a frequency of at least two nonconsecutive days per week for weight training. Allow your muscles at least one day of rest between workouts; if you train too often, your muscles won't be able to work with enough intensity to improve their fitness, and soreness and injury are more likely to result. One technique, called split routines, works different muscle groups on alternate days. For example, work your arms and upper body one day, work your lower body the next day, and then return to upper-body exercises on the third day. Recent studies found, however, that training the same muscle groups three times a week was more effective than split routines.

Intensity of Exercise: Amount of Resistance The amount of weight (resistance) you lift in weight training exercises is equivalent to intensity in cardiorespiratory endurance training. It determines how your body will adapt to weight training and how quickly these adaptations will occur.

Choose weights based on your current level of muscular fitness and your fitness goals. The weight should be heavy enough to fatigue your muscles but light enough for you to complete the repetitions with good form. (For tips on perfecting your form,

WELLNESS IN THE DIGITAL AGE
Improving Your Technique with Video

Want to get stronger? Then you need to focus on developing your skills at least as much as you focus on lifting more weight. Improving skill is the best way to increase strength during movements such as hitting a tennis ball or baseball, performing a bench press, driving a golf ball, skiing down a slope, or carrying a bag of groceries up a flight of stairs. In the world of weight training, skill means lifting weights with proper form; the better your form, the better your results.

The brain develops precise neural pathways as you learn a skill. As you improve, the pathways conduct nervous impulses faster and more precisely until the movement becomes almost reflexive. The best way to learn a skill is through focused practice that involves identifying mistakes, correcting them, and practicing the refined movement many times. However, simply practicing the skill is not enough if you want to improve and perform more powerful movements. You must perform the movements correctly instead of practicing mistakes or poor form over and over again.

Here's where technology can help. Watch videos of people performing weight training movements correctly. You may be able to borrow videos from your instructor, purchase low-cost training videos through magazines and sporting goods stores, or find them on the Internet. If you watch training videos online, however, make sure they were produced by an authoritative source on weight training. Otherwise, you may be learning someone else's mistakes.

Film your movements using a phone camera or inexpensive video camera. Compare your movements with those of a more skilled person performing them correctly. Make a note of movement patterns that need work and try to change your technique to make it more mechanically correct. Share your videos with your instructor or a certified personal trainer, who can help you identify poor form and teach you ways to correct your form. Smartphone apps such as Coach's Eye, Hudl Technique, and Dartfish allow you to analyze movements in slow motion, compare movements side by side, and share your videos with others.

Box icon: ©Hong Li/Getty Images RF

---

see the box "Improving Your Technique with Video.") To build strength rapidly, you should lift weights as heavy as 80% of your maximum capacity (1 RM). If you're more interested in building endurance, choose a lighter weight (perhaps 40–60% of 1 RM), and do more repetitions.

For example, if your maximum capacity for the leg press is 160 pounds, you might lift 130 pounds to build strength and 80 pounds with more repetitions to build endurance. For a general fitness program to develop both muscular strength and endurance, choose a weight in the middle of this range, perhaps 70% of 1 RM. Or you can create a program that includes both higher-intensity exercise (80% of 1 RM for 8–10 repetitions) and lower-intensity exercise (60% of 1 RM for 15–20 repetitions); this routine will develop both fast-twitch and slow-twitch muscle fibers.

Time of Exercise: Repetitions and Sets To improve fitness, you must do enough repetitions of each exercise to fatigue your muscles. The number of repetitions needed to cause fatigue depends on the amount of resistance: The heavier the weight, the fewer repetitions to reach fatigue. In general, a heavy weight and a low number of repetitions (1–5) build strength and overload primarily fast-twitch fibers, whereas a light weight and a high number of repetitions (15–20) build endurance and overload primarily slow-twitch fibers.

For a general fitness program to build both strength and endurance, try to do about 8–12 repetitions of each exercise; a few exercises, such as abdominal crunches and calf raises, may require more. To avoid injury, older (approximately age 50–60 and above) and frailer people should perform more repetitions (10–15) using a lighter weight.

In weight training, a **set** refers to a group of repetitions of an exercise followed by a rest period. To develop strength and endurance for general fitness, you can make gains doing a single set of each exercise, provided you use enough resistance to fatigue your muscles. (You should just barely be able to complete the 8–12 repetitions—using good form—for each exercise.) Doing more than one set of each exercise will increase strength development; most serious weight trainers do at least three sets of each exercise (see the section "More Advanced Strength Training Programs" for guidelines).

If you perform more than one set of an exercise, you need to rest long enough between sets to allow your muscles to work with enough intensity to increase fitness. The length of the rest interval depends on the amount of resistance. In a program to develop a combination of strength and endurance for wellness, a rest period of 1–3 minutes between sets is appropriate. If you are lifting heavier loads to build strength, rest 3–5 minutes between sets. You can save time in your workouts by alternating sets of different exercises. One muscle group can rest between sets while you work on another group.

Overtraining—doing more exercise than your body can recover from—can occur in response to heavy resistance training. Possible signs of overtraining include lack of progress or decreased performance, chronic fatigue, decreased coordination, and chronic muscle soreness. The best remedy for overtraining is rest; add more days of recovery between workouts. With extra rest, chances are you'll be refreshed and ready to train again. Adding variety to your program, as discussed later in the chapter, can also help you avoid overtraining with resistance exercise.

set A group of repetitions followed by a rest period.   TERMS

Type or Mode of Exercise   For overall fitness, you need to include exercises for your neck, upper back, shoulders, arms, chest, abdomen, lower back, thighs, buttocks, and calves—about 8–10 exercises in all. If you are also training for a particular sport, include exercises to strengthen the muscles important for optimal performance *and* the muscles most likely to be injured. Weight training exercises for general fitness are presented later in this chapter.

BALANCE EXERCISES FOR OPPOSING MUSCLE GROUPS   It is important to balance exercises between antagonistic muscle groups. When a muscle contracts, the opposing muscle must relax. Whenever you do an exercise that moves a joint in one direction, also select an exercise that works the joint in the opposite direction. For example, if you do knee extensions to develop the muscles on the front of your thighs, also do leg curls to develop the antagonistic muscles on the back of your thighs.

SETTING ORDER OF EXERCISES   The order of exercises can also be important. Do exercises for large-muscle groups such as the chest and shoulders before you do exercises that use small-muscle groups such as the upper and lower arms. Alternate pushing and pulling exercises. This allows for more effective overload of the larger, more powerful muscle groups. Small-muscle groups fatigue more easily than larger ones, and small-muscle fatigue limits your capacity to overload large-muscle groups. For example, lateral raises, which work the shoulder muscles, should be performed after bench presses, which work the chest and arms in addition to the shoulders. If you fatigue your shoulder muscles by doing lateral raises first, you won't be able to lift as much weight and effectively fatigue all the key muscle groups used during the bench press.

Also, order exercises so that you work opposing muscle groups in sequence, one after the other. For example, follow biceps curls, which work the biceps, with triceps extensions, which exercise the triceps—the antagonistic muscle to the biceps.

Volume   Volume is the product of frequency, intensity, and time. For weight training, the volume of a specific exercise during a workout would be the amount of weight lifted multiplied by the number of reps and sets. Choose a training volume that promotes progress and that you will do consistently. And change the components from time to time—that is, increase the weight on some days and the sets and reps on other days. Changing the training volume prevents the body from adapting to exercise stress and results in more consistent improvements in fitness.

Progression   Training intensity is the most important factor promoting improvements in strength and power. You will progress rapidly when you begin training, but progress slows as you become more fit. Set fitness goals and progress systematically by adding weight or sets as you gain strength and power; see the section "Getting Started and Making Progress" for specific recommendations for adjusting training intensity in response to fitness improvements. After achieving your goal, maintain strength by training one to three times per week.

The Warm-Up and Cool-Down

As with cardiorespiratory endurance exercise, you should warm up before every weight training session and cool down afterward (Figure 4.4). You should do both a general warm-up—several minutes of walking or easy jogging and a warm-up for the weight training exercises you plan to perform. For example, if you plan to do one or more sets of 10 repetitions of bench presses with 125 pounds, you might do one set of 10 repetitions with 50 pounds as a warm-up. Do similar warm-up exercises for each exercise in your program.

To cool down, perform 5–10 minutes of increasingly less intense aerobic and muscular endurance activity so that your body transitions to a resting state. Although controversial, a few

Warm-up 5–10 minutes	Strength training exercises for major muscle groups (8–10 exercises)		Cool-down 5–10 minutes
	Sample program		
	Exercise	*Muscle group(s) developed*	
	Bench press	Chest, shoulders, triceps	
	Lat-Pulls	Lats, biceps	
	Shoulder press	Shoulders, trapezius, triceps	
	Upright rowing	Deltoids, trapezius	
	Biceps curls	Biceps	
	Lateral raises	Shoulders	
	Squats	Gluteals, quadriceps	
	Heel raises	Calves	
	McGill curl-ups	Abdominals	
	Spine extensions	Low- and mid-back spine extensors	
Start	Side bridges	Obliques, quadratus lumborum	*Stop*

Frequency: 2–3 nonconsecutive days per week

Intensity/resistance: Use weights heavy enough to cause muscle fatigue when exercises are performed with good form for the selected number of repetitions

Time: repetitions: 8–12 of each exercise (10–15 with a lower weight for people over age 50–60); **sets:** 1 (doing more than 1 set per exercise may result in faster and greater strength gains); rest 1–2 minutes between exercises.

Type of activity: 8–10 strength training exercises that focus on major muscle groups

Volume: An example might be 3 sets of 8-12 repetitions of each exercise with 1 minute rest between sets.

Progression: As you progress, add weight according to the "two-for-two" rule: When you can perform two additional repetitions with a given weight on two consecutive training sessions, increase the load. For example, if your target is to perform 8–10 repetitions per exercise, and you performed 12 repetitions in your previous two workouts, it would be appropriate to increase your load.

FIGURE 4.4   The FITT-VP principle for a strength training workout.

studies have suggested that including a period of post-exercise stretching may help prevent muscle soreness; warmed-up muscles and joints make the cool-down period a particularly good time to work on flexibility.

Getting Started and Making Progress

The first few sessions of weight training should be devoted to learning the movements and allowing your nervous system to practice communicating with your muscles so that you can develop strength effectively. To start, choose a weight that you can move easily through 8–12 repetitions, do only one set of each exercise, and rest 1–2 minutes between exercises. Gradually add weight and (if you want) sets to your program over the first few weeks until you are doing one to three sets of 8–12 repetitions of each exercise. If adding weight means you can do only 7 or 8 repetitions, stay with that weight until you can again complete 12 repetitions per set. If you can do only 4–6 repetitions after adding weight, or if you can't maintain good form, you've added too much and should take some off.

You can add more resistance in large-muscle exercises, such as squats and bench presses, than you can in small-muscle exercises, such as curls. For example, when you can complete 12 repetitions of squats with good form, you may be able to add 10–20 pounds of additional resistance; for curls, by contrast, you might add only 3–5 pounds. As a general guideline, try increases of approximately 5%, which is half a pound of additional weight for each 10 pounds you are currently lifting.

You can expect to improve rapidly during the first 6–10 weeks of training—a 10–30% increase in the amount of weight lifted. Gains will then come more slowly. Your rate of improvement will depend on how hard you work and how your body responds to resistance training. Factors such as age, gender, motivation, and heredity also will affect your progress.

After you achieve the level of strength and muscularity you want, you can maintain your gains by training two or three days per week. You can monitor the progress of your program by recording the amount of resistance and the number of repetitions and sets you perform on a workout card like the one shown in Figure 4.5.

More Advanced Strength Training Programs

The program just described is sufficient to develop and maintain muscular strength and endurance for general fitness. Performing more sets and fewer repetitions with a heavier load will cause greater increases in strength. Such a program might include three to five sets of 4–6 repetitions each; the load should be heavy enough to cause fatigue with the smaller number of repetitions. Rest long enough after a set (3–5 minutes) to allow your muscles to recover and work intensely during the next set. Train purposefully when lifting heavy weights—that is, make an effort to train explosively, no matter how much weight you are lifting. This increases the capacity of the nervous system to recruit motor units and maximize strength and power output.

Experienced weight trainers often practice some form of cycle training, also called *periodization*, in which the exercises, number of sets and repetitions, and intensity vary within a

	LTE	7:41 AM		
Session date: March 5				
Exercise	**Wt**	**Sets**	**Reps or Secs**	
Bench press	45	2	10	
Lat pulls	40	2	10	
Shoulder press	25	2	10	
Upright rowing	10	2	10	
Biceps curls	15	2	8	
Lateral raise	5	2	12	
Squats	45	2	12	
Heel raises	45	2	11	
McGill curl-ups	0	2	25	
Spine extensions	0	2	10	
Side bridge	0	2	65	

FIGURE 4.5 **A sample workout log for a general fitness strength training program.**

workout and/or between workouts. For example, you might do a particular exercise more intensely during some sets or on some days than others. You might also vary the exercises you perform for particular muscle groups. For more detailed information on these more advanced training techniques, consult a certified strength coach. If you decide to adopt a more advanced training regimen, start off slowly to give your body a chance to adjust and to minimize the risk of injury.

Weight Training Safety

Injuries happen in weight training. Maximum physical effort, elaborate machinery, rapid movements, and heavy weights can combine to make the weight room a dangerous place if proper precautions aren't taken. To help ensure that your workouts are safe and productive, follow the guidelines in the box "Safe Weight Training" and the suggestions that follow.

Use Proper Lifting Technique Every exercise has a proper technique that is important for obtaining maximum benefits and preventing injury. Your instructor or weight room

TAKE CHARGE
Safe Weight Training

General Guidelines

- When beginning a program or trying new exercises or equipment, ask a qualified trainer or instructor to show you how to do exercises safely and correctly.

- Lift weights from a stabilized body position; keep weights as close to your body as possible. **Hinge** at the hips, and use the large gluteal and quadriceps muscles, rather than fragile back muscles, to lift heavy loads.

- Protect your back by maintaining control of your spine and stiff core muscles. Don't twist your body while lifting.

- Observe proper lifting techniques and good form at all times. Don't lift beyond the limits of your strength.

- Don't hold your breath while doing weight training exercises. Doing so causes a decrease in blood returning to the heart and can make you dizzy and faint. It can also increase blood pressure to dangerous levels. Exhale when exerting the greatest force, and inhale when moving the weight into position for the active phase of the lift. Breathe smoothly and steadily.

- Don't use defective equipment. Be aware of broken collars or bolts, frayed cables, broken chains, or loose cushions.

- Don't exercise if you are ill, injured, or overtrained. Do not try to work through the pain.

Free Weights

- Make sure the bar is loaded evenly on both sides and weights are secured with collars or spring clips.

- When you pick up a weight from the ground, keep your back straight and your head level. Don't bend at the waist with straight legs.

- Lift weights smoothly; don't jerk them. Control the weight through the entire range of motion.

- Maximize lifting strength by hinging at the hips rather than rounding the back. When doing standing lifts, maintain a good posture so that you protect your back. Feet should be shoulder-width apart, heels and balls of the feet in contact with the floor, and knees slightly bent.

- Don't bounce weights against your body during an exercise.

Spotting

- Use spotters for free-weight exercises in which the bar crosses the face or head (e.g., the bench press), is placed on the back (e.g., squats), or is racked in front of the chest (e.g., overhead press from the rack holding the weight).

- If one spotter is used, the spotter should stand behind the lifter; if two spotters are used, one spotter should stand at each end of the barbell.

- For squats with heavy resistance, use at least three spotters—one behind the lifter (hands near lifter's hips, waist, or torso) and one at each end of the bar. Squatting in a power rack will increase safety during this exercise. A power rack consists of four vertical posts with two movable horizontal bar catchers on each side.

- Spot dumbbell exercises at the forearms, as close to the weights as possible.

- For over-the-face and over-the-head lifts, the spotter should hold the bar with an alternate grip (one palm up and one palm down) inside the lifter's grip.

- Spotter and lifter should ensure good communication by agreeing on verbal signals before the exercise.

©Neil Tanner Photography

Box icon: ©VisualCommunications/Getty Images RF

---

attendant can help explain the specific techniques for different exercises and weight machines.

Perform exercises smoothly and with good form. Lift or push the weight forcefully during the active phase of the lift

> **hinge**   A powerful movement in the lower body involving first hip flexion and then hip extension; the hip hinge maximizes the use of the gluteal and quadriceps muscles while maintaining a stiff core to keep the spine in a neutral position.
>
> TERMS

and then lower it with control. Perform all lifts through the full range of motion and strive to maintain a neutral spine position during each exercise.

Use Spotters and Collars with Free Weights Spotters are necessary when an exercise has potential for danger; a weight that is out of control or falls can cause a serious injury. A spotter can assist you if you cannot complete a lift or if the weight tilts. A spotter can also help you move a weight into position before a lift and provide help or additional resistance during a lift. Spotting requires practice and coordination between the lifter and the spotter(s).

Collars are devices that secure weight disks or plates to a barbell or dumbbell; they may have a coiled spring mechanism or a clamp or bolt. Although people lift weights without collars, doing so is dangerous. It is easy to lose your balance or to raise one side of the weight faster than the other. Without collars, the weights can slip off and crash to the floor. If you use spring clip collars, make sure they fit the bar tightly. Worn spring collars can slide off the bar easily.

Be Alert for Injuries Report any obvious muscle or joint injuries to your instructor or physician, and stop exercising the affected area. Training with an injured joint or muscle can lead to a more serious injury. Make sure you get the necessary first aid. Even minor injuries heal faster if you use the R-I-C-E principle of treating injuries described in Chapter 3.

Consult a physician if you have any unusual symptoms during exercise or if you're uncertain whether weight training is a proper activity for you. Weight training can aggravate conditions such as heart disease and high blood pressure. Immediately report symptoms such as headaches; dizziness; labored breathing; numbness; vision disturbances; and chest, neck, or arm pain. Pushing muscles to failure can sometimes result in **rhabdomyolysis** (destruction of muscle cells), which can cause serious illness or even death.

Supplements and Drugs

Active people may use nutritional supplements and drugs—called **ergogenic aids**—in the quest to improve performance and appearance, and more specifically, for these reasons:

- To enhance muscle hypertrophy, strength, power, and endurance
- To speed recovery and prevent the effects of overtraining
- To increase training intensity and aggressiveness
- To control fat, body water, and appetite

This section discusses a selection of "performance aids" along with their potential side effects. Although some of these substances improve performance, most are ineffective and expensive, and some are dangerous. Also keep in mind that dietary supplements are not regulated in the same way that drugs are. A balanced diet should be your primary nutritional strategy.

Drug scandals involving Olympic or professional athletes may lead people to believe that only elite athletes use performance-enhancing drugs. In fact, recreationally active young adults (18–35 years old) are the principle users of sports supplements such as protein and creatine monohydrate and muscle-building drugs such as anabolic steroids and growth hormone. Nonathletes also use performance aids to improve physical appearance and improve fitness.

Anabolic-Androgenic Steroids People take anabolic steroids (AS) for much the same reasons they take other ergogenic aids, but AS have many undesirable and dangerous side effects, including the following:

- Liver toxicity and tumors
- Decreased high-density lipoproteins (good cholesterol)
- Cardiac **arrhythmia**
- Reduced sperm count
- Lowered testosterone production
- High blood pressure
- Increased risk of HIV infection (from shared needles)
- Depressed immune function
- **Glucose intolerance**
- Psychological disturbances
- Masculinization in women and children
- Premature closure of the bone growth centers
- Increased cancer risk

Creatine Monohydrate Creatine monohydrate (i.e., creatine) is among the most popular and widely used supplements taken by athletes to build strength and muscle mass, enhance recovery, and improve exercise capacity. Taking creatine increases the creatine phosphate content of the muscles by about 20%. Creatine phosphate is an important high-energy chemical that maintains ATP levels. Recall from the discussion of exercise physiology in Chapter 3 that ATP supplies the energy for most of the body's hundreds of physiological functions.

Research shows that creatine supplementation improves performance in short-term, high-intensity, repetitive exercise, which might make it a valuable supplement for some physically active people. It may improve performance by augmenting creatine phosphate availability and possibly by regulating the rate of muscle sugar breakdown. It may also increase muscle-building capacity during resistance exercise by allowing athletes to train more intensely.

The long-term safety or effectiveness is currently unknown, however. More than 100 studies on this supplement have failed to report any significant side effects. Creatine monohydrate should be used with caution, especially in youth.

Protein, Amino Acid, and Polypeptide Supplements Athletes may take amino acids and polypeptide supplements in an effort to promote muscle hypertrophy, decrease body fat,

---

rhabdomyolysis Destruction of muscle tissue **TERMS** resulting in the release of enzymes and electrolytes from the cell contents, which can cause kidney damage and even death. This usually occurs during traumatic injuries such as automobile accidents. Overzealous training programs can also cause "rhabdo."

ergogenic aids Substances consumed to improve athletic performance.

arrhythmia A change in the normal pattern of the heartbeat.

glucose intolerance Elevated blood glucose (blood sugar) levels caused by metabolic problems.

and stimulate growth hormone release. Little scientific proof exists to support a benefit to taking amino acid or polypeptide supplementation. The protein requirement for active athletes is not much greater than for the average person—0.8–1.5 grams of protein per kilogram body weight per day. However, the timing of protein and amino acid ingestion may be important for stimulating muscle growth. Radioactive tracer studies that precisely chronicle the metabolism of various fuels reported that taking a protein supplement either 30 minutes before weight training or immediately after speeds the movement of amino acids into muscle and stimulates protein synthesis.

Other Supplements Carbohydrate beverages consumed during and immediately following physical activity enhance recovery from intense training, speeding the replenishment of liver and muscle glycogen. Benefits of other substances used to speed recovery—N-acetyl-L-cysteine (NAC), inosine, and beta-hydroxy beta-methylbutyrate (HMB)—are not consistently supported by research.

Caffeine is found in coffee, cola, tea, energy drinks, plants, beans and seeds, some over-the-counter medicines, and chocolate. It is a favorite stimulant of physically active people and is the principle ingredient in energy drinks. Its stimulates the central nervous system to release adrenaline (epinephrine). In athletics, caffeine is used as a stimulant and to mobilize fatty acids. Caffeine may improve endurance, strength, and power, and promote recovery from intense exercise. However, caffeine increases the risk of heart arrhythmias and insomnia. It is a controlled substance in the National Collegiate Athletic Association but is not controlled in Olympic or professional sports.

Popular ergogenic aids appear in Table 4.3.

> **caffeine**   A central nervous system stimulant found in coffee, tea, chocolate, and energy drinks; it increases energy level and alertness.   **TERMS**

Table 4.3	Performance Aids Marketed to Weight Trainers		
SUBSTANCE	SUPPOSED EFFECTS	ACTUAL EFFECTS	SELECTED POTENTIAL SIDE EFFECTS
Adrenal androgens, such as dehydroepiandrosterone (DHEA), androstenedione	Increased testosterone, muscle mass, and strength; decreased body fat	Increased testosterone, strength, and fat-free mass; decreased fat in older subjects (more studies needed in younger people)	Gonadal suppression, prostate hypertrophy, breast development in males, masculinization in women and children; long-term effects unknown
Amphetamines	Prevention of fatigue; increased confidence and training intensity	Increased arousal, wakefulness, and confidence; feeling of enhanced decision-making ability	Depression and fatigue, extreme confusion; aggressiveness, paranoia, hallucinations, restlessness, irritability, heart arrhythmia, high blood pressure, and chest pain
Anabolic steroids (steroids are controlled substances*)	Increased muscle mass, strength, power, psychological aggressiveness, and endurance	Increased strength, power, fat-free mass, and aggression; no effects on endurance	Liver damage and tumors, abnormal blood lipids, impaired reproductive health, hypertension, depressed immunity, insulin resistance, psychological disturbances, acne, breast development in males, masculinization in women and children, heart disease, thicker blood, and increased risk of cancer
Caffeine	Weight loss; improved endurance, strength, and power output; stimulant effect	Improves sports performance in low to moderate doses (3–6 mg/kg body weight); improves endurance and high-intensity exercise capacity	Abnormal heart rhythm and insomnia in some people; caffeine is addictive
Creatine monohydrate	Increased creatine phosphate levels in muscles, muscle mass, and capacity for high-intensity exercise	Increased muscle mass and performance in some types of high-intensity exercise	Minimal side effects; long-term effects unknown
Diuretics	Promote loss of body fluid	Promote loss of body fluid to accentuate muscle definition; often taken with potassium supplements and very low-calorie diets	Muscle cell destruction, low blood pressure, blood chemistry abnormalities, and heart problems
Energy drinks	Increased energy, strength, power	Increased training volume; caffeine and carbohydrates are main ingredients; products are overpriced	Insomnia, increased blood pressure, heart palpitations
Erythropoietin	Enhanced performance during endurance events	Stimulated growth of red blood cells; enhanced oxygen uptake and endurance	Increased blood viscosity (thickness), can cause potentially fatal blood clots
			(Continued)

SUBSTANCE	SUPPOSED EFFECTS	ACTUAL EFFECTS	SELECTED POTENTIAL SIDE EFFECTS
Ginseng	Decreased effects of physical and emotional stress; increased oxygen consumption	Most well-controlled studies show no effect on performance	No serious side effects; high doses can cause high blood pressure, nervousness, and insomnia
Growth hormone (extremely expensive controlled substance*)	Increased muscle mass, strength, and power; decreased body fat	Increased muscle mass and strength; decreased fat mass; little effect on exercise performance	Elevated blood sugar, high insulin levels, and carpal tunnel and tarsal syndrome; enlargement of the heart and other organs
Insulin	Increased muscle mass	Effectiveness in stimulating muscle growth unknown	Insulin shock (characterized by extremely low blood sugar), which can lead to unconsciousness and death
"Metabolic-optimizing" meals for athletes	Increased muscle mass and energy supply; decreased body fat	No proven effects beyond those of balanced meals	No reported side effects, extremely expensive
Nitric oxide boosters (arginine, beet root)	Increased blood flow by stimulating nitric oxide production in blood vessels	Might increase endurance (beet root); little evidence that they promote muscle hypertrophy	Generally safe; could lower blood pressure in some people and make herpes infections worse
Protein, amino acids such as leucine and their metabolites (beta-hydroxy beta-methylbutyrate (HMB)	Increased muscle mass and growth hormone release; accelerated muscle development and protein synthesis; decreased body fat	No effects if dietary protein intake is adequate; may promote protein synthesis if taken immediately before or after weight training	Can be dangerous for people with liver or kidney disease; substituting amino acid or polypeptide supplements for protein-rich food can cause nutrient deficiencies; protein supplements and sports foods such as bars and gels are more expensive than whole foods

*Possession of a controlled substance is illegal without a prescription, and physicians are not allowed to prescribe controlled substances for the improvement of athletic performance. In addition, the use of anabolic steroids, growth hormone, or any of several other substances listed in this table is banned for athletic competition. Some apparently safe supplements may contain substances banned for use in sports.

SOURCES: Fahey, T., et al. 2015. "Sport and exercise physiology: Performance-enhancing substances—anabolic steroids, in Sports Science and Physical Education," ed., L. Georgescu, *Encyclopedia of Life Support Systems (EOLSS),* developed under the auspices of UNESCO. Oxford, UK: EOLSS Publishers; Brooks, G. A., et al. 2005. *Exercise Physiology: Human Bioenergetics and Its Applications,* 4th ed. New York: McGraw-Hill; Pasiakos, S. M., et al. 2015. "The effects of protein supplements on muscle mass, strength, and aerobic and anaerobic power in healthy adults: A systematic review," *Sports Medicine,* vol. 45, no. 1, 111–131; American College of Sports Medicine, Academy of Nutrition and Dietetics, and Dietitians of Canada, "Position Statement: Nutrition and Athletic Performance," *Medicine and Science in Sports and Exercise* DOI: 10.1249/MSS.0000000000000852, 2016.

TIPS FOR TODAY AND THE FUTURE

To improve and maintain your muscle fitness, perform strength training exercise for major muscle groups at least twice a week.

RIGHT NOW YOU CAN

- Stand up and do some body weight exercises—air squats, lunges, side bridges, and planks.
- Identify your current options for equipment and facilities for strength training. If you are interested in a machine weight-training program, research low-cost facility options on your campus or in your community.

IN THE FUTURE YOU CAN

- Add variety to your strength training workouts by trying different equipment and types of exercises; for example, if you normally use machines, try free weights. Also make changes in the specific exercises you do for major muscle groups.
- Reassess your muscular strength and endurance by repeating tests from the lab activities. Evaluate the progress of your program to date, and make changes to your FITT-VP factors. For example, you might start training less frequently but with heavier weights and/or more sets.

WEIGHT TRAINING EXERCISES

A general book on fitness and wellness cannot include a detailed description of all weight training exercises. The following pages present a basic program for developing muscular strength and endurance for general fitness using body weight (no equipment), free weights, and weight machines. Photographs and a list of the muscles being trained accompany instructions for each exercise; Table 4.4 lists exercises and major muscles and functions for the major muscle groups that you should train in your program. See Figure 4.6 for a clear illustration of the deep and superficial muscles referenced in the exercises.

Labs 4.2 and 4.3 will help you assess your current level of muscular endurance and design your own weight training program. If you want to develop strength for a particular activity, your program should contain exercises for general fitness, exercises for the muscle groups most important for the activity, and exercises for muscle groups most often injured. Regardless of the goals of your program or the type of equipment you use, your program should be structured so that you obtain maximum results without risking injury.

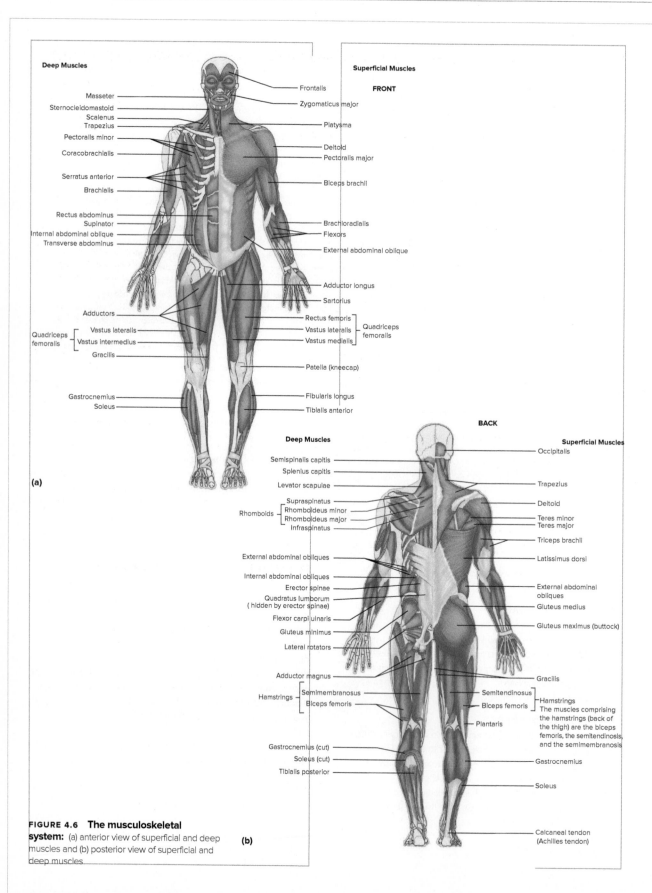

Deep Muscles

- Masseter
- Sternocleidomastoid
- Scalenus
- Trapezius
- Pectoralis minor
- Coracobrachialis
- Serratus anterior
- Brachialis
- Rectus abdominus
- Supinator
- Internal abdominal oblique
- Transverse abdominus
- Adductors
- Vastus lateralis — Quadriceps
- Vastus intermedius — femoralis
- Gracilis
- Gastrocnemius
- Soleus

Superficial Muscles

FRONT

- Frontalis
- Zygomaticus major
- Platysma
- Deltoid
- Pectoralis major
- Biceps brachii
- Brachioradialis
- Flexors
- External abdominal oblique
- Adductor longus
- Sartorius
- Rectus femoris
- Vastus lateralis — Quadriceps
- Vastus medialis — femoralis
- Patella (kneecap)
- Fibularis longus
- Tibialis anterior

(a)

Deep Muscles

- Semispinalis capitis
- Splenius capitis
- Levator scapulae
- Supraspinatus
- Rhomboideus minor — Rhomboids
- Rhomboideus major
- Infraspinatus
- External abdominal obliques
- Internal abdominal obliques
- Erector spinae
- Quadratus lumborum (hidden by erector spinae)
- Flexor carpi ulnaris
- Gluteus minimus
- Lateral rotators
- Adductor magnus
- Semimembranosus — Hamstrings
- Biceps femoris
- Gastrocnemius (cut)
- Soleus (cut)
- Tibialis posterior

BACK

Superficial Muscles

- Occipitalis
- Trapezius
- Deltoid
- Teres minor
- Teres major
- Triceps brachii
- Latissimus dorsi
- External abdominal obliques
- Gluteus medius
- Gluteus maximus (buttock)
- Gracilis
- Semitendinosus
- Biceps femoris — Hamstrings
- Plantaris

The muscles comprising the hamstrings (back of the thigh) are the biceps femoris, the semitendinosis, and the semimembranosis

- Gastrocnemius
- Soleus
- Calcaneal tendon (Achilles tendon)

(b)

FIGURE 4.6   The musculoskeletal system: (a) anterior view of superficial and deep muscles and (b) posterior view of superficial and deep muscles.

Table 4.4	Muscle Groups, Major Muscles and Functions, and Strength Training Exercises	
MUSCLE GROUP	MAJOR MUSCLES AND FUNCTIONS	STRENGTH TRAINING EXERCISES
Neck and upper back	Trapezius: A large muscle in the upper back and neck that moves the shoulder blades. Latissimus dorsi: A large muscle in the back that extends, adducts (lowers) the shoulder down and to the side, and helps stabilize the shoulder. Rhomboids: Moves (retracts and elevate) the shoulder blades.	Front plank, pull-up, shoulder press, upright rowing, kettlebell swing, horizontal rowing, kettlebell one-arm snatch, kettlebell carry, lat pull, assisted pull-up, overhead press, pullover, lateral raise
Shoulders	Deltoids: Large round shoulder muscles that lift the arm to the front (flexion) and to the side (abduction). Rhomboids: Moves and stabilizes the shoulder blades; assists during rowing motions. Rotator cuff: Internally and externally rotates the shoulder; consists of the supraspinatus, infraspinatus, teres minor, and subscapularis.	Burpees with a push-up, spine extension, thrusters, front plank, push-ups, bench press, shoulder press, upright rowing, lateral raise, kettlebell one-arm snatch, overhead press, lateral raise, assisted dip
Arms	Biceps: Muscle on the front of the upper arm that bends the elbow (elbow flexion) and lifts the shoulder (shoulder flexion). Triceps: A muscle on the back of the arm that extends (straightens) the elbow. Brachialis: Muscle in the upper arm that bends (flexes) the elbows.	Thrusters, push-ups, bench press, pull-up, shoulder press, upright rowing , biceps curl, lat pull, assisted pull-up, overhead press, pullover, triceps extension, assisted dip
Chest	Pectoralis major and minor: Large chest muscles that move the shoulder (flexion, adduction, and rotation)	Burpees with a push-up, thrusters, front plank, push-ups, bench press, pullover, assisted dip
Abdomen	Rectus abdominis: A large muscle on the front part of the abdomen that flexes the spine and stabilizes the core. Sometimes called the "six-pack" muscle. Obliques: Muscles on the side of the abdomen that stabilize the core and bend the trunk to the side (lateral flexion). Transversus abdominis: A muscle that stabilizes the core.	Curl-up, isometric side bridge, front plank, kettlebell carry, pullover
Lower back	Erector spinae: Muscles running along the spinal column that straighten and rotate the back and stabilize the core. Quadratus lumborum: A deep core muscle connecting the spine, hip, and ribs. It stabilizes the core, bends the trunk to the side, and rotates the hip.	Spine extension, isometric side bridge, front plank, kettlebell carry
Thighs	Quadriceps: Muscle group on the front of the thighs consisting of the vastus lateralis, vastus intermedius, vastus medialis, and rectus femoris. Hamstrings: Muscle group on the back of the thigh consisting of the semimembranosis, semitendinosis, biceps femoris.	Squats (all types), lunges, burpees with a push-up, spine extension, thrusters, kettlebell swing, kettlebell one-arm snatch, kettlebell carry, leg press, leg extension, seated leg curl
Buttocks	Gluteals: Muscles of the buttocks, consisting of the gluteus maximus, gluteus minimus, and gluteus medius.	Squats (all types), lunges, burpees with a push-up, spine extension, thrusters, front plank, kettlebell swing, kettlebell one-arm snatch, leg press
Calves	Calf muscles: Muscles on the back of the lower leg consisting of the gastrocnemius, soleus, and plantaris.	Squats, lunges, burpees with a push-up, thrusters, heel raise, seated leg curl, heel raise

WEIGHT TRAINING EXERCISES Body Weight

EXERCISE 1

Air Squats

Instructions: (a) Keep your back straight and head level; stand with feet slightly more than shoulder-width apart and toes pointed slightly outward. Hold your hands out in front of you. (b) Squat down until your thighs are below parallel with the floor. Let your thighs move laterally (outward) so that you "squat between your legs." Hinge at your hips and don't let your back sag. This will help keep your back straight and your heels on the floor. Drive upward toward the starting position, hinging at the hips and keeping your back in a fixed position throughout the exercise.

Muscles developed: Quadriceps, gluteals, hamstrings, calf

Front   Back

Back

a

b

(a-b): ©Taylor Robertson Photography

EXERCISE 2

Lunges

Instructions: (a) Stand with one foot about two feet in front of the other. (b) Lunge forward with the front leg, bending it until the thigh is parallel to the floor. The heel of the lead leg should stay on the ground. Do not shift your weight so far forward that the knee moves out past the toes. Repeat the exercise using the other leg. Keep your back and head as straight as possible and maintain control while performing the exercise.

Muscles developed: Quadriceps, gluteals, hamstrings, calf

Front   Back

Back

a   b

(a-b): ©Taylor Robertson Photography

EXERCISE 3

Burpees with a Push-up

a

b

c

Front   Back

Back

Front   Back

(a-c): ©Taylor Robertson Photography

Instructions: From a standing position, squat down and place your hands on the floor; and then (a) kick your legs behind you and land in the "up" push-up position. Do a push-up. (b) Then move your knees forward returning to the squat position; (c) spring up as high as you can into a full jump. Repeat.

Muscles developed: Quadriceps, gluteals, hamstrings, calf, deltoids, pectoralis major, triceps

| **EXERCISE 4** | **McGill Curl-Up** |

Instructions: (a) Lie on your back on the floor with one leg bent, foot placed flat on the floor, and the other leg straight. Place your hands under the small of your back or fold your arms across your chest. **(b)** Slowly raise the chest, shoulders, and head as a unit while maintaining a neutral spine. Try to isolate the rectus abdominis. Do not grasp your hands around your head when doing crunches because you might injure your neck.

Muscles developed: Rectus abdominis, obliques

Front

Courtesy Tom Fahey

| **EXERCISE 5** | **Spine Extension ("Bird Dog") (Isometric Exercise)** |

Instructions: Begin on all fours with your knees below your hips and your hands below your shoulders.

Unilateral spine extension: (a) Extend your right leg to the rear and reach forward with your right arm. Keep your spine neutral and your raised arm and leg in line with your torso. Don't arch your back or let your hip or shoulder sag. Hold this position for 10–30 seconds. Repeat with your left leg and left arm.

Bilateral spine extension: (b) Extend your left leg to the rear and reach forward with your right arm. Keep your spine neutral and your raised arm and leg in line with your torso. Don't arch your back or let your hip or shoulder sag. Hold this position for 10–30 seconds. Repeat with your right leg and left arm.

You can make this exercise more difficult by making box patterns with your arms and legs.

Muscles developed: Erector spinae, gluteus maximus, hamstrings, deltoids

Front   Back   Back

a

b

(a-b): ©Wayne Glusker

EXERCISE 6 — Isometric Side Bridge

Courtesy Joseph Quever

Instructions: Lie on the floor on your side with your knees bent and your top arm lying alongside your body. Lift and drive your hips forward so that your weight is supported by your forearm and knee. Hold this position for 3–10 seconds, breathing normally. Repeat on the other side. Perform 3–10 repetitions on each side.

Variation: You can make the exercise more difficult by keeping your legs straight and supporting yourself with your feet and forearm (see Lab 5.3) or with your feet and hand (with elbow straight). An advanced version of this exercise that builds the core and shoulder muscles is to do a side bridge on the right side, rotate to a front plank, and then rotate to a side bridge on the left side. Hold each position for 3 seconds.

Muscles developed: Obliques, quadratus lumborum

Front   Back

EXERCISE 7 — Thrusters

(a-c): ©Taylor Robertson Photography

Instructions: (a) From a standing position, hold stones, soup cans, dumbbells, or barbells (or a single rock with both hands) at chest level with palms facing outward. (b) Squat down until your thighs are parallel with the floor. (c) Immediately stand and press the objects overhead in one continuous motion. Lower the objects to the starting position and immediately repeat the exercise.

Muscles developed: Quadriceps, gluteus maximus, hamstrings, gastrocnemius, deltoids, pectoralis major, triceps

Front   Back

Back

Front   Back

EXERCISE 8 — Overhead squats

Instructions: **(a)** Stand holding a broom handle, stones, barbell, or soup cans overhead with straight arms, feet placed slightly more than shoulder-width apart, toes pointed out slightly, head neutral, and back straight. Center your weight over your arches or slightly behind. **(b)** Squat down, keeping your weight centered over your arches, and actively flex the hips (hinge at the hips with buttocks back) until your legs break parallel (hips below knees). During the movement, keep your spine neutral, shoulders back, and chest out, and let your thighs part to the side so that you are "squatting between your legs." Try to "spread the floor" with your feet. Push up to the starting position, maximizing the use of the posterior hip and thigh muscles, and maintaining a straight back and neutral head position.

Front   Back
Front   Back

(a-b): ©Taylor Robertson Photography

Muscles developed: Quadriceps, hamstrings, gluteal muscles, core muscles

EXERCISE 9 — Front Plank

Instructions: Lying on your front with body straight, raise your body upward, supporting your weight on forearms and toes. Hold the position. Begin with 10-second holds and progress until you can hold the plank for at least two minutes. Breathe normally. Tighten your abs, glutes, and quads as you do this exercise.

Muscles developed: Rectus abdominis, erector spinae, trapezius, rhomboids, deltoids, pectorals, gluteal muscles

Front

Back

©Taylor Robertson Photography

EXERCISE 10 — Push-ups

Instructions: **(a)** Start in the push-up position with your body weight supported by your hands and feet. Your arms and back should be straight and your fingers pointed forward. Lower your chest to the floor with your back straight, and then return to the starting position.

Variation: **(b)** Do modified push-ups if you can't do at least 10 regular push-ups. Start with your body weight supported by your hands and knees. Your arms and back should be straight and your fingers pointed forward. Lower your chest to the floor with your back straight, and then return to the starting position.

Muscles developed: Pectorals, triceps, deltoids

Front   Back

©Taylor Robertson Photography

WEIGHT TRAINING EXERCISES Free Weights

EXERCISE 1   Bench Press

Instructions: (a) Lying on a bench on your back with your feet on the floor, grasp the bar with palms upward and hands shoulder-width apart. If the weight is on a rack, move the bar carefully from the supports to a point over the middle of your chest or slightly above it (at the lower part of the sternum). **(b)** Lower the bar to your chest. Then press it in a straight line to the starting position. Don't arch your back or bounce the bar off your chest. You can also do this exercise with dumbbells or one arm at a time (unilateral training).

(a-b): ©Wayne Glusker

Front   Back

Muscles developed: Pectoralis major, triceps, deltoids

Note: *To allow an optimal view of exercise technique, a spotter does not appear in these demonstration photographs; however, spotters should be used for this exercise.*

EXERCISE 2   Pull-Up

Instructions: (a) Begin by grasping the pull-up bar with both hands, palms facing forward and elbows extended fully. **(b)** Pull yourself upward until your chin goes above the bar. Then return to the starting position.

Assisted pull-up: (c) This is done as described for a pull-up, except that a spotter assists the person by pushing upward at the waist, hips, or legs during the exercise.

Muscles developed: Latissimus dorsi, biceps

(a-c): ©Neil Tanner Photography

Front   Back

| EXERCISE 3 | Shoulder Press (Overhead or Military Press) |

Instructions: This exercise can be done standing or seated, with dumbbells or a barbell. The shoulder press begins with the weight at your chest, preferably on a rack. **(a)** Grasp the weight with your palms facing away from you. **(b)** Push the weight overhead until your arms are extended. Then return to the starting position (weight at chest). Be careful not to arch your back excessively.

If you are a more advanced weight trainer, you can "clean" the weight (lift it from the floor to your chest). The clean should be attempted only after instruction from a knowledgeable coach; otherwise, it can lead to injury.

Muscles developed:
Deltoids, triceps, trapezius

Front   Back

a   b

(a-b): Courtesy Joseph Quever

| EXERCISE 4 | Upright Rowing |

Instructions: (a) From a standing position with arms extended fully, grasp a barbell with a close grip (hands about 6–12 inches apart) and palms facing the body. **(b)** Raise the bar to about the level of your collarbone, keeping your elbows above bar level at all times. Return to the starting position.

This exercise can be done using dumbbells, a weighted bar (shown), or a barbell.

Muscles developed:
Trapezius, deltoids, biceps

Front   Back

a   b

(a-b): ©Wayne Glusker

| EXERCISE 5 | Biceps Curl |

Instructions: (a) From a standing position, grasp the bar with your palms facing away from you and your hands shoulder-width apart. **(b)** Keeping your upper body rigid, flex (bend) your elbows until the bar reaches a level slightly below the collarbone. Return the bar to the starting position.

This exercise can be done using dumbbells, a curl bar (shown), or a barbell; some people find that using a curl bar places less stress on the wrists.

Muscles developed:
Biceps, brachialis

Front

a   b

(a-b): Courtesy Joseph Quever

EXERCISE 6   Lateral Raise

Instructions: (a) Stand with feet shoulder-width apart and a dumbbell in each hand. Hold the dumbbells in front of you and parallel to each other. **(b)** With elbows slightly bent, slowly lift both weights to the side until they reach shoulder level. Keep your wrists in a neutral position, in line with your forearms. Return to the starting position.

Muscles developed: Deltoids

Front   Back

(a-b): Courtesy Neil A. Tanner

EXERCISE 7   Squat

Instructions: (a) If the bar is racked, place the bar on the fleshy part of your upper back and grasp the bar at shoulder width. Keeping your back straight and head level, remove the bar from the rack and take a step back. Stand with feet slightly more than shoulder-width apart and toes pointed slightly outward. Rest the bar on the back of your shoulders, holding it there with palms facing forward. **(b)** Keeping your head level and lower back straight and pelvis back, squat down until your thighs are below parallel with the floor. Let your thighs move laterally (outward) so that you "squat between your legs." This will help keep your back straight and keep your heels on the floor. Drive upward toward the starting position, hinging at the hips and keeping your back in a fixed position throughout the exercise.

Muscles developed: Quadriceps, gluteals, hamstrings, calf

Front   Back

Back

(a-b): ©Taylor Robertson Photography

EXERCISE 8   Heel Raise

Instructions: Stand with feet shoulder-width apart and toes pointed straight ahead. **(a)** Rest the bar on the back of your shoulders, holding it there with palms facing forward. **(b)** Press down with your toes while lifting your heels. Return to the starting position.

Muscle developed: Calf

Back

(a-b): Courtesy Neil Tanner

EXERCISE 9 — Kettlebell Swing

Instructions: (a) Begin by holding the kettlebell in both hands with palms facing toward you, in a standing position with knees bent, feet placed slightly more than shoulder-width apart, hips flexed, back straight, chest out, and head in a neutral position. **(b)** Holding the kettlebell at knee level, swing the weight to a horizontal position by initiating the motion with the hips, thighs, and abs (tighten the quads, glutes, and ab muscles as hard as you can), keeping your arm straight and relaxed during the movement. Let the weight swing back between your legs in a "football hiking motion" and then repeat the exercise. During the movement, hinge at the hips and not at the spine.

Front Back

Front Back

a

b

(a-b): ©Taylor Robertson Photography

Muscles developed: Quadriceps, hamstrings, lattisimus dorsi, erector spinae, gluteals, core

EXERCISE 10 — Kettlebell One-Arm Snatch

Instructions: (a) Begin by holding the kettlebell in one hand with your palm facing toward you, in a standing position with knees bent, feet placed slightly more than shoulder-width apart, hips flexed, back straight, chest out, and head in a neutral position.

Hold the kettlebell at knee level. **(b)** Swing the weight to a horizontal position by initiating the motion with the hips, thighs, and abs (tighten the quads, glutes, and ab muscles as hard as you can), bending your arm as it approaches the chest and continuing the motion until straightening it overhead.

a

b

c

(a-c): ©Taylor Robertson Photography

The kettlebell should rotate from the front of your hand to the back during the motion. Use an upward punching motion at the top of the movement to prevent injuring your forearm. **(c)** Let the weight swing back between your legs in a "football hiking motion" and then repeat the exercise. During the movement, hinge at the hips and not at the spine.

Muscles developed: Quadriceps, gluteals, hamstrings, core, deltoids, trapezius, erector spinae, latissimus dorsi, pectoralis major

Front Back

Front Back

EXERCISE 11 — Kettlebell or Dumbbell Carry ("Suitcase Carry")

Instructions: This is an excellent exercise for building the core muscles. Pick up a dumbbell or kettlebell in one or both hands. Maintaining good posture, walk 20 to 100 yards carrying the weight. Carry 10 to several hundred pounds, depending on your fitness.

Muscles developed: Core, trapezius, quadriceps, gluteals

Front

©Taylor Robertson Photography

WEIGHT TRAINING EXERCISES Weight Machines

EXERCISE 1

Instructions: Sit or lie on the seat or bench, depending on the type of machine and the manufacturer's instructions. Your back, hips, and buttocks should be pressed against the machine pads. Place your feet on the floor or the foot supports.

(a) Grasp the handles with your palms facing away from you; the handles should be aligned with your armpits.

(b) Push the bars until your arms are fully extended, but don't lock your elbows. Return to the starting position.

Front   Back

Bench Press (Chest or Vertical Press) Weight Machines

(a-b): ©Taylor Robertson Photography

Muscles developed: Pectoralis major, anterior deltoids, triceps

EXERCISE 2   Lat Pull

Instructions: Begin in a seated or kneeling position, depending on the type of lat machine and the manufacturer's instructions.

(a) Grasp the bar of the machine with arms fully extended.

(b) Slowly pull the weight down until it reaches the top of your chest. Slowly return to the starting position.

Muscles developed: Latissimus dorsi, biceps

Front   Back

Note: *This exercise focuses on the same major muscles as the assisted pull-up (Exercise 3); choose an appropriate exercise for your program based on your preferences and equipment availability.*

(a-b): Courtesy Neil A. Tanner

EXERCISE 3   **Assisted Pull-Up**

Instructions: Set the weight according to the amount of assistance you need to complete a set of pull-ups—the heavier the weight, the more assistance provided.

(a) Stand or kneel on the assist platform, and grasp the pull-up bar with your elbows fully extended and your palms facing away.

(b) Pull up until your chin goes above the bar, and then return to the starting position.

Muscles developed: Latissimus dorsi, biceps

Front   Back

(a-b): ©Wayne Glusker

EXERCISE 4   **Overhead Press (Shoulder Press)**

Instructions: Adjust the seat so that your feet are flat on the ground and the hand grips are slightly above your shoulders. **(a)** Sit down, facing away from the machine, and grasp the hand grips with your palms facing forward. **(b)** Press the weight upward until your arms are extended. Return to the starting position.

Muscles developed: Trapezius, triceps, deltoids, pectoralis major, rotator cuff

Front   Back

(a-b): Courtesy Joseph Quever

EXERCISE 5   **Biceps Curl**

Instructions: (a) Adjust the seat so that your back is straight and your arms rest comfortably against the top and side pads. Place your arms on the support cushions and grasp the hand grips with your palms facing up. **(b)** Keeping your upper body still, flex (bend) your elbows until the hand grips almost reach your collarbone. Return to the starting position.

Muscles developed: Biceps, brachialis

Front

(a-b): Courtesy Joseph Quever

EXERCISE 6   Pullover

Instructions: Adjust the seat so that your shoulders are aligned with the cams. Push down on the foot pads with your feet to bring the bar forward until you can place your elbows on the pads. Rest your hands lightly on the bar. If possible, place your feet flat on the floor. **(a)** To get into the starting position, let your arms go backward as far as possible. **(b)** Pull your elbows forward until the bar almost touches your abdomen. Return to the starting position.

Muscles developed: Latissimus dorsi, pectorals, triceps, rectus abdominis

Front   Back

(a-b): Courtesy Nell A. Tanner

EXERCISE 7   Lateral Raise

Instructions: **(a)** Adjust the seat so that the pads rest just above your elbows when your upper arms are at your sides, your elbows are bent, and your forearms are parallel to the floor. Lightly grasp the handles. **(b)** Push outward and up with your arms until the pads are at shoulder height. Lead with your elbows rather than trying to lift the bars with your hands. Return to the starting position.

Muscles developed: Deltoids, trapezius

Front   Back

(a-b): Courtesy Joseph Quever

EXERCISE 8   Triceps Extension

Instructions: **(a)** Adjust the seat so that your back is straight and your arms rest comfortably against the top and side pads. Place your arms on the support cushions and grasp the hand grips with palms facing inward. **(b)** Keeping your upper body still, extend your elbows as much as possible. Return to the starting position.

Muscles developed: Triceps

Back

(a-b): Courtesy Joseph Quever

Note: *This exercise focuses on some of the same muscles as the Assisted Dip (Exercise 9); choose an appropriate exercise for your program based on your preferences and equipment availability.*

EXERCISE 9

Assisted Dip

Instructions: Set the weight according to the amount of assistance you need to complete a set of dips—the heavier the weight, the more assistance provided. **(a)** Stand or kneel on the assist platform with your body between the dip bars. With your elbows fully extended and palms facing your body, support your weight on your hands. **(b)** Lower your body until your upper arms are almost parallel with the bars. Then push up until you reach the starting position.

Muscles developed: Triceps, deltoids, pectoralis major

Front   Back

(a-b): ©Taylor Robertson Photography

EXERCISE 10

Leg Press

Instructions: Sit or lie on the seat or bench, depending on the type of machine and the manufacturer's instructions. Your head, back, hips, and buttocks should be pressed against the machine pads. Loosely grasp the handles at the side of the machine. **(a)** Begin with your feet flat on the foot platform about shoulder-width apart. Extend your legs, but do not forcefully lock your knees. **(b)** Slowly lower the weight by bending your knees and flexing your hips until your knees are bent at about a 90-degree angle or your heels start to lift off the foot platform. Keep your lower back flat against the support pad. Then extend your knees and return to the starting position.

Muscles developed: Gluteals, quadriceps, hamstrings

Front   Back

(a-b): ©Taylor Robertson Photography

EXERCISE 11

Leg Extension (Knee Extension)

Instructions: (a) Adjust the seat so that the pads rest comfortably on top of your lower shins. Loosely grasp the handles. **(b)** Extend your knees until they are almost straight. Return to the starting position.

Knee extensions cause kneecap pain in some people. If you have kneecap pain during this exercise, check with an orthopedic specialist before repeating it.

Muscles developed: Quadriceps

Front

(a-b): Courtesy Joseph Quever

EXERCISE 12 — Seated Leg Curl

Instructions: **(a)** Sit on the seat with your back against the back pad and the leg pad below your calf muscles. **(b)** Flex your knees until your lower and upper legs form a 90-degree angle. Return to the starting position.

Muscles developed: Hamstrings, calf

Back   Back

(a-b): ©Wayne Glusker

EXERCISE 13 — Heel Raise

Instructions: **(a)** Stand with your head between the pads and one pad on each shoulder. The balls of your feet should be on the platform. Lightly grasp the handles. **(b)** Press down with your toes while lifting your heels. Return to the starting position. Changing the direction your feet are pointing (straight ahead, inward, and outward) will work different portions of your calf muscles.

Muscle developed: Calf

Back

(a-b): Courtesy Joseph Quever

Note: *Abdominal machines, low-back machines, and trunk rotation machines are not recommended because of injury risk. Refer to the "Body Weight" and "Free Weights" exercise sections for appropriate exercises to strengthen the abdominal and low-back muscles. For the rectus abdominis, obliques, and transverse abdominis, perform curl-ups (Exercise 4 in the "Body Weight" section) and the stir-the-pot exercise (Exercise 11 in the "Flexibility and Low-Back Health" chapter), and for the erector spinae and quadratus lumborum, perform the spine extension and the isometric side bridge (Exercises 5 and 6 in the "Body Weight" section).*

COMMON QUESTIONS ANSWERED

Q Will I gain weight if I do resistance exercises?

A Your weight probably will not change significantly as a result of a general fitness program: one set of 8–12 repetitions of 8–10 exercises, performed on at least two nonconsecutive days per week. You will lose body fat but also increase muscle mass, so your weight will stay about the same. You may notice a change in how your clothes fit, however, because muscle is denser than fat. Increased muscle mass will help you control body fat. Muscle increases your metabolism, which means you burn more calories every day. If you combine resistance exercises with endurance exercises, you will be on your way to developing a healthier body composition. Concentrate on fat loss rather than weight loss.

Q Do I need more protein in my diet when I train with weights?

A No. Although some evidence indicates that power athletes involved in heavy training have a higher-than-normal protein requirement, there is no reason for most people to consume extra protein. Most Americans take in more protein than they need, so even if there is an increased protein need during heavy training, the average diet probably supplies it. However, recent studies from Canada showed that the combination of high-intensity training (high-intensity interval training and weight training), caloric restriction, and high protein intake (2.4 grams per kilogram body weight per day) resulted in substantial increases in lean mass and decreases in body fat. Consuming a protein-rich snack before or after training may promote muscle hypertrophy. You may find protein bars and shakes to be convenient, but keep in mind that they are more expensive than whole foods and do not contain all the nutrients found in a well-rounded diet.

Q What causes muscle soreness the day or two following a weight training workout?

A The muscle pain you feel a day or two after a heavy weight training workout is caused by injury to the muscle fibers and surrounding connective tissue. Contrary to popular belief, delayed-onset muscle soreness is not caused by lactic acid buildup. Scientists believe that injury to muscle fibers causes inflammation, which in turn causes the release of chemicals that break down part of the muscle tissue and cause pain. After a bout of intense exercise that causes muscle injury and delayed-onset muscle soreness, the muscles produce protective proteins that prevent soreness during future workouts. If you don't work out regularly, you lose these protective proteins and become susceptible to soreness again.

Q Will strength training improve my sports performance?

A Strength developed in the weight room does not automatically increase your power in sports such as skiing, tennis, or cycling. Hitting a forehand in tennis and making a turn on skis are precise skills that require coordination between your nervous system and muscles. For skilled people, movements become reflex; you don't think about them when you do them. Increasing strength can disturb this coordination. Only by simultaneously practicing a sport and improving fitness can you expect to become more powerful in the skill. Practice helps you integrate your new strength with your skills, which makes you more powerful. Consequently, you can hit the ball harder in tennis or make more forceful turns on the ski slopes. (Refer to Chapter 2 for more on the concept of specificity in physical training.)

Q Will I improve faster if I train every day?

A No. Your muscles need time to recover between training sessions. Doing resistance exercises every day will cause you to become overtrained, which will increase your chance of injury and impede your progress. If your strength training program reaches a plateau, try one of these strategies:

- Vary the number of sets. If you have been performing one set of each exercise, add sets.
- Train less frequently. If you are currently training the same muscle groups three or more times per week, you may not be allowing your muscles to fully recover from intense workouts.
- Change exercises. Using different exercises for the same muscle group may stimulate further strength development.
- Vary the load and number of repetitions. Try increasing or decreasing the loads you are using and changing the number of repetitions accordingly.
- If you are training alone, find a motivated training partner. A partner can encourage you and assist you with difficult lifts, forcing you to work harder.
- Train explosively (purposefully). This trains the nervous system and the muscles, which results in greater improvements in strength and power than training more slowly.

Q If I stop training, will my muscles turn to fat?

A No. Fat and muscle are two different kinds of tissue, and one cannot turn into the other. Muscles that aren't used become smaller (atrophy), and body fat may increase if caloric intake exceeds calories burned. Although the result of inactivity may be smaller muscles and more fat, the change is caused by two separate processes.

Q **Should I wear a weight belt when I lift?**

A Until recently, most experts advised people to wear weight belts. However, several studies have shown that weight belts do not prevent back injuries and may, in fact, increase the risk of injury by encouraging people to lift more weight than they are capable of lifting with good form. Although wearing a belt may allow you to lift more weight in some lifts, you may not get the full benefit of your program because use of a weight belt reduces the effectiveness of the workout on the muscles that help support your spine.

SUMMARY

• Hypertrophy (increased muscle fiber size) occurs when weight training causes the size and number of myofibrils to increase, thereby increasing total muscle size. Strength also increases through muscle learning. Most women do not develop large muscles from weight training.

• Improvements in muscular strength and endurance lead to enhanced physical performance, protection against injury, improved body composition, better self-image, improved muscle and bone health with aging, reduced risk of chronic disease, and decreased risk of premature death.

• Muscular strength can be assessed by determining the amount of weight that can be lifted in one repetition of an exercise. Muscular endurance can be assessed by determining the number of repetitions of a particular exercise that can be performed.

• Static (isometric) exercises involve contraction without movement. They are most useful when a person is recovering from an injury or surgery or needs to overcome weak points in a range of motion.

• Dynamic (isotonic) exercises involve contraction that results in movement. The two most common types are constant resistance (free weights and body weight) and variable resistance (many weight machines).

• Free weights and weight machines have pluses and minuses for developing fitness, although machines tend to be safer.

• Lifting heavy weights for only a few repetitions helps develop strength. Lifting lighter weights for more repetitions helps develop muscular endurance.

• A strength training program for general fitness includes at least one set of 8–12 repetitions (enough to cause fatigue) of 8–10 exercises, along with warm-up and cool-down periods. The program should be carried out at least two nonconsecutive days per week.

• Safety guidelines for strength training include using proper technique, using spotters and collars when necessary, and taking care of injuries.

• Supplements or drugs that are promoted as instant or quick "cures" usually don't work and are either dangerous, expensive, or both. Although some elite athletes take performance-enhancing drugs, the largest consumers are physically active young adults (18–35 years old) who want to improve appearance and physical performance.

FOR FURTHER EXPLORATION

American College of Sports Medicine Position Stand: Progression Models in Resistance Training for Healthy Adults. Provides an in-depth look at strategies for setting up a strength training program and making progress based on individual program goals.

http://journals.lww.com/acsm-msse/Fulltext/2009/03000/Progression_Models_in_Resistance_Training_for.26.aspx

Crossfit. Extensive written and video resources for people interested in cross-training and resistive exercise.

https://www.crossfit.com/

Dan John. An excellent website for people serious about improving strength and fitness, written by a world-class athlete and coach in track and field and Highland games.

http://danjohn.net

InnerBody. Provides text, illustrations, and animations about the muscular system, nerve-muscle connections, muscular contraction, and other topics.

http://www.innerbody.com/htm/body.html

Mayo Clinic: Weight Training: Improve Your Muscular Fitness. Provides a basic overview of weight training essentials along with links to many other articles on specific weight-training-related topics.

http://www.mayoclinic.com/health/weight-training/HQ01627

National Strength and Conditioning Association. A professional organization that focuses on strength development for fitness and athletic performance.

http://www.nsca.com

Pilates Method Alliance. Provides information about Pilates and about instructor certification; includes a directory of instructors.

http://www.pilatesmethodalliance.org

Strong First: A website hosted by kettlebell master Pavel Tsatsouline that presents excellent information on strength training.

http://www.strongfirst.com/

University of California, San Diego: Muscle Physiology Home Page. Provides an introduction to muscle physiology, including information about types of muscle fibers and energy cycles.

http://muscle.ucsd.edu/index.html

University of Michigan: Muscles in Action. Interactive descriptions of muscle movements.

http://www.med.umich.edu/lrc/Hypermuscle/Hyper.html

Yoga Alliance. A resource site for yoga instructors and people interested in yoga.

http://www.yogaalliance.org

See also the listings in Chapter 2.

SELECTED BIBLIOGRAPHY

Alfini, A. J., et al. 2016. Hippocampal and cerebral blood flow after exercise cessation in masters athletes. *Frontiers in Aging Neuroscience.* doi: 10.3389/fnagi.2016.00184

American College of Sports Medicine. 2013. *ACSM's Resource Manual for Guidelines for Exercise Testing and Prescription,* 7th ed. Philadelphia: Lippincott Williams and Wilkins.

American College of Sports Medicine. 2011. American College of Sports Medicine position stand: Progression models in resistance training for healthy adults. *Medicine and Science in Sports and Exercise* 43(7): 1334–1359.

American College of Sports Medicine. 2018. *ACSM's Guidelines for Exercise Testing and Prescription,* 10th ed. Philadelphia: Wolters Kluwer.

Andersen, V., et al. 2016. Core muscle activation in one-armed and two-armed kettlebell swing. *Journal of Strength and Conditioning Research* 30: 1196–1204.

Baechle, T., and R. W. Earl. 2016. *National Strength and Conditioning Association's Essentials of Strength and Conditioning,* 4th ed. Champaign, Ill.: Human Kinetics.

Beck, B. R., et al. 2016. Exercise and Sports Science Australia (ESSA) position statement on exercise prescription for the prevention and management of osteoporosis. *Journal of Science and Medicine in Sport* S1440-2440(16)30217-1.

Behm, D. G., et al. 2010. Canadian Society for Exercise Physiology position stand: The use of instability to train the core in athletic and nonathletic conditioning. *Applied Physiology, Nutrition and Metabolism* 35(1): 109–112.

Bompa, T., M. Di Pasquale, and L. Cornacchia. 2013. *Serious Strength Training.* Champaign, Ill.: Human Kinetics.

Brennan, R., et al. 2016. The injecting use of image and performance-enhancing drugs (IPED) in the general population: A systematic review. *Health and Social Care in the Community.* doi:10.1111/hsc.12326

Brooks, G. A., et al. 2005. *Exercise Physiology: Human Bioenergetics and Its Applications,* 4th ed. New York: McGraw-Hill.

Campbell, B. 2013. International Society of Sports Nutrition position stand: Energy drinks. *Journal of the International Society of Sports Nutrition* 10: 1.

Cermak, N. M., et al. 2013. Perspective: Protein supplementation during prolonged resistance type exercise training augments skeletal muscle mass and strength gains. *Journal of the American Medical Directors Association* 14(1): 71–72.

Deutz, N. E., et al. 2014. Protein intake and exercise for optimal muscle function with aging: Recommendations from the ESPEN Expert Group. *Clinical Nutrition* 33(6): 929–936.

Earnest, C. P., et al. 2013. Cardiometabolic risk factors and metabolic syndrome in the Aerobics Center Longitudinal Study. *Mayo Clinics Proceedings* 88(3): 259–270.

Fahey, T. D. 2011. *Basic Weight Training for Men and Women,* 8th ed. New York: McGraw-Hill.

Farrar, R. E., et al. 2010. Oxygen cost of kettlebell swings. *Journal of Strength and Conditioning Research* 24(4): 1034–1036.

Goldstein, E. R., et al. 2010. International Society of Sports Nutrition position stand: Caffeine. *Journal of the International Society of Sports Nutrition* 7: 5.

Hackett, D., et al. 2016. Olympic weightlifting training improves vertical jump height in sportspeople: A systematic review with meta-analysis. *British Journal Sports Medicine* 50: 865–872.

Halperin, I., et al. 2016. The mind-muscle connection in resistance training: Friend or foe? *European Journal of Applied Physiology* 116: 863–864.

Hill, K. 2015. The value of resistance training for individuals with common lifestyle diseases. *ACSM's Health & Fitness Journal* 19(2): 9–13.

Hill, M., et al. 2016. Predicted maximal heart rate for upper body exercise testing. *Clinical Physiology and Functional Imaging* 36(2):155–158.

Jimenez-Reyes, P., et al. 2016. Maximal velocity as a discriminating factor in the performance of loaded squat jumps. *International Journal of Sports Physiology and Performance* 11: 227–234.

Jones, M. T. 2014. Effect of compensatory acceleration training in combination with accommodating resistance on upper body strength in collegiate athletes. *Open Access Journal of Sports Medicine* 5: 183–189.

Kang, D. Y., et al. 2015. The effects of bodyweight-based exercise with blood flow restriction on isokinetic knee muscular function and thigh circumference in college students. *Journal of Physical Therapy Science* 27: 2709–2712.

Kilgour, A. H., et al. 2014. A systematic review of the evidence that brain structure is related to muscle structure and their relationship to brain and muscle function in humans over the life-course. *Biomedical Central (BMC) Geriatrics* 14: 85.

Laine, M. K., et al. 2016. Former male elite athletes have better metabolic health in late life than their controls. *Scandinavian Journal of Medicine Science in Sports* 26: 284–290.

Landi, F., et al. 2017. Age-related variations of muscle mass, strength, and physical performance in community-dwellers: Results from the Milan EXPO Survey. *Journal of the American Medical Directors Association* 88(1): e17–88.

Lee, B., and S. McGill. 2015. The effect of long term isometric training on core/ torso stiffness. *Journal of Strength and Conditioning Research* 29(6): 1515–1526.

Lee, G. 2014. Exercise-induced rhabdomyolysis. *Rhode Island Medical Journal* (http://www.rimed.org/rimedicaljournal/2014/11/2014-11-22-sportsmed-lee.pdf).

Leopoldino, A. A., et al. 2013. Effect of Pilates on sleep quality and quality of life of sedentary population. *Journal of Bodyworks and Movement Therapy* 17(1): 5–10.

Longland, T. M., et al. 2016. Higher compared with lower dietary protein during an energy deficit combined with intense exercise promotes greater lean mass gain and fat mass loss: A randomized trial. *American Journal Clinical Nutrition* 2103(3): 738–746.

McKendry, J., et al. 2016. Short inter-set rest blunts resistance exercise-induced increases in myofibrillar protein synthesis and intracellular signaling in young males. *Experimental Physiology* 101(7): 866–882.

Metter, E. J. 1997. Age-associated loss of power and strength in the upper extremities in women and men. *Journal of Gerontology: Biological Sciences.* 52A(5): 8267–8276.

Nakahara, H., et al. 2015. Low-frequency severe-intensity interval training improves cardiorespiratory functions. *Medicine and Science in Sports and Exercise* 47(4): 789–798.

Ostry, D. J., et al. 2016. Sensory plasticity in human motor learning. *Trends in Neuroscience* 39: 114–123.

Outram, S., and B. Stewart. 2015. Doping through supplement use: A review of the available empirical data. *International Journal of Sports Nutrition and Exercise Metabolism* 25(1): 54–59.

Pasiakos, S. M., et al. 2015. The effects of protein supplements on muscle mass, strength, and aerobic and anaerobic power in healthy adults: a systematic review. *Sports Medicine* 45(1): 111–131.

Roshanravan, B., et al. 2017. Association of muscle endurance, fatigability, and strength with functional limitation and mortality in the Health Aging and Body Composition Study. *Journal of Gerontology Series A: Biological Sciences and Medical Sciences* 72(2): 284–291.

Saeterbakken, A. H., and M. S. Fimland. 2013. Electromyographic activity and 6RM strength in bench press on stable and unstable surfaces. *Journal of Strength and Conditioning Research* 27(4): 1101–1107.

Sanchis-Gomar, F., et al. 2014. 'Olympic' centenarians: Are they just biologically exceptional? *International Journal of Cardiology* 175(1): 216–217.

Sattler, F. R. 2013. Growth hormone in the aging male. *Best Practices & Research in Clinical Endocrinology and Metabolism* 27(4): 541–555.

Sawyer, B. J., et al. 2015. Predictors of fat mass changes in response to aerobic exercise training in women. *Journal of Strength Conditioning Research* 29(2): 297–304.

Schmidt, D., et al. 2016. The effect of high-intensity circuit training on physical fitness. *Journal of Sports Medicine and Physical Fitness* 56: 534–540.

Seery, S., et al. A metered intake of milk following exercise and thermal dehydration restores whole-body net fluid balance better than a carbohydrate-electrolyte solution or water in healthy young men. *British Journal of Nutrition* 116: 1013–1021.

Tafuri, S., et al. 2016. CrossFit athletes exhibit high symmetry of fundamental movement patterns. A cross-sectional study. *Muscles, Ligaments and Tendons Journal* 6:157–160.

Tsatsouline, P. 2010. *Enter the Kettlebell.* Minneapolis, MN: Dragon Door Publications.

Tucker, M. A., et al. 2013. The effect of caffeine on maximal oxygen uptake and vertical jump performance in male basketball players. *Journal of Strength and Conditioning Research* 27(2): 382–387.

Van de Vijver, P. L., et al. 2016. Early and extraordinary peaks in physical performance come with a longevity cost. *Aging* 8: 1822–1829.

Vechin, F. C., et al. 2015. Comparisons between low-intensity resistance training with blood flow restriction and high-intensity resistance training on quadriceps muscle mass and strength in elderly. *Journal of Strength and Conditioning Research* 29(4): 1071–1076.

Vikmoen, O., et al. 2016. Effects of heavy strength training on running performance and determinants of running performance in female endurance athletes. *PLoS One* 11: e0150799.

Villanueva, M. G., et al. 2015. Short rest interval lengths between sets optimally enhance body composition and performance with 8 weeks of strength resistance training in older men. *European Journal Applied Physiology* 115(2): 295–308.

Name _____ Section _____ Date _____

LAB 4.1 Assessing Your Current Level of Muscular Strength

For best results, don't do any strenuous weight training within 48 hours of any test. Use great caution when completing 1-RM tests; do not take the maximum bench press test if you have any injuries to your shoulders, elbows, back, hips, or knees. In addition, do not take these tests until you have had at least one month of weight training experience and competent instruction in the techniques.

The Maximum Bench Press Test

Equipment

The free weights bench press test uses the following equipment

1. Flat bench (with or without racks)
2. Barbell
3. Assorted weight plates with collars to hold them in place
4. One or two spotters
5. Weight scale

If a weight machine is preferred, use the following equipment:

1. Bench press machine
2. Weight scale

Preparation

Try a few bench presses with a small amount of weight so that you can practice your technique, warm up your muscles, and, if you use free weights, coordinate your movements with those of your spotters. Weigh yourself and record the results.

Body weight: _____ lb.

©Wayne Glusker

Instructions

1. Use a weight that is lower than the amount you believe you can lift. For free weights, men should begin with a weight about two-thirds of their body weight; women should begin with the weight of just the bar (45 lb).

2. Lie on the bench with your feet firmly on the floor. If you are using a weight machine, grasp the handles with palms away from you; the tops of the handles should be aligned with the tops of your armpits.

    If you are using free weights, grasp the bar slightly wider than shoulder width with your palms away from you. If you have one spotter, she or he should stand directly behind the bench; if you have two spotters, they should stand to the side, one at each end of the barbell. Signal to the spotter when you are ready to begin the test by saying, "1, 2, 3." On "3," the spotter should help you lift the weight to a point over your mid-chest (nipple line).

3. Push the handles or barbell until your arms are fully extended. Exhale as you lift. If you are using free weights, the weight moves from a low point at the chest straight up. Keep your feet firmly on the floor, don't arch your back, and push the weight evenly with your right and left arms. Don't bounce the weight on your chest.

4. Rest for several minutes, then repeat the lift with a heavier weight. It will probably take several attempts to determine the maximum amount of weight you can lift (1 RM).

    1 RM: _____ lb

    Check one: _____ Free weights _____ Universal _____ Other

5. If you used free weights, convert your free weights bench press score to an estimated value for 1 RM on the Universal bench press or other bench press machine using the appropriate formula:

    Males: Estimated Universal 1 RM = (1.016 × free weights 1 RM _____ lb) + 18.41 = _____ lb

    Females: Estimated Universal 1 RM = (0.848 × free weights 1 RM _____ lb) + 21.37 = _____ lb

(Note: this formula might not be accurate on other bench press machines.)

LABORATORY ACTIVITIES

Rating Your Bench Press Result

1. Divide your 1-RM value by your body weight.

    1 RM _____ lb ÷ body weight _____ lb = _____

2. Find this ratio in the table to determine your bench press strength rating. Record the rating here and in the chart at the end of this lab.

    Bench press strength rating: _____

Strength Ratings for the Maximum Bench Press Test

	Pounds Lifted/Body Weight (lb)					
Men	*Very Poor*	*Poor*	*Fair*	*Good*	*Excellent*	*Superior*
Age: Under 20	Below 0.89	0.89–1.05	1.06–1.18	1.19–1.33	1.34–1.75	Above 1.75
20–29	Below 0.88	0.88–0.98	0.99–1.13	1.14–1.31	1.32–1.62	Above 1.62
30–39	Below 0.78	0.78–0.87	0.88–0.97	0.98–1.11	1.12–1.34	Above 1.34
40–49	Below 0.72	0.72–0.79	0.80–0.87	0.88–0.99	1.00–1.19	Above 1.19
50–59	Below 0.63	0.63–0.70	0.71–0.78	0.79–0.89	0.90–1.04	Above 1.04
60 and over	Below 0.57	0.57–0.65	0.66–0.71	0.72–0.81	0.82–0.93	Above 0.93
Women						
Age: Under 20	Below 0.53	0.53–0.57	0.58–0.64	0.65–0.76	0.77–0.87	Above 0.87
20–29	Below 0.51	0.51–0.58	0.59–0.69	0.70–0.79	0.80–1.00	Above 1.00
30–39	Below 0.47	0.47–0.52	0.53–0.59	0.60–0.69	0.70–0.81	Above 0.81
40–49	Below 0.43	0.43–0.49	0.50–0.53	0.54–0.61	0.62–0.76	Above 0.76
50–59	Below 0.39	0.39–0.43	0.44–0.47	0.48–0.54	0.55–0.67	Above 0.67
60 and over	Below 0.38	0.38–0.42	0.43–0.46	0.47–0.53	0.54–0.71	Above 0.71

SOURCES: The Cooper Institute of Aerobic Research, Dallas, Tex; from *The Physical Fitness Specialist Manual,* revised 2005.

Predicting 1 RM from Multiple-Repetition Lifts Using Free Weights

Instead of doing the 1-RM maximum strength bench press test, you can predict your 1 RM from multiple-repetition lifts.

Instructions

1. Choose a weight you think you can bench press five times.

2. Follow the instructions for lifting the weight given in the maximum bench press test.

3. Do as many repetitions of the bench press as you can. A repetition counts only if done correctly

4. Refer to the chart below, or calculate predicted 1 RM using the Brzycki equation:

    1 RM = *weight* ÷ (1.0278 – [0.0278 × *number of repetitions*])

    1 RM = _____ lb ÷ (1.0278 – [0.0278 × _____ repetitions]) = _____

5. Divide your predicted 1-RM value by your body weight.

    1 RM _____ lb ÷ body weight _____ lb = _____

6. Find this ratio in the table above to determine your bench press strength rating. Record the rating here and in the chart at the end of the lab.

    Bench press strength rating: _____

RMs from the Multiple-Repetitions Bench Press Test

	Repetitions											
Weight Lifted (lb.)	*1*	*2*	*3*	*4*	*5*	*6*	*7*	*8*	*9*	*10*	*11*	*12*
66	66	68	70	72	74	77	79	82	85	88	91	95
77	77	79	82	84	87	89	92	96	99	103	107	111
88	88	91	93	96	99	102	106	109	113	117	122	127
99	99	102	105	108	111	115	119	123	127	132	137	143
110	110	113	116	120	124	128	132	137	141	147	152	158
121	121	124	128	132	136	141	145	150	156	161	168	174
132	132	136	140	144	149	153	158	164	170	176	183	190
143	143	147	151	156	161	166	172	178	184	191	198	206
154	154	158	163	168	173	179	185	191	198	205	213	222
165	165	170	175	180	186	192	198	205	212	220	229	238
176	176	181	186	192	198	204	211	219	226	235	244	254
187	187	192	198	204	210	217	224	232	240	249	259	269
198	198	204	210	216	223	230	238	246	255	264	274	285
209	209	215	221	228	235	243	251	259	269	279	289	301
220	220	226	233	240	248	256	264	273	283	293	305	317
231	231	238	245	252	260	268	277	287	297	308	320	333
242	242	249	256	264	272	281	290	300	311	323	335	349
253	253	260	268	276	285	294	304	314	325	337	350	364
264	264	272	280	288	297	307	317	328	340	352	366	380
275	275	283	291	300	309	319	330	341	354	367	381	396
286	286	294	303	312	322	332	343	355	368	381	396	412
297	297	305	314	324	334	345	356	369	382	396	411	428
308	308	317	326	336	347	358	370	382	396	411	427	444

SOURCES: Brzycki, M. January 1993. "Strength testing—predicting a one-rep max from reps to fatigue," *The Journal of Physical Education, Recreation and Dance*, vol. 64, , 88–90.

Functional Lower Body Movement Tests

The following tests assess functional leg movement skills using squats. Most people do squats improperly, increasing their risk of knee and back pain. Before you add weight-bearing squats to your weight training program, you should determine your functional leg movement skills, check your ability to squat properly, and give yourself a chance to master squatting movements. The following leg strength tests will help you in each of these areas.

These tests are progressively more difficult, so do not move to the next test until you have scored at least a 3 on the current test. On each test, give yourself a rating of 0, 1, 3, or 5, as described in the instructions that follow the last test.

1. Chair Squat

Instructions

1. Sit up straight in a chair with your back resting against the backrest and your arms at your sides. Your feet should be placed more than shoulder-width apart so that you can get them under the body.

2. Begin the motion of rising out of the chair by flexing (bending) at the hips—not the back. Then squat up using a hip hinge movement (no spine movement). Stand without rocking forward, bending your back, or using external support, and keep your head in a neutral position.

3. Return to the sitting position while maintaining a straight back and keeping your weight centered over your feet. Your thighs should abduct (spread) as you sit back in the chair. Use your rear hip and thigh muscles as much as possible as you sit.

Courtesy Tom Fahey

LABORATORY ACTIVITIES

Do five repetitions.

Your rating: _____

(See rating instructions that follow.)

2. Single-Leg Step-Up

Instructions

1. Stand facing a bench, with your right foot placed on the middle of the bench, right knee bent at 90 degrees, and arms at your sides.

2. Step up on the bench until your right leg is straight, maximizing the use of the hip muscles.

3. Return to the starting position. Keep your hips stable, back straight, chest up, shoulders back, and head neutral during the entire movement.

Do five repetitions for each leg.

Your rating: _____

(See rating instructions that follow.)

©Wayne Glusker

3. Unweighted Squat

Instructions

1. Stand with your feet placed slightly more than shoulder-width apart, toes pointed out slightly, hands on hips or across your chest, head neutral, and back straight. Center your weight over your arches or slightly behind.

2. Squat down, keeping your weight centered over your arches and actively flexing (bending) your hips until your legs break parallel. During the movement, keep your back straight, shoulders back, and chest out, and let your thighs part to the side so that you are "squatting between your legs."

3. Push back up to the starting position, hinging at the hips and not with the spine, maximizing the use of the rear hip and thigh muscles, and maintaining a straight back and neutral head position.

Do five repetitions.

Your rating: _____

(See rating instructions that follow.)

©Wayne Glusker

4. Single-Leg Lunge-Squat with Rear-Foot Support

Instructions

1. Stand about three feet in front of a bench (with your back to the bench).
2. Place the top of your left foot on the bench, and put most of your weight on your right leg (your left leg should be bent), with your hands at your sides.
3. Squat on your right leg until your thigh is parallel with the floor. Keep your back straight, chest up, shoulders back, and head neutral.
4. Return to the starting position.

Do three repetitions for each leg.
Your rating: _____
(See rating instructions that follow.)

©Wayne Glusker

Rating Your Functional Leg Strength Test Results

5 points: Performed the exercise properly with good back and thigh position, weight centered over the middle or rear of the foot, chest out, and shoulders back; good use of hip muscles on the way down and on the way up, with head in a neutral position throughout the movement; maintained good form during all repetitions; abducted (spread) the thighs on the way down during chair squats and double-leg squats; for single-leg exercises, showed good strength on both sides; for single-leg lunge-squat with rear-foot support, maintained straight back, and knees stayed behind toes.

3 points: Weight was forward on the toes, with some rounding of the back; used thigh muscles excessively, with little use of hip muscles; head and chest were too far forward; showed little abduction of the thighs during double-leg squats; when going down for single-leg exercises, one side was stronger than the other; form deteriorated with repetitions; for single-leg lunge-squat with rear-foot support, could not reach parallel (thigh parallel with floor).

1 point: Had difficulty performing the movement, rocking forward and rounding back badly; used thigh muscles excessively, with little use of hip muscles on the way up or on the way down; chest and head were forward; on unweighted squats, had difficulty reaching parallel and showed little abduction of the thighs; on single-leg exercises, one leg was markedly stronger than the other; could not perform multiple repetitions.

0 points: Could not perform the exercise.

Summary of Results

Maximum bench press test from either the 1-RM test or the multiple-repetition test: Weight pressed: _____ lb   Rating: _____
Functional leg strength tests (0–5): Chair squat: _____ Single-leg step-up: _____ Unweighted squat: _____
Single-leg lunge-squat with rear-foot support: _____
Remember that muscular strength is specific: Your ratings may vary considerably for different parts of your body.

LABORATORY ACTIVITIES

Using Your Results

How did you score? Are you surprised by your ratings for muscular strength? Are you satisfied with your current ratings?

If you're not satisfied, set realistic goals for improvement:

Are you satisfied with your current level of muscular strength as evidenced in your daily life—for example, your ability to lift objects, climb stairs, and engage in sports and recreational activities?

If you're not satisfied, set realistic goals for improvement:

What should you do next? Enter the results of this lab in the Preprogram Assessment column in Appendix B. If you've set goals for improvement, begin planning your strength training program by completing the plan in Lab 4.3. After several weeks of your program, complete this lab again and enter the results in the Postprogram Assessment column of Appendix B. How do the results compare?

Name_____ Section _____ Date _____

LAB 4.2 Assessing Your Current Level of Muscular Endurance

For best results, don't do any strenuous weight training within 48 hours of any test. To assess endurance of the abdominal muscles, perform the curl-up test. To assess endurance of muscles in the upper body, perform the push-up test. To assess endurance of the muscles in the lower body, perform the squat endurance test.

The Curl-Up Test

Equipment

1. Two six-inch strips of self-stick Velcro or heavy tape
2. Ruler
3. Partner
4. Mat (optional)

Preparation

Affix the strips of Velcro or long strips of tape on the mat or testing surface. Place the strips 3 inches apart.

Instructions

1. Start by lying on your back on the floor or mat, arms straight and by your sides, shoulders relaxed, palms down and on the floor, and fingers straight. Adjust your position so that the longest fingertip of each hand touches the end of the near strip of Velcro or tape. Your knees should be bent about 90 degrees, with your feet about 12–18 inches from your buttocks.

2. To perform a curl-up, flex your spine while sliding your fingers across the floor until the fingertips of each hand reach the second strip of Velcro or tape. Then return to the starting position; the shoulders must be returned to touch the mat between curl-ups, but the head need not touch. Shoulders must remain relaxed throughout the curl-up, and feet and buttocks must stay on the floor. Breathe easily, exhaling during the lift phase of the curl-up; do not hold your breath.

3. Once your partner says "go," perform as many curl-ups as you can at a steady pace with correct form. Your partner counts the curl-ups you perform and calls a stop to the test if she or he notices any incorrect form or drop in your pace.

   Number of curl-ups: _____

Both photos courtesy of Neil A. Tanner

LABORATORY ACTIVITIES

Rating Your Curl-Up Test Result

Your score is the number of completed curl-ups. Refer to the appropriate portion of the table for a rating of your abdominal muscular endurance. Record your rating below and in the summary at the end of this lab.

Rating: _____

Ratings for the Curl-Up Test

	Number of Curl-Ups					
Men	*Very Poor*	*Poor*	*Average*	*Good*	*Excellent*	*Superior*
Age: 16–19	Below 48	48–57	58–64	65–74	75–93	Above 93
20–29	Below 46	46–54	55–63	64–74	75–93	Above 93
30–39	Below 40	40–47	48–55	56–64	65–81	Above 81
40–49	Below 38	38–45	46–53	54–62	63–79	Above 79
50–59	Below 36	36–43	44–51	52–60	61–77	Above 77
60–69	Below 33	33–40	41–48	49–57	58–74	Above 74
Women						
Age: 16–19	Below 42	42–50	51–58	59–67	68–84	Above 84
20–29	Below 41	41–51	52–57	58–66	67–83	Above 83
30–39	Below 38	38–47	48–56	57–66	67–83	Above 83
40–49	Below 36	36–45	46–54	55–64	65–83	Above 83
50–59	Below 34	34–43	44–52	53–62	63–81	Above 81
60–69	Below 31	31–40	41–49	50–59	60–78	Above 78

SOURCE: Ratings based on norms calculated from data collected by Robert Lualhati on 4545 college students, 16–80 years of age, at Skyline College, San Bruno, Calif.

The Push-Up Test

Equipment:

Mat or towel (optional)

Preparation

In this test, you will perform either standard push-ups or modified push-ups, in which you support yourself with your knees. The Cooper Institute developed the ratings for this test with men performing push-ups and women performing modified push-ups. Biologically, males tend to be stronger than females; the modified technique reduces the need for upper-body strength in a test of muscular endurance. Therefore, for an accurate assessment of upper-body endurance, men should perform standard push-ups and women should perform modified push-ups. However, in using push-ups as part of a strength training program, individuals should choose the technique most appropriate for increasing their level of strength and endurance—regardless of gender.

Instructions

1. *For push-ups:* Start in the push-up position with your body supported by your hands and feet. *For modified push-ups:* Start in the modified push-up position with your body supported by your hands and knees. *For both positions,* keep your arms and your back straight and your fingers pointed forward.

2. Lower your chest to the floor with your back straight, and then return to the starting position.

Both photos courtesy of Neil A. Tanner

3. Perform as many push-ups or modified push-ups as you can without stopping.

Number of push-ups: _____ Number of modified push-ups: _____

Rating Your Push-Up Test Result

Your score is the number of completed push-ups or modified push-ups. Refer to the appropriate portion of the table for a rating of your upper-body endurance. Record your rating below and in the summary at the end of this lab.

Rating: _____

Ratings for the Push-Up and Modified Push-Up Tests

	Number of Push-Ups					
Men	*Very Poor*	*Poor*	*Fair*	*Good*	*Excellent*	*Superior*
Age: 18–29	Below 22	22–28	29–36	37–46	47–61	Above 61
30–39	Below 17	17–23	24–29	30–38	39–51	Above 51
40–49	Below 11	11–17	18–23	24–29	30–39	Above 39
50–59	Below 9	9–12	13–18	19–24	25–38	Above 38
60 and over	Below 6	6–9	10–17	18–22	23–27	Above 27
	Number of Modified Push-Ups					
Women	*Very Poor*	*Poor*	*Fair*	*Good*	*Excellent*	*Superior*
Age: 18–29	Below 17	17–22	23–29	30–35	36–44	Above 44
30–39	Below 11	11–18	19–23	24–30	31–38	Above 38
40–49	Below 6	6–12	13–17	18–23	24–32	Above 32
50–59	Below 6	6–11	12–16	17–20	21–27	Above 27
60 and over	Below 2	2–4	5–11	12–14	15–19	Above 19

SOURCE: *The Physical Fitness Specialist Manual,* The Cooper Institute of Aerobic Research: Dallas, TX, revised 2002.

The Squat Endurance Test

Instructions

1. Stand with your feet placed slightly more than shoulder-width apart, toes pointed out slightly hands on hips or across your chest, head neutral, and back straight. Center your weight over your arches or slightly behind.

2. Squat down, keeping your weight centered over your arches, until your thighs are parallel with the floor. Push back up to the starting position, maintaining a straight back and neutral head position.

3. Perform as many squats as you can without stopping.

    Number of squats: _____

Rating Your Squat Endurance Test Result

Your score is the number of completed squats. Refer to the appropriate portion of the table for a rating of your leg muscular endurance. Record your rating below and in the summary at the end of this lab.

Rating: _____

©Wayne Glusker

LABORATORY ACTIVITIES

Ratings for the Squat Endurance Test

Number of Squats Performed

Men	Very Poor	Poor	Below Average	Average	Above Average	Good	Excellent
Age: 18–25	<25	25–30	31–34	35–38	39–43	44–49	>49
26–35	<22	22–28	29–30	31–34	35–39	40–45	>45
36–45	<17	17–22	23–26	27–29	30–34	35–41	>41
46–55	<13	13–17	18–21	22–24	25–28	29–35	>35
56–65	<9	9–12	13–16	17–20	21–24	25–31	>31
65+	<7	7–10	11–14	15–18	19–21	22–28	>28
Women	**Very Poor**	**Poor**	**Below Average**	**Average**	**Above Average**	**Good**	**Excellent**
Age: 18–25	<18	18–24	25–28	29–32	33–36	37–43	>43
26–35	<13	13–20	21–24	25–28	29–32	33–39	>39
36–45	<7	7–14	15–18	19–22	23–26	27–33	>33
46–55	<5	5–9	10–13	14–17	18–21	22–27	>27
56–65	<3	3–6	7–9	10–12	13–17	18–24	>24
65+	<2	2–4	5–10	11–13	14–16	17–23	>23

SOURCE: www.topendsports.com/testing/tests/home-squat.htm

Summary of Results

Curl-up test: Number of curl-ups: _____ Rating: _____

Push-up test: Number of push-ups: _____ Rating: _____

Squat endurance test: Number of squats: _____ Rating: _____

Remember that muscular endurance is specific: Your ratings may vary considerably for different parts of your body.

Using Your Results

How did you score? Are you surprised by your ratings for muscular endurance? Are you satisfied with your current ratings?

If you're not satisfied, set realistic goals for improvement:

Are you satisfied with your current level of muscular endurance as evidenced in your daily life—for example, your ability to carry groceries or your books, hike, and do yard work?

If you're not satisfied, set realistic goals for improvement:

What should you do next? Enter the results of this lab in the Preprogram Assessment column in Appendix B. If you've set goals for improvement, begin planning your strength training program by completing the plan in Lab 4.3. After several weeks of your program, complete this lab again and enter the results in the Postprogram Assessment column of Appendix B. How do the results compare?

Name _____   Section _____   Date _____

LAB 4.3   Designing and Monitoring a Strength Training Program

1. *Set goals.* List goals for your strength training program. Your goals can be specific or general, short or long term. In the first section, include specific, measurable goals that you can use to track the progress of your fitness program—for example, raising your upper-body muscular strength rating from fair to good or being able to complete 10 repetitions of a lat pull with 125 pounds of resistance. In the second section, include long-term and more qualitative goals, such as improving self-confidence and reducing your risk for back pain.

Specific Goals: Current Status   Final Goals

_____   _____

_____   _____

_____   _____

Other goals: _____

_____

2. *Choose exercises.* Based on your goals, choose 8–10 exercises to perform during each weight training session. If your goal is general training for wellness, use the sample program in Figure 4.4. List your exercises and the muscles they develop in your program plan.

3. *Frequency: Choose the number of training sessions per week.* Work out at least two nonconsecutive days per week. Indicate the days you will train in your program plan; be sure to include days of rest to allow your body to recover.

4. *Intensity: Choose starting weights.* Experiment with different amounts of weight until you settle on a good starting weight, one that you can lift easily for 10–12 repetitions. As you progress in your program, add more weight. Fill in the starting weight for each exercise in your program plan.

5. *Time: Choose a starting number of sets and repetitions.* Include at least one set of 8–12 repetitions of each exercise. (When you add weight, you may have to decrease the number of repetitions slightly until your muscles adapt to the heavier load.) If your program is focusing on strength alone, your sets can contain fewer repetitions using a heavier load. If you are over approximately age 50–60, your sets should contain more repetitions (10–15) using a lighter load. Fill in the starting number of sets and repetitions of each exercise in your program plan.

6. *Volume.* Choose a training volume (weight lifted multiplied by number of reps and sets) that promotes progress and that you will do consistently. Vary the components from time to time—for example, increase the weight on some days and the sets and reps on other days.

7. *Monitor your progress.* Use a phone app or the workout card here to monitor your progress and keep track of exercises, weights, sets, and repetitions.

Many excellent weight training program apps, such as the Beast Sensor, Strong, and Stronger are available for smartphones. The Beast Sensor includes a wearable accelerometer that tracks power and strength and stores workout data on the cloud. Though sophisticated and motivating, it is fairly expensive. Strong and Stronger are low-cost apps that serve as online workout cards and can also store data on the cloud.

Program Plan for Weight Training											
Exercise	Muscle(s) Developed	Frequency (✓)							Intensity: Weight (lb.)	Time	
		M	T	W	Th	F	Sa	Su		Repetitions	Sets

LABORATORY ACTIVITIES

WORKOUT CARD FOR _____

Exercise/Date																																							
Wt																																								
Sets																																								
Reps																																								

5 Flexibility and Low-Back Health

LOOKING AHEAD...

After reading this chapter, you should be able to

- Identify the potential benefits of flexibility and stretching exercises.
- List the factors that affect a joint's flexibility.
- Describe the types of stretching exercises and how they affect muscles.
- Describe the frequency, intensity, duration, volume, and progression for a successful flexibility program.
- List safe stretching exercises for major joints.
- Explain how low-back pain can be prevented and managed.

TEST YOUR KNOWLEDGE

1. Static stretching exercises should be performed
   a. at the start of a warm-up.
   b. first thing in the morning.
   c. after endurance exercise or strength training.

2. If you injure your back, it's usually best to rest in bed until the pain is completely gone. True or false?

3. It is better to hold a stretch for a short time than to "bounce" while stretching. True or false?

See answers on the next page.

©Sebastian Gauert/123RF

lexibility—the ability of a joint to move through its normal, full **range of motion**—is important for general fitness and wellness. Flexibility is a highly adaptable physical fitness component: It increases in response to a regular program of stretching exercises and decreases with inactivity. Flexibility is also specific: Good flexibility in one joint doesn't necessarily mean good flexibility in another. You can increase your overall flexibility by doing regular stretching exercises for all your major joints.

This chapter describes the factors that affect flexibility and the benefits of maintaining good flexibility. It provides guidelines for assessing your current level of flexibility and putting together a successful stretching program. It also examines the common problem of low-back pain.

TYPES OF FLEXIBILITY

There are two types of flexibility:

- *Static flexibility* is the ability to hold an extended position at one end or point in a joint's range of motion. For example, static flexibility determines how far you can extend your arm across the front of your body or out to the side. Static flexibility depends on your ability to tolerate stretched muscles, the structure of your joints, and the elasticity of muscles.

- *Dynamic flexibility* is the ability to move a joint through its range of motion with little resistance. It would affect your ability to pitch a ball or swing a golf club. Dynamic flexibility depends on static flexibility, but it also involves strength, coordination, and resistance to movement.

Dynamic flexibility is important for daily activities and sports. But because static flexibility is easier to measure and better researched, most assessment tests and stretching programs target that type of flexibility.

WHAT DETERMINES FLEXIBILITY?

The flexibility of a joint is affected by its structure, by muscle elasticity and length, and by nervous system regulation. Joint structure can't be changed, but other factors, such as the length of resting muscle fibers, can be changed through exercise; these factors should be the focus of a program to develop flexibility.

Joint Structure

How flexible a joint is depends partly on the nature and structure of the joint (Figure 5.1). Hinge joints such as those in your fingers and knees allow only limited forward and backward movement; they lock when fully extended. Ball-and-socket joints like the hip enable movement in many directions and provide for a greater range of motion. **Joint capsules**, semielastic structures that give joints strength and stability but limit movement, surround the major joints. The bone surfaces within the joint are lined with cartilage and separated by a joint cavity containing *synovial fluid,* which cushions the bones and reduces friction as the joint moves. Breakdown in joint cartilage from injury or aging leads to **arthritis**, which severely limits joint flexibility. Ligaments, both inside and outside the joint capsule, strengthen and reinforce the joint.

Heredity plays a part in joint structure and flexibility. For example, although everyone has a broad range of motion in the hip joint, not everyone can do a split. Gender may also play a role. Some studies have found that women have greater flexibility in certain joints.

Muscle Elasticity and Length

Soft tissues—including skin, muscles, tendons, and ligaments—also affect the flexibility of a joint. Muscle tissue is the key to developing flexibility because regular stretching can lengthen it. The most important component of muscle tissue related to flexibility is the connective tissue that envelops every part of muscle

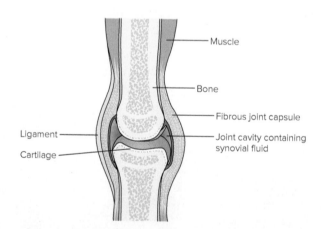

Muscle

Bone

Fibrous joint capsule

Joint cavity containing synovial fluid

Ligament

Cartilage

FIGURE 5.1   Basic joint structures.

range of motion   The full motion possible in a joint.   **TERMS**

joint capsules   Semielastic structures, composed primarily of connective tissue, that surround major joints.

arthritis   A disorder of the joints characterized by joint pain, stiffness, and inflammation. Osteoarthritis, the most common form, is a degenerative joint disease. Rheumatoid arthritis is an autoimmune disease that typically affects the hands and feet.

soft tissues   Tissues of the human body that include skin, fat, linings of internal organs and blood vessels, connective tissues, tendons, ligaments, muscles, and nerves.

tissue, from individual muscle fibers to entire muscles. Connective tissue provides structure, elasticity, and bulk and makes up about 30% of muscle mass. Two principal types of connective tissue are **collagen**—white fibers that provide structure and support—and **elastin**—yellow fibers that are elastic and flexible. The collagen and elastin are closely intertwined, so muscle tissue exhibits the properties of both types of fibers. A structural protein in muscles called *titin* also has elastic properties and contributes to flexibility.

When a muscle is stretched, the wavelike elastin fibers straighten; when the stretch is relieved, they rapidly snap back to their resting position. This temporary lengthening is called **elastic elongation**. If stretched gently and regularly, connective tissues may lengthen and flexibility may improve. This long-term lengthening is called **plastic elongation**. Without regular stretching, the process reverses: These tissues shorten, resulting in decreased flexibility. Regular stretching may contribute to flexibility by lengthening muscle fibers through the addition of contractile units called *sarcomeres.*

A muscle can tolerate a limited amount of stretch. As the limits of its flexibility are reached, connective tissue becomes more brittle and may rupture if overstretched. A safe and effective program stretches muscles enough to slightly elongate the tissues but not so much that they are damaged. Research has shown that flexibility is improved best by stretching when muscles are warm (following exercise or the application of heat) and the stretch is applied gradually and conservatively. Sudden, high-stress stretching is less effective and can lead to muscle damage.

Nervous System Regulation

Proprioceptors are nerves that send information about changes in the muscular and skeletal systems to the nervous system, which responds with signals to help control the speed, strength, and coordination of muscle contractions. When a muscle is stretched (lengthened), proprioceptors detect the amount and rate of the change in muscle length. The nerves send a signal to the spinal cord, which then sends a signal back to the muscle, triggering a muscle contraction that resists the change in muscle length. Another signal is sent to the opposing muscle (**antagonist**), causing it to relax and facilitate contraction of the stretched (agonist) muscle. These reflexes occur frequently in active muscles and allow for fine control of muscle length and movement. Muscle flexibility is linked to strength. Practicing lower-body eccentric exercise (lengthening contractions) increases strength and flexibility and might decrease the risk of lower-body muscle injury.

Small movements that only slightly stimulate the nerves cause small reflex actions. Rapid, powerful, and sudden changes in muscle length strongly stimulate the nerve receptors and can cause large and powerful reflex muscle contractions. Thus, stretches that involve rapid, bouncy movements can be dangerous and cause injury. Each bounce causes a reflex contraction, which means a muscle might be stretching at the same time it is contracting. Performing a gradual stretch and then holding it allows the proprioceptors to adjust to the new muscle length and to reduce the signals sent to the spine, thereby allowing muscles to lengthen and, over time, improving flexibility.

The stretching technique called *proprioceptive neuromuscular facilitation (PNF),* described later, takes advantage of

nerve activity to improve flexibility. For example, contracting a muscle prior to stretching it can help allow the muscle to stretch farther. The advanced strength training technique called plyometrics (Chapter 4) also takes advantage of the nervous system action in stretching and contracting muscles.

Modifying nervous control through movement and specific exercises is the best way to improve the functional range of motion. Regular stretching trains the proprioceptors to allow the muscles to lengthen. Proprioceptors adapt quickly to stretching (or lack of stretching), so frequent stretching helps develop flexibility. Stretching before exercising, however, can disturb proprioceptors and interfere with motor control during exercise. This is another good reason to stretch *after* exercising.

BENEFITS OF FLEXIBILITY

Good flexibility provides benefits for the entire musculoskeletal system. Flexibility training increases range of motion, and it may prevent muscle strains. As long as you don't overstretch, flexibility training will increase strength and the quality of movement, which might decrease the risk of some sports injuries. Most studies, however, show that stretching does not prevent overuse injuries.

Joint Health

Good flexibility is essential to good joint health. When the muscles and other tissues that support a joint are tight, the joint is subject to abnormal stresses that can cause joint deterioration. For example, tight thigh muscles cause excessive pressure on the kneecap, leading to pain in the knee joint. Poor joint flexibility can also cause abnormalities in joint lubrication, leading to deterioration of the sensitive cartilage cells lining the joint; pain and further joint injury can result.

Improved flexibility can greatly improve your quality of life, particularly as you get older. People tend to exercise less as they age, leading to loss of joint mobility and increased incidence of joint pain. Aging also decreases the natural elasticity of muscles, tendons, and joints, resulting in stiffness. The problem is often compounded by arthritis (see the box "Does Physical Activity Increase or Decrease the Risk of Bone and Joint Disease?"). Good joint flexibility may help prevent arthritis, and stretching

---

collagen   White fibers that provide structure and support in connective tissue.   **TERMS**

elastin   Yellow fibers that make connective tissue flexible.

elastic elongation   Temporary change in the length of muscles, tendons, and supporting connective tissues.

plastic elongation   Long-term change in the length of muscles, tendons, and supporting connective tissues.

proprioceptor   A nerve that sends information about the muscular and skeletal systems to the nervous system.

antagonist muscle   A muscle that opposes the action of another. For example, the biceps brachii muscle (agonist) flexes the elbow, while the triceps brachius (antagonist) extends the elbow.

THE EVIDENCE FOR EXERCISE
Does Physical Activity Increase or Decrease the Risk of Bone and Joint Disease?

Most college students don't worry much about fall-related fractures or chronic bone-related illnesses, such as **osteoporosis** (loss of bone mass) or osteoarthritis (degeneration of the cartilage inside joints). Even so, bone health should be a concern throughout life. This is because girls amass 85% of their adult bone mass by age 18, and boys build the same amount by age 20, but most people begin losing bone mass around age 30. For many people, poor diet and lack of exercise accelerate bone loss. According to the National Osteoporosis Foundation, 10 million Americans have osteoporosis. Meanwhile, 34 million Americans are at risk of the disease because of low bone mass. Overall, osteoporosis is a health threat for about 55% of Americans age 50 and older.

Getting enough nutrients is important for bone health (see Chapter 8), but there is mounting evidence that exercise can also help preserve or improve bone health. For example, several studies have shown an inverse relationship between physical activity and the risk for bone fractures. That is, the more you exercise, the less likely you are to suffer fractures, especially of the upper leg and hip. Research has not determined conclusively how much exercise is required to reduce fracture risk, but people who walk at least four hours per week and devote at least one hour per week to other forms of physical activity appear to reduce that risk. These findings seem to be consistent for women and men, but because some studies disagree on this point, further research is needed.

One way that exercise helps both men and women is by increasing the mineral density of bones, or at least by decreasing the loss of mineral density over time. Several one-year-long studies found that exercise can increase bone mineral density by 1–2% per year, which is significant—especially considering that the same amount of bone mineral density can be lost every one to four years in older persons. Currently, the American College of Sports Medicine recommends that adults perform weight-bearing physical activities (such as walking) three to five days per week and strength training exercises two or three days per week to increase bone mass or avoid loss of mineral density. They also recommend that adults practice neuromotor exercise training exercises, such as yoga or tai chi, to prevent falls and bone fractures. Exercise is particularly important in lactating (breastfeeding) women for preventing bone loss.

The evidence is less conclusive for the effect of exercise on osteoarthritis but still fairly positive. All experts agree that regular, moderate-intensity exercise is necessary for joint health. However, they also warn that vigorous or too-frequent

©Tim Platt/Iconica/Getty Images

exercise may contribute to joint damage and encourage the onset of osteoarthritis. For this reason, experts try to strike a balance in their exercise recommendations, especially for those with a family history of osteoarthritis. Research seems to support this cautious approach. Some studies have found that regular physical activity (as recommended for general health) at least does not increase osteoarthritis risk. Other studies show that moderate activity may provide some protection against the disease, but this evidence is limited.

A few studies also reveal that the type of exercise you do may increase your risk. For example, competitive or strenuous sports such as ballet, orienteering, football, basketball, soccer, and tennis have been associated with the disease, whereas sports such as cross-country skiing, running, swimming, biking, and walking have not.

The bottom line is that the earlier in life you become physically active, the greater your protection against bone loss and bone-related diseases. However, if you have a family history of osteoporosis or osteoarthritis, or if you have already developed symptoms of one of these ailments, be sure to talk to your physician before beginning an exercise program.

SOURCE: American College of Sports Medicine. 2018. *ACSM's Guidelines for Exercise Testing and Prescription,* 10th ed. Philadelphia: Wolters Kluwer; Giangregorio, L. M., et al. 2015. "Too Fit to Fracture: Outcomes of a Delphi consensus process on physical activity and exercise recommendations for adults with osteoporosis with or without vertebral fractures," *Osteoporosis International* 26(3), 891–910; American College of Sports Medicine. 2004. "ACSM position stand: Physical activity and bone health," *Medicine and Science in Sports and Exercise* 36(11), 1985–1996.

Box icon: ©Vstock LLC/Getty Images RF

may lessen pain in people who have the condition. Another benefit of good joint flexibility for older adults is that it increases balance and stability.

osteoporosis   A condition in which the bones become extremely thin and brittle and break easily; due largely to insufficient calcium intake.

TERMS

Prevention of Low-Back Pain and Injuries

Poor spinal stability puts pressure on the nerves leading out from the spinal column and can lead to low-back pain. Strength and flexibility in the back, pelvis, and thighs may help prevent this type of back pain but may or may not improve back health or reduce the risk of injury. Good hip an d knee flexibility protects the spine from excessive motion during the tasks of daily living.

Although scientific evidence is limited, people with either high or low flexibility seem to have an increased risk of injury. Extreme flexibility reduces joint stability, and poor flexibility limits a joint's range of motion. Persons of average fitness should try to attain normal flexibility in joints throughout the body, meaning each joint can move through its normal range of motion with no difficulty. Stretching programs are particularly important for older adults, people engaged in high-power sports that require rapid changes in direction (such as football and tennis), workers involved in brief bouts of intense exertion (such as police officers and firefighters), and people who sit for prolonged periods (such as office workers and students).

However, as we have seen, static stretching *before* a high-intensity activity (such as sprinting or basketball) may increase the risk of injury by interfering with neuromuscular control and reducing muscles' natural ability to stretch and contract. When injuries occur, flexibility exercises can reduce symptoms and help restore normal range of motion in affected joints.

Additional Potential Benefits of Flexibility

- *Relief of aches and pains.* Studying or working in one place for a long time can make your muscles tense. Stretching helps relieve tension and joint stiffness, so that you can go back to work refreshed and effective. Stretching reduces the symptoms of exercise-induced muscle damage, and flexible muscles are less susceptible to the damage.
- *Relief of muscle cramps.* Recent research suggests that exercise-related muscle cramps are caused by increased electrical activity within the affected muscle. The best treatment for muscle cramps is gentle stretching, which reduces the electrical activity and allows the muscle to relax.
- *Improved body position and strength for sports (and life).* Good flexibility lets you assume more efficient body positions and exert force through a greater range of motion. For example, swimmers with more flexible shoulders have stronger strokes because they can pull their arms through the water in the optimal position. Some studies also suggest that flexibility training enhances strength development.
- *Maintenance of good posture and balance.* Good flexibility also contributes to body symmetry and good posture. Bad posture can gradually change your body structures. Sitting in a slumped position, for example, can lead to tightness in the muscles in the front of your chest and overstretching and looseness in the upper spine, causing a rounding of the upper back. This condition, called *kyphosis,* is common in older people. Stretching regularly may prevent it.
- *Relaxation.* Flexibility exercises, particularly when practiced in combination with yoga or tai chi, reduce mental tension, slow your breathing rate, and reduce blood pressure.
- *Improving impaired mobility.* Stretching often decreases pain and improves functional capacity in people with arthritis, stroke, or muscle and nerve diseases and in people who are recovering from surgery or injury.

Wellness Tip Flexibility training helps maintain pain-free joints as you age. You don't have to be at the gym to stretch. There are lots of simple, small-movement stretches you can do anywhere—whether at your desk or on the go. For some examples, visit a good health website such as http://www.MayoClinic.com and search for "stretching exercises."
©Image Source/Alamy Stock Photo RF

ASSESSING FLEXIBILITY

Because flexibility is specific to each joint, there are no tests of general flexibility. The most commonly used flexibility test is the sit-and-reach test, which rates the flexibility of the muscles in the lower back and hamstrings. To assess your flexibility and identify inflexible joints, complete Lab 5.1.

CREATING A SUCCESSFUL PROGRAM TO DEVELOP FLEXIBILITY

A successful program for developing flexibility includes safe exercises executed with the most effective techniques. Your goal should be to attain normal flexibility in the major joints. Balanced flexibility (not too much or too little) provides joint stability and facilitates smooth, economical movement patterns. You can achieve balanced flexibility by performing stretching exercises regularly and by using a variety of stretches and stretching techniques.

Applying the FITT-VP Principle

As with other programs, the acronym FITT-VP can be used to remember key components of a stretching program: **F**requency, **I**ntensity, **T**ime, **T**ype, **V**olume, and **P**rogression of exercise.

Frequency The American College of Sports Medicine (ACSM) recommends that stretching exercises be performed at least two or three days per week, but more often is even better. To prevent injury and improve flexibility, it's best to stretch when your muscles are warm, either after a warm-up or after cardiorespiratory endurance exercise or weight training.

As described earlier, static stretching can adversely affect muscle performance in the short term. So, if you are planning a workout for which high performance is important, it is best to perform static stretches after your workout but while your muscles are still warm and your joints are lubricated. Stretching isn't the same thing as a cool-down, so be sure to do the cardiorespiratory cool-down first, so that you can transition to a lower level of intensity before stretching. If the plan for your workout includes a moderate activity like walking, then static stretching prior to your workout isn't likely to impact performance in a significant way.

Dynamic stretching, described in the next section, may have less of an impact on muscle performance and so is sometimes included as part of an active warm-up. However, dynamic stretching is more challenging to learn and perform.

Intensity and Time (Duration) For each exercise, slowly stretch your muscles to the point of slight tension or mild discomfort—but not to the point of pain. Hold the stretch for 10–30 seconds. As you hold the stretch, the feeling of slight tension should subside slowly; at that point, try to stretch a bit farther. Throughout the stretch, try to relax and breathe easily. Rest for about 30–60 seconds between each stretch, and do 2–4 repetitions of each stretch for a total of 60 seconds per exercise. A complete flexibility workout usually takes about 10–30 minutes (Figure 5.2).

Types of Stretching Techniques Stretching techniques vary from simply stretching the muscles during the course of normal activities to sophisticated methods based on patterns of muscle reflexes. Improper stretching can do more harm than good, so it's important to understand the different types of stretching exercises and how they affect the muscles. Four common techniques are static stretches, ballistic stretches, dynamic stretches, and proprioceptive neuromuscular facilitation (PNF).

STATIC STRETCHING   In **static stretching**, each muscle is gradually stretched, and the stretch is held for 10–30 seconds. A slow stretch prompts less reaction from proprioceptors, and the muscles can safely stretch farther than usual. Static stretching is the type most often recommended by fitness experts because it is safe and effective.

The key to this technique is to stretch the muscles and joints to the point where a pull is felt, but not to the point of pain.

---

static stretching   A technique in which a muscle is slowly and gently stretched and then held in the stretched position.

ballistic stretching   A technique in which muscles are stretched by the force generated as a body part is repeatedly bounced, swung, or jerked.

dynamic stretching   A technique in which muscles are stretched by moving joints slowly and fluidly through their range of motion in a controlled manner; also called *functional stretching*.

passive stretching   A technique in which muscles are stretched by force applied by an outside source.

active stretching   A technique in which muscles are stretched by the contraction of the opposing muscles.

Warm-up 5–10 minutes or following an endurance or strength training workout	Stretching exercises for major joints **Sample program**	
	Exercise	*Areas stretched*
	Head turns and tilts	Neck
	Towel stretch	Triceps, shoulders, chest
	Across-the-body and overhead stretches	Shoulders, upper back, back of arm
	Upper-back stretch	Upper back
	Lateral stretch	Trunk muscles
	Step stretch	Hip, front of thigh
	Side lunge	Inner thigh, hip, calf
	Inner-thigh stretch	Inner thigh, hip
	Hip and trunk stretch	Trunk, outer thigh, hip, buttocks, lower back
	Modified hurdler stretch	Back of thigh, lower back
	Alternate leg stretcher	Back of thigh, hip, knee, ankle, buttocks
	Lower-leg stretch	Calf, soleus, Achilles tendon

Frequency: 2 or 3 days per week (minimum); 5–7 days per week (ideal).

Intensity: Stretch to the point of mild discomfort, not pain.

Time (duration): Hold static stretches for 10–30 seconds.

Type of activity: Stretching exercises that focus on major joints.

Volume: Perform 2–4 repetitions for a total stretching time of 60 seconds for each exercise.

Progression: Progressively build flexibility, striving for a normal range of motion; avoid excessive flexibility.

FIGURE 5.2   The FITT-VP principle for a flexibility program.

(One note of caution: Excess static stretching can decrease joint stability and increase the risk of injury. This may be a particular concern for women, whose joints are less stable and more flexible than are men's.) The sample stretching program presented later in this chapter features static stretching exercises.

BALLISTIC STRETCHING   In **ballistic stretching**, the muscles are stretched suddenly in a forceful bouncing movement. For example, touching the toes repeatedly in rapid succession is a ballistic stretch for the hamstrings. A problem with this technique is that the heightened activity of proprioceptors caused by the rapid stretches can continue for some time, possibly causing injuries during any physical activities that follow. Another concern is that triggering strong responses from the nerves can cause a reflex muscle contraction that makes it harder to stretch. For these reasons, ballistic stretching is usually not recommended, especially for people of average fitness.

Ballistic stretching trains the muscle dynamically, so it can be an appropriate stretching technique for some well-trained athletes. For example, tennis players stretch their hamstrings and quadriceps ballistically when they lunge for a ball during a tennis match. Because this movement is part of their sport, they might benefit from ballistic training of these muscle groups.

DYNAMIC (FUNCTIONAL) STRETCHING   The emphasis in **dynamic stretching** is on functional movements. Dynamic stretching is similar to ballistic stretching in that it includes movement, but it differs in that it does not involve rapid bouncing. Instead, dynamic stretching moves the joints in an exaggerated but controlled manner through the range of motion used in a specific exercise or sport; movements are fluid rather than jerky. An example of a dynamic stretch is the lunge walk, in which a person takes slow steps with an exaggerated stride length and reaches a lunge stretch position with each step.

Slow dynamic stretches can lengthen the muscles in many directions without developing high tension in the tissues. These stretches elongate the tissues and train the neuromuscular system. Because dynamic stretches are based on sports movements or movements used in daily life, they develop functional flexibility that translates well into activities.

Dynamic stretches are more challenging than static stretches because they require balance and coordination and may carry a greater risk of muscle soreness and injury. People just beginning a flexibility program might want to start off with static stretches and try dynamic stretches only after they are comfortable with static stretching and have improved their flexibility. It is also a good idea to seek expert advice on dynamic stretching technique and program development.

Functional flexibility training can be combined with functional strength training. For example, lunge curls, which combine dynamic lunges with free weights biceps curls, stretch the hip, thigh, and calf muscles; stabilize the core muscles in the trunk; and build strength in the arm muscles. Many activities build functional flexibility and strength at the same time, including yoga, Pilates, tai chi, Olympic weight lifting, plyometrics, stability training (including Swiss and Bosu ball exercises), medicine ball exercises, and functional training machines (for example, Life Fitness and Cybex).

PROPRIOCEPTIVE NEUROMUSCULAR FACILITATION (PNF)
PNF techniques use reflexes initiated by both muscle and joint nerves to cause greater training effects. The most popular PNF stretching technique is the contract-relax stretching method, in which a muscle is contracted before it is stretched. The contraction activates proprioceptors, causing relaxation in the muscle about to be stretched. For example, in a seated stretch of calf muscles, the first step in PNF is to contract the calf muscles. The individual or a partner can provide resistance for an isometric contraction. Following a brief period of relaxation, the next step is to stretch the calf muscles by pulling the tops of the feet toward the body. A duration of 3–6 seconds for the contraction at 20–75% of maximum effort and 10–30 seconds for the stretch is recommended. PNF appears to be most effective if the individual pushes hard during the isometric contraction.

Another example of a PNF stretch is the contract-relax-contract pattern. In this technique, begin by contracting the muscle to be stretched and then relaxing it. Next, contract the opposing muscle (the antagonist). Finally, stretch the first muscle. For example, using this technique to stretch the hamstrings (the muscles in the back of the thigh) would require the following steps: Contract the hamstrings, relax the hamstrings, contract the quadriceps (the muscles in the front of the thigh), and then stretch the hamstrings.

PNF appears to allow more effective stretching and greater increases in flexibility than static stretching, but it tends to cause more muscle stiffness and soreness. It also usually requires a partner and takes more time.

PASSIVE VERSUS ACTIVE STRETCHING   Stretches can be done either passively or actively. In **passive stretching**, an outside force or resistance provided by yourself, a partner, gravity, or a weight helps your joints move through their range of motion. For example, a seated stretch of the hamstring and back muscles can be done by reaching the hands toward the feet until a pull is felt in those muscles. You can achieve a greater range of motion (a more intense stretch) using passive stretching. However, because the stretch is not controlled by the muscles themselves, there is a greater risk of injury. Communication between partners in passive stretching is important to ensure that joints aren't forced outside their normal functional range of motion.

In **active stretching**, a muscle is stretched by a contraction of the opposing muscle (the muscle on the opposite side of the limb). For example, an active seated stretch of the calf muscles occurs when a person actively contracts the muscles on the top of the shin. The contraction of this opposing muscle produces a reflex that relaxes the muscles to be stretched. The muscle can be stretched farther with a low risk of injury. The only disadvantage of active stretching is that a person may not be able to produce enough stress (enough stretch) to increase flexibility using only the contraction of opposing muscle groups.

The safest and most convenient technique is *active static stretching,* with an occasional passive assist. For example, you might stretch your calves both by contracting the muscles on the top of your shin and by pulling your feet toward you. This

Fitness Tip In passive stretching (top), an outside force—such as pressure exerted by another person—helps move the joint and stretch the muscles. In active stretching (bottom), the force to move the joint and stretch the muscles is provided by a contraction of the opposing muscles.
(top and bottom): Courtesy Shirlee Stevens

way you combine the advantages of active stretching—safety and the relaxation reflex—with those of passive stretching—greater range of motion. People who are just beginning flexibility training may be better off doing active rather than passive stretches. For PNF techniques, it is particularly important to have a knowledgeable partner.

Making Progress

As with any type of training, you will make progress and improve your flexibility if you stick with your program. Judge your progress by noting your body position while stretching. For example, note how far you can lean forward during a modified hurdler stretch. Repeat the assessment tests that appear in Lab 5.1 periodically and be sure to take the test at the same time of day each time. You will likely notice some improvement after only two to three weeks of stretching, but you may need at least two months to attain significant improvements. By then, you can expect flexibility increases of about 10–20% in

many joints. Don't continue to try to increase flexibility once you have achieved a normal range of motion in your joints; excessive flexibility can cause joint instability.

EXERCISES TO IMPROVE FLEXIBILITY: A SAMPLE PROGRAM

There are hundreds of exercises that can improve flexibility. Your program should include exercises that work all the major joints of the body by stretching their associated muscle groups (refer back to Figure 5.2). The exercises on the following pages are simple to do and pose a minimum risk of injury. Use these exercises to create a well-rounded program for developing flexibility. Be sure to perform each stretch using the proper technique. Hold each position for 10–30 seconds and perform 2–4 repetitions of each exercise. Complete Lab 5.2 when you're ready to start your program.

FLEXIBILITY EXERCISES

EXERCISE 1

Head Turns and Tilts

Instructions:

Head turns: Turn your head to the right and hold the stretch. Repeat to the left.

Head tilts: Tilt your head to the right and left side. Hold the stretch. Repeat to the left. Do not hyperextend the neck (bend it backward) because this can cause injury.

Area stretched: Neck

Variation: Place your right palm on your right cheek; try to turn your head to the right as you resist with your hand. Repeat on the left side.

©Taylor Robertson Photography

EXERCISE 2

Towel Stretch

Instructions: Roll up a towel and grasp it with both hands, palms down. With your arms straight, slowly lift the towel back over your head as far as possible. The closer together your hands are, the greater the stretch.

Areas stretched: Triceps, shoulders, chest (pectorals)

Variation: Repeat the stretch with your arms down and the towel behind your back. Grasp the towel with your palms forward and thumbs pointing out. Gently raise your arms behind your back. This exercise can also be done without a towel.

©Wayne Glusker

EXERCISE 3

Instructions: (**a**) Keeping your back straight, cross your right arm in front of your body and grasp it with your left hand. Stretch your arm, shoulders, and back by gently pulling your arm as close to your body as possible. Hold. (**b**) Bend your right arm over your head, placing your right elbow as close to your right ear as possible. Grasp your right elbow with your left hand over your head. Stretch the back of your arm by gently pulling your right elbow back and toward your head. Hold. Repeat both stretches on your left side.

Across-the-Body and Overhead Stretches

Areas stretched: Shoulders, upper back, back of the arm (triceps)

(a-b): ©Taylor Robertson Photography

EXERCISE 4

Instructions: Stand with your feet shoulder-width apart, knees slightly bent, and pelvis tucked under. Lace your fingers in front of your body and press your palms forward.

Upper-Back Stretch

Area stretched: Upper back

Variation: In the same position, wrap your arms around your body as if you were giving yourself a hug.

©Taylor Robertson Photography

EXERCISE 5

Instructions: Stand with your feet shoulder-width apart, knees slightly bent, and pelvis tucked under. Raise one arm over your head and bend sideways from the waist. Support your trunk by placing the hand or forearm of your other arm on your thigh or hip for support. Be sure you bend directly sideways and don't move your body below the waist. Repeat on the other side.

Lateral Stretch

Areas stretched: Core muscles

Variation: Perform the same exercise in a seated position.

©Taylor Robertson Photography

EXERCISE 6

Step Stretch

Instructions: Step forward and bend your forward knee, keeping it directly above your ankle. Stretch your other leg back so that your shin is parallel to the floor. Press your hips forward and down to stretch. Your arms can be at your sides, on top of your knee, or on the ground for balance. Repeat on the other side.

Areas stretched: Hip flexors and quadriceps

Courtesy Neil A. Tanner

EXERCISE 7

Side Lunge

Instructions: Stand in a wide straddle with your legs turned out from your hip joints and your hands on your thighs. Lunge to one side by bending one knee and keeping the other leg straight. Keep your bent knee directly over your ankle; do not bend it more than 90 degrees. Repeat on the other side.

Areas stretched: Inner thigh, hip, calf

Variation: In the same position, lift the heel of the bent knee to provide additional stretch. The exercise may also be performed with your hands on the floor for balance.

Courtesy Neil A. Tanner

EXERCISE 8

Inner-Thigh Stretch

Instructions: Sit on the floor with the soles of your feet together. Push your knees toward the floor using your hands or forearms.

Areas stretched: Inner thigh, hip

Variation: When you first begin to push your knees toward the floor, use your legs to resist the movement. Then relax and press your knees down as far as they will go.

©Taylor Robertson Photography

EXERCISE 9

Hip and Trunk Stretch

Instructions: Sit on the floor with your left leg straight, right leg bent and crossed over the left knee, and right hand on the floor next to your right hip. Turn your trunk as far as possible to the right by pushing against your right leg with your left forearm or elbow. Keep your right foot on the floor. Repeat on the other side.

Areas stretched: Core, outer thigh, gluteal muscles, lower back

©Wayne Glusker

| **EXERCISE 10** | **Modified Hurdler Stretch (Seated Single-Leg Hamstring)** |

Instructions: Sit on the floor with your left leg straight and your right leg tucked close to your body. Reach toward your left ankle as far as possible. Repeat for the other leg.

Areas stretched: Hamstrings, lower back

Variation: As you stretch forward, point your toe as much as possible. Repeat for the other leg. Alternately flex and point the foot of your extended leg.

©Wayne Glusker

| **EXERCISE 11** | **Leg Stretcher** |

Instructions: Lie flat on your back with both legs straight. **(a)** Grasp your left leg behind the thigh, and pull it in to your chest. **(b)** Hold this position, and then extend your left leg toward the ceiling. **(c)** Hold this position, and then bring your left knee back to your chest and pull your toes toward your shin (hamstring), hip, knee, ankle, and buttocks with your left hand. Stretch the back of the leg by attempting to straighten your knee. Repeat for the other leg.

Areas stretched: Hamstrings, gluteal muscles, calf

Variation: Perform the stretch on both legs at the same time.

(a–c): Courtesy Shirlee Stevens

| **EXERCISE 12** | **Lower-Leg Stretch** |

Instructions: Stand with one foot about 1–2 feet in front of the other, with both feet pointing forward. **(a)** Keeping your back leg straight, lunge forward by bending your front knee and pushing your rear heel backward. Hold. **(b)** Then pull your back foot in slightly and bend your back knee. Shift your weight to your back leg. Hold. Repeat on the other side.

Areas stretched: Hamstrings, calf

Variation: Place your hands on a wall and extend one foot back, pressing your heel down to stretch, or stand with the balls of your feet on a step or bench and allow your heels to drop below the level of your toes.

(a-b): Courtesy Neil A. Tanner

| **EXERCISE 13** | **Single-Leg Deadlift** |

Instructions: Start with a dumbbell or kettlebell placed slightly outside the foot of one leg. Bend down to the weight by hinging at the hips and bending at the knee. Your other leg should be bent and relaxed. Pick up the weight and tighten your body and extend the hip and knee as you stand straight, locking out your hip and contracting your glute. Repeat with the other leg.

Areas stretched: This exercise stretches and loads the hamstrings and gluteal muscles both eccentrically and concentrically (lengthening and shortening contractions).

©Taylor Robertson Photography

PREVENTING AND MANAGING LOW-BACK PAIN

More than 85% of Americans experience back pain by age 50. Low-back pain is the second most common ailment in the United States—headache tops the list—and the second most common reason for absences from work and visits to a physician. Low-back pain is estimated to cost as much as $50 billion a year in lost productivity, medical and legal fees, and disability insurance and compensation.

Back pain can result from sudden traumatic injuries, but it is more often the long-term result of weak and inflexible muscles, poor posture, or poor body mechanics during activities like lifting and carrying. Any abnormal strain on the back can result in pain. Most cases of low-back pain clear up within a few weeks or months, but some people have recurrences or suffer from chronic pain.

Function and Structure of the Spine

The spinal column performs many important functions in the body:

- It provides structural support for the body, especially the thorax (upper-body cavity).
- It surrounds and protects the spinal cord.
- It supports much of the body's weight.

TERMS

vertebrae Bony segments composing the spinal column that provide structural support for the body and protect the spinal cord.

intervertebral disk An elastic disk located between adjoining vertebrae, consisting of a gel- and water-filled nucleus surrounded by fibrous rings; serves as a shock absorber for the spinal column.

nerve roots The bases of the 31 pairs of spinal nerves that branch off the spinal cord through spaces between vertebrae.

core muscles The trunk muscles extending from the hips to the upper back.

- It serves as an attachment site for a large number of muscles, tendons, and ligaments.
- It allows movement of the neck and back in all directions.

The spinal column is made up of bones called **vertebrae** that provide structural support to the body and protect the spinal cord (Figure 5.3). The spine consists of 7 cervical vertebrae in the neck, 12 thoracic vertebrae in the upper back, and 5 lumbar vertebrae in the lower back. The 9 vertebrae at the base of the spine are fused into two sections and form the sacrum and the coccyx (tailbone). The spine has four curves: the cervical, thoracic, lumbar, and sacral curves (see Figure 5.3). These curves help bring the body weight supported by the spine in line with the axis of the body.

Although the structure of vertebrae depends on their location on the spine, the types of vertebrae share common characteristics. Each consists of a body, an arch, and several bony processes (Figure 5.4). The vertebral body is cylindrical, with flattened surfaces where **intervertebral disks** are attached. The vertebral body is designed to carry the stress of body weight and physical activity. The vertebral arch surrounds and protects the spinal cord. Irregularly shaped bony outgrowths serve as joints for adjacent vertebrae and attachment sites for muscles and ligaments. **Nerve roots** from the spinal cord pass through notches in the vertebral arch.

Intervertebral disks are shock absorbers that disperse the stresses placed on the spine and separate vertebrae from one another. Disks are made up of a gel- and water-filled nucleus surrounded by a series of fibrous rings. The liquid nucleus can change shape when it is compressed, allowing the disk to absorb shock. The intervertebral disks also help maintain the spaces between vertebrae where the spinal nerve roots are located.

Core Muscle Fitness

The **core muscles** are the trunk muscles in the middle of the body extending from the hips to the upper back, including those in the abdomen, pelvic floor, sides of the trunk, back, buttocks, hip, and pelvis (Figure 5.5). These muscles are attached to the ribs, hips, spinal column, and other bones in the trunk of the body. The core muscles stabilize the spine and help transfer of your trunk support your spine when you sit in a chair and fix your midsection as you use your legs to stand up. When hitting a forehand in tennis or batting a softball, most of the force is transferred from the legs and hips, across the core muscles, to the arms. Strong core muscles make movements more forceful and help prevent back pain.

During any dynamic movement, the core muscles work together. Some shorten to cause movement, while others contract and hold to provide stability, lengthen to brake the movement, or send signals to the brain about the movements and positions of the muscles and bones (proprioception). When specific core muscles are weak or tired, the nervous system steps in and uses other muscles. This substitution causes abnormal stresses on the joints, decreases power, and increases the risk of injury.

The best exercises for low-back health are whole-body exercises that force the core muscles to stabilize and support the spine in many directions. The low-back exercises presented later in this chapter include several exercises that focus on the core muscles, including the step stretch (lunge), side bridges, and spine extensions. These exercises are generally safe for beginning exercisers and, with physician approval, people who have some back pain. More challenging core exercises utilize stability balls or free weights. Stability ball exercises require the core muscles to stabilize the ball (and the body) while performing nearly any type of exercise. Many traditional exercises with free weights can strengthen the core muscles if you do them in a standing position. Weight machines train muscles in isolation, while exercises with free weights done while standing help train the body for real-world movements—an essential principle of core training.

Causes of Back Pain

Back pain can occur at any point along your spine. The lumbar area, because it bears the majority of your weight, is the most common site. Any movement that puts excessive stress on the spinal column can cause injury and pain. The spine is well equipped to bear body weight and the force or stress of body movements along its long axis. However, it is less capable of bearing loads at an angle to its long axis or when the trunk is flexed (bent). You do not have to carry a heavy load or participate in a vigorous contact sport to injure your back. Picking up a pencil from the floor while using poor body mechanics—reaching too far out in front of you or bending over with your knees straight, for example—can also result in back pain.

Risk factors associated with low-back pain include age greater than 34 years, degenerative diseases such as arthritis or osteoporosis, a family or personal history of back pain or trauma, a sedentary lifestyle, low job satisfaction, low socio-economic status, excess body weight, smoking (which appears to hasten degenerative changes in the spine), and psychological stress or depression (which can cause muscle tension and back pain). Occupations and activities associated with low-back pain are those requiring physically hard work, such as frequent lifting, twisting, bending, standing up, or straining in forced

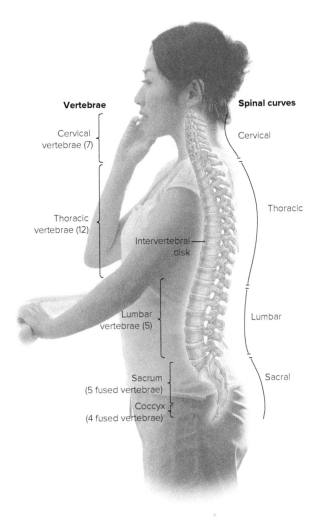

FIGURE 5.3 The spinal column. The spine is made up of five separate regions and has four distinct curves. An intervertebral disk is located between adjoining vertebrae.
©Image Source/Photo Disc/Getty Images RF

FIGURE 5.4 Vertebrae and an intervertebral disk.

force between the upper body and lower body. They stabilize the midsection when you sit, stand, reach, walk, jump, twist, squat, throw, or bend. The muscles on the front, back, and sides

Front

Deep Muscles

Abdominal muscles:
internal obliques, transversus abdominis

Hip muscles:
adductor brevis, adductor magnus, gemellus superior, gemellus inferior, obturator internus, periformis

Superficial Muscles

Abdominal muscles:
rectus abdominis, external obliques

Hip muscles:
rectus femoris, Iliopsoas, tensor fascia lata, sartorius, pectineus, adductor longus, gracilis

Back

Deep Muscles

Spinal muscles:
quadratus lumborum, paraspinals, rotatores

Hip muscles:
quadratus femoris, obturator externus, gluteus medius, gluteus minimus

Superficial Muscles

Spinal muscles:
erector spinae, iliocostalis thoracis, iliocostalis lumborum, latissimus dorsi, trapezius, serratus anterior

Hip muscles:
gluteus maximus, hamstrings (biceps femoris, semimembranosus, semitendinosus)

FIGURE 5.5   Major core muscles.

positions; those requiring high concentration demands while seated (such as computer programming); and those involving vibrations affecting the entire body (such as truck driving).

Underlying causes of back pain include poor muscle endurance and strength in the core muscles; excess body weight; poor posture or body position when standing, sitting, or sleeping; and poor body mechanics when performing actions like lifting and carrying or sports movements. Strained muscles, tendons, or ligaments can cause pain and, over time, lead to injuries to vertebrae, intervertebral disks, and surrounding muscles and ligaments.

Physical stress can cause disks to break down and lose some of their ability to absorb shock. A damaged disk may bulge out between vertebrae and put pressure on a nerve root, which causes pain. Painful pressure on nerves can also occur if damage to a disk narrows the space between two vertebrae. With age, you lose fluid from the disks, making them more likely to bulge and put pressure on nerve roots. Depending on the amount of pressure on a nerve, symptoms may include numbness in the back, hip, leg, or foot; radiating pain; loss of muscle function; depressed reflexes; and muscle spasm. If the pressure is severe enough, loss of function can be permanent.

Preventing Low-Back Pain

Incorrect posture is responsible for many back injuries. Strategies for maintaining good posture are presented in the box "Good Posture and Low-Back Health." Follow the same guidelines when you engage in sports or recreational activities. Control your movements, and warm up thoroughly before you exercise. Take special care when lifting weights.

The role of exercise in preventing and treating back pain is still being investigated. However, many experts recommend exercise, especially for people who have already experienced an episode of low-back pain. The exercise can take the form of a workout aimed at increasing muscle endurance and strength in the back and abdomen or just regular lifestyle physical activity such as walking. Movement helps lubricate your spinal joints and increases muscle fitness in your trunk and legs. Other lifestyle recommendations for preventing back pain include the following:

- Maintain a healthy weight. Excess fat contributes to poor posture, which can place harmful stresses on the spine.

- Stop smoking, and reduce stress.

- Avoid sitting, standing, or working in the same position for too long. Stand up every hour or half-hour and move around.

- Use a supportive seat and a medium-firm mattress.

- Use lumbar support when driving, particularly for long distances, to prevent muscle fatigue and pain.

- Warm up thoroughly before exercising.

- Progress gradually when attempting to improve strength or fitness.

Managing Acute Back Pain

Sudden (acute) back pain usually involves tissue injury. Symptoms may include pain, muscle spasms, stiffness, and inflammation. Many cases of acute back pain go away by themselves within a few days or weeks. You may be able to reduce pain and inflammation by applying cold and then heat (see Chapter 3). Apply ice several times a day; once inflammation and spasms subside, you can apply heat using a heating pad or a warm bath. If the pain is bothersome, an over-the-counter nonsteroidal anti-inflammatory medication such as ibuprofen or naproxen may be helpful. Stronger pain medications and muscle relaxants are available by prescription.

TAKE CHARGE
Good Posture and Low-Back Health

Changes in everyday posture and behavior can help prevent and alleviate low-back pain.

- **Lying down.** When resting or sleeping, lie on your side with your knees and hips bent. If you lie on your back, place a pillow under your knees. However, do not elevate your knees so much that the curve in your lower spine is flattened. Don't lie on your stomach. Use a medium-firm mattress.

- **Sitting at a computer.** Sit in a slightly reclined position of 100–110 degrees, not an upright 90-degree position. Adjust your chair so your knees are slightly lower than your hips. If your back flattens as you sit, try using a lumbar roll to maintain your back's natural curvature. Place your feet flat on the floor or on a footrest. Place the monitor directly in front of you and adjust it so your eyes are level with the top of the screen; you should be looking slightly downward at the middle of the screen. Adjust the keyboard and mouse so your forearms and wrists are in a neutral position, parallel with the floor. Stand up and walk a short distance at least once every hour.

- **Lifting.** If you need to bend down to grasp an object, hinge at the hips and bend at the knees rather than at the waist. Your feet should be about shoulder-width apart. Lift gradually, keeping your arms straight, by standing up or by pushing with your hip muscles. Keep the object close to your body. Don't twist; if you have to turn with the object, change the position of your feet so that you pivot your body as a whole rather than twisting at your waist or shoulders. Maintain a stiff core and neutral spine (natural spinal curves).

- **Standing.** When you are standing, a straight line should run from the top of your ear through the center of your shoulder, the center of your hip, the back of your kneecap, and the front of your ankle bone. Support your weight mainly on your heels, with one or both knees slightly bent. Don't let your pelvis tip forward or your back arch. Shift your weight back and forth from foot to foot. Avoid prolonged standing.

To check your posture, stand normally with your back to a wall. Your upper back and buttocks should touch the wall; your heels may be a few inches away. Slide one hand into the space between your lower back and the wall. It should slide in easily but should almost touch both your back and the wall. Adjust your posture as needed, and try to hold this position as you walk away from the wall.

- **Walking.** Walk with your toes pointed straight ahead. Keep your back flat, head up and centered over your body, and chin in. Swing your arms freely. Don't wear tight or high-heeled shoes. Walking briskly is better for back health than walking slowly.

Box icon: ©VisualCommunications/Getty Images RF

Bed rest immediately following the onset of back pain may make you feel better, but it should be of very short duration. Prolonged bed rest—five days or more—was once thought to be an effective treatment for back pain, but most physicians now advise against it because it may weaken muscles and actually worsen pain. Limit bed rest to one day and begin moderate physical activity as soon as possible. Exercise can increase muscular endurance and flexibility and protect disks from loss of fluid. Three of the back exercises discussed later in the chapter may be particularly helpful following an episode of acute back pain: McGill curl-ups, side bridges, and spine extensions ("bird dogs").

See your physician if acute back pain doesn't resolve within a short time. Other warning signals of a more severe problem that requires a professional evaluation include severe pain, numbness, pain that radiates down one or both legs, problems with bladder or bowel control, fever, and rapid weight loss.

Managing Chronic Back Pain

Low-back pain is considered chronic if it persists for more than three months. Symptoms vary—some people experience stabbing or shooting pain, and others a steady ache accompanied by stiffness. Sometimes pain is localized; in other cases, it radiates to another part of the body. Underlying causes of chronic back pain include injuries, infection, muscle or ligament strains, and disk herniations.

Because symptoms and causes are so varied, different people benefit from different treatment strategies, and researchers have found that many treatments have only limited benefits. Potential treatments include over-the-counter or prescription medications; exercise; physical therapy, massage, yoga, or chiropractic care; acupuncture; percutaneous electrical nerve stimulation (PENS), in which acupuncture-like needles deliver an electrical current; education and advice about posture, exercise, and body mechanics; and surgery (see the box "Yoga for Relaxation and Pain Relief").

Psychological therapy may also be beneficial in some cases. Reducing emotional stress that causes muscle tension can provide direct benefits, and other therapies can help people deal better with chronic pain and its effects on their daily lives. Support groups and expressive writing are beneficial for people with chronic pain and other conditions.

EXERCISES FOR THE PREVENTION AND MANAGEMENT OF LOW-BACK PAIN

The tests in Lab 5.3 can help you assess low-back muscular endurance. The exercises that follow are designed to help you maintain a healthy back by stretching and strengthening the major muscle groups that affect the back—the abdominal muscles, the muscles along your spine and sides, and the muscles of your hips and thighs. If you have back problems, check with your physician before beginning any exercise program. Perform the exercises slowly and progress very gradually. Stop and consult your physician if any exercise causes back pain. General guidelines for back exercise programs include the following:

- Do low-back exercises at least three days per week. Most experts recommend daily back exercises.

- Emphasize muscular endurance rather than muscular strength—endurance is more protective.

- Don't do spine exercises involving a full range of motion early in the morning. Because your disks have a high fluid content early in the day, injuries may result.

- Engage in regular endurance exercise such as cycling or walking in addition to performing exercises that specifically build muscular endurance and flexibility. Brisk walking with a natural arm swing may help relieve back pain. Start with fast walking if your core muscles are weak or you have back pain.

- Be patient and stick with your program. Increased back fitness and pain relief may require as long as three months of regular exercise.

- The adage "no pain, no gain" does not apply to back exercises. Always use good form and stop if you feel pain.

- Build core stiffness through stabilization exercises because they strengthen muscles, improve muscular endurance, reduce low back pain, and boost sports performance. Greater core stiffness transfers strength and speed to the limbs, increases the load-bearing capacity of the spine, and protects the internal organs during sports movements. When working on abdominal muscles, emphasize stabilization exercises, such as side bridges, carry exercises, planks, bird dogs, and the stir-the-pot exercise rather than spinal flexion exercises such as sit-ups. Poor performance on the spinal endurance labs means that you are not training your abdominal muscles correctly.

TIPS FOR TODAY AND THE FUTURE

To improve and maintain your flexibility, perform stretches that work the major joints at least twice a week.

RIGHT NOW YOU CAN

- Stand up and stretch—do either the upper-back stretch or the across-the-body stretch shown in the chapter.
- Practice the recommended sitting and standing postures described in the chapter. If needed, adjust your chair or find something to use as a footrest.

IN THE FUTURE YOU CAN

- Build up your flexibility by incorporating more sophisticated stretching exercises into your routine. Increase the frequency of your flexibility workouts to five or more days per week.
- Increase the efficiency of your workouts by adding stretching exercises to the cool-down period of your endurance or strength workouts.
- Incorporate low-back exercises into your daily routine.

TAKE CHARGE
Yoga for Relaxation and Pain Relief

Exercise, such as yoga and tai chi, can provide relief from back pain, depending on the pain's underlying cause. Effective exercises stretch the muscles and connective tissue in the hips, stabilize the spine, and strengthen and build endurance in the core muscles of the back and abdomen.

Yoga may be an option for many back pain sufferers because it offers a variety of exercises that target the spine and the core muscles. Yoga is an ancient practice involving slow, gentle movements performed with controlled breathing and focused attention. Yoga practitioners slowly move into a specific posture (called an *asana*) and hold the posture for up to 60 seconds. There are hundreds of asanas, many of which are easy to do and provide good stretches.

Yoga also involves simple breathing exercises that gently stretch the muscles of the upper back while helping the practitioner focus. Yoga experts say that breathing exercises not only encourage relaxation but also clear the mind and

can help relieve mild to moderate pain. Yoga enthusiasts end their workouts energized and refreshed but calm and relaxed.

Many medical professionals now recommend yoga for patients with back pain, particularly asanas that arch and gently stretch the back, such as the cat pose (similar to the cat stretch shown in the "Low-Back Exercises" section) and the child pose (shown below). These are basic asanas that most people can perform repeatedly and hold for a relatively long time.

Because asanas must be performed correctly to be beneficial, qualified instruction is recommended. For those with back pain, physicians advise choosing an instructor who is not only accomplished in yoga but also knowledgeable about back pain and its causes. Such instructors can steer students away from exercises that do more harm than good. It is especially important to choose postures that will benefit the back without worsening the

underlying problem. Some asanas can aggravate an injured or painful back if they are performed incorrectly or too aggressively. In fact, people with back pain should avoid a few yoga postures, such as a standing forward bend.

If you have back pain, see your physician to determine its cause before beginning any type of exercise program. Even gentle exercise or stretching can be bad for an already injured back, especially if the spinal disks or nerves are involved. For some back conditions, rest or therapy may be a better option than exercise, at least in the short term.

©Wavebreakmedia Ltd/Getty Images RF

SUMMARY

• Flexibility, the ability of a joint to move through its full range of motion, is highly adaptable and specific to each joint.

• Range of motion can be limited by joint structure, muscle inelasticity, and proprioceptor activity.

• Developing flexibility depends on stretching the elastic tissues within muscles regularly and gently until they lengthen. Overstretching can make connective tissue brittle and lead to rupture.

• Signals sent between muscle and tendon nerves and the spinal cord can enhance flexibility.

• The benefits of flexibility include preventing abnormal stresses that lead to joint deterioration and possibly reducing the risk of injuries.

• Static stretches should be held for 10–30 seconds and performed with 2–4 repetitions for a total stretching time of 60 seconds per exercise. Flexibility training should be done a minimum of two or three days per week, preferably following activity, when muscles are warm.

• Static stretching is slow and held to the point of mild tension; ballistic stretching, consisting of bouncing stretches, can lead to injury. Dynamic stretching moves joints slowly and fluidly through their range of motions. Proprioceptive neuromuscular facilitation uses muscle receptors in contracting and relaxing a muscle.

• Passive stretching, using an outside force to move muscles and joints, achieves a greater range of motion (and has a higher injury risk) than active stretching, which uses opposing muscles to initiate a stretch.

• The spinal column consists of vertebrae separated by intervertebral disks. It provides structure and support for the body and protects the spinal cord. The core muscles stabilize the spine and transfer force between the upper and lower body.

• Acute back pain can be treated as a soft tissue injury, with cold treatment followed by application of heat (once swelling subsides); prolonged bed rest is not recommended. A variety of treatments have been suggested for chronic back pain, including regular exercise, physical therapy, acupuncture, education, and psychological therapy.

• In addition to good posture, proper body mechanics, and regular physical activity, a program for preventing low-back pain includes exercises that develop flexibility, strength, and endurance in the muscle groups that affect the lower back.

• Build core stiffness through stabilization exercises because they strengthen muscles, improve muscular endurance, reduce low-back pain, and boost sports performance. Greater core stiffness transfers strength and speed to the limbs, increases the load-bearing capacity of the spine, and protects the internal organs during sports movements.

LOW-BACK EXERCISES

| EXERCISE 1 | Cat Stretch |

Instructions: Begin on all fours with your knees below your hips and your hands below your shoulders. Slowly and deliberately move through a cycle of extension and flexion of your spine. **(a)** Begin by slowly pushing your back up and dropping your head slightly until your spine is extended (rounded). **(b)** Then slowly lower your back and lift your chin slightly until your spine is flexed (relaxed and slightly arched). *Do not press at the ends of the range of motion.* Stop if you feel pain. Do 10 slow, continuous cycles of the movement.

Target: Improved strength and flexibility in the erector spinae, relaxation, and reduced stiffness in the spine.

(a-b): ©Wayne Glusker

| EXERCISE 2 | Step Stretch (see Exercise 6 in the flexibility program) |

Instructions: Hold each stretch for 10–30 seconds and do 2–4 repetitions on each side.

Target: Improved flexibility, strength, and endurance in the hip flexors and hip extensors and stiffens the core.

| EXERCISE 3 | Leg Stretcher (see Exercise 11 in the flexibility program) |

Instructions: Hold each stretch for 10–30 seconds and do 2–4 repetitions on each side.

Target: Improved flexibility in the hip extensors and hamstrings.

| EXERCISE 4 | Trunk Twist |

Instructions: Lie on your side with top knee bent, lower leg straight, lower arm extended in front of you on the floor, and upper arm at your side. Push down with your upper knee while you twist your trunk to the opposite side. Try to get your shoulders and upper body flat on the floor, turning your head as well. Return to the starting position, and then repeat on the other side. Hold the stretch for 10–30 seconds and do 2–4 repetitions on each side.

Target: Improved flexibility in the lower back and core muscles.

©Taylor Robertson Photography

| **EXERCISE 5** | **McGill Curl-Up (see Exercise 4 in the body weight program in Chapter 4)** |

Instructions: Lie on your back with one knee bent and arms crossed on your chest or hands under your lower back. Maintain a neutral spine. Tuck your chin in and slowly curl up, one vertebra at a time, as you use your abdominal muscles to lift your head first and then your shoulders. Stop when you can see your knees and hold for 5–10 seconds before returning to the starting position. Do 10 or more repetitions.

Target: Improved strength, endurance, and stiffness in the abdomen.

| **EXERCISE 6** | **Isometric Side Bridge (see Exercise 6 in the body weight program in Chapter 4)** |

Instructions: Hold the bridge position for 10 seconds, breathing normally. Build up to five or more repetitions on each side.

Target: Increased strength and endurance in the muscles along the sides of the abdomen and deep lateral muscles that support the spine.

Variation: You can make the exercise more difficult by keeping your legs straight and supporting yourself with your feet and forearm (see Lab 5.3) or with your feet and hand (with elbow straight).

| **EXERCISE 7** | **Spine Extensions ("Bird Dogs"; see Exercise 5 in the body weight program in Chapter 4)** |

Instructions: Hold each position for 5–15 seconds. Begin with one repetition on each side, and work up to five or more repetitions.

Target: Increased strength and endurance in the back, gluteal muscles, and hamstrings.

Variation: If you have experienced back pain in the past or if this exercise is difficult for you, do the exercise with both hands on the ground rather than with one arm lifted. You can make this exercise more difficult by doing it balancing on an exercise ball. Find a balance point on your chest while lying face down on the ball with one arm and the opposite leg on the ground. Tense your abdominal muscles while reaching and extending with one arm and reaching and extending with the opposite leg. Repeat this exercise using the other arm and leg.

| **EXERCISE 8** | **Wall Squat (Phantom Chair)** |

Instructions: Lean against a wall and bend your knees as though you are sitting in a chair. Support your weight with your legs. Begin by holding the position for 5–10 seconds. Squeeze your gluteal muscles together as you do the exercise. Build up to one minute or more. Perform one or more repetitions.

Target: Increased strength and endurance in the lower back, quadriceps, gluteal muscles, and core muscles.

Courtesy Neil A. Tanner

EXERCISE 9   Pelvic Tilt

Instructions: Lie on your back with knees bent and arms extended to the side. Tilt your pelvis under and try to flatten your lower back against the floor. Tighten your buttock and abdominal muscles while you hold this position for 5–10 seconds. Don't hold your breath. Work up to 10 repetitions of the exercise. Pelvic tilts can also be done standing or leaning against a wall. *Note:* Although this is a popular exercise with many therapists, some experts question the safety of pelvic tilts. Stop if you feel pain in your back at any time during the exercise.

Target: Increased strength and endurance in the gluteal muscles and core muscles.

©Taylor Robertson Photography

EXERCISE 10   Back Bridge

Instructions: Lie on your back with knees bent and arms extended to the side. Tuck your pelvis under; contract your gluteal muscles; then lift your tailbone, buttocks, and lower back from the floor. Hold this position for 5–10 seconds with your weight resting on your feet, arms, and shoulders, and then return to the starting position. Work up to 10 repetitions of the exercise.

Target: Increased strength and endurance in quadriceps, gluteal muscles, and core muscles.

©Taylor Robertson Photography

EXERCISE 11   Stir the Pot

Instructions: Assume a plank position on an exercise ball, with forearms on the ball and legs extended to the rear. Maintaining a stiff torso and neutral spine, rotate on the ball in a clockwise direction for 10 repetitions and then repeat in a counterclockwise direction for 10 repetitions.

Target: Increased strength and endurance in the core muscles and shoulders.

©Taylor Robertson Photography

EXERCISE 12   Kettlebell or Dumbbell Carry ("Suitcase Carry"; see Exercise 11 in the body weight program in Chapter 4)

Instructions: This is an excellent exercise for building the core muscles. Pick up a dumbbell or kettlebell in one or both hands. Maintaining good posture, walk 20 to 100 yards carrying the weights. Carry 10 to several hundred pounds, depending on your fitness.

Target: Core muscles, trapezius, quadriceps and gluteal muscles.

COMMON QUESTIONS ANSWERED

Q **Is stretching the same as warming up?**

A No. They are two distinct activities. A warm-up is light exercise that involves moving the joints through the same motions used during a more intense activity; it increases body temperature so that your metabolism works better when you're exercising at high intensity. Stretching increases the movement capability of your joints, so that you can move more easily with less risk of injury. It is best to stretch when your muscles are warm. Warmed muscles stretch better than cold ones and are less prone to injury.

Q **How much flexibility do I need?**

A This question is not always easy to answer. If you're involved in a sport such as gymnastics, figure skating, or ballet, you are often required to reach extreme joint motions to achieve success.

However, nonathletes do not need to reach these extreme joint positions. In fact, too much flexibility may, in some cases, create joint instability and increase your risk of injury. As with other types of fitness, moderation is the key. You should regularly stretch your major joints and muscle groups but not aspire to reach extreme flexibility.

Q **Can I stretch too far?**

A Yes. As muscle tissue is progressively stretched, it reaches a point where it becomes damaged and may rupture. The greatest danger occurs during passive stretching when a partner is doing the stretching for you. It is critical that your stretching partner not force your joint outside its normal functional range of motion.

Q **Can physical training limit flexibility?**

A When done properly, weight training increases flexibility.

However, because of the limited range of motion used during the running stride, jogging tends to compromise flexibility. It is important for runners to do flexibility exercises for the hamstrings and quadriceps regularly.

Q **Does static stretching affect muscular strength?**

A Flexibility training increases muscle strength over time, but many recent studies have found that stretching causes short-term decreases in strength, power, and motor control. This is one reason some experts suggest that people not stretch as part of their exercise warm-up, particularly if they plan to engage in a high-performance activity. It is important to warm up before any workout by engaging in 5–10 minutes of light exercise such as walking or slow jogging.

FOR FURTHER EXPLORATION

American Academy of Orthopaedic Surgeons. Provides information about a variety of joint problems.

http://orthoinfo.aaos.org

Back Fit Pro. A website maintained by Dr. Stuart McGill, a professor of spine biomechanics at the University of Waterloo, which provides evidence-based information on preventing and treating back pain.

http://www.backfitpro.com

CUErgo: Cornell University Ergonomics Website. Provides information about how to arrange a computer workstation to prevent back pain and repetitive strain injuries, as well as other topics related to ergonomics.

http://ergo.human.cornell.edu

Georgia State University: Flexibility. Provides information about the benefits of stretching and ways to develop a safe and effective program; includes illustrations of stretches.

http://www2.gsu.edu/~wwwfit/flexibility.html

International Fitness Association: Stretching and Flexibility. Provides information on the physiology of stretching and different types of stretching exercises.

http://www.ifafitness.com/stretch/stretch5.htm

International Yoga Alliance. A good resource for yoga organizations around the world.

https://www.yogaalliance.org/

Mayo Clinic: Focus on Flexibility. Presents an easy-to-use program of basic stretching exercises for beginners, with a focus on the benefits of greater flexibility.

http://www.mayoclinic.org/healthy-lifestyle/fitness/in-depth/stretching/art-20047931

NIH Back Pain Fact Sheet. Provides basic information on the prevention and treatment of back pain.

http://www.ninds.nih.gov/disorders/backpain/backpain.htm

Southern California Orthopedic Institute. Provides information on a variety of orthopedic problems, including back injuries; also has illustrations of spinal anatomy.

http://www.scoi.com

See also the listings for Chapters 2 and 4.

SELECTED BIBLIOGRAPHY

Aguilar, A. J., et al. 2012. A dynamic warm-up model increases quadriceps strength and hamstring flexibility. *Journal of Strength and Conditioning Research* 26(4): 1130–1141.

American College of Sports Medicine. 2018. *ACSM's Guidelines for Exercise Testing and Prescription,* 10th ed. Philadelphia: Wolters Kluwer.

Armiger, P., and M. A. Martyn. 2010. *Stretching for Functional Flexibility.* Philadelphia: Lippincott Williams & Wilkins.

Avloniti, A., et al. 2016. The effects of static stretching on speed and agility: One or multiple repetition protocols? *European Journal of Sport Science* 16(4): 402–408.

Ayala, C.A., et al. 2017. Acute effects of three neuromuscular warm-up strategies on several physical performance measures in football players. *PlosOne* 12(1): e0169660.

Barengo, N. C., et al. 2014. The impact of the FIFA 11+ training program on injury prevention in football players: A systematic review. *International Journal of Environmental Research and Public Health* 11(11): 1198–2000.

Baxter, C., et al. 2017. Impact of stretching on the performance and injury risk of long-distance runners. *Research in Sports Medicine* 25(1): 78–90.

Chang, D. G., et al. 2016. Yoga as a treatment for chronic low back pain: A systematic review of the literature. *Journal of Orthopedics and Rheumatology* 3(1): 1–8.

Chatzopoulos, D., et al. 2014. Acute effects of static and dynamic stretching on balance, agility, reaction time and movement time. *Journal of Sports Science and Medicine* 13(2): 403–409.

Costa, P. B., et al. 2014. Effects of dynamic stretching on strength, muscle imbalance, and muscle activation. *Medicine and Science in Sports and Exercise* 46(3): 586–593.

Gonzalez-Rave, J. M., et al. 2012. Efficacy of two different stretch training programs (passive vs. proprioceptive neuromuscular facilitation) on shoulder and hip range of motion in older people. *Journal of Strength and Conditioning Research* 26(4): 1045–1051.

Grande, G. H., et al. 2016. Effect of Pilates exercise for improving balance in older adults. *British Journal of Sports Medicine.* Published online November 4.

Haddad, M., et al. 2014. Static stretching can impair explosive performance for at least 24 hours. *Journal of Strength and Conditioning Research* 28(1): 140–146.

Haladay, D. E., et al. 2013. Quality of systematic reviews on specific spinal stabilization exercise for chronic low back pain. *Journal of Orthopedic Sports Physical Therapy* 43(4): 242–250.

Howley, E., and D. Thompson. 2017. *Fitness Professional's Handbook,* 7th ed. Champaign, Ill.: Human Kinetics.

Inami, T., et al. 2015. Acute changes in peripheral vascular tonus and systemic circulation during static stretching. *Research in Sports Medicine* 23(2): 167–178.

Judge, L. W., et al. 2013. An examination of pre-activity and post-activity stretching practices of cross country and track and field distance coaches. *Journal of Strength and Conditioning Research* 27(9): 2456–2464.

Kirmizigil, B., et al. 2014. Effects of three different stretching techniques on vertical jumping performance. *Journal of Strength and Conditioning Research* 28(5): 1263–1271.

Konrad, A., and M. Tilp. 2014. Increased range of motion after static stretching is not due to changes in muscle and tendon structures. *Clinical Biomechanics* 29(6): 636–642.

Konrad A., et al. 2016. The effects of acute static, ballistic, and PNF stretching exercise on the muscle and tendon tissue properties. *Scandinavian Journal of Medicine and Science in Sports.* doi:10.1111/sms.12725

Lee, B. C. Y., and S. M. McGill. 2015. Effect of long-term isometric training on core/torso stiffness. *Journal of Strength and Conditioning Research* 29(6): 1515–1526.

Lima, C. D., et al. 2016. Acute effects of static vs. ballistic stretching on strength and muscular fatigue between ballet dancers and resistance-trained women. *Journal of Strength and Conditioning Research* 30(11): 3220–3227.

Lowery, R. P., et al. 2014. Effects of static stretching on 1-mile uphill run performance. *Journal of Strength and Conditioning Research* 28(1): 161–167.

Matsuo, S., et al. 2015. Changes in force and stiffness after static stretching of eccentrically damaged hamstrings. *European Journal of Applied Physiology* 115(5): 981–991.

McGill, S. 2007. *Low Back Disorders: Evidence-Based Prevention and Rehabilitation,* 2nd ed. Champaign, Ill.: Human Kinetics.

McGill, S. 2014. *Ultimate Back Fitness and Performance,* 5th ed. Waterloo, Canada: Backfit Pro.

McGill, S. 2015. *Back Mechanics.* Waterloo, Canada: Backfit Pro.

McGill, S., et al. 2013. Movement quality and links to measures of fitness in firefighters. *Work* 45(3): 357–366.

McGill, S. M., and L. W. Marshall. 2012. Kettlebell swing, snatch, and bottoms-up carry: back and hip muscle activation, motion, and low back loads. *Journal of Strength and Conditioning Research* 26(1): 16–27.

McGill, S. M., et al. 2013. Low back loads while walking and carrying: Comparing the load carried in one hand or in both hands. *Ergonomics* 56(2): 293–302.

McGill, S. M., et al. 2014. Analysis of pushing exercises: Muscle activity and spine load while contrasting techniques on stable surfaces with a labile suspension strap training system. *Journal of Strength and Conditioning Research* 28(1): 105–116.

Miller, K. C., and J. A. Burne. 2014. Golgi tendon organ reflex inhibition following manually applied acute static stretching. *Journal of Sports Science* 32(15): 1491–1497.

Mizuno, T., et al. 2014. Stretching-induced deficit of maximal isometric torque is restored within 10 minutes. *Journal of Strength and Conditioning Research* 28(1): 147–153.

Nieman, D. C. 2011. *Exercise Testing and Prescription: A Health-Related Approach,* 7th ed. New York: McGraw-Hill.

O'Sullivan, K., et al. 2012. The effects of eccentric training on lower limb flexibility: A systematic review. *British Journal of Sports Medicine* 46(12): 838–845.

Plouvier, S., et al. 2015. Occupational biomechanical exposure predicts low back pain in older age among men in the Gazel Cohort. *International Archives of Occupational and Environmental Health* 88: 501–510.

Ribeiro, A. S., et al. 2014. Static stretching and performance in multiple sets in the bench press exercise. *Journal of Strength and Conditioning Research* 28(4): 1158–1163.

Ryan, E. D., et al. 2014. Acute effects of different volumes of dynamic stretching on vertical jump performance, flexibility and muscular endurance. *Clinical Physiology and Functional Imaging* 34(6): 485–492.

Samuel, M. N., et al. 2008. Acute effects of static and ballistic stretching on measures of strength and power. *Journal of Strength and Conditioning Research* 22(5): 1422–1428.

Shnayderman, I., and M. Katz-Leurer. 2013. An aerobic walking programme versus muscle strengthening programme for chronic low back pain: A randomized controlled trial. *Clinical Rehabilitation* 27(3): 207–214.

Taniguchi, K., et al. 2015. Acute decrease in the stiffness of resting muscle belly due to static stretching. *Scandinavian Journal of Medicine and Science in Sports* 25(1): 32–40.

Trajano, G., et al. 2015. Static stretching increases muscle fatigue during submaximal sustained isometric contractions. *Journal of Sports Medicine and Physical Fitness* 55(1–2): 43–50.

Wells, C., et al. 2013. Effectiveness of Pilates exercise in treating people with chronic low back pain: a systematic review of systematic reviews. *BMC Medical Research Methodology* 13: 7.

Wieland, L. S., et al. 2017. Yoga treatment for chronic non-specific low back pain. *Cochrane Database System Review.* Published online January 12.

Wirth, K. 2016. Core stability in athletes: A critical analysis of current guidelines. *Sports Medicine.* Published online July 16.

Yamaguchi, T., et al. 2015. Acute effect of dynamic stretching on endurance running performance in well-trained male runners. *Journal of Strength and Conditioning Research* 29 (11): 3045–3052.

Name _____ Section _____ Date _____

LAB 5.1   Assessing Your Current Level of Flexibility

Part I Sit-and-Reach Test

Equipment
Use a modified Wells and Dillon flexometer or construct your own measuring device using a firm box or two pieces of wood about 30 centimeters (12 inches) high attached at right angles to each other. Attach a metric ruler to measure the extent of reach. With the low numbers of the ruler toward the person being tested, set the 26-centimeter mark of the ruler at the footline of the box. Individuals who cannot reach as far as the footline will have scores below 26 centimeters; those who can reach past their feet will have scores above 26 centimeters. Most studies show no relationship between performance on the sit-and-reach test and the incidence of back pain.

Preparation
Warm up your muscles with a low-intensity activity such as walking or easy jogging. Then perform slow stretching movements.

Instructions
1. Remove your shoes and sit facing the flexibility measuring device with your knees fully extended and your feet flat against the device about 10 centimeters (4 inches) apart.
2. Reach as far forward as you can, with palms down, arms evenly stretched, and knees fully extended; hold the position of maximum reach for about two seconds.
3. Perform the stretch 2 times, recording the distance of maximum reach to the nearest 0.5 centimeters:
   _____ cm

Courtesy Shirlee Stevens

Rating Your Flexibility
Find the score in the table below to determine your flexibility rating. Record it here and on the final page of this lab.
Rating: _____

Ratings for Sit-and-Reach Test

	Rating/Score (cm)*				
Men	*Needs Improvement*	*Fair*	*Good*	*Very Good*	*Excellent*
Age: 15–19	Below 24	24–28	29–33	34–38	Above 38
20–29	Below 25	25–29	30–33	34–39	Above 39
30–39	Below 23	23–27	28–32	33–37	Above 37
40–49	Below 18	18–23	24–28	29–34	Above 34
50–59	Below 16	16–23	24–27	28–34	Above 34
60–69	Below 15	15–19	20–24	25–32	Above 32
Women					
Age: 15–19	Below 29	29–33	34–37	38–42	Above 42
20–29	Below 28	28–32	33–36	37–40	Above 40
30–39	Below 27	27–31	32–35	36–40	Above 40
40–49	Below 25	25–29	30–33	34–37	Above 37
50–59	Below 25	25–29	30–32	34–38	Above 38
60–69	Below 23	23–26	27–30	31–34	Above 34

*Footline is set at 26 cm.

SOURCE: *The Canadian Physical Activity, Fitness & Lifestyle Approach: CSEP-Health & Fitness Program's Health-Related Appraisal and Counseling Strategy,* 3rd ed. Canadian Society for Exercise Physiology, 2003.

LABORATORY ACTIVITIES

Part II Range-of-Motion Assessment

This portion of the lab can be completed by doing visual comparisons or by measuring joint range of motion with a goniometer or other instrument.

Equipment

1. A partner to do visual comparisons or to measure the range of motion of your joints. (You can also use a mirror to perform your own visual comparisons.)
2. For the measurement method, you need a goniometer, flexometer, or other instrument to measure range of motion.

Preparation

Warm up your muscles with some low-intensity activity such as walking or easy jogging.

Instructions

On the following pages, the average range of motion is illustrated and listed quantitatively for some of the major joints. Visually assess the range of motion in your joints, and compare it to that shown in the illustrations. For each joint, note (with a check mark) whether your range of motion is above average, average, or below average and in need of improvement. Average values for range of motion are given in degrees for each joint in the assessment. You can also complete the assessment by measuring your range of motion with a goniometer, flexometer, or other instrument. If you are using this measurement method, identify your rating (above average, average, or below average) and record your range of motion in degrees next to the appropriate category. Although the measurement method is more time-consuming, it allows you to track the progress of your stretching program more precisely and to note changes within the broader ratings categories (below average, above average).

Record your ratings on the following pages and on the chart on the final page of this lab. (Ratings were derived from several published sources.)

Assessment of range of motion using a goniometer
©Wayne Glusker

1. Shoulder Abduction and Adduction

For each position and arm, check one of the following; fill in degrees if using the measurement method.

Shoulder abduction—raise arm up to the side.

Right	Left	
_____	_____	Below average/needs improvement
_____	_____	Average (92–95°)
_____	_____	Above average

Shoulder adduction—move arm down and in front of body.

Right	Left	
_____	_____	Below average/needs improvement
_____	_____	Average (124–127°)
_____	_____	Above average

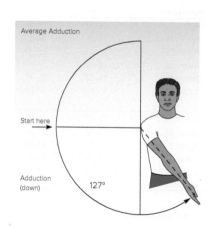

LABORATORY ACTIVITIES

2. Shoulder Flexion and Extension

For each position and arm, check one of the following; fill in degrees if using the measurement method.

Shoulder flexion—raise arm up in front of the body.

Right	Left	
_____	_____	Below average/needs improvement
_____	_____	Average (92–95°)
_____	_____	Above average

Shoulder extension—move arm down and behind the body.

Right	Left	
_____	_____	Below average/needs improvement
_____	_____	Average (145–150°)
_____	_____	Above average

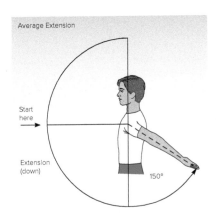

3. Trunk/Low-Back Lateral Flexion

Bend directly sideways at your waist. To prevent injury, keep your knees slightly bent, and support your trunk by placing your hand or forearm on your thigh. Check one of the following for each side; fill in degrees if using the measurement method.

Right	Left	
_____	_____	Below average/needs improvement
_____	_____	Average (36–40°)
_____	_____	Above average

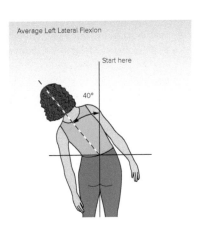

LABORATORY ACTIVITIES

4. Hip Abduction

Raise your leg to the side at the hip. Check one of the following for each leg; fill in degrees if using the measurement method.

Right   *Left*

_____   _____   Below average/needs improvement

_____   _____   Average (40–45°)

_____   _____   Above average

5. Hip Flexion (Bent Knee)

With one leg flat on the floor, bend the other knee and lift the leg up at the hip. Check one of the following for each leg; fill in degrees if using the measurement method.

Right   *Left*

_____   _____   Below average/needs improvement

_____   _____   Average (121–125°)

_____   _____   Above average

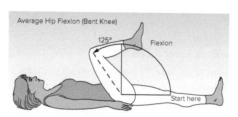

6. Hip Flexion (Straight Leg)

With one leg flat on the floor, raise the other leg at the hip, keeping both legs straight. Take care not to put excess strain on your back. Check one of the following for each leg; fill in degrees if using the measurement method.

Right   *Left*

_____   _____   Below average/needs improvement

_____   _____   Average (79–81°)

_____   _____   Above average

7. Ankle Dorsiflexion and Plantar Flexion

For each position and foot, check one of the following; fill in degrees if using the measurement method.

Ankle dorsiflexion—pull your toes toward your shin.

Right	Left	
_____	_____	Below average/needs improvement
_____	_____	Average (9–13)
_____	_____	Above average

Right	Left	
_____	_____	Below average/needs improvement
_____	_____	Average (50–55)
_____	_____	Above average

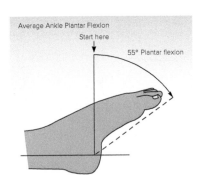

Plantar flexion—point your toes.

Rating Your Flexibility

Sit–and–reach test: Score: _____ cm Rating: _____

Range-of-Motion Assessment

Identify your rating for each joint on each side of the body. If you used the comparison method, put check marks in the appropriate categories; if you measured range of motion, enter the degrees for each joint in the appropriate category.

Joint/Assessment		Right			Left		
		Below Average	Average	Above Average	Below Average	Average	Above Average
1. Shoulder abduction and adduction	Abduction						
	Adduction						
2. Shoulder flexion and extension	Flexion						
	Extension						
3. Trunk/low-back lateral flexion	Flexion						
4. Hip abduction	Abduction						
5. Hip flexion (bent knee)	Flexion						
6. Hip flexion (straight leg)	Flexion						
7. Ankle dorsiflexion and plantar flexion	Dorsiflexion						
	Plantar flexion						

LABORATORY ACTIVITIES

Using Your Results

How did you score? Do your scores for the flexibility tests surprise you? Are you satisfied with your current ratings?

If you're not satisfied, set a realistic goal for improvement:

Are you satisfied with your current level of flexibility as expressed in your daily life—for example, your ability to maintain good posture and move easily and without pain?

If you're not satisfied, set some realistic goals for improvement:

What should you do next? Enter the results of this lab in the Preprogram Assessment column in Appendix B. If you've set goals for improvement, begin planning your flexibility program by completing the plan in Lab 5.2. After several weeks of your program, complete this lab again and enter the results in the Postprogram Assessment column of Appendix B. How do the results compare?

Name _____   Section _____   Date _____

LAB 5.2 Creating a Personalized Program for Developing Flexibility

1. *Goals.* List goals for your flexibility program. On the left, include specific, measurable goals that you can use to track the progress of your fitness program. These goals might be things like raising your sit-and-reach score from fair to good or your bent-leg hip flexion rating from below average to average. On the right, include long-term and more qualitative goals, such as reducing your risk for back pain.

Specific Goals: Current Status   Final Goals

_____   _____

_____   _____

_____   _____

Other Goals: _____

_____

2. *Exercises.* The exercises in the program plan below are from the general stretching program presented in Chapter 5. You can add or delete exercises depending on your needs, goals, and preferences. For any exercises you add, fill in the areas of the body affected.

3. *Frequency.* A minimum frequency of two or three days per week is recommended; five–seven days per week is ideal. You may want to do your stretching exercises the same days you plan to do cardiorespiratory endurance exercise or weight training because muscles stretch better following exercise, when they are warm.

4. *Intensity.* All stretches should be done to the point of mild discomfort, not pain.

5. *Time/duration.* All stretches should be held for 10–30 seconds. (PNF techniques should include a 6-second contraction followed by a 10- to 30-second assisted stretch.) All stretches should be performed 2–4 times, for a total volume of 60 seconds per exercise.

Program Plan for Flexibility

Exercise	Areas Stretched	Frequency (check ✓)						
		M	T	W	Th	F	Sa	Su
Head turns and tilts	Neck							
Towel stretch	Triceps, shoulders, chest							
Across-the-body and overhead stretches	Shoulders, upper back, back of the arm							
Upper-back stretch	Upper back							
Lateral stretch	Trunk muscles							
Step stretch	Hip, front of thigh							
Side lunge	Inner thigh, hip, calf							
Inner-thigh stretch	Inner thigh, hip							
Hip and trunk stretch	Trunk, outer thigh and hip, lower back							
Modified hurdler stretch	Back of the thigh, lower back							
Leg stretcher	Back of the thigh, hip, knee, ankle, buttocks							
Lower-leg stretch	Back of the lower leg							
Single-leg deadlift	Hamstrings and gluteal muscles							

LABORATORY ACTIVITIES

You can monitor your program using a chart like the one below.

Flexibility Program Chart

Fill in the dates you perform each stretch, the number of seconds you hold each stretch (should be 10–30), and the number of repetitions of each (should be 2–4). For an easy check on the duration of your stretches, count "one thousand one, one thousand two," and so on. You will probably find that over time you'll be able to hold each stretch longer (in addition to being able to stretch farther).

Exercise/Date																						
	Duration																					
	Reps																					
	Duration																					
	Reps																					
	Duration																					
	Reps																					
	Duration																					
	Reps																					
	Duration																					
	Reps																					
	Duration																					
	Reps																					
	Duration																					
	Reps																					
	Duration																					
	Reps																					
	Duration																					
	Reps																					
	Duration																					
	Reps																					
	Duration																					
	Reps																					
	Duration																					
	Reps																					
	Duration																					
	Reps																					
	Duration																					
	Reps																					
	Duration																					
	Reps																					
	Duration																					
	Reps																					
	Duration																					
	Reps																					
	Duration																					
	Reps																					

Name _____   Section _____   Date _____

LAB 5.3   Assessing Muscular Endurance for Low-Back Health

The four tests in this lab evaluate the muscular endurance of major spine-stabilizing muscles. These tests are the trunk flexor endurance test, back extensor endurance test, side bridge endurance test, and the front plank endurance test.

Trunk Flexor Endurance Test (also called the V-Sit Flexor Endurance Test)

©Taylor Robertson Photography

Equipment

1. Stopwatch or clock with a second hand
2. Exercise mat or padded exercise table
3. Two helpers
4. A wedge angled at 55 degrees from the floor or padded bench (optional)

Preparation
Warm up with some low-intensity activity such as walking or easy jogging.

Instructions

1. To start, assume a sit-up posture with your back supported at an angle of 55 degrees from the floor; support can be provided by a wedge, a padded bench, or a spotter (see photos). Your knees and hips should both be flexed at 90 degrees, and your arms should be folded across your chest with your hands placed on the opposite shoulders. Your toes should be secured under a toe strap or held by a partner.

2. Your goal is to hold the starting position (isometric contraction) as long as possible after the support is pulled away. To begin the test, a helper should pull the wedge or other support back about 10 centimeters (4 inches). The helper should keep track of the time; if a spotter is acting as your support, she or he should be ready to support your weight as soon as your torso begins to move back. Your final score is the total time you are able to hold the contraction—from the time the support is removed until any part of your back touches the support or you request to discontinue the test. Remember to breathe normally throughout the test.

3. Record your time here and on the chart at the end of the lab. Trunk flexors endurance time: _____ sec

Back Extensor Endurance Test (also called the Biering-Sorensen extension test)

©Taylor Robertson Photography

Equipment

1. Stopwatch or clock with a second hand
2. Extension bench with padded ankle and hip support or any padded bench
3. Partner

Preparation
Warm up with some low-intensity activity such as walking or easy jogging.

Instructions

1. Lie face down on the test bench with your upper body extending out over the end of the bench and your pelvis, hips, and knees flat on the bench. Your arms should be folded across your chest with your hands placed on the opposite shoulders. Your legs and hips should be secured under padded straps or held by a partner.

LABORATORY ACTIVITIES

2. Your goal is to hold your upper body in a straight horizontal line with your lower body as long as possible. Keep your neck straight and neutral; don't raise your head and don't arch your back. Breathe normally. Your partner should keep track of the time and watch your form. Your final score is the total time you are able to hold the horizontal position—from the time you assume the position until your upper body drops from the horizontal position.

3. Record your time here and on the chart at the end of the lab. Back extensor endurance time: _____ sec

Side Bridge Endurance Test

Equipment

1. Stopwatch or clock with a second hand

2. Exercise mat

3. Partner

Preparation

Warm up your muscles with some low-intensity activity such as walking or easy jogging. Practice assuming the side bridge position described below.

Courtesy Joseph Quever

Instructions

1. Lie on the mat on your side with your legs extended. Place your top foot in front of your lower foot for support. Lift your hips off the mat so that you are supporting yourself on one elbow and your feet (see photo). Your body should maintain a straight line. Breathe normally; don't hold your breath.

2. Hold the position as long as possible. Your partner should keep track of the time and make sure that you maintain the correct position. Your final score is the total time you are able to hold the side bridge with correct form—from the time you lift your hips until your hips return to the mat.

3. Rest for five minutes and then repeat the test on the other side. Record your times here and on the chart at the end of the lab.

    Right side bridge time: _____ sec

    Left side bridge time: _____ sec

Front Plank Test

Equipment

1. Stopwatch or clock with a second hand

2. Exercise mat

3. Partner

Preparation

Warm up your muscles with some low-intensity activity such as walking or easy jogging. Practice assuming the front plank position described below.

Instructions

1. Assume a front plank position by lying on your front and then lifting your hips, supporting your weight on your forearms and toes and keeping the torso rigid (see photo). Your body should maintain a straight line; keep your hands together and elbows directly under your shoulders. Breathe normally and don't hold your breath.

©Taylor Robertson Photography

2. Hold the position as long as possible. Your partner should keep track of the time and make sure that you maintain the correct position. Your final score is the total time you are able to hold the front plank with correct form—from the time you lift your hips until your hips return to the mat.

3. Record your time here and on the chart at the end of the lab.

    Front plank time: _____ sec

LABORATORY ACTIVITIES

Rating Your Test Results for Muscular Endurance for Low-Back Health

The table below shows percentiles for torso endurance tests for healthy young college students, ages 17–25, based on a study of 181 university students. Compare your scores with the times shown in the table. Your percentile on each test tells you the percentage of the students in the study who scored at or below your score.

Percentiles Ranks for Torso Muscle Endurance Tests for College-Age Men and Women (age 17–25)

Percentiles	Trunk flexor test (sec)		Back extensor test (sec)		Side bridge test, right (sec)		Side bridge test, left (sec)		Front plank test (sec)	
	Men	Women	Men	Women	Men	Women	Men	Women	Men	Women
99%	276	246	246	265	193	130	187	133	400	213
95%	234	208	215	232	164	112	160	114	336	181
90%	211	188	199	215	149	102	146	104	302	165
85%	196	174	188	204	140	96	137	97	280	154
80%	184	163	179	194	131	91	129	92	261	145
75%	174	154	171	186	124	86	122	87	245	137
70%	164	145	164	179	118	83	116	83	231	130
65%	156	138	159	173	113	79	111	79	219	124
60%	148	130	152	167	107	76	106	75	206	118
55%	140	123	147	161	102	72	101	72	195	112
50%	132	116	141	155	97	69	96	68	183	106
45%	124	109	135	149	92	66	91	64	171	100
40%	117	102	130	143	87	63	86	61	160	95
35%	108	94	123	137	81	59	81	57	147	88
30%	100	87	118	131	76	55	76	53	135	82
25%	90	78	111	124	70	52	70	49	121	75
20%	80	69	103	116	63	47	63	44	105	67
15%	68	58	94	106	54	42	55	39	86	58
10%	53	44	83	95	45	36	46	32	64	47
5%	30	24	67	78	30	26	32	22	30	31
1%	0	0	36	45	1	8	5	3	0	0

NOTE: The percentiles were based on data collected on 181 university kinesiology students ages 17–25. The results might not be representative of other populations.
Source: Percentile charts calculated from the data of McGill, S., M. Belore, I. Crosby, and C. Russell, 2010, "Clinical tools to quantify torso flexion endurance: Normative data from student and firefighter populations," *Occupational Ergonomics*, vol. 9, no. 1, 55–61.

Record Your Scores

Test	Time	Percentile
Trunk Flexor Endurance Test		
Back Extensor Endurance Test		
Side Bridge Endurance Test, right side		
Side Bridge Endurance Test, left side		
Front Plank Test		

LABORATORY ACTIVITIES

Using Your Results

How did you score? Are you surprised by your scores for the low-back tests? Are you satisfied with your current ratings?

If you're not satisfied, set a realistic goal for improvement. The norms in this lab are based on healthy young adults, so a score above the mean may or may not be realistic for you. Instead, you may want to set a specific goal based on time rather than rating; for example, set a goal of improving your time by 10%. Imbalances in muscular endurance have been linked with back problems, so if your rating is significantly lower for one of the three tests, you should focus particular attention on that area of your body.

Goal:

What should you do next? Enter the results of this lab in the Preprogram Assessment column in Appendix B. If you've set a goal for improvement, begin a program of low-back exercises such as that suggested in this chapter. After several weeks of your program, complete this lab again and enter the results in the Postprogram Assessment column of Appendix B. How do the results compare?

6 Body Composition

LOOKING AHEAD...

After reading this chapter, you should be able to

- Define fat-free mass and body fat, and describe their functions in the body.

- Explain how body composition affects overall health and wellness.

- Describe how body mass index, body composition, and body fat distribution are measured and assessed.

- Explain how to determine recommended body weight and body fat distribution.

TEST YOUR KNOWLEDGE

1. Exercise helps reduce the risks associated with overweight and obesity even if it doesn't result in improvements in body composition. True or false?

2. Which of the following is the most significant controllable risk factor for the most common type of diabetes (type 2 diabetes)?
   a. smoking
   b. low-fiber diet
   c. overweight or obesity
   d. inactivity

3. In women, excessive exercise and low energy (calorie) intake can cause which of the following?
   a. unhealthy reduction in body fat levels
   b. amenorrhea (absent menstruation)
   c. bone density loss and osteoporosis
   d. muscle wasting and fatigue
   e. all of these

See answers on the next page.

©EVOK/S.Nolte/Getty Images RF

ody composition, the body's relative amounts of fat and fat-free mass, is an important component of fitness for health and wellness. People with an optimal body composition tend to be healthier, to move more efficiently, and to feel better about themselves. They also have a lower risk of many chronic diseases.

Many people, however, don't succeed in their efforts to obtain a fit and healthy body because they set unrealistic goals and emphasize short-term weight loss rather than permanent lifestyle changes that lead to fat loss and a healthy body composition. Successful management of body composition requires the long-term, consistent coordination of many aspects of a wellness program. Even in the absence of changes in body composition, an active lifestyle improves wellness and decreases the risk of disease and premature death (later in the chapter, see the box "Why Is Physical Activity Important Even If Body Composition Doesn't Change?").

This chapter focuses on defining and measuring body composition. The aspects of lifestyle that affect body composition—physical activity and exercise, nutrition, weight management, and stress management—are discussed in detail in other chapters.

WHAT IS BODY COMPOSITION, AND WHY IS IT IMPORTANT?

The human body can be divided into fat-free mass and body fat. As defined in Chapter 2, fat-free mass comprises all the body's nonfat tissues: bone, water, muscle, connective tissue, organ tissues, and teeth.

Body fat is incorporated into the nerves, brain, heart, lungs, liver, mammary glands, and other body organs and tissues. A certain amount of body fat is necessary for the body to function. It is the main source of stored energy in the body; it also cushions body organs and helps regulate body temperature. This **essential fat** makes up about 3–5% of total body weight in men and about 8–12% in women (Figure 6.1). The percentage is higher in women due to fat deposits in the breasts, uterus, and other gender-specific sites.

Most of the fat in the body is stored in fat cells, or **adipose tissue**, located under the skin (**subcutaneous fat**) and around major organs (**visceral fat** or *intra-abdominal fat*). People have a genetically determined number of fat cells, but these cells can become larger or smaller depending on how much fat is being stored. The amount of stored fat depends on several factors, including age, gender, metabolism, diet, and activity level.

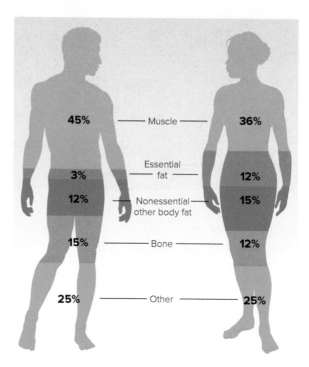

FIGURE 6.1 Body composition of a typical man and woman, 20–24 years old. Each number represents each component's contribution to total body mass.
SOURCES: Brooks, G. A., et al. 2005. *Exercise Physiology: Human Bioenergetics and Its Applications*, 4th ed. New York: McGraw-Hill; Santos, D.A., et al. 2014. "Reference Values for body composition and anthropometric measurements in athletes," *PLoS ONE*, vol. 9, no. 5, e97846.

The primary source of excess body fat is excess calories consumed in the diet—that is, calories consumed beyond what are expended in metabolism, physical activity, and exercise. A pound of body fat is equivalent to 3,500 calories. Over the short term, consuming 3,500 more or fewer calories would result in a gain or loss of about one pound. Over the long term, the relationship between changes in calorie intake and body weight is more complex, as metabolism and calorie needs change as body weight changes; see Chapter 9 for more on strategies for making changes in body composition. Excess stored body fat is associated with increased risk of chronic diseases like diabetes and cardiovascular disease, as described later in this chapter.

Overweight and Obesity Defined

When looking at body composition, the most important consideration is the proportion of the body's total weight that is fat—the **percent body fat**. For example, two women may be 5 feet 5 inches tall and weigh 130 pounds. But one woman may have only 15% of her body weight as fat, whereas the other woman could have 34% body fat. Although neither woman is overweight by most standards, the second woman is considered overfat. Too much body fat (not just total weight) has a negative effect on health and well-being. Just as the proportion of body fat is important, so is its location on your body. Visceral fat is more harmful to health than subcutaneous fat.

Answers (Test Your Knowledge)
1. **True.** Regular physical activity provides protection against the health risks of overweight and obesity. It lowers the risk of death for people who are overweight or obese as well as for those at a normal weight.
2. **c.** All four are risk factors for diabetes, but overweight/obesity is the most significant. It's estimated that 90% of cases of type 2 diabetes could be prevented if people adopted healthy lifestyle behaviors.
3. **e. all of these.** Very low levels of body fat, and the behaviors used to achieve them, have serious health consequences for both men and women.

Overweight is usually defined as total body weight above the recommended range for good health as determined by large-scale population surveys. **Obesity** is defined as a more serious degree of overweight that carries multiple major health risks. The cutoff point for obesity may be set in terms of percent body fat or in terms of some measure of total body weight.

Prevalence of Overweight and Obesity among Americans

Americans are getting fatter. Since 1960, the average American man's weight has increased from 166 to 196 pounds, and the average American woman's weight has increased from 140 to 166 pounds. The prevalence of obesity has increased from about 13% in 1960 to 36.5% in 2014. Today, 62–69% of Americans are obese or overweight (Figures 6.2 and 6.3). In 2015, according to the National Center for Health Statistics, about 34.3% of adult men and 38.3% of adult women were obese. Since 1960, overweight and obesity rates have increased in both men and women, in every age and socioeconomic group, and in people living in every part of the country. Obesity rates are particularly high in blacks, in low-income Americans, and in the South and Midwest; between 2008 and 2014, obesity rates increased most among middle-aged and older adults.

Possible explanations for this increase include more time spent in sedentary work and leisure activities, fewer short trips on foot and more by automobile, fewer daily gym classes for students, more meals eaten outside the home, greater consumption of fast food, increased portion sizes, and increased consumption of soft drinks and convenience foods. According to National Health and Nutrition Examination Survey (NHANES), energy intake increased from 1,955 calories per day in 1971 to 2,269 calories per day in 2003 and then declined to 2,195 calories per day in 2010. In spite of this decline, overweight and obesity rates have continued to increase. People are not losing weight because they are doing less daily physical activity.

Excess Body Fat and Wellness

As rates of overweight and obesity increase, so do the problems associated with them. Obesity doubles mortality rates and can reduce life expectancy by 10–20 years. In fact, if the current trends in overweight and obesity (and their related health problems) continue, scientists believe the average American's life expectancy may soon decline by as much as several years.

Diabetes *Diabetes* is a disease that disrupts normal metabolism. The pancreas normally secretes the hormone insulin, which stimulates cells to take up glucose (blood sugar) to produce energy. Diabetes interferes with this process, causing a buildup of glucose in the bloodstream. Diabetes is associated with kidney failure; nerve damage; erectile dysfunction; circulation problems; retinal damage and blindness; and increased rates of heart attack, stroke, and hypertension. Diabetes is currently the seventh leading cause of death in the United States.

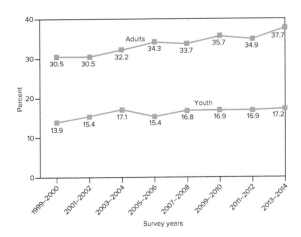

FIGURE 6.2 Obesity trends for U.S. adults age 20 and over and youth ages 2–19, 1999–2014. Since 1999, the proportion of American adults who are obese (body mass index ≥ 30) has increased substantially.

SOURCE: Ogden, C.L., et al, "Prevalence of Obesity Among Adults and Youth: United States, 2011–2014," *National Center Health Statistics Data Brief*, No. 219, November 2015.

Even mild to moderate overweight is associated with a substantial increase in the risk of type 2 diabetes, the most common form, and excess body fat is the key controllable risk factor for diabetes. Obese people are more than three times as likely as nonobese people to develop type 2 diabetes. The incidence of this disease among Americans has increased dramatically as the rate of obesity has climbed, more than doubling between 1995 and 2015.

See Chapter 11 for more on types, diagnosis, treatment, and prevention of diabetes.

Metabolic Syndrome and Premature Death Many overweight and obese people—especially those who are sedentary and eat a poor diet—suffer from a group of symptoms

TERMS

essential fat Fat incorporated in various tissues of the body that is critical for normal body functioning.

adipose tissue Tissue in which fat is stored; fat cells.

subcutaneous fat Fat located under the skin.

visceral fat Fat located around major organs; also called *intra-abdominal fat*.

percent body fat The percentage of total body weight that is composed of fat.

overweight Body weight above the recommended range for good health; sometimes defined as a body mass index between 25 and 29.9, a measure of the proportion of weight to height.

obesity Severely overweight, characterized by an excessive accumulation of body fat; may also be defined in terms of some measure of total body weight or a body mass index of 30 or more.

called **metabolic syndrome** (or *insulin resistance syndrome*). Metabolic syndrome is diagnosed if a person has at least three out of five of these key factors: large waistline (fat deposits in the abdominal region), high blood pressure, high fasting blood sugar (due to **insulin resistance**), high triglycerides, and low HDL ("good") cholesterol. Associated conditions include **chronic inflammation**, **erectile dysfunction**, and **fatty liver** disease. Metabolic syndrome increases the risk of heart disease, more so in men than in women. According to the American Heart Association, about 34% of adult Americans have metabolic syndrome.

Obesity is also associated with increased risk of death from many types of cancer. Other health problems associated with obesity include hypertension, impaired immune function, gallbladder and kidney diseases, skin problems, sleep and breathing disorders, erectile dysfunction, pregnancy complications, back pain, arthritis, and other bone and joint disorders.

Body Fat Distribution and Health The distribution of body fat (the locations of fat on the body) is also an important indicator of health. Men and postmenopausal women tend to store fat in the upper regions of their bodies, particularly in the abdominal area (the "apple shape"). Premenopausal women usually store fat in the hips, buttocks, and thighs (the "pear shape"). Excess fat in the abdominal area increases risk of high blood pressure, diabetes, early-onset heart disease, stroke, certain cancers, and mortality. The reason for this increase in risk is not entirely clear, but it appears that abdominal fat is more easily mobilized and sent into the bloodstream, increasing disease-related blood fat levels.

A measure of waist circumference helps assess the risks of unhealthy body fat distribution. A total waist measurement of more than 40 inches (102 cm) for men and more than 35 inches (88 cm) for women is associated with a significantly increased risk of disease. Waist circumference tends to be higher in taller

Percentage Obese

	2008	2014	Difference (% points)
All adults	25.5	27.7	2.2
Ages 18–29	17.4	17.7	0.3
Ages 30–44	27.0	29.3	2.3
Ages 45–64	29.5	33.0	3.5
Ages 65+	23.4	27.4	4.0
Women	23.9	26.7	2.8
Men	27.0	28.7	1.7
Whites	24.3	26.7	2.4
Hispanics	28.8	28.3	–0.5
Blacks	35.0	35.5	0.5
Annual income less than $36,000	30.0	32.3	2.3
Annual income $36,000 – $89,999	25.8	27.7	1.9
Annual income $90,000+	21.1	23.1	2.0
Midwest	26.8	29.7	2.9
South	26.9	29.2	2.3
East	24.7	26.6	1.9
West	22.8	24.6	1.8

FIGURE 6.3 **Percentage of self-reported obesity (body mass index ≥ 30) among various demographic groups, adults 18 and older, in the United States, 2008 and 2014.** The self-reported values differ from those collected by the Centers for Disease Control and Prevention, but the trend toward increasing obesity in nearly all groups is clear. The association between obesity and lower income is particularly strong. Since 2008, the largest increases in obesity rates were among older adults, adults aged 45–64, those living in the Midwest, and women.
sources: Data from Levy, Jenna, "U.S. obesity rate inches up to 27.7% in 2014," *Gallup-Healthways Well-Being Index,* January 26, 2015. (http://www.gallup.com/poll/181271/obesity-rate-inches-2014.aspx).

metabolic syndrome A cluster of symptoms present in many overweight and obese people that greatly increases their risk of heart disease, diabetes, and other chronic illnesses; symptoms include insulin resistance, abnormal blood fats, abdominal fat deposition, type 2 diabetes, high blood pressure, and high blood glucose.

insulin resistance A condition in which body cells do not respond normally to insulin and cannot easily absorb glucose from the bloodstream; excess glucose can build up in the blood.

chronic inflammation A response of blood vessels to harmful substances, such as germs, damaged cells, or irritants; can lead to heart disease, cancer, allergies, and muscle degeneration.

erectile dysfunction (ED) Inability of a man to develop an erection firm enough for sex. ED is a risk factor of coronary artery disease.

fatty liver Increased fat storage in the liver that can lead to liver inflammation and failure.

TERMS

people, so waist-to-height ratio can be a more accurate measure than waist circumference alone. Your waist measurement should be less than half your height. Using this index, a person who is 5 feet 8 inches (68 inches) tall should have a waist circumference of less than 34 inches. A person who is 6 feet 4 inches (76 inches) tall should have a waist circumference of less than 38 inches.

Performance of Physical Activities Too much body fat makes physical activity difficult because moving the body through everyday activities entails working harder and using more energy. In general, overfat people are less fit than others and don't have the muscular strength, endurance, and flexibility that make normal activity easy. Because exercise is more difficult, they do less of it, depriving themselves of an effective way to improve body composition.

Emotional Wellness and Self-Image Obesity can affect psychological as well as physical wellness. Being perceived as fat can be a source of judgment, ostracism, and sometimes discrimination by others; it can contribute to psychological problems such as depression, anxiety, and low self-esteem.

The popular image of the "ideal" body has changed greatly in the past 50 years, evolving from slightly plump to unhealthily thin. The ideal body—as presented by the media—is an unrealistic goal for most Americans. This is because one's ability to change body composition depends on heredity as well as diet and exercise. Body image, problems with body image, and unhealthy ways of dealing with a negative body image are discussed in Chapter 9. We need to change popular perceptions so that active obese people are regarded as more fit, and normal-weight sedentary people as less fit.

Problems Associated with Very Low Levels of Body Fat

Though not as prevalent a problem as overweight or obesity, having too little body fat is also dangerous. Essential fat is necessary for the functioning of the body, and health experts generally view too little body fat—less than 8–12% for women and 3–5% for men—as a threat to health. Extreme leanness is linked with reproductive, respiratory, circulatory, and immune system disorders and with premature death. Extremely lean people may experience muscle wasting and fatigue. They are also more likely to have eating disorders (described in more detail in Chapter 9). For women, an extremely low percentage of body fat is associated with loss of bone mass and **amenorrhea**—absent or infrequent menstruation (see the box "The Female Athlete Triad"). In older adults, having a low level of lean body mass and muscle strength are better predictors of premature death than body mass index (BMI).

ASSESSING BODY MASS INDEX, BODY COMPOSITION, AND BODY FAT DISTRIBUTION

Although a scale can tell your total weight, it can't reveal whether a fluctuation in weight is due to a change in muscle, body water, or fat. Most important, a scale can't differentiate between overweight and overfat. Some methods of assessing and classifying body composition are based on body fat and others on total body weight. Methods based on total body weight are less accurate, but they are commonly used because body weight is easier to measure than body fat. (Various methods of assessing body composition are described later in the chapter.)

In the past, many people relied on height-weight tables (which were based on insurance company mortality statistics) to determine whether they were at a healthy weight. Such tables, however, can be highly inaccurate for some people. Because muscle tissue is denser and heavier than fat, a fit person can easily weigh more than the recommended weight on a height-weight table. For the same reason, an unfit person may weigh less than the table's recommended weight.

There are a number of simple, inexpensive ways to estimate healthy body weight and healthy body composition. These assessments can provide you with information about the health risks associated with your current body weight and body composition. They can also help you establish reasonable goals and set a starting point for current and future decisions about weight loss and weight gain.

Calculating Body Mass Index

Body mass index (BMI) is useful for classifying the health risks of body weight if you don't have access to more sophisticated methods. Though more accurate than height-weight tables, body mass index is also based on the concept that weight should be proportional to height. BMI is easy to calculate and rate. Researchers frequently use BMI in conjunction with waist circumference in studies that examine the health risks associated with body weight.

BMI is calculated by dividing your body weight (expressed in kilograms) by the square of your height (expressed in meters). The following example is for a person who is 5 feet 3 inches tall (63 inches) and weighs 130 pounds:

1. Divide body weight in pounds by 2.2 to convert weight to kilograms: $130 \div 2.2 = 59.1$

2. Multiply height in inches by 0.0254 to convert height to meters: $63 \times 0.0254 = 1.6$

3. Multiply the result of step 2 by itself to get the square of the height measurement: $1.6 \times 1.6 = 2.56$

4. Divide the result of step 1 by the result of step 3 to determine BMI: $59.1 \div 2.56 = 23$

An alternative equation, based on pounds and inches, is

$$BMI = [weight/(height \times height)] \times 703$$

Space for your own calculations can be found in Lab 6.1, and a complete BMI chart appears in Lab 6.2. The online CDC Adult BMI calculator (https://www.cdc.gov/healthyweight/assessing/bmi/adult_bmi/english_bmi_calculator/bmi_calculator.html) and many apps can also be used to calculate BMI.

---

amenorrhea Absent or infrequent menstruation, sometimes related to unhealthily low levels of body fat and excessive quantity or intensity of exercise. **TERMS**

body mass index (BMI) A measure of relative body weight correlating highly with more direct measures of body fat, calculated by dividing total body weight (in kilograms) by the square of body height (in meters).

DIVERSITY MATTERS
The Female Athlete Triad

Even though obesity is at epidemic levels in the United States, many girls and women strive for unrealistic thinness in response to pressure from peers and a society obsessed with appearance. This quest for thinness has led to an increasingly common, under-reported condition called the **female athlete triad**.

The triad consists of three interrelated disorders: abnormal eating patterns (and excessive exercising), followed by lack of menstrual periods (amenorrhea), followed by decreased bone density (premature osteoporosis). Left untreated, the triad can lead to decreased physical performance, reproductive problems, increased incidence of bone fractures, disturbances of heart rhythm and metabolism, and even death.

Abnormal eating leads to the other two components of the triad. Abnormal eating ranges from moderately restricting food intake, to binge eating and purging (bulimia), to severely restricting food intake (anorexia nervosa). Whether serious or relatively mild, eating disorders prevent women from getting enough calories to meet their bodies' needs.

Disordered eating, combined with intense exercise and emotional stress, can suppress the hormones that control the menstrual cycle. If the menstrual cycle stops for three consecutive months, the condition is called amenorrhea. Chronic disruption of the menstrual cycle can lead to osteoporosis. Bone

Excess exercise and disordered eating

Decreased bone density

Absent or infrequent menstruation

©EyeWire Collection/Getty Images RF

density may erode to the point that a woman in her 20s has the bone density of a woman in her 60s. Women with osteoporosis have fragile, easily fractured bones. Some researchers have found that even a few missed menstrual periods can decrease bone density.

All physically active women and girls have the potential to develop one or more components of the female athlete triad. For example, it is estimated that 5–20% of women who exercise regularly and vigorously may develop amenorrhea. But the triad is most prevalent among athletes who participate in certain sports: those in which appearance is highly important, those that emphasize a prepubertal body shape, those that require contour-revealing clothing for competition, those that require endurance, and those that use weight categories for participation. Such sports include

gymnastics, figure skating, swimming, distance running, cycling, cross-country skiing, track, volleyball, rowing, horse racing, and cheerleading.

The female athlete triad can be life threatening. Typical signs of the eating disorders that trigger the condition are extreme weight loss, dry skin, loss of hair, brittle fingernails, cold hands and feet, low blood pressure and heart rate, swelling around the ankles and hands, and weakening of the bones. Female athletes who have repeated stress fractures may be suffering from the condition.

Early intervention is the key to stopping this series of interrelated conditions. Unfortunately, once the condition has progressed, long-term consequences, especially bone loss, are unavoidable. Teenagers may need only to learn about good eating habits; college-age women with a long-standing problem may require psychological counseling.

SOURCES: Tenforde, A. S., et al. 2017. "Association of the female athlete triad risk assessment stratification to the development of bone stress injuries in collegiate athletes," *American Journal of Sports Medicine* 45(2), 302–310; Mountjoy, M., et al. 2014. "The IOC consensus statement: Beyond the female athlete triad–relative energy deficiency in sport," *British Journal Sports Medicine* 48(7), 491–497; Goolsby, M. A., and N. Boniquit, "Bone health in athletes: The role of exercise, nutrition, and hormones," *Sports Health* 9(2), 2017, 108–117.

Box Icon: ©Rawpixel Ltd/Getty Images RF

A BMI between 18.5 and 24.9 is considered normal and desirable under separate standards from the National Institutes of Health (NIH) and the World Health Organization (WHO). A person with a BMI of 25 or above is classified as overweight, and someone with a BMI of 30 or above is classified as obese (Table 6.1). A person with a BMI below 18.5 is classified as underweight, although low BMI values may be healthy in some cases if they are not the result of smoking, an eating disorder, or an underlying disease. A BMI of 17.5 or less is sometimes used as a diagnostic criterion for the eating disorder anorexia nervosa.

A meta-analysis from the National Center for Health Statistics, pooling data from studies of nearly 3 million people,

> **female athlete triad**   A condition consisting of three interrelated disorders: abnormal eating patterns (and excessive exercising) followed by lack of menstrual periods (amenorrhea) and decreased bone density (premature osteoporosis).
>
> **TERMS**

found that those with severe obesity (BMI greater than 34.9) had a higher death rate from all causes than did people with normal weight (BMI = 18.5–24.9). However, overweight people (BMI = 25–29.9) had a *lower* all-cause death rate than normal weight people, and moderately obese people (BMI = 30–34.9) had similar death rates to normal-weight people. These controversial results showed that there are problems associated with using a one-time measure of BMI to predict health and longevity. Other factors, such as amount of physical activity, lean body mass, body fat changes over time, level of stress, dietary composition, and social factors, might account for the results.

Fat percentage varies for people with a given BMI. In the NHANES, for example, people with BMIs less than 25 had fat percentages ranging from 10% to nearly 32%. Factors influencing fat percentage at a given BMI included age, race, gender, and physical activity.

In classifying the health risks associated with overweight and obesity, the NIH and WHO guidelines consider body fat distribution and other disease risk factors in addition to BMI. As described earlier, excess fat in the abdomen is of greater concern than excess fat in other areas. Measurement of waist circumference (see Table 6.1) is one method of assessing body fat distribution. At a given level of overweight, people with a large waist circumference and/or additional disease risk factors are at risk for health problems. For example, a man with a BMI of 27, a waist circumference of more than 40 inches, and high blood pressure is at greater risk for health problems than another man who has a BMI of 27 but a smaller waist circumference and no other risk factors.

Table 6.1	Classifications from the World Health Organization

BODY MASS INDEX (BMI) CLASSIFICATIONS

WEIGHT STATUS CLASSIFICATION	BODY MASS INDEX
Underweight	<18.5
Severe thinness	<16.0
Moderate thinness	16.0–16.9
Mild thinness	17.0–18.4
Normal	18.5–24.9
Overweight	25.0–29.9
Obese, Class I	30.0–34.9
Obese, Class II	35.0–39.9
Obese, Class III	≥40.0

WAIST CIRCUMFERENCE CLASSIFICATIONS

RISK CLASSIFICATION	WAIST CIRCUMFERENCE IN INCHES (CENTIMETERS) WOMEN	MEN
Normal	<32 in. (80 cm)	<37 in. (94 cm)
Increased	≥32 in. (80 cm)	≥37 in. (94 cm)
Substantially increased	≥35 in. (88 cm)	≥40 in. (102 cm)

SOURCE: World Health Organization. 2008. *Waist Circumference and Waist-to-Hip Ratio. Report of a WHO Expert Consultation.* Geneva: WHO.

Thus, optimal BMI for good health depends on many factors; if your BMI is 25 or above, consult a physician for help in determining a healthy BMI for you. While BMI and waist circumference are important measures of health, they must be considered with other factors such as high blood pressure, diabetes, blood fats, and insulin resistance.

Because BMI doesn't distinguish between fat weight and fat-free weight, it is only an indirect indicator of body fatness and so will not accurately classify all individuals. Factors including muscle mass, age, sex, and race/ethnicity, and height influence the relationship between BMI and actual percent body fat:

- *Muscle mass:* An athlete who weight trains will have more muscle mass than a less trained person of the same height and weight. Although both might be classified as overweight by the BMI scale, that classification would be inaccurate for the athlete because her or his "excess" weight is in the form of muscle, and it is healthy.

- *Age:* Older adults tend to have more body fat than younger adults for an equivalent BMI.

- *Sex:* Women are likely to have more body fat at a given BMI than men, although among healthy adults, women naturally have a higher percent body fat than men.

- *Race/ethnicity:* BMI measurements have over- and underestimated the prevalence of obesity in several groups, such as Hispanics and blacks, because of racial and ethnic differences in muscle mass and muscle density.

- *Height:* BMI is a poor predictor of health in people of **short stature**, whose gene function may have been altered by environmental factors early in life.

If you are an athlete, a serious weight trainer, or a person of short stature, do not use BMI as your primary means of assessing whether your current weight is healthy. Instead, try one of the methods described in the next section for estimating percent body fat. Further, BMI is not particularly useful for tracking changes in body composition over time—gains in muscle mass and losses of fat.

Estimating Percent Body Fat

Assessing body composition involves estimating percent body fat. The dissection and chemical analysis of the body is the only method for directly measuring the percentage of body weight that is fat. However, there are indirect techniques that can provide an *estimate* of percent body fat. One of the most accurate is underwater weighing. Other techniques include the Bod Pod, skinfold measurements, bioelectrical impedance analysis, and dual-energy X-ray absorptiometry.

All of these methods have a margin of error, so it is important not to focus too much on precise values. For example,

short stature Women less than 5 ft 0 in (153 centimeters) tall and men less than 5 ft 5 in (166 centimeters)   TERMS underwater weighing has a margin of error of about ±3%, meaning that if a person's percent body fat is actually 17%, the test result could range from 14% to 20%. The results of different methods may also vary. If you plan to track changes in body composition over time, be sure to perform the assessment using the same method each time. See Table 6.2 for body composition ratings based on percent body fat as a criterion for obesity. It should be noted, however, that the NIH has not developed an official standard linking body fat percentage with obesity.

Underwater Weighing

In hydrostatic (underwater) weighing, an individual is submerged and weighed under water. The percentages of fat and fat-free weight are calculated from body density. Muscle has a higher density and fat a lower density than water. Therefore, people with more body fat tend to float and weigh less under water, and lean people tend to sink and weigh more under water. Many university exercise physiology departments or sports medicine laboratories have an underwater weighing facility. For an accurate assessment of your body composition, find a place that does underwater weighing or has a BodPod (described in the next section).

The Bod Pod

The Bod Pod, a small chamber containing computerized sensors, measures body composition by air displacement. The technique's technical name is *plethysmography*. It determines the percentage of fat by calculating body density from how much air is displaced by the person sitting inside the chamber. The Bod Pod has an error rate of about ±2–4% in determining percent body fat.

> **caliper** A pressure-sensitive measuring instrument with two jaws that can be adjusted to determine thickness of the skinfold.
>
> **TERMS**

Skinfold Measurements

Skinfold measurement is a simple, inexpensive, and practical way to assess body composition. Equations can link the thickness of skinfolds at various sites to percent body fat calculations from more precise laboratory techniques.

Skinfold assessment typically involves measuring the thickness of skinfolds at several different places on the body. You can sum the skinfold values as an indirect measure of body fatness. For example, if you plan to create a fitness (and dietary change) program to improve body composition, you can compare the sum of skinfold values over time as an indicator of your program's progress and of improvements in body composition. You can also plug your skinfold values into equations like those in Lab 6.1 that predict percent body fat. When using these equations, however, remember that they have a fairly substantial margin of error (±4% if performed by a skilled technician), so don't focus too much on specific values. The sum represents only a relative measure of body fatness.

Skinfolds are measured with a device called a **caliper**, which is a pair of spring-loaded, calibrated jaws. High-quality calipers are made of metal and have parallel jaw surfaces and constant spring tension. Inexpensive plastic calipers are also available, but you need to make sure they are spring-loaded and have metal jaws to ensure accuracy. Refer to Lab 6.1 for instructions on how to take skinfold measurements.

Taking accurate measurements with calipers requires patience, experience, and considerable practice. It's best to take several measurements at each site (or have several different people take each measurement). Be sure to take the measurements in the exact location called for in the procedure. Because the amount of water in your body changes during the day, skinfold measurements taken in the morning and evening often differ. If you repeat the measurements in the future to track changes in

---

Table 6.2	Percent Body Fat Classification

	PERCENT BODY FAT (%)				PERCENT BODY FAT (%)		
	20–39 YEARS	*40–59* YEARS	*60–79* YEARS		*20–39* YEARS	*40–59* YEARS	*60–79* YEARS
Women				**Men**			
Essential*	8–12	8–12	8–12	Essential*	3–5	3–5	3–5
Low/athletic**	13–20	13–22	13–23	Low/athletic**	6–7	6–10	6–12
Recommended	21–32	23–33	24–35	Recommended	8–19	11–21	13–24
Over fat†	33–38	34–39	36–41	Overfat†	20–24	22–27	25–29
Obese†	≥39	≥40	≥42	Obese†	≥25	≥28	≥30

NOTE: The cutoffs for recommended, overfat, and obese ranges in this table are based on a study that linked BMI classifications from the NIH with predicted percent body fat (measured using dual-energy X-ray absorptiometry).

*Essential body fat is necessary for the basic functioning of the body.

**Percent body fat in the low/athletic range may be appropriate for some people as long as it is not the result of illness or disordered eating habits.

†Health risks increase as percent body fat exceeds the recommended range.

SOURCES: American College of Sports Medicine. 2018. *ACSM's Guidelines for Exercise Testing and Prescription*, 10th ed. Philadelphia: Wolters Kluwer. Borrud, L.G., et al. 2010. "Body composition data for individuals 8 years of age and older: U.S. population, 1999–2004," *Vital Health Stat*, vol. 11, no. 250; Gallagher, D., et al. 2009. "Healthy percentage body fat ranges: An approach for developing guidelines based on body mass index," *American Journal of Clinical Nutrition*, vol. 72, 694–701.

©BOD POD® Body Composition Tracking System photo provided courtesy of COSMED USA, Inc.

Fitness Tip If you plan to track body composition, be sure to use the same assessment method each time. In addition, don't become overly focused on precise values, because even the most accurate methods have a margin of error. The Bod Pod estimates body composition by air displacement and has a margin of error of about ±2–4%. Skinfold assessment is based on measurement of the thickness of several skinfolds, including the back of the arm, as shown here; equations translate these measurements into a percent body fat estimate, with about a ±4% margin of error.
©Zefrog/Alamy Stock Photo

your body composition, measure skinfolds at approximately the same time of day.

Bioelectrical Impedance Analysis (BIA) The BIA technique works by sending a small electrical current through the body and measuring the body's resistance to it. Fat-free tissues, where most body water is located, are good conductors of

electrical current, whereas fat is not (see the box "Using BIA at Home"). Thus, the amount of resistance to electrical current is related to the amount of fat-free tissue in the body (the lower the resistance, the greater the fat-free mass) and can be used to estimate percent body fat.

Bioelectrical impedance analysis has an error rate of about ±4–5%. To reduce error, follow the manufacturer's instructions carefully and avoid overhydration or underhydration (having more or less body water than normal). Because measurement varies with the type of analyzer, use the same instrument to compare measurements over time.

Advanced Techniques: DEXA and TOBEC Dual-energy X-ray absorptiometry (DEXA) works by measuring the tissue absorption of high- and low-energy X-ray beams. The procedure has an error rate of about ±2%. Total body electrical conductivity (TOBEC) estimates lean body mass by passing a body through a magnetic field. These methods are often used in sophisticated research projects but are seldom available to the average person. We mention them because they are often used for comparison with some of the field tests described in this chapter.

Assessing Body Fat Distribution

Researchers have studied many different methods for measuring body fat distribution. Two of the simplest to perform are waist circumference measurement and waist-to-hip ratio calculation. In the first method, you measure your waist circumference; in the second, you divide your waist circumference by your hip circumference. Waist circumference has been found to be a better indicator of abdominal fat than waist-to-hip ratio. More research is needed to determine the precise degree of risk associated with specific values for these two assessments of body fat distribution. However, as noted earlier, a total waist measurement of more than 40 inches (102 cm) for men and 35 inches (88 cm) for women and a waist-to-hip ratio above 0.94 for young men and 0.82 for young women are associated with a significantly increased risk of heart disease and diabetes. Lab 6.1 shows you how to measure your body fat distribution.

Somatotype

Somatotype describes your basic body build. The three somatotypes are endomorph, mesomorph, and ectomorph:

- *Endomorphs* are round and pear shaped, with wide hips and shoulders. They gain weight easily and will typically regain weight rapidly if they resume their normal lifestyle after losing weight. Endomorphs often excel at weight lifting and might enjoy weight-supported aerobic exercises such as swimming or cycling. Conversely, they might find distance running difficult and painful.

- *Mesomorphs* are lean and muscular and respond well to exercise. They have wedged-shaped bodies, broad shoulders, narrow hips, and little body fat. They gain fitness easily and usually excel at almost any kind of physical activity or sport.

WELLNESS IN THE DIGITAL AGE
Using BIA at Home

Scientists can use several techniques to accurately measure body composition. As described in the chapter, these techniques include underwater weighing, air displacement, and more advanced methods such as dual-energy X-ray absorptiometry (DEXA) and total body electrical conductivity (TOBEC). These methods, however, are costly and require technical expertise.

You can estimate your body fat and fat-free weight simply and accurately, at home, without the help of a technician. All you need is a digital home scale with a built-in bioelectrical impedance analyzer or a hand-held BIA unit. BIA works by measuring the resistance in the body to a small electric current. Electricity flows more slowly through fat tissue than through muscle, so the more fat you have, the more slowly such a current will flow through your body. Conversely, a current will pass through your body more quickly if you have more fat-free (muscle) weight.

To use a BIA scale or hand-held unit, just stand on the scale with bare feet or grasp the handles with each hand. As it checks your weight, the BIA unit sends a low-voltage electrical current through your body and analyzes the speed at which the current travels. Checking your weight and body composition takes no longer than checking your weight alone. Most BIA units can remember your last weight and body composition measurement, making it easy to compare the measurements from day to day or week to week. Some scales can remember measurements for multiple people, as well.

©Lebazele/Getty Images RF

A study of 22 weight-trained men showed that BIA compared favorably to underwater weighing for measuring body composition. Measurements of fat and lean mass are most valuable for measuring changes in body composition during diet and exercise programs.

Popular BIA scales and hand-held BIA devices are manufactured by Taylor, Whynter, Omron, Remedy, and Tanita. These scales and devices are available in most department stores and online, and cost between $30 and $200, depending on features.

Box icon: ©Hong Li/Getty Images RF

- *Ectomorphs* are thin and linear, with narrow hips and shoulders. They typically have little muscle or fat. Their light frame helps make them successful in activities such as distance running and gymnastics.

Few people have extreme body types—most of us are a mixture of all three. People with every body type can benefit from some form of physical activity.

Wellness Tip Many body shapes and sizes are associated with good health. Focus on positive lifestyle behaviors rather than on unrealistic goals related to body weight or shape.
©FredFroese/Getty Images RF

SETTING BODY COMPOSITION GOALS

If assessment tests indicate that fat loss would be beneficial for your health, your first step is to establish a goal. You can use the ratings in Table 6.1 or Table 6.2 to choose a target value for BMI or percent body fat (depending on which assessment you completed).

Set a realistic goal that will ensure good health. Heredity limits your capacity to change your body composition, and few people can expect to develop the body of a fashion model or competitive bodybuilder. However, you can improve your body composition through a program of regular exercise and a healthy diet. If your body composition is in or close to the recommended range, you may want to set a lifestyle goal rather than a specific percent body fat or BMI goal. For example, you might set a goal of increasing your daily physical activity from 20 to 60 minutes or beginning a program of weight training, and then let any improvements in body composition occur as a secondary result of your primary target (physical activity). Remember, a lifestyle that includes regular exercise may be more important for health than trying to reach any ideal weight.

If you are significantly overfat or if you have known risk factors for disease (such as high blood pressure or high cholesterol), consult your physician to determine a body composition goal for your individual risk profile. For people who are obese, even small losses of body weight (5–15%) over a 6- to 12-month period can result in significant health improvements.

After you've established a body composition goal, you can then set a target range for body weight. Although body weight is not an accurate method of assessing body composition, it's a useful method for tracking progress in a program to change body composition. If you're losing a small or moderate amount of weight and exercising, you're probably losing fat while building muscle mass. Lab 6.2 will help you determine a range for recommended body weight.

Using percent body fat or BMI will generate a fairly accurate target body weight for most people. However, it's best not to stick rigidly to a recommended body weight calculated from any formula; individual genetic, cultural, and lifestyle factors are also important. Decide whether the body weight that the formulas generate for you is realistic, meets all your goals, is healthy, *and* is reasonable for you to maintain.

MAKING CHANGES IN BODY COMPOSITION

Chapter 9 includes specific strategies for losing or gaining weight and improving body composition. In general, lifestyle should be your focus—regular physical activity, endurance exercise, strength training, and a moderate energy intake. Making significant cuts in food intake in order to lose weight and body fat is a difficult strategy to maintain; focusing on increased physical activity is a better approach for many people. In studies of people who have lost weight and maintained the loss, physical activity was the key to long-term success. But even in the absence of significant changes in body composition, an active lifestyle improves wellness and decreases the risk of disease and premature death; see the box "Why Is Physical Activity Important Even If Body Composition Doesn't Change?"

You can track your progress toward your target body composition by checking your body weight regularly. Also, focus on how much energy you have and how your clothes fit. To get a more accurate idea of your progress, reassess your body composition occasionally during your program: Body composition changes as weight changes, although body composition can change even if your weight remains the same. If you lose a significant amount of weight, you will usually lose both body fat and some muscle weight because muscles don't have to work as hard to move a lighter body. However, the decline in weight will favor fat loss, and the proportion of body fat will decline, meaning an improvement in body composition.

SUMMARY

- The human body is composed of fat-free mass (which includes bone, muscle, organ tissues, and connective tissues) and body fat.

TIPS FOR TODAY AND THE FUTURE

A wellness lifestyle can lead naturally to a body composition that is healthy and appropriate for you.

RIGHT NOW YOU CAN

- Find out what types of body composition assessment techniques are available at facilities on your campus or in your community.
- Do 30 minutes of physical activity five days per week—walk, jog, bike, swim, or climb stairs.
- Drink a glass of water instead of a soda, and include a high-fiber food such as whole-grain bread or cereal, popcorn, apples, berries, or beans in your next snack or meal.

IN THE FUTURE YOU CAN

- Think about your image of the ideal body type for your sex. Consider where your idea comes from, whether you use this image to judge your own body, and whether it is a realistic goal for you.
- Be aware of media messages (especially visual images) that make you feel embarrassed or insecure about your body. Remind yourself that these messages are usually designed to sell a product; they should not form the basis of your body image.

- Having too much body fat has negative health consequences, especially in terms of cardiovascular disease and diabetes. Distribution of fat is also a significant factor in health.

- A fit and healthy looking body, with the right body composition for a particular person, develops from habits of proper nutrition and exercise.

- Measuring body weight alone is not an accurate way to assess body composition because this measure does not differentiate between muscle weight and fat weight.

- Body mass index (calculated from weight and height measurements) and waist circumference can help classify the health risks associated with being overweight. BMI is sometimes inaccurate, however, particularly in muscular people.

- Techniques for estimating percent body fat include underwater weighing, the Bod Pod, skinfold measurements, bioelectrical impedance analysis (BIA), dual-energy X-ray absorptiometry (DEXA), and total body electrical conductivity (TOBEC).

- Body fat distribution can be assessed through waist measurement or the waist-to-hip ratio.

- Somatotype—endomorph (round), mesomorph (muscular), ectomorph (linear)—is a useful tool for describing basic body characteristics.

- You can determine a recommended body composition and weight by choosing a target BMI or target body fat percentage. Keep heredity in mind when setting a goal, and focus on positive changes in lifestyle.

THE EVIDENCE FOR EXERCISE
Why Is Physical Activity Important Even If Body Composition Doesn't Change?

Physical activity is important for health even if it produces little or no change in body composition—that is, even if a person remains overweight or obese. Physical activity confers benefits no matter how much you weigh; conversely, physical inactivity operates as a risk factor for health problems independently of body composition.

Regular physical activity and exercise block many of the destructive effects of obesity. For example, physical activity improves blood pressure, blood glucose levels, cholesterol levels, and body fat distribution. It also lowers the risk of cardiovascular disease, diabetes, and premature death. Although physical activity and exercise produce these improvements quickly in some people and slowly in others, due to genetic differences, the improvements do occur. Physical activity is particularly important for the many people who have *metabolic syndrome* or *prediabetes*, both of which are characterized by *insulin resistance*. Exercise encourages the body's cells to take up and use insulin efficiently for converting nutrients into usable energy. Being physically inactive for just one day decreases the capacity of the cells to take up and use blood sugar. Exercise makes fat cells fit by improving the function of their mitochondria (powerhouses of the cell) and decreasing inflammation.

Although being physically active and not being sedentary may sound identical, experts describe them as different dimensions of the same health issue. Data suggest that it is important not only to be physically active but also to avoid prolonged sitting. In one study, people who watched TV or used a computer four or more hours a day had twice the risk of having metabolic syndrome as those who spent less

©imtmphoto/Alamy Stock Photo RF

than one hour a day in these activities; other studies reported similar results. Thus, in addition to increasing physical activity, avoiding or reducing sedentary behavior is an important—and challenging—health goal.

Physical activity, then, is important even if it doesn't change body composition. But at a certain level, physical activity and exercise do improve body composition (meaning less fat and more lean muscle mass). Evidence supports a *dose-response* relation between exercise and fat loss: The more you exercise, the more fat you will lose. This includes both total body fat and abdominal fat. In addition, the more body fat a person has, the greater the loss of abdominal fat with exercise. Studies show that, even without calorie reduction, walking 150 minutes per week at a pace of four miles per hour, or jogging 75 minutes a week at six miles per hour, decreases total fat and abdominal fat and improves *metabolic health*.

Studies also show, however, that combining exercise with an appropriate reduction in calories is an even better way to reduce levels of body fat and increase lean muscle mass. The results of combining exercise and calorie reduction may not show up as expected on the scale because the weight of body fat lost is partially offset by the weight of muscle mass gained. Still, your body composition, physical fitness, and overall health have improved.

The question is sometimes asked: Which is more important in combating the adverse health effects of obesity—physical activity or physical fitness? Many studies suggest that both are important; the more active and fit you are, the lower your risk of having health problems and dying prematurely. Of the two, however, physical activity appears to be more important for health than physical fitness.

SOURCES: Silva, D.R., et al. 2016. "Cardiorespiratory fitness effect may be under-estimated in 'fat but fit' hypothesis studies," *Annals of Human Biology* published online; Loprinzi, P., et al. 2014. "The "fit but fat" paradigm addressed using accelerometer-determined physical activity data," *North American Journal of Medical Sciences* 6(7), 295–301; Vieira-Potter, V. J., et al. 2015. "Exercise (and estrogen) make fat cells 'fit'," *Exercise Sport Sciences Reviews*, 43(3), 172–178.

Box Icon: ©Vstock LLC/Getty Images RF

FOR FURTHER EXPLORATION

American Heart Association: Body Composition Tests. Offers detailed information about body composition, testing and analysis, and the impact of body composition on heart health.

http://www.heart.org/HEARTORG/GettingHealthy/NutritionCenter/Body-CompositionTests_UCM_305883_Article.jsp

Methods of Body Composition Analysis Tutorials. Provides information about body composition assessment techniques, including underwater weighing, BIA, and DEXA.

http://nutrition.uvm.edu/bodycomp

National Health and Nutrition Examination Survey (NHANES). Ongoing survey and assessment of health status and practices in the United States.

http://www.cdc.gov/nchs/nhanes/new_nhanes.htm

National Heart, Lung, and Blood Institute: Obesity Education Initiative. Provides information on the latest federal obesity standards and a BMI calculator.

http://www.nhlbi.nih.gov/about/oei/index.htm

National Institute of Diabetes and Digestive and Kidney Diseases: Weight-control Information Network. Provides information about adult obesity: how it is defined and assessed, the risk factors associated with it, and its causes.

http://win.niddk.nih.gov

COMMON QUESTIONS ANSWERED

Skin

Adipose tissue (fat)

Muscle tissue

Before training

After training

Effects of Exercise on Body Composition. Endurance exercise and strength training both reduce body fat and increase muscle mass.

Q Is spot reducing effective?

A *Spot reducing* refers to attempts to lose body fat in specific parts of the body by doing exercises for those parts. Danish researchers have shown that fat use increases in adipose tissue surrounding active muscle, but it is not known if short-term fat use helps reduce fat in specific sites. Most studies show that spot-reducing exercises contribute to fat loss only to the extent that they burn calories. The best way to reduce fat in any specific area is to create an overall negative energy balance: Take in less energy (food) than you use through exercise and metabolism.

Q How does exercise affect body composition?

A Cardiorespiratory endurance exercise burns calories, thereby helping create a negative energy balance. Weight training does not use many calories and therefore is of little use in creating a negative energy balance. However, weight training increases muscle mass, which maintains a higher metabolic rate (the body's rate of energy use) and helps improve body composition. To minimize body fat and increase muscle mass, thereby improving body composition, combine cardiorespiratory

endurance exercise and weight training (see figure above).

Q Are people who have a desirable body composition physically fit?

A Having a healthy body composition is not necessarily associated with overall fitness. For example, many bodybuilders have very little body fat but have poor cardiorespiratory capacity and flexibility. Some athletes, such as NFL linemen, weigh 300 pounds or more; they have to lose the weight when they retire if they don't want to jeopardize their health. To be fit, you must rate high on all the components of fitness.

Q What is liposuction, and will it help me lose body fat?

A Suction lipectomy, popularly known as *liposuction,* has become the most popular type of elective surgery in the world. The procedure involves removing limited amounts of fat from specific areas. Typically, no more than 2.5 kilograms (5.5 pounds) of adipose tissue are removed at a time. The procedure is usually

successful if the amount of excess fat is limited and skin elasticity is good. The procedure is most effective if integrated into a program of dietary restriction and exercise. Side effects include infection, dimpling, and wavy skin contours. Liposuction has a death rate of 1 in 5,000 patients, primarily from pulmonary thromboembolism (a blood clot in the lungs) or fat embolism (circulatory blockage caused by a dislodged piece of fat). In contrast, the death rate for all other surgeries performed in the United States is 1 in 100,000. Other serious complications include shock, bleeding, and impaired blood flow to vital organs.

Q What is cellulite, and how do I get rid of it?

A *Cellulite* is the name commonly given to rippling, wavy fat deposits that collect just under the skin. The "cottage cheese" appearance stems from the breakdown of tissues supporting the fat. These rippling fat deposits are really the same as fat deposited anywhere else in the body. The only way to control them is to create a negative energy balance—that is, burn more calories than you take in. There are no creams or lotions that will rub away surface (subcutaneous) fat deposits, and spot reducing is also ineffective. The solution is sensible eating habits and exercise.

Robert Wood Johnson Foundation. Promotes the health and health care of Americans through research and distribution of information on healthy lifestyles. The foundation publishes an annual report on the status of the national obesity problem.

> http://www.rwjf.org

USDA Food and Nutrition Information Center: Weight and Obesity. Provides links to recent reports and studies on the issue of obesity among Americans.

> http://fnic.nal.usda.gov/weight-and-obesity

See also the listings for Chapters 2, 8, and 9.

SELECTED BIBLIOGRAPHY

Aatashak, S., et al. 2016. Cardiovascular risk factors adaptation to concurrent training in overweight sedentary middle-aged men. *Journal of Sports Medicine and Physical Fitness* 56(5): 624–630.

American College of Sports Medicine. 2018. *ACSM's Guidelines for Exercise Testing and Prescription,* 10th ed. Philadelphia: Wolters Kluwer.

Ashwell, M., and S. Gibson. 2014. A proposal for a primary screening tool: "Keep your waist circumference to less than half your height." *BMC Medicine* 12: 207.

Aune, D., et al. 2016. BMI and all cause mortality: Systematic review and non-linear dose-response meta-analysis of 230 cohort studies with 3.74 million deaths amont 30.3 million participants. *BMJ* 353:i2156. doi:10.1136/bmj.i2156

Buckinx, F., et al. 2015. Concordance between muscle mass assessed by bioelectrical impedance analysis and by dual energy X-ray absorptiometry: A cross-sectional study. *BMC Musculoskeletal Disorders* 16: 60.

Campisi, J., et al. 2015. Sex and age-related differences in perceived, desired and measured percentage body fat among adults. *Journal of Human Nutrition and Dietetics* 28(5): 486–492.

Chuang, S. Y., et al. 2014. Skeletal muscle mass and risk of death in an elderly population. *Nutrition, Metabolism, and Cardiovascular Diseases* 24(7): 784–791.

Dagan, S. S., et al. 2013. Waist circumference vs body mass index in association with cardiorespiratory fitness in healthy men and women: A cross sectional analysis of 403 subjects. *Nutrition Journal* 12: 12.

Dixon, J. B., et al. 2015. Fat-free mass loss generated with weight loss in overweight and obese adults: What may we expect? *Diabetes, Obesity, and Metabolism* 17(1): 91–93.

Ellefsen, S., et al. 2014. Irisin and FNDC5: Effects of 12-week strength training, and relations to muscle phenotype and body mass composition in untrained women. *European Journal of Applied Physiology* 114(9): 1875–1888.

Fahey, T., and M. Fahey. 2014. Nutrition, physical activity, and the obesity epidemic: Issues, policies, and solutions (1960s–present). In T. Oliver, ed., *The Guide to U.S. Health and Health Care Policy,* pp. 363–374. New York: DWJ Books.

Farrell, S. W., et al. 2010. Cardiorespiratory fitness, adiposity, and all-cause mortality in women. *Medicine and Science in Sports and Exercise* 42(11): 2006–2012.

Fosbol, M. O., and B. Zerahn. 2015. Contemporary methods of body composition measurement. *Clinical Physiology and Functional Imaging* 35(2): 81–97.

Fothergill, E., et al. 2016. Persistent metabolic adaptation 6 years after "The Biggest Loser" competition. *Obesity* 24(8): 1612–1619.

Funk, L. M., et al. 2017. Electronic health record data versus the National Health and Nutrition Examination Survey (NHANES); a comparison of overweight and obesity rates. Medical Care. Published online.

Gallagher, K. M., et al. 2011. When "fit" leads to fit, and when "fit" leads to fat: How message framing and intrinsic vs. extrinsic exercise outcomes interact in promoting physical activity. *Psychological Health* 26: (7): 819–834.

Gill, J. M., et al. 2014. Physical activity, ethnicity and cardio-metabolic health: Does one size fit all? *Atherosclerosis* 232(2): 319–333.

Goyal, A., et al. 2014. Is there a paradox in obesity? *Cardiology Reviews* 22(4): 163–170.

Graf, C. E., et al. 2015. Body composition and all-cause mortality in subjects older than 65 y. *American Journal of Clinical Nutrition* 101(4): 760–767.

Heo, M., et al. 2012. Percentage of body fat cutoffs by sex, age, and race-ethnicity in the US adult population from NHANES, 1999–2004. *American Journal of Clinical Nutrition* 95(3): 594–602.

Heymsfield, S. B., et al. 2015. Skeletal muscle mass and quality: Evolution of modern measurement concepts in the context of sarcopenia. *Proceedings of the Nutrition Society* 74(4): 355–366.

Heyward, V. H. 2014. *Advanced Fitness Assessment and Exercise Prescription,* 7th ed. Champaign, Ill.: Human Kinetics.

Hong, H. O., and B. A. Lee. 2016. The effects of the academic performance of college students whose major is sports on body composition and abdominal fat rates. *Journal of Exercise Rehabilitation* 12(4): 328–332.

Hopkins, M., and J. E. Blundell. 2016. Energy balance, body composition, sedentariness and appetite regulation: Pathways to obesity. *Clinical Science* 130(18): 1615–1628.

Joy, E., et al. 2014. 2014 Female Athlete Triad Coalition consensus statement on treatment and return to play of the female athlete triad. *Current Sports Medicine Reports* 13(4): 219–232.

Katchunga, P. B., et al. 2015. Bioelectrical impedance outperforms waist circumference for predicting cardiometabolic risk in Congolese hypertensive subjects: A cross-sectional study. *BMC Cardiovascular Disorders* 15(1): 17.

Kee, C. C., et al. 2017. Association of BMI with risk of CVD mortality and all-cause mortality. *Public Health Nutrition* 12: 1–9.

Kim, S., et al. 2014. Combined impact of cardiorespiratory fitness and visceral adiposity on metabolic syndrome in overweight and obese adults in Korea. *PLoS One* 9(1): e85742.

Kim, S., et al. 2016. Reappraisal of waist circumference cutoff value according to general obesity. *Nutrition & Metabolism* 13: 26.

Kiviruusu, O., et al. 2016. Self-esteem and body mass index from adolescence to mid-adulthood. A 26-year follow-up. *International Journal of Behavioral Medicine* 23(3): 355–363.

Lang, P. O., et al. 2015. Markers of metabolic and cardiovascular health in adults: Comparative analysis of DEXA-based body composition components and BMI categories. *Journal of Cardiology* 65(1): 42–49.

Longland, T. M., et al. 2016. Higher compared to lower dietary protein during an energy deficit combined with intense exercise promotes greater lean mass gain and fat mass loss: A randomized trial. *American Journal of Clinical Nutrition* 103: 738–746.

Nichols, G. A., et al. 2017. Cardiometabolic risk factors among 1.3 million adults with overweight or obesity, but not diabetes, in 10 geographically diverse regions of the United States, 2012–2013. *Preventing Chronic Diseases* 14: E22.

Porto, L. G., et al. 2016. Agreement between BMI and body fat obesity definitions in a physically active population. *Archives of Endocrinology and Metabolism* 60(6): 515–525.

Tian, S., et al. 2016: Age-related changes in segmental body composition by ethnicity and history of weight change across the lifespan. *International Journal of Environmental Research and Public Health* 13: 821–838.

Vieira-Potter, V. J., et al. 2015. Exercise (and estrogen) make fat cells "fit." *Exercise and Sport Sciences Reviews* 43(3): 172–178.

Wick, K., et al. 2016. Deviation between self-reported and measured occupational physical activity levels in office employees: Effects of age and body composition. *International Archives of Occupational and Environment Health* 89: 575–582.

LABORATORY ACTIVITIES

Name _____ Section _____ Date _____

LAB 6.1   Assessing Body Mass Index and Body Composition

Body Mass Index

Equipment

1. Weight scale
2. Tape measure or other means of measuring height

Instructions

Measure your height and weight, and record the results. Be sure to record the unit of measurement.

Height: _____ Weight: _____

Calculating BMI (see also the shortcut chart of BMI values in Lab 6.2)

1. Convert your body weight to kilograms by dividing your weight in pounds by 2.2.

   Body weight_____ lb ÷ 2.2 lb/kg = body weight_____kg

2. Convert your height measurement to meters by multiplying your height in inches by 0.0254.

   Height_____in. × 0.0254 m/in. = height_____m

3. Square your height measurement.

   Height_____m × height_____m = height m^2

4. BMI equals body weight in kilograms divided by height in meters squared (kg/m^2).

   Body weight _____ kg ÷ height _____ m^2 = BMI _____ kg/m^2
   _____(from step 1)_____ _____(from step 3)_____

Rating Your BMI

Refer to the table for a rating of your BMI. Record the results below and on the final page of this lab.

Classification	BMI(kg/m^2)
Underweight	<18.5
Normal	18.5–24.9
Overweight	25.0–29.9
Obesity (I)	30.0–34.9
Obesity (II)	35.0–39.9
Extreme obesity (III)	≥40.0

BMI _____ kg/m^2

Classification _____

Skinfold Measurements

Equipment

1. Skinfold caliper
2. Partner to take measurements
3. Marking pen (optional)

LABORATORY ACTIVITIES

Instructions

1. *Select and locate the correct sites for measurement.* All measurements should be taken on the right side of the body with the subject standing. Skinfolds are normally measured on the natural fold line of the skin, either vertically or at a slight angle. The skinfold measurement sites for males are chest, abdomen, and thigh; for females, triceps, suprailium, and thigh. If the person taking skinfold measurements is inexperienced, it may be helpful to mark the correct sites with a marking pen.

(a) Chest   (b) Abdomen   (c) Thigh   (d) Triceps   (e) Suprailium
(all): Courtesy Shirlee Stevens

   (a) *Chest.* Pinch a diagonal fold halfway between the nipple and the shoulder crease. (b) *Abdomen.* Pinch a vertical fold about 1 inch to the right of the umbilicus (navel). (c) *Thigh.* Pinch a vertical fold midway between the top of the hipbone and the kneecap. (d) *Triceps.* Pinch a vertical skinfold on the back of the right arm midway between the shoulder and elbow. The arm should be straight and should hang naturally. (e) *Suprailium.* Pinch a fold at the top front of the right hipbone. The skinfold here is taken slightly diagonally according to the natural fold tendency of the skin.

2. *Measure the appropriate skinfolds.* Pinch a fold of skin between your thumb and forefinger. Pull the fold up so that no muscular tissue is included; don't pinch the skinfold too hard. Hold the calipers perpendicular to the fold and measure the skinfold about 0.25 inch away from your fingers. Allow the tips of the calipers to close on the skinfold and let the reading settle before marking it down. Take readings to the nearest half-millimeter. Continue to repeat the measurements until two consecutive measurements match, releasing and repinching the skinfold between each measurement. Make a note of the final measurement for each site.

   Time of day of measurements: _____

Courtesy Wayne Glusker

Men	Women
Chest: _____ mm	Triceps: _____ mm
Abdomen: _____ mm	Suprailium: _____ mm
Thigh: _____ mm	Thigh: _____ mm

Determining Percent Body Fat

Add the measurements of your three skinfolds. Use this sum as a point of comparison for future assessments and/or to find the percent body fat that corresponds to your total in the appropriate table. For example, a 20-year-old female with measurements of 17 mm, 21 mm, and 22 mm would have a skinfold sum of 60 mm; according to the following table, her percent body fat is 23.5. The table lists ages in increments of five. If your age is not listed on the table, use the column for the age closest to your own.

Sum of three skinfolds: _____mm   Percent body fat: _____%

Prediction of Fat Percentage in Females from the Sum of Three Skinfolds

Sum of Skinfolds (mm)	Age (Years)								
	20	25	30	35	40	45	50	55	60 and over
20	9.3	9.6	9.9	10.2	10.5	10.8	11.1	11.4	11.7
25	11.2	11.5	11.8	12.1	12.4	12.7	13.0	13.3	13.6
30	13.1	13.4	13.7	14.0	14.3	14.6	14.9	15.2	15.5
35	14.9	15.2	15.5	15.8	16.1	16.4	16.7	17.0	17.3
40	16.7	17.0	17.3	17.6	17.9	18.2	18.5	18.8	19.1
45	18.4	18.8	19.1	19.4	19.7	20.0	20.3	20.6	20.9
50	20.2	20.5	20.8	21.1	21.4	21.7	22.0	22.4	22.7
55	21.9	22.2	22.5	22.8	23.1	23.4	23.7	24.1	24.4
60	23.5	23.8	24.1	24.4	24.8	25.1	25.4	25.7	26.0
65	25.1	25.4	25.7	26.1	26.4	26.7	27.0	27.3	27.7
70	26.7	27.0	27.3	27.6	27.9	28.3	28.6	28.9	29.2
75	28.2	28.5	28.8	29.1	29.5	29.8	30.1	30.4	30.8
80	29.7	30.0	30.3	30.6	31.0	31.3	31.6	31.9	32.3
85	31.1	31.4	31.7	32.1	32.4	32.7	33.0	33.4	33.7
90	32.5	32.8	33.1	33.5	33.8	34.1	34.4	34.8	35.1
95	33.8	34.1	34.5	34.8	35.1	35.5	35.8	36.1	36.5
100	35.1	35.4	35.8	36.1	36.4	36.8	37.1	37.4	37.8
105	36.3	36.7	37.0	37.3	37.7	38.0	38.3	38.7	39.0
110	37.5	37.9	38.2	38.5	38.9	39.2	39.5	39.9	40.2
115	38.7	39.0	39.3	39.7	40.0	40.4	40.7	41.0	41.4
120	39.8	40.1	40.4	40.8	41.1	41.5	41.8	42.1	42.5
125	40.8	41.2	41.5	41.8	42.2	42.5	42.9	43.2	43.5
130	41.8	42.1	42.5	42.8	43.2	43.5	43.9	44.2	44.5
135	42.7	43.1	43.4	43.8	44.1	44.5	44.8	45.1	45.5

NOTE: Find the value on the chart that most closely corresponds to your age and the sum of measurement skinfolds. To calculate the value more precisely, plug your age and sum of skinfolds into the appropriate formula:

% Body Fat = ([4.95 ÷ [1.0994921 − (.0009929 × sum of skinfolds) + (.0000023 × the square of sum of skinfolds) − (.0001392 × age)] − 4.5} × 100), where the skinfold sites (measured in mm) are triceps, suprailium, and thigh

SOURCES: Table generated from equations in Jackson, A. S., M. L. Pollock, and A. Ward. 1980. "Generalized equations for predicting body density in women," *Medicine and Science in Sports and Exercise*, vol. 12, 175–182; Seri, W. E. 1956. "Gross composition of the body," *Advances in Biological and Medical Physics*, 4ed, ed. J. H. Lawrence and C. A. Tobias. New York: Academic Press.

LABORATORY ACTIVITIES

Prediction of Fat Percentage in Males from the Sum of Three Skinfolds

Sum of Skinfolds (mm)	Age (Years)								
	20	25	30	35	40	45	50	55	60 and over
10	1.6	2.1	2.7	3.2	3.7	4.3	4.8	5.3	5.9
15	3.2	3.8	4.3	4.8	5.4	5.9	6.4	7.0	7.5
20	4.8	5.4	5.9	6.4	7.0	7.5	8.1	8.6	9.2
25	6.4	6.9	7.5	8.0	8.6	9.1	9.7	10.2	10.8
30	8.0	8.5	9.1	9.6	10.2	10.7	11.3	11.8	12.4
35	9.5	10.0	10.6	11.2	11.7	12.3	12.8	13.4	13.9
40	11.0	11.6	12.1	12.7	13.2	13.8	14.4	14.9	15.5
45	12.5	13.1	13.6	14.2	14.7	15.3	15.9	16.4	17.0
50	14.0	14.5	15.1	15.6	16.2	16.8	17.3	17.9	18.5
55	15.4	16.0	16.5	17.1	17.7	18.2	18.8	19.4	19.9
60	16.8	17.4	17.9	18.5	19.1	19.7	20.2	20.8	21.4
65	18.2	18.8	19.3	19.9	20.5	21.1	21.6	22.2	22.8
70	19.5	20.1	20.7	21.3	21.9	22.4	23.0	23.6	24.2
75	20.9	21.5	22.0	22.6	23.2	23.8	24.4	24.9	25.5
80	22.2	22.8	23.3	23.9	24.5	25.1	25.7	26.3	26.9
85	23.4	24.0	24.6	25.2	25.8	26.4	27.0	27.6	28.2
90	24.7	25.3	25.9	26.5	27.0	27.6	28.2	28.8	29.4
95	25.9	26.5	27.1	27.7	28.3	28.9	29.5	30.1	30.7
100	27.1	27.7	28.3	28.9	29.5	30.1	30.7	31.3	31.9
105	28.2	28.8	29.4	30.0	30.6	31.2	31.8	32.4	33.0
110	29.3	29.9	30.5	31.1	31.7	32.4	33.0	33.6	34.2
115	30.4	31.0	31.6	32.2	32.8	33.5	34.1	34.7	35.3
120	31.5	32.1	32.7	33.3	33.9	34.5	35.1	35.7	36.4
125	32.5	33.1	33.7	34.3	34.9	35.6	36.2	36.8	37.4

NOTE: Find the value on the chart that most closely corresponds to your age and the sum of measurement skinfolds. To calculate the value more precisely, plug your age and sum of skinfolds into the appropriate formula:

% Body Fat = ([4.95 ÷ [1.109380 − (.0008267 x sum of skinfolds) + (.0000016 x square of the sum of skinfolds) − (.0002574 x age)] − 4.5] x 100), where the skinfold sites (measured in mm) are chest, abdomen, and thigh

SOURCES: Table generated from equations in Jackson, A. S., and M. L. Pollock. 1978. "Generalized equations for predicting body density in men," *British Journal of Nutrition*, vol. 40, 497–504; Jackson, A. S., M. L. Pollock, and A. Ward. 1980. "Generalized equations for predicting body density in women," *Medicine and Science in Sports and Exercise*, vol. 12, 175–182; Seri, W. E. 1956. "Gross composition of the body," *Advances in Biological and Medical Physics*, 4ed, ed. J. H. Lawrence and C. A. Tobias. New York: Academic Press.

Bioelectrical Impedance Analysis (BIA)

Equipment

A bioelectrical impedance analyzer such as Omron Body Fat Analyzer: The BIA device sends an extremely weak electrical current through your body to determine the amount of total body water. You will not feel the current during the test. The body fat percentage is calculated from a formula that uses body water, electric resistance, height, weight, age, and gender.

Instructions

1. Enter your height, weight, gender, and age into the BIA device.

2. Grasp the left and right handles and wrap your middle finger around the groove in the handle. With your thumbs facing up and resting on the unit, place the palms of your hands on the top and bottom electrodes.

3. Hold your arms straight out at a 90-degree angle to your body.

4. Confirm the ready to measure display and the **READY** indicator turns on. Push the start button and the display **START** turns on. The unit automatically detects that it is held and starts measurement. Do not move during measurement.

5. Record your fat, percent fat, and fat-free weight.

    Fat: _____

    Percent fat: _____

    Fat-free weight: _____

6. Compare the BIA measurements with other techniques of assessing body composition.

U.S. Navy Circumference Method of Measuring Percent Fat

This method measures fat percentage from abdominal circumference, neck circumference, and height in men, and from abdominal circumference, hip circumference, neck circumference, and height in women.

Equipment

1. Measuring tape

2. Stadiometer or tape on wall to measure height

Instructions

1. Measure height without shoes using a stadiometer or tape measure. A stadiometer is a height-measuring device that is often part of a scale found in a gym or physician's office.

    Height (inches): _____

2. Measure neck circumference below the larynx (Adam's apple), with the tape sloping slightly downward at the front.

    Neck circumference (inches): _____

3. Measure waist circumference at navel level for men and at the smallest point for women.

    Waist circumference (inches): _____

4. Measure hip circumference (women only) at the largest point.

    Hip circumference (inches): _____

Calculating percent fat using charts developed by the U.S. Navy

Men:

Calculate circumference value: Abdominal circumference − neck circumference: _____

Read percent fat from the chart from where the circumference value intersects with height. Enter fat percentage: _____

Women:

Calculate circumference value: Abdominal circumference + hip circumference − neck circumference (in inches): _____

Read percent fat from the chart from where the circumference value intersects with height. Enter fat percentage: _____

LABORATORY ACTIVITIES

U.S. Navy Circumference Chart for Predicting Percent Fat in Men

Circumference	Height (inches)																				
	60	61	62	63	64	65	66	67	68	69	70	71	72	73	74	75	76	77	78	79	80
13	8	8	7	7	6	6	5	5	4	4	3	3									
14	11	10	10	9	9	8	8	7	7	7	6	6	5	5	4	4	4	3	3		
15	13	13	12	12	11	11	10	10	10	9	9	8	8	7	7	7	6	6	5	5	5
16	16	15	15	14	14	13	13	12	12	12	11	11	10	10	9	9	9	8	8	7	7
17	18	18	17	17	16	16	15	15	14	14	13	13	13	12	12	11	11	10	10	10	9
18	20	20	19	19	18	18	17	17	16	16	15	15	15	14	14	13	13	13	12	12	11
19	22	22	21	21	20	20	19	19	18	18	18	17	17	16	16	15	15	15	14	14	13
20	24	24	23	23	22	22	21	21	20	20	19	19	19	18	18	17	17	17	16	16	15
21	26	25	25	24	24	24	23	23	22	22	21	21	20	20	20	19	19	18	18	18	17
22	28	27	27	26	26	25	25	24	24	23	23	23	22	22	21	21	20	20	20	19	19
23	29	29	28	28	27	27	26	26	26	25	25	24	24	23	23	23	22	22	21	21	21
24	31	30	30	29	29	28	28	28	27	27	26	26	25	25	25	24	24	23	23	23	22
25	32	32	31	31	30	30	30	29	29	28	28	27	27	26	26	26	25	25	24	24	24
26	34	33	33	32	32	31	31	31	30	30	29	29	28	28	28	27	27	26	26	26	25
27	35	35	34	34	33	33	32	32	32	31	31	30	30	29	29	29	28	28	27	27	27
28	37	36	36	35	35	34	34	33	33	32	32	32	31	31	30	30	29	29	29	28	28
29	38	37	37	37	36	36	35	35	34	34	33	33	32	32	32	31	31	30	30	30	29
30	39	39	38	38	37	37	36	36	35	35	35	34	34	33	33	32	32	32	31	31	31
31	40	40	39	39	39	38	38	37	37	36	36	35	35	35	34	34	33	33	33	32	32
32	42	41	41	40	40	39	39	38	38	37	37	37	36	36	35	35	34	34	34	33	33
33	43	42	42	41	41	40	40	39	39	39	38	38	37	37	36	36	36	35	35	34	34
34	44	43	43	42	42	42	41	41	40	40	39	39	38	38	38	37	37	36	36	36	35
35	45	45	44	44	43	43	42	42	41	41	40	40	39	39	39	38	38	37	37	37	36

U.S. Navy Circumference Chart for Predicting Percent Fat in Women

Circumference	Height (inches)																				
	58	59	60	61	62	63	64	65	66	67	68	69	70	71	72	73	74	75	76	77	78
45	19	18	18	17	16	16	15	14	14	13	12	12	11	11	10	9	9	8	8		
46	21	20	19	19	18	17	17	16	15	15	14	13	13	12	12	11	10	10	9	9	8
47	22	22	21	20	19	19	18	17	17	16	16	15	14	14	13	12	12	11	11	10	10
48	24	23	22	22	21	20	20	19	18	18	17	16	16	15	15	14	13	13	12	12	11
49	25	24	24	23	22	22	21	20	20	19	18	18	17	17	16	15	15	14	14	13	13
50	27	26	25	24	24	23	22	22	21	21	20	19	19	18	17	17	16	16	15	15	14
51	28	27	27	26	25	25	24	23	23	22	21	21	20	19	19	18	18	17	17	16	15
52	29	29	28	27	27	26	25	25	24	23	23	22	21	21	20	20	19	19	18	17	17
53	31	30	29	28	27	27	26	25	25	24	24	23	22	22	21	20	20	19	19	18	18
54	32	31	31	30	29	29	28	27	27	26	25	25	24	24	23	22	22	21	21	20	20
55	33	33	32	31	31	30	29	29	28	27	27	26	25	25	24	24	23	22	22	21	21
56	35	34	33	33	32	31	30	30	29	29	28	27	27	26	25	25	24	24	23	23	22
57	36	35	34	34	33	32	32	31	30	30	29	29	28	27	27	26	26	25	24	24	23
58	37	36	36	35	34	34	33	32	32	31	30	30	29	29	28	27	27	26	26	25	25
59	38	38	37	36	36	35	34	34	33	32	32	31	30	30	29	29	28	27	27	26	26
60	40	39	38	37	37	36	35	35	34	33	33	32	32	31	30	30	29	29	28	28	27
61	41	40	39	39	38	37	37	36	35	35	34	33	33	32	32	31	30	30	29	29	28
62	42	41	40	40	39	38	38	37	36	36	35	35	34	33	33	32	32	31	30	30	29
63	43	42	42	41	40	40	39	38	38	37	36	36	35	34	34	33	33	32	32	31	30
64	44	43	43	42	41	41	40	39	39	38	37	37	36	36	35	34	34	33	33	32	32
65	45	45	44	43	42	42	41	40	40	39	38	38	37	37	36	35	35	34	34	33	33
66	46	46	45	44	43	43	42	41	41	40	40	39	38	38	37	37	36	35	35	34	34
67	47	47	46	45	45	44	43	43	42	41	41	40	39	39	38	38	37	36	36	35	35
68	48	48	47	46	46	45	44	44	43	42	42	41	40	40	39	39	38	38	37	36	36
69	49	49	48	47	47	46	45	45	44	43	43	42	41	41	40	40	39	39	38	37	37
70	50	50	49	48	48	47	46	46	45	44	44	43	43	42	41	41	40	40	39	38	38
71	51	51	50	49	49	48	47	47	46	45	45	44	44	43	42	42	41	41	40	39	39
72	52	52	51	50	50	49	48	48	47	46	46	45	45	44	43	43	42	42	41	40	40
73	53	53	52	51	51	50	49	49	48	47	47	46	45	45	44	44	43	43	42	41	41
74	54	54	53	52	52	51	50	50	49	48	48	47	46	46	45	45	44	44	43	42	42
75	55	55	54	53	53	52	51	51	50	49	49	48	47	47	46	46	45	44	44	43	43

SOURCE: Hodgdon, J. A., and K. Friedl, *Development of the DoD body composition estimation equations.* Washington, D.C.: Bureau of Medicine and Surgery, Naval Health Research Center. Technical Document 99–2B, 1998.

Rating Your Body Composition

Refer to the chart below to rate your percent body fat. Record it below and in the chart at the end of this lab.

Rating: _____

Percent Body Fat Classification

	Percent Body Fat (%)				Percent Body Fat (%)		
	20–39 Years	40–59 Years	60–79 Years		20–39 Years	40–59 Years	60–79 Years
Women				**Men**			
Essential*	8–12	8–12	8–12	Essential*	3–5	3–5	3–5
Low/athletic**	13–20	13–22	13–23	Low/athletic**	6–7	6–10	6–12
Recommended	21–32	23–33	24–35	Recommended	8–19	11–21	13–24
Overfat[†]	33–38	34–39	36–41	Overfat[†]	20–24	22–27	25–29
Obese[†]	≥39	≥40	≥42	Obese[†]	≥25	≥28	≥30

NOTE: The cutoffs for recommended, overfat, and obese ranges in this table are based on a study that linked BMI classifications from the NIH with predicted percent body fat (measured using dual-energy X-ray absorptiometry).

*Essential body fat is necessary for the basic functioning of the body.

**Percent body fat in the low/athletic range may be appropriate for some people as long as it is not the result of illness or disordered eating habits.

[†]Health risks increase as percent body fat exceeds the recommended range.

SOURCES: Gallagher, D., et al. 2009. "Healthy percentage body fat ranges: An approach for developing guidelines based on body mass index," *American Journal of Clinical Nutrition,* vol 72, 694–701; Swain, D. P. 2013. *ACSM's Resource Manual for Guidelines for Exercise Testing and Prescription,* 7th ed. Philadelphia: Wolters Kluwer/Lippincott Williams & Wilkins Health.

Other Methods of Assessing Percent Body Fat

If you use a different method, record the name of the method and the result below and in the chart at the end of this lab. Find your body composition rating on the chart above.

Method used: _____ Percent body fat: _____

% Rating (from chart above): _____

Body Fat Distribution

Waist Circumference and Waist-to-Hip Ratio

Equipment

1. Tape measure
2. Partner to take measurements

Preparation

Wear clothes that will not add significantly to your measurements.

Instructions

Stand with your feet together and your arms at your sides. Raise your arms only high enough to allow for taking the measurements. Your partner should make sure the tape is horizontal around the entire circumference and pulled snugly against your skin. The tape shouldn't be pulled so tight that it causes indentations in your skin. Record measurements to the nearest millimeter or one-sixteenth of an inch.

Waist. Measure at the smallest waist circumference. If you don't have a natural waist, measure at the level of your navel.

Waist measurement: _____

Hip. Measure at the largest hip circumference. Hip measurement: _____

Waist-to-Hip Ratio: You can use any unit of measurement (e.g., inches or centimeters) as long as you are consistent. Waist-to-hip ratio equals waist measurement divided by hip measurement.

Waist-to-hip ratio: ÷ _____ = _____ _____
              (hip measurement)   **(waist measurement)**

LABORATORY ACTIVITIES

Determining Your Risk

The table below indicates values for waist circumference and waist-to-hip ratio above which the risk of health problems increases significantly. If your measurement or ratio is above either cutoff point, put a check on the appropriate line below and in the chart at the end of this lab.

Waist circumference: _____(✓ high risk) Waist-to-hip ratio: _____(✓ high risk)

Body Fat Distribution

Cutoff Points for High Risk

	Waist Circumference	Waist-to-Hip Ratio
Men	More than 40 in. (102 cm)	More than 0.94
Women	More than 35 in. (88 cm)	More than 0.82

SOURCE: National Heart, Lung, and Blood Institute. 1998. *Clinical Guidelines on the Identification, Evaluation, and Treatment of Overweight and Obesity in Adults: The Evidence Report.* Bethesda, Md.: National Institutes of Health; Heyward, V. H., and D. R. Wagner. 2004. *Applied Body Composition Assessment,* 2nd ed. Champaign, Ill.: Human Kinetics.

Rating Your Body Mass Index, Body Composition, and Body Fat Distribution

Assessment	Value	Classification
BMI	_____ kg/m^2	_____
Skinfold measurements or alternative method of determining percent body fat. Specify method: _____	_____ % body fat	_____
Bioelectrical Impedance Analysis (BIA)	_____ % body fat	_____
U.S. Navy Circumference Method	_____ % body fat	_____
Waist circumference Waist-to-hip ratio	_____ in. or cm _____ (ratio)	_____ (✓ high risk) _____ (✓ high risk)

Using Your Results

How did you score? Are you surprised by your ratings for body composition and body fat distribution? Are your current ratings in the range for good health? Are you satisfied with your current body composition? Why or why not?

If you're not satisfied, set a realistic goal for improvement:

What should you do next? Enter the results of this lab in the Preprogram Assessment column in Appendix B. If you've determined that you need to improve your body composition, set a specific goal by completing Lab 6.2, and then plan your program using the labs in Chapters 8 and 9. After several weeks or months of an exercise and/or dietary change program, complete this lab again and enter the results in the Postprogram Assessment column of Appendix B. How do the results compare?

Name _____   Section _____   Date _____

LAB 6.2   Setting Goals for Target Body Weight

This lab is designed to help you set body weight goals based on a target BMI or percent body fat. If the results of Lab 6.1 indicate that a change in body composition would be beneficial for your health, you may want to complete this lab to help you set goals.

Remember, though, that a wellness lifestyle—including a balanced diet and regular exercise—is more important for your health than achieving any specific body weight, BMI, or percent body fat. You may want to set goals for improving your diet and increasing physical activity and let your body composition change as a result. If so, use the labs in Chapters 3, 4, 8, and 9 as your guides.

Equipment

Calculator (or pencil and paper for calculations)

Preparation

Determine percent body fat and/or calculate BMI as described in Lab 6.1. Keep track of height and weight as measured for these calculations.

Height: _____   Weight: _____

Instructions: Target Body Weight from Target BMI

Use the chart below to find the target body weight that corresponds to your target BMI. Find your height in the left column, and then move across the appropriate row until you find the weight that corresponds to your target BMI. Remember, BMI is only an indirect measurement of body composition. It is possible to improve body composition without any significant change in weight. For example, a weight training program may result in increased muscle mass and decreased fat mass without any change in overall weight. For this reason, you may want to set alternative or additional goals, such as improving the fit of your clothes or decreasing your waist measurement.

	<18.5 Underweight		18.5–24.9 Normal						25–29.9 Overweight					30–34.9 Obesity (Class I)					35–39.9 Obesity (Class II)					≥40 Extreme Obesity
BMI	17	18	19	20	21	22	23	24	25	26	27	28	29	30	31	32	33	34	35	36	37	38	39	40
Height									Body Weight (pounds)															
4' 10"	81	86	91	96	101	105	110	115	120	124	129	134	139	144	148	153	158	163	168	172	177	182	187	192
4' 11"	84	89	94	99	104	109	114	119	124	129	134	139	144	149	154	159	163	168	173	178	183	188	193	198
5'	87	92	97	102	108	113	118	123	128	133	138	143	149	154	159	164	169	174	179	184	190	195	200	205
5' 1"	90	95	101	106	111	117	122	127	132	138	143	148	154	159	164	169	175	180	185	191	196	201	207	212
5' 2"	93	98	104	109	115	120	126	131	137	142	148	153	159	164	170	175	181	186	191	197	202	208	213	219
5' 3"	96	102	107	113	119	124	130	136	141	147	153	158	164	169	175	181	186	192	198	203	209	215	220	226
5' 4"	99	105	111	117	122	128	134	140	146	152	157	163	169	175	181	187	192	198	204	210	216	222	227	233
5' 5"	102	108	114	120	126	132	138	144	150	156	162	168	174	180	186	192	198	204	210	216	222	229	235	241
5' 6"	105	112	118	124	130	136	143	149	155	161	167	174	180	186	192	198	205	211	217	223	229	236	242	248
5' 7"	109	115	121	128	134	141	147	153	160	166	173	179	185	192	198	204	211	217	224	230	236	243	249	256
5' 8"	112	118	125	132	138	145	151	158	165	171	178	184	191	197	204	211	217	224	230	237	244	250	257	263
5' 9"	115	122	129	136	142	149	156	163	169	176	183	190	197	203	210	217	224	230	237	244	251	258	264	271
5' 10"	119	126	133	139	146	153	160	167	174	181	188	195	202	209	216	223	230	237	244	251	258	265	272	279
5' 11"	122	129	136	143	151	158	165	172	179	187	194	201	208	215	222	230	237	244	251	258	265	273	280	287
6'	125	133	140	148	155	162	170	177	184	192	199	207	214	221	229	236	243	251	258	266	273	280	288	295
6' 1"	129	137	144	152	159	167	174	182	190	197	205	212	220	228	235	243	250	258	265	273	281	288	296	303
6' 2"	132	140	148	156	164	171	179	187	195	203	210	218	226	234	242	249	257	265	273	281	288	296	304	312
6' 3"	136	144	152	160	168	176	184	192	200	208	216	224	232	240	248	256	264	272	280	288	296	304	312	320
6' 4"	140	148	156	164	173	181	189	197	206	214	222	230	238	247	255	263	271	280	288	296	304	312	321	329

SOURCE: Ratings from the National Heart, Lung, and Blood Institute. 1998. *Clinical Guidelines on the Identification, Evaluation, and Treatment of Overweight and Obesity in Adults.* Bethesda, Md.: National Institutes of Health.

LABORATORY ACTIVITIES

Current BMI: _____ Target BMI: _____ Target body weight (from chart): _____
Alternative/additional goals:

Note: You can calculate target body weight from target BMI more precisely by using the following formula: (1) convert your height measurement to meters, (2) square your height measurement, (3) multiply this number by your target BMI to get your target weight in kilograms, and (4) convert your target weight from kilograms to pounds:

1. Height _____ in. × 0.0254 m/in. = height _____ m

2. Height _____ m × height _____ m = _____ m^2

3. Target BMI _____ × height _____ m = target weight _____ kg

4. Target weight _____ kg × 2.2 lb/kg = target weight _____ lb

Instructions: Target Body Weight from Target Body Fat Percentages
Use the formula below to determine the target body weight that corresponds to your target percent body fat.
Current percent body fat: _____ Target percent body fat: _____

Formula	*Example: 180-lb male,* *current percent body fat of 24%, goal of 21%*
1. To determine the fat weight in your body, multiply your current weight by percent body fat (determined through skinfold measurements and expressed as a decimal).	180 lb × 0.24 = 43.2 lb
2. Subtract the fat weight from your current weight to get your current fat-free weight.	180 lb − 43.2 lb = 136.8 lb
3. Subtract your target percent body fat from 1 to get target percent fat-free weight.	1 − 0.21 = 0.79
4. To get your target body weight, divide your fat-free weight by your target percent fat-free weight.	136.8 lb ÷ 0.79 = 173 lb

Note: You can express weight in either pounds or kilograms, as long as you use the unit of measurement consistently.

1. Current body weight _____ × percent body fat _____ = fat weight _____

2. Current body weight _____ − fat weight _____ = fat-free weight _____

3. 1 − target percent body fat _____ = target percent fat-free weight _____

4. Fat-free weight _____ ÷ target percent fat-free weight _____ = target body weight _____

Setting a Goal

Based on these calculations and other factors (including heredity, individual preference, and current health status), select a target weight or range of weights for yourself.

Target body weight: _____

7 Putting Together a Complete Fitness Program

LOOKING AHEAD...

After reading this chapter, you should be able to

- List the steps for putting together a personal fitness program.

- Describe strategies for maintaining a fitness program over the long term.

- Tailor a fitness program to accommodate different life stages and special health concerns.

TEST YOUR KNOWLEDGE

1. Which of the following physical activities is considered a high-intensity exercise?
   a. hiking uphill
   b. singles tennis
   c. jumping rope

2. Older adults should avoid exercise to protect themselves against falls and injuries. True or false?

3. Swimming is a total fitness activity that develops all the components of health-related fitness. True or false?

See answers on the next page.

©andresr/E+/Getty Images RF

Understanding the benefits of physical fitness, as explained in earlier chapters, is the first step toward creating a well-rounded exercise program. The next challenge is to choose activities and combine them into a program that develops all the components of fitness and helps you stay motivated. This chapter presents a step-by-step plan for creating and maintaining a well-rounded fitness program. At the end of this chapter, you'll find sample programs based on popular activities. These programs provide structure that can be helpful if you're beginning an exercise program for the first time.

DEVELOPING A PERSONAL FITNESS PLAN

If you're ready to create a complete fitness program based on the activities you enjoy most, begin by preparing the program plan and agreement in Lab 7.1. By carefully developing your plan and signing an agreement, you'll increase your chances of success. The step-by-step procedure outlined here will guide you through the steps of Lab 7.1 to create an exercise program that's right for you. (See Figure 7.1 for a sample personal fitness program plan and agreement.)

If you'd like additional help in setting up your program, choose one of the sample programs at the end of this chapter. Sample programs are provided for walking/jogging, bicycling, swimming, and rowing. They include detailed instructions for starting a program and developing and maintaining fitness.

1. Set Goals

Ask yourself, "What do I want from my fitness program?" Develop different types of goals—general and specific, long term and short term. General or long-term goals might include lowering your risk for chronic disease, improving posture, having more energy, or improving the fit of your clothes.

It's also a good idea to develop some specific, short-term goals based on measurable factors. Specific goals might be

- Raising cardiorespiratory capacity ($\dot{V}O_{2max}$) by 10%
- Reducing the time it takes you to jog two miles from 22 minutes to 19 minutes
- Increasing the number of push-ups you can do from 15 to 25
- Lowering your BMI from 26 to 24.5

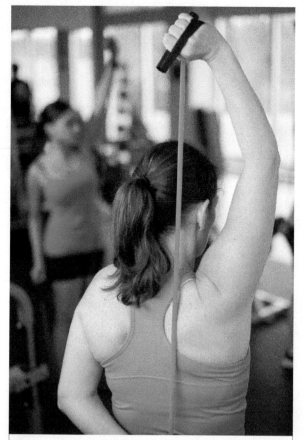

Fitness Tip An overall fitness program includes activities to develop all the components of physical fitness. Remember that you don't need to go to the gym for all your fitness activities. For example, research shows that, especially for young women, resistance bands are just as effective as weight machines or free weights for increasing muscular strength.
©yellowdog/Getty Images RF

Having specific goals will allow you to track your progress and enjoy the measurable changes brought about by your fitness program. Break your specific goals into several smaller steps (mini-goals), such as those shown in Figure 7.1. For example, instead of dwelling on losing 20 or 30 pounds, try losing 2 pounds. Remember, yard by yard is hard; inch by inch is a cinch. (For detailed discussions of goals and goal setting in a behavior change or fitness program, refer back to Chapters 1 and 2.)

Physical fitness assessment tests—as described in Chapters 3, 4, 5, and 6—are essential to determining your goals. They help you decide which types of exercise you should emphasize, and they help you understand the relative difficulty of attaining specific goals. If you have health problems, such as high blood pressure, heart disease, obesity, or serious joint or muscle disabilities, see your physician before taking assessment tests. Measure your progress by taking these tests about every three months.

2. Select Activities

If you have already chosen activities and created separate program plans for different fitness components in Chapters 3, 4, and 5,

A. I [Tracie Kaufman] am contracting with myself to follow a physical
(name)
fitness program to work toward the following goals:

Specific or short-term goals

1. Improving cardiorespiratory fitness by raising my $\dot{V}O_{2max}$ from 34 to 37 ml/kg/min
2. Improving upper body muscular strength and endurance rating from fair to good
3. Improving body composition (from 28% to 25% body fat)
4. Improving my tennis game (hitting 20 playable shots in a row against the ball machine)

General or long-term goals

1. Developing a more positive attitude about myself
2. Improving the fit of my clothes
3. Building and maintaining bone mass to reduce my risk of osteoporosis
4. Increasing my life expectancy and reducing my risk for diabetes and heart disease

B. **My program plan is as follows:**

	Components (Check X)						Frequency (Check X)							Intensity*
Activities	CRE	MS	ME	F	BC	Time	M	Tu	W	Th	F	S	S	
Swimming	X	X	X	X	X	35min	X		X		X			140–170 bpm
Tennis	X	X	X	X	X	90min					X			RPE } 4–6
Weight training		X	X	X	X	30min		X		X		X		see Lab 4.3
Stretching				X		25min	X		X		X	X		—

*List your target heart rate range or an RPE value if appropriate.

C. My program will begin on [Sept.] [21]. My program includes the following schedule
of mini-goals. For each step in my program, I will give myself the reward listed.

Completing 2 full weeks of program (mini-goal 1)	Oct. 5	movie with friends (reward)
$\dot{V}O_{2max}$ of 35 ml/kg/min (mini-goal 2)	Nov. 2	new app or game (reward)
Completing 10 full weeks of program (mini-goal 3)	Nov. 30	new sweater (reward)
Percent body fat of 27% (mini-goal 4)	Dec. 22	weekend away (reward)
$\dot{V}O_{2max}$ of 36 ml/kg/min (mini-goal 5)	Jan. 18	new app or game (reward)

D. My program will include the addition of physical activity to my daily routine (such
as climbing stairs or walking to class):

1. Walking to and from campus job
2. Taking the stairs to dorm room instead of elevator
3. Bicycling to the library instead of driving
4. Taking a drop-in fitness class at the campus recreation center

E. My program will include the following strategies for reducing sedentary time:

1. Setting "move" reminders on phone and laptop
2. Moving during television commercial breaks or between programs
3. Standing or walking during phone calls

F. I will use the following tools to monitor my program and my progress toward
my goals:

I'll use a chart that lists the number of laps and minutes I swim and the

charts for strength and flexibility from Labs 4.3 & 5.2.

I sign this contract as an indication of my personal commitment to reach my goal.

Tracie Kaufman   Sep. 10
(your signature)

I have recruited a helper who will witness my contract and

swim with me three days per week

(list any way your helper will participate in your program)

Russell Walker   Sep. 10
(witness's signature)

FIGURE 7.1   A sample personal fitness program plan and agreement.

Table 7.1	Examples of Aerobic Activities and Their Intensities

MODERATE-INTENSITY ACTIVITIES	VIGOROUS-INTENSITY ACTIVITIES
• Walking briskly (3 miles per hour or faster, but not race-walking)	• Race-walking, jogging, or running
• Water aerobics	• Swimming laps
• Bicycling slower than 10 miles per hour	• Singles tennis
• Doubles tennis	• Cardio dance and other group fitness
• Social dancing	• Bicycling 10 miles per hour or faster
• General gardening	• Jumping rope
• Washing car	• Heavy gardening (continuous digging or hoeing)
• Fly fishing	• Hiking uphill or with a heavy backpack
• Round of golf	• **Interval training**, **Arc Trainer**, or **elliptical trainer**: 4 to 6 intervals of
• Frisbee	30 seconds at maximum intensity, 3 minutes rest between intervals

SOURCE: Adapted from the Centers for Disease Control and Prevention, 2017, https://www.cdc.gov/physicalactivity/resources/recommendations.html

you can put those plans together into a single program. It's usually best to include exercises to develop each of the health-related components of fitness. The components (with abbreviations used in Figure 7.1, section B) are as follows:

- Cardiorespiratory endurance (CRE) is developed by activities that use continuous rhythmic movements of large-muscle groups, like those in the legs (see Chapter 3).
- Muscular strength and endurance (MS and ME) are developed by strength training against resistance (see Chapter 4).
- Flexibility (F) is developed by stretching the major muscle groups (see Chapter 5).
- Healthy body composition (BC) can be developed by combining a sensible diet and a program of regular exercise, including cardiorespiratory endurance exercise to burn calories and resistance training to build muscle mass (see Chapter 6).

Table 7.1 shows the intensity levels of several popular activities that promote health. Check the intensity levels of the activities you're considering to make sure the program you put together will help you achieve your goals.

If you select activities you enjoy and that support your commitment rather than activities that turn exercise into a chore, your program will provide plenty of incentive for continuing. Consider the following factors in making your choices:

- *Fun and interest.* Your fitness program is much more likely to be successful if you choose activities that you currently engage in and enjoy. Often you can modify your

current activities to fit your fitness program. If you want to add a new activity to your program, try it for a while before committing to it.

- *Your current skill and fitness level.* Although many activities are appropriate for beginners, some sports and activities require a certain level of skill to obtain fitness benefits. For example, if you are a beginning tennis player, you will probably not be able to sustain rallies long enough to develop cardiorespiratory endurance. A better choice might be a walking program while you improve your tennis game. To build skill for a particular activity, consider taking a class or getting some instruction from a physical activity coach or fellow participant.

- *Time and convenience.* You are more likely to maintain a long-term exercise program if you can easily fit exercise into your daily routine. As you consider activities, think about whether a special location or facility is required. Can you participate in the activity close to your home, school, or job? Are the necessary facilities available at convenient times (see Lab 7.2)? Can you participate in the activity year-round, or will you need to find an alternative during the summer or winter? Would a home treadmill make you more likely to exercise regularly?

- *Cost.* Some sports and activities require equipment, fees, or some type of membership investment. If you are on a tight budget, limit your choices to free or inexpensive activities. Investigate the facilities on your campus, which you may be able to use at little or no cost. Many activities require no equipment beyond an appropriate pair of shoes. Chapter 4 provides examples of resistance exercises you can do at home without equipment.

- *Special health needs.* If you have a particular health problem, choose activities that will conform to your needs and enhance your ability to cope. Ask your physician how to tailor an exercise program to your needs and goals. See the section "Exercise Guidelines for Life Stages and People with Special Health Concerns" later in this chapter.

TERMS

interval training Repeated bouts of intense exercise followed by rest (e.g., on a running track, sprint the straightaways and walk the turns for one to two miles).

Arc Trainer A weight-bearing, stationary exercise device that exercises the lower body muscles in a crescent-shape pattern.

elliptical trainer A weight-bearing stationary exercise device that works the lower body muscles in an elliptical pattern.

3. Set a Target Frequency, Intensity, and Time (Duration) for Each Activity

The next step is to apply the FITT-VP principle and set a starting frequency, intensity, and time (duration), volume, and progression for each type of activity you've chosen (see the summary in Figure 7.2 and the sample in Figure 7.1).

Cardiorespiratory Endurance Exercise As noted in earlier chapters, based on more than 50 years of research on exercise and health, the U.S. Department of Health and Human Services concluded that most health benefits occur with at least 150 minutes per week of moderate-intensity physical activity (such as brisk walking) or 75 minutes per week of vigorous-intensity activity (such as jogging). Additional benefits occur with more exercise. An appropriate frequency for cardiorespiratory endurance exercise is three to five days per week. For intensity, note your target heart rate zone or RPE (rating of perceived exertion) value. Your target total workout time (duration) should be about 20–60 minutes per day, depending on the intensity of the activity. You can exercise in a single session or in multiple sessions of 10 or more minutes. New research on high-intensity interval training suggests that you can exercise for shorter durations if you train at maximal intensities; be sure to choose an intensity and volume of activity that is safe and appropriate for you.

Muscular Strength and Endurance Training At least two nonconsecutive days per week of strength training is recommended. As described in Chapter 4, a general fitness strength training program includes one or more sets of 8–12 repetitions of 8–10 exercises that work all major muscle groups. For intensity, choose a weight that is heavy enough to fatigue your muscles but not so heavy that you cannot complete the full number of repetitions with proper form. Exercises that use body weight for resistance also build strength and muscle endurance. A note of caution: Years of weight training can lead to stiffer blood vessels. Some studies show that doing aerobics after weight training helps to prevent blood vessel stiffening.

Flexibility Training Stretches should be performed at least two or three days per week (daily is most effective), when the muscles are warm. The stretches should work all major muscle groups. For each exercise, stretch to the point of slight tension or mild discomfort, and hold the stretch for 10–30 seconds; do 2–4 repetitions of each exercise.

4. Set Up a System of Mini-Goals and Rewards

To keep your program on track, set up a system of goals and rewards. Break your specific goals into several steps, and set a target date for each step. For example, if one of the goals of an 18-year-old male student's program is to improve upper-body strength and endurance, he could use the push-up test in Lab 4.2 to set intermediate goals. If he can currently perform 15 push-ups (for a rating of "very poor"), he might set intermediate goals of 17, 20, 25, and 30 push-ups (for a final rating of "fair"). By allowing several weeks between mini-goals and by specifying rewards, he'll be able to track his progress and reward himself as he moves toward his final goal. Reaching a series of small goals

	Cardiorespiratory endurance training	Strength training	Flexibility training
Frequency	3–5 days per week	2–3 nonconsecutive days per week	2–3 days per week (minimum); 5–7 days per week (ideal)
Intensity	55/65–90% of maximum heart rate	Sufficient resistance to fatigue muscles	Stretch to the point of tension
Time	20–60 minutes in sessions lasting 10 minutes or more	Duration of training sufficient to reach target volume	Hold static stretches for 10–30 seconds
Type	Continuous rhythmic activities using large muscle groups	Resistance exercises for all major muscle groups	Stretching exercises for all major joints
Volume	Equivalent of at least 150 minutes or 1,000 or more calories per week of moderate-intensity activity, consistent with individual fitness status and goals	8–12 repetitions of each exercise, 1 or more sets (2–4 sets recommended for most adults), with rest intervals of 2–3 minutes between sets (volume = resistance × sets × reps)	2–4 repetitions for a total stretching time of 60 seconds for each exercise
Progression	Gradually increase volume (frequency, intensity, and/or time) to achieve health and fitness goals; increasing intensity is most important for increasing fitness	Gradually increase resistance, number of sets, or frequency of training to achieve goals; intensity is the most important factor promoting improvements in strength and power	Stretch regularly to build and maintain normal range of motion; avoid excessive flexibility

FIGURE 7.2 A summary of the FITT-VP principle for the health-related components of fitness.
SOURCE: Adapted from American College of Sports Medicine. 2018. *ACSM's Guidelines for Exercise Testing and Prescription*, 10th ed. Philadelphia, PA: Wolters Kluwer Health.

THE EVIDENCE FOR EXERCISE
The Importance of Reducing Sedentary Time

Does a 45-minute workout make up for the effects of 8 hours of sitting time? The answer to this question appears to be no. A complete exercise program focused on the health-related components of fitness provides many benefits. But researchers have found that too much sedentary time—sitting too much—is detrimental to health regardless of whether an individual meets the goals set by the Physical Activity Guidelines for Americans. A 2015 review found that sedentary time was associated with the following, independent of participation in physical activity:

- Deaths from all causes

- Cardiovascular disease

- Cancer (breast, colon, colorectal, endometrial, and certain types of ovarian cancers)

- Type 2 diabetes

The risk of negative outcomes from sedentary time was lower among people with higher levels of physical activity, but they were not eliminated.

How does sedentary time impact health? Although not completely understood, sedentary time is associated with markers of poor metabolic functioning, including unhealthy levels of blood glucose, insulin, and blood fats, as well as a large waist circumference. A study that looked at the impact of increased sedentary time in moderately active individuals found that sitting for more than 30 or 60 minutes at a time resulted in significantly elevated glucose and insulin levels. Sedentary time also affects blood fats and markers for inflammation. All these factors have the potential to contribute to the development of type 2 diabetes, metabolic syndrome, heart disease, and cancer.

What does this mean for an individual? Studies have found that the average American adult spends more than half her or his waking day in sedentary activities, such as using a computer or watching television. Luckily, evidence so far suggests that frequent breaks from sedentary time—2 minutes every 20 or 30 minutes, for example—are protective against some of the impacts of sedentary time. So, it is important to take frequent breaks when you are engaged in sedentary activities, whether at work, at school, or during leisure time. Try some of the strategies suggested in Chapter 2, "Move More, Sit Less" and invent your own. To help stick with your plan, include your strategies as part of your overall fitness program plan.

©blue jean images/Getty Images RF

SOURCES: Tigbe, W. W., et al. 2017. "Time spent in sedentary posture is associated with waist circumference and cardiovascular risk," *International Journal of Obesity*. doi:10.1038/ijo. 30; Evenson, K. R., A. H. Herring, and F. Wen. 2017. "Accelerometry-assessed latent class patterns of physical activity and sedentary behavior with mortality," *American Journal of Preventive Medicine* 52(2), 135–143; Biswas, A., et al. 2015. "Sedentary time and its association with risk for disease incidence, mortality, and hospitalization in adults: A systematic review and meta-analysis," *Annals of Internal Medicine* 162, 123–132; Lyden, K., et al. 2015. "Discrete features of sedentary behaviors impact cardiometabolic risk factors," *Medicine and Science in Sports and Exercise* 47(5), 1079–1086.

Box Icon: ©Vstock LLC/Getty Images RF

is more satisfying than working toward a single, more challenging goal that may take months to achieve. For more on choosing appropriate rewards, see Chapter 1 and Activity 4 in the Behavior Change Workbook at the end of the text.

5. Include Lifestyle Physical Activity and Strategies to Reduce Sedentary Time in Your Program

Daily physical activity is a simple but important way to improve your overall wellness. As part of your fitness program plan, specify ways to be more active during your daily routine, say, by taking the stairs up to class rather than taking an elevator. In addition, develop specific strategies to reduce the amount of time you spend being sedentary (see the box "The Importance of Reducing Sedentary Time"). You may find it helpful to first use a health journal to track your activities for several days. Review the records in your journal, identify routine opportunities to be more active, and add these to your program plan in Lab 7.1.

6. Develop Tools for Monitoring Your Progress

A record that tracks your daily progress will help remind you of your ongoing commitment to your program and give you a sense of accomplishment. Figure 7.3 shows you how to create a general program log and record the activity type, frequency, and times (durations). Or you can complete specific activity logs like those in Labs 3.2, 4.3, and 5.2 in addition to, or instead of, a general log. Post your log in a place where you'll see it often as a reminder and as an incentive for improvement. If you have specific, measurable goals, you can also graph your

Name	Tracie Kaufman															

Enter time, distance, or another factor (such as heart rate or perceived exertion) to track your progress.

Activity/Date	M	Tu	W	Th	F	S	S	Weekly Total	M	Tu	W	Th	F	S	S	Weekly Total
1 Swimming	800 yd		725 yd		800 yd			2325 yd	800 yd		800 yd		850 yd			2450 yd
2 Tennis					90 min			90 min							95 min	95 min
3 Weight Training		X		X		X				X		X			X	
4 Stretching	X		X		X	X					X		X	X	X	X

FIGURE 7.3 A sample program log.

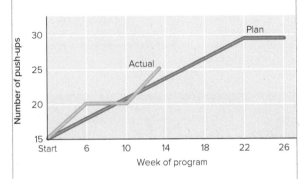

FIGURE 7.4 A sample program progress chart.

weekly or monthly progress toward each goal (Figure 7.4). To monitor the overall progress of your fitness program, you may choose to reassess your fitness every three months or so during the improvement phase of your program. Because the results of different fitness tests vary, be sure to compare results for the same assessments over time.

7. Make a Commitment

Your final step in planning your program is to make a commitment by signing an agreement. Find a witness for your agreement—preferably someone who will be actively involved in your program. Keep your agreement in a visible spot to remind you of your commitment.

PUTTING YOUR PLAN INTO ACTION

After you've developed a detailed plan and signed your agreement, you are ready to begin your fitness program. Refer to the specific training suggestions provided in Chapters 2, 3, 4, and 5 for advice on beginning and maintaining your program. Many people find it easier to plan a program than to put their plan into action and stick with it over time. For that reason, adherence to healthy lifestyle programs has become an important area of study for psychologists and health researchers. The guidelines below and in the next section reflect research into strategies that help people stick with an exercise program.

- *Start slowly and increase fitness gradually.* Overzealous exercising can result in discouraging discomforts and injuries. Your program is meant to last a lifetime. The important first step is to break your established pattern of inactivity. Be patient and realistic. After your body has adjusted to your starting level of exercise, slowly increase the amount of overload. Small increases are the key—achieving a large number of small improvements will eventually result in substantial gains in fitness. It's usually best to increase duration and frequency before increasing intensity.

- *Find an exercise buddy.* The social side of exercise is an important factor for many regular exercisers. Working out with a friend will make exercise more enjoyable and increase your chances of sticking with your program. Find an exercise partner who shares your goals and general fitness level. On days when a partner isn't available, a smartphone or MP3 player can be your workout buddy; see the box "Digital Motivation" for more information.

- *Ask for support from others.* Consistent exercise requires the support of important people in your life, such as parents, spouse, partner, and friends. Talk with them about your program, and let them know the importance of exercise and wellness in your life. Exercise needs to be a critical component of your day (just like sleeping and eating). Good communication will help others become more supportive of and enthusiastic about the time you spend on your wellness program.

- *Vary your activities.* You can make your program more fun over the long term if you participate in a variety of activities that you enjoy. You can also add interest by varying the routes you take when walking, playing with different tennis partners, or switching to a new volleyball or basketball court. Varying your activities, a strategy known as *cross-training,* has other benefits. It can help you develop balanced, total-body fitness. For example, by alternating running with swimming, you build both upper- and lower-body strength. Cross-training can reduce the risk of injury and overtraining because the same muscles, bones, and joints are not continuously subjected to the stresses of the same activity. You can cross-train either by choosing different activities on different days or by alternating activities within a single workout.

WELLNESS IN THE DIGITAL AGE
Digital Motivation

If you ever have trouble getting inspired to work out, motivation may be as close as your smartphone.

Since the iPhone's advent, dozens of interactive motivational applications ("apps") have been developed for use on smart cell phones. Coaching and motivational recordings are available for use on MP3 players, as well. These apps and recordings can substitute for an exercise partner when your workout buddy isn't around and can inspire you to keep your program on track. Some smartphone apps can monitor your workouts, track your progress, and even provide on-the-spot coaching to help you keep going.

Here are just a few examples of low-cost or free smartphone apps that can help you keep exercising:

- **Nike Training Club (http://www.nike.com/us/en_us/c/ nike-plus/training-app).** This training app designs programs according to your goals and experience. Goals include "get lean"—high-intensity cardio exercise to promote weight loss; "get toned"—lightweight training and interval training; "get strong"—weight training to build strength and muscle mass; and "get focused"—15-minute workouts that target specific areas of the body. The app shows specific exercises, paces, and repetitions for the person exercising. It also has tools for motivating you to exercise, such as workout music and a clock that keeps track of the workout time. It is a digital personal trainer at an affordable price.

- **The Beast Sensor (https://www.thisisbeast.com/).** The Beast combines a wearable accelerometer with a smartphone app that tracks sets, reps, acceleration, force, and power. This is an excellent system for monitoring and promoting intense weight-training workouts.

- **Cyclemeter (https://abvio.com/cyclemeter/).** Use this highly motivational app for cycling, running, and walking. It brings detailed statistics to your workouts by keeping track of peak and average speed, caloric expenditure, rest times, elevation changes, and environmental conditions. You can store the results on the cloud or e-mail them to yourself, friends, or social media. You can also integrate the app with a heart rate monitor. The GPS function gives you a map or satellite view of your route.

- **Endomondo (https://www.endomondo.com).** This app uses GPS to keep track of routes used during running, walking, cycling, skating, or cross-country skiing. It also helps people share their workouts with social media, which promotes social accountability as a way to stick with the program.

- **Fitbit (https://www.fitbit.com/app).** This wearable device tracks daily step count, heart rate, sleep quality, nutrition, and energy expenditure and is compatible with a wide variety of devices. It also keeps track of your progress and encourages you to reach your goals.

©YUSUKE SAITO/123RF

Box Icon: ©Hong Li/Getty Images RF

- *Cycle the duration and intensity of your workouts.* Olympic athletes use a technique called periodization of training, meaning that they vary the duration and intensity of their workouts. Sometimes they exercise very intensely; other times they train lightly or rest. You can use the same technique to improve fitness more quickly and make your training program more varied and enjoyable. For example, if your program consists of walking, weight training, and stretching, pick one day a week for each activity to train a little harder or longer than you normally do. If you usually walk two miles at 16 minutes per mile, increase the pace to 15 minutes per mile once a week. If you lift weights twice a week, train more intensely during one of the workouts by using more resistance or performing multiple sets.

- *Adapt to changing environments and schedules.* Most people are creatures of habit and have trouble adjusting to change. Don't use bad weather or a new job as an excuse to give up your exercise program. If you walk in the summer, put on a warm coat and walk in the winter as well. If you can't go out because of darkness, join a gym and walk on a treadmill. Review the results of Lab 2.2 on overcoming barriers to activity to develop additional strategies.

- *Expect fluctuations and lapses.* On some days, your progress will be excellent, but on others, you'll barely be able to drag yourself through your scheduled activities. Don't let off-days or lapses discourage you or make you feel guilty (see the box "Getting Your Fitness Program Back on Track").

- *Choose other healthy lifestyle behaviors.* Exercise provides huge benefits for your health, but other behaviors are also important. Choose a nutritious diet, and avoid harmful habits like smoking and overconsumption of alcohol. Be sure to stay hydrated with water or other healthy beverages (see the box "Choosing Healthy Beverages"). Don't skimp on sleep, which has a mutually beneficial relationship with exercise. Physical activity improves sleep, and adequate sleep can improve physical performance.

TAKE CHARGE
Getting Your Fitness Program Back on Track

Lapses are a normal part of any behavior change program. The important point is to move on and avoid becoming discouraged. Try again and keep trying. Know that continued effort will lead to success. Here are some tips to help you keep going:

- Don't judge yourself too harshly, especially in comparison with others. Some people make faster gains in fitness than others. Focus on the improvements you've already made from your program and how good you feel after exercise—both physically and mentally.

- Visualize what it will be like to reach your goals. Keep these images in mind as an incentive to stick with your program.

- Use your exercise journal to identify thoughts and behaviors that are causing noncompliance. Devise strategies to combat these problematic patterns. If needed, make additional changes in your environment or find more social support. For example, call a friend to walk with you, or keep exercise clothes in your car or backpack.

- Make changes in your plan and your reward system to help renew enthusiasm for and commitment to your program. Try changing fitness activities or your exercise schedule. Build in more opportunities to reward yourself.

- Plan ahead for difficult situations. Think about what circumstances might make it tough to keep up your fitness routine. Develop strategies to increase your chances of sticking with your program. For example, figure out ways to continue your program during vacation, travel, bad weather, and so on.

- If you're in a bad mood or just don't feel like exercising, remind yourself that physical activity is probably the one thing you can do that will make you feel better. Even if you can only do half your scheduled workout, you'll boost your energy, improve your mood, and help keep your program on track.

Box Icon: ©VisualCommunications/Getty Images RF

EXERCISE GUIDELINES FOR LIFE STAGES AND PEOPLE WITH SPECIAL HEALTH CONCERNS

Physical activity is beneficial for people of all ages and for many people with special health concerns.

Exercise Guidelines for Life Stages

A fitness program may need to be adjusted to accommodate the requirements of different life stages.

Children and Adolescents Lack of physical activity has led to alarming increases in overweight and obesity in children and adolescents. If you have children or are in a position to influence children, keep these guidelines in mind:

- Provide opportunities for children and adolescents to exercise every day. Minimize sedentary activities, such as watching television. Children and adolescents should aim for at least 60 minutes of moderate activity every day. Less fit kids should start with 30 minutes a day until their fitness improves and they can exercise longer.

- During family outings, choose dynamic activities. For example, go for a walk or park away from a mall and then walk to the stores.

- For children younger than 12, emphasize skill development and fitness rather than excellence in competitive sports. For adolescents, combine participation and training in lifetime sports with traditional, competitive sports.

- Make sure children are developmentally capable of participating in an activity. For example, catching skills

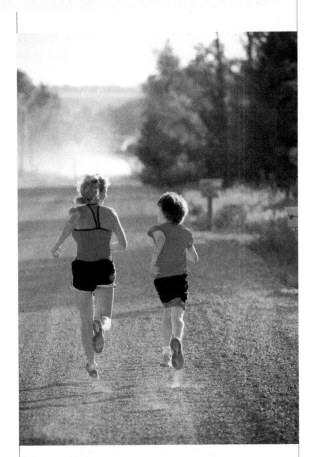

Fitness Tip People of all ages benefit from exercise. By including their children, not only do parents set a positive example that can lead to a lifetime of physical activity, but both parent and child also will have an exercise buddy.

©Zia Soleil/Iconica/Getty Images

CRITICAL CONSUMER
Choosing Healthy Beverages

It's important to stay hydrated at all times, but especially when you are exercising. Too little water intake can leave you feeling fatigued, reduce your body's performance, and leave you vulnerable to heat-related sicknesses in hot weather. But *what* you drink is as significant as how much you drink, both when you are exercising and when you are going about your normal routine.

The Great Water Controversy

Wherever you see people exercising, you will see bottled water in abundance. For several years, a debate has been raging about the quality and safety of commercially bottled water. Manufacturing, bottling, shipping, and disposal processes pollute. Moreover, bottled water is no better for you than regular tap water. Some bottled waters may actually be bad for you, as explained below. To make matters worse, bottled water costs up to 1,900 times more than tap water.

In a 2011 analysis of 173 bottled water products, the Environmental Working Group found 38 contaminants in 10 popular brands of bottled water. Contaminants included heavy metals such as arsenic, pharmaceutical residues and other pollutants commonly found in urban wastewater, as well as a variety of industrial chemicals. Bottled-water companies are notoriously secretive about their products. Overall, 18% of bottled waters failed to list the location of their source, and 32% disclosed nothing about the treatment or purity of the water.

Many commercially bottled water products are, in fact, tap water drawn from municipal water systems. Such revelations have caused the Food and Drug Administration (FDA) to require bottlers to put statements on their products' labels, identifying them as having been drawn from a standard water supply. These products, priced many times higher than water from a residential tap, provide no benefit over standard tap water.

An even bigger issue is that plastic water bottles have become a huge environmental problem: Billions of bottles now pile up in landfills and float in the world's oceans. Some types of plastic take years to biodegrade, and many kinds of plastic bottles will never decompose at all. Newer types of plastic bottles can decompose significantly faster than older bottles, but fast-degrading plastics have not yet come into widespread use in the bottled-water industry.

Experts say that when you're exercising, the cheapest and safest way to stay hydrated is to drink filtered tap water. If you need to carry water with you, buy a reusable container (preferably made of stainless steel) that you can clean after each use. If you drink from plastic bottles, be sure they are recyclable and dispose of them by recycling.

Other Choices

Instead of water, many people choose to drink sodas, juice, tea, or flavored water. While these kinds of beverages have their place, it's important not to drink them too often or in large amounts, especially if they are high in sugar or caffeine. Sugary drinks add empty calories to your diet, and caffeine is a psychoactive drug with a variety of side effects.

Regular (nondiet) sodas are now the leading source of calories in the American diet; most people don't count the calories from beverages as part of their daily caloric intake, leading them to underestimate their total intake. For this reason and others, many experts believe that soda consumption is a major factor in the increasing levels of obesity, metabolic syndrome, diabetes, and other chronic diseases among Americans.

If you're concerned that the liquid portion of your diet is not as healthy as it should be, choose water, fat-free milk, or unsweetened herbal tea more often. Avoid regular soda, sweetened bottled iced tea, flavored water, and fruit beverages made with little fruit juice. To make water more appealing, try adding slices of citrus fruit with sparkling water. With some imagination, you can make sure you stay hydrated without consuming excess calories, spending money unnecessarily, or hurting the environment.

SOURCE: Environmental Working Group, "Bottled water scorecard," 2017. http://www.ewg.org/health/report/Bottled Water/Bottled-Water-Scorecard/Search.

Box icon: ©sam74100/Getty Images RF

are difficult for young children because their nervous system is not developed enough to fully master the skill. Gradually increase the complexity of the skill once the child has mastered the simpler skill.

- Make sure children get plenty of water when exercising in the heat. Make sure they are dressed properly when exercising in the cold.

Pregnant Women   Exercise is important during pregnancy, but women should be cautious because some types of exercise can pose increased risk to the mother and the unborn child. The following guidelines are consistent with the recommendations of the American College of Obstetrics and Gynecology:

- See your physician about possible modifications needed for your particular pregnancy.

- Continue mild to moderate exercise routines at least three times a week. (For most women, this means maintaining an exercise heart rate of 100–160 beats per minute.) Avoid exercising vigorously or to exhaustion, especially in the third trimester. Monitor exercise intensity by assessing how you feel rather than by monitoring your heart rate; ratings of perceived exertion (RPE) levels of 2–4 (fairly light to somewhat hard) are appropriate.

- Favor non- or low-weight-bearing exercises such as swimming or cycling over weight-bearing exercises, which can carry increased risk of injury.

- Avoid exercise in a supine position—lying on your back—after the first trimester. This position restricts blood flow to the uterus. Also avoid prolonged periods of motionless standing.

- Avoid exercise that could cause loss of balance, especially in the third trimester, and exercise that might injure the abdomen, stress the joints, or carry a risk of falling (such as contact sports, vigorous racquet sports, skiing, and in-line skating).

- Avoid activities involving extremes in barometric pressure, such as scuba diving and mountain climbing.

- Especially during the first trimester, drink plenty of fluids and exercise in well-ventilated areas to avoid heat stress.

- Do three to five sets of 10 Kegel exercises daily. These exercises call for tightening the muscles of the pelvic floor for 5–15 seconds per repetition. Kegel exercises are thought to help prevent incontinence (involuntary loss of urine) and speed recovery after giving birth.

- After giving birth, resume prepregnancy exercise routines gradually, based on how you feel.

Older Adults   Older people readily adapt to endurance exercise and strength training. Exercise principles are the same as for younger people, but some specific guidelines apply:

- Follow the same guidelines for aerobic exercise as younger adults, but judge intensity on a 10-point scale of perceived exertion rather than by heart rate.

- For strength training, use a lighter weight and perform more (10–15) repetitions than young adults.

- Perform flexibility exercises at least two days per week for at least 10 minutes. Exercises that improve balance should also be performed two days per week.

- Drink plenty of water and avoid exercising in excessively hot or cold environments. Wear clothes that speed heat loss in warm environments and prevent heat loss in cold environments.

- Warm up slowly and carefully. Increase intensity and duration of exercise gradually.

- Cool down slowly, continuing very light exercise until the heart rate is below 100.

- If you have physical disabilities or limitations and cannot meet the recommendation of at least 150 minutes per week of moderate-intensity exercise, do as much exercise as you can.

Exercise Guidelines for People with Special Health Concerns

As emphasized throughout the text, regular, appropriate exercise is safe and beneficial for everyone. In fact, for many people with special health concerns, the risks associated with not exercising are far greater than those associated with a moderate program of regular exercise.

The fitness recommendations made throughout this book are intended for the general population and can serve as basic guidelines for any exercise program. If you have a chronic health condition, however, you may need to modify your exercise program to accommodate your situation. This section presents precautions and recommendations for people with a variety of special health concerns.

These recommendations, however, are not intended to replace a physician's advice. If you have a special health concern, talk to your physician before starting any exercise program. For additional information about these and other health concerns, visit the website for Exercise Is Medicine: Your Rx for Health Series (http://www.exerciseismedicine.org/support_page.php/your-rx-for-health-series).

Arthritis

- Begin an exercise program as early as possible in the course of the disease.

- Warm up thoroughly before each workout to loosen stiff muscles and lower the risk of injury.

- For cardiorespiratory endurance exercise, avoid high-impact activities that may damage arthritic joints. Consider swimming, water walking, or other exercise that can be done in a warm pool.

- Strength train the whole body. Pay special attention to muscles that support and protect affected joints. For example, build the quadriceps, hamstrings, and calf muscles to support and protect arthritic knees. Start with small amounts of weight and gradually increase the intensity of your workouts.

- Perform flexibility exercises daily to maintain joint mobility.

Asthma

- Exercise regularly. Acute attacks are more likely to occur if you exercise only occasionally.

- Carry medication during workouts and avoid exercising alone. Use your inhaler as recommended by your physician.

- Warm up and cool down slowly to reduce the risk of acute attacks.

- When starting an exercise program, choose self-paced endurance activities, especially those involving interval training (short bouts of exercise followed by a rest period). Gradually increase the intensity of your cardiorespiratory endurance workouts.

- Educate yourself about situations that can trigger an asthma attack and act accordingly when exercising. For example, cold, dry air can trigger or worsen an attack, as can pollen, dust, and polluted air. To avoid attacks in dry air, drink water before, during, and after a workout to moisten your airways. In cold weather, cover your mouth with a mask or scarf to warm and humidify the air you breathe. Also, avoid outdoor activities during pollen season or when the air is polluted or dusty.

Diabetes

- Don't begin an exercise program unless your diabetes is under control and you have discussed exercise safety with your physician. Because people with diabetes have an increased risk for heart disease, an exercise stress test may be recommended.

- Don't exercise alone. Wear a bracelet that identifies you as someone with diabetes.

- If you take insulin or another medication, adjust the timing and amount of each dose as needed. Work with your physician and check your blood sugar level regularly so that you can learn to balance your energy intake and output and your medication dosage.

- To prevent abnormally rapid absorption of injected insulin, inject it over a muscle that will not be exercised, and wait at least an hour before exercising.

- Check your blood sugar before, during, and after exercise. Adjust your diet and insulin dosage as needed. Keep high-carbohydrate foods on hand during a workout. Avoid exercise if your blood sugar level is above 250 mg/dl; if your blood sugar level is below 100 mg/dl, eat some carbohydrate-rich food before exercising.

- If you have poor circulation or numbness in your extremities, check your skin regularly for blisters and abrasions, especially on your feet. Avoid high-impact activities and wear comfortable shoes.

- For maximum benefit and minimum risk, choose moderate-intensity activities.

Heart Disease and Hypertension

- Check with your physician about exercise safety before increasing your activity level. Your doctor may recommend that you take an exercise stress test before starting your program.

- Exercise at moderate intensity rather than high intensity. Keep your heart rate below the level at which abnormalities appear on an exercise stress test.

- Warm up and cool down gradually. Every warm-up and cool-down session should last at least 10 minutes.

- Monitor your heart rate during exercise, and stop if you experience dizziness or chest pain.

- If your physician prescribes nitroglycerin, carry it with you during exercise. If you take a beta-blocker to manage hypertension, use RPE rather than heart rate to monitor your exercise intensity (beta-blockers reduce heart rate). Exercise at an RPE level of "fairly light" to "somewhat hard." Your breathing should be unlabored, and you should be able to talk during exercise.

- Don't hold your breath when exercising. Doing so can cause sudden, steep increases in blood pressure. Take special care during weight training and do not lift heavy loads. Exhale during the exertion phase of each lift.

- Increase exercise frequency, intensity, and time very gradually.

Obesity

- For maximum benefit and minimum risk, begin by choosing low- to moderate-intensity activities. Increase intensity slowly as your fitness improves. Studies of overweight people show that exercising at moderate to high intensities causes more fat loss than training at low intensities.

- People who want to lose weight or maintain weight loss should exercise moderately for 60 minutes or more every day. To get the benefit of 60 minutes of exercise, you can exercise all at once or divide your total activity time into sessions of 10, 20, or 30 minutes.

- Choose non- or low-weight-bearing activities such as swimming, water exercises, cycling, or walking. Low-impact activities are less likely to cause joint problems or injuries.

- Stay alert for symptoms of heat-related problems during exercise (as described in Chapter 3). Obese people are vulnerable to heat intolerance.

- Ease into your exercise program, and increase overload gradually. Increase time and frequency of exercise before increasing intensity.

- Include strength training in your fitness program to build or maintain muscle mass.

- Include as much lifestyle physical activity in your daily routine as possible.

Osteoporosis

- For cardiorespiratory endurance activities, exercise at the maximum intensity that causes no significant discomfort. If possible, choose low-impact, weight-bearing exercises to help safely maintain bone density. (See Chapter 8 for strategies for building and maintaining bone density.)

- To prevent fractures, avoid any activity or movement that stresses the back or carries a risk of falling.

- Include weight training in your exercise program to improve strength and balance and to reduce the risk of falls and fractures. Always use proper exercise technique and avoid lifting heavy loads.

- Include muscle-strengthening exercises three days per week.

- Include bone-strengthening exercises, such as jumping, at least three days per week, if they are safe for you. If you already have bone loss, avoid high-impact activities. Also include balance exercises such as tai chi, which can help prevent falls.

COMMON QUESTIONS ANSWERED

Q Should I exercise every day?

A Some daily exercise is beneficial, but if you train intensely every day without giving yourself a rest, you will likely injure yourself or overtrain. When strength training, for example, rest at least 48 hours between workouts before exercising the same muscle group. For cardiorespiratory endurance exercise, rest or exercise lightly the day after an intense or lengthy workout. Balancing the proper amount of rest and exercise will help you feel better and improve your fitness faster.

Q If exercise is so good for my health, why hasn't my physician ever mentioned it to me?

A A recent study by the American College of Sports Medicine (ACSM) suggests that most people would benefit from getting a physician's advice about exercising. According to the study, 65% of patients said they would be more interested in exercising if their physicians suggested it. About 40% of physicians said they talk to their patients about exercise.

To encourage physicians and patients to talk more often about exercise and its benefits, the ACSM and the American Medical Association have launched the Exercise Is Medicine program. The program advises physicians to give more guidance to patients about exercise and suggests that everyone try to exercise at least five days each week. For more information on the program, visit www.exerciseismedicine.org.

SUMMARY

- Steps for putting together a complete fitness program include (1) setting realistic goals; (2) selecting activities to develop all the health-related components of fitness; (3) setting a target frequency, intensity, and time (duration) for each activity; (4) setting up a system of mini-goals and rewards; (5) making lifestyle physical activity and strategies to reduce sedentary time a part of the daily routine; (6) developing tools for monitoring progress; and (7) making a commitment.

- In selecting activities, consider fun and interest, your current skill and fitness levels, time and convenience, cost, and any special health concerns.

- Keys to beginning and maintaining a successful program include starting slowly, increasing intensity and duration gradually, finding a buddy, varying the activities and intensity of the program, and expecting fluctuations and lapses.

- Regular exercise is appropriate and beneficial for people in all stages of life, although program modifications may be necessary for safety.

- Regular exercise is also appropriate and beneficial for people with special health concerns such as arthritis, asthma, diabetes, heart disease and hypertension, obesity, and osteoporosis, if adapted to the particular condition.

FOR FURTHER EXPLORATION

American Academy of Orthopaedic Surgeons. Provides information about injuries, treatment, and rehabilitation, along with exercise guidelines for people with bone, muscle, and joint pain.

http://www.aaos.org

American Congress of Obstetricians and Gynecologists. Provides guidelines for promoting a healthy pregnancy and postpartum recovery, including exercise during pregnancy.

http://www.acog.org

American Diabetes Association. Promotes diabetes education, research, and advocacy; includes guidelines for diet and exercise for people with diabetes.

http://www.diabetes.org

American Heart Association. Includes information on fitness for kids as well as diet, exercise, fitness, and weight management for adults.

http://www.americanheart.org

For additional listings, see Chapters 2, 3, 4, 5, and 6.

SELECTED BIBLIOGRAPHY

American College of Sports Medicine. 2018. *ACSM's Guidelines for Exercise Testing and Prescription,* 10th ed. Philadelphia: Wolters Kluwer.

American College of Sports Medicine. 2013. *ACSM's Resource Manual for Guidelines for Exercise Testing and Prescription,* 7th ed. Philadelphia: Wolters Kluwer/ Lippincott Williams & Wilkins Health.

Behm, D. G., et al. 2010. Canadian Society for Exercise Physiology position stand: The use of instability to train the core in athletic and nonathletic conditioning. *Applied Physiology, Nutrition and Metabolism* 35(1): 109–112.

Biswas, A., et al. 2015. Sedentary time and its association with risk for disease incidence, mortality, and hospitalization in adults: A systematic review and meta-analysis. *Annals of Internal Medicine* 162: 123–132.

Brody, L., and C. Hall. 2017. *Therapeutic Exercise,* 4th ed. Philadelphia: Wolters Kluwer.

Canadian Society for Exercise Physiology. 2011. *Public Health Agency of Canada Physical Activity Guidelines* (www.publichealth.gc.ca5).

Carlson, S. A., et al. 2015. Inadequate physical activity and health care expenditures in the United States. *Progress in Cardiovascular Diseases* 57(4): 315–323.

Centers for Disease Control and Prevention. 2014. *State Indicator Report on Physical Activity, 2014.* Atlanta, GA: U.S. Department of Health and Human Services.

DeFina, L. F., et al. 2015. Physical activity versus cardiorespiratory fitness: Two (partly) distinct components of cardiovascular health? *Progress in Cardiovascular Diseases* 57(4): 324–329.

Fahey, T., and M. Fahey. 2014. Nutrition, physical activity, and the obesity epidemic: Issues, policies, and solutions (1960s–present). In T. Oliver, ed., *The Guide to U.S. Health and Health Care Policy,* pp. 363–374. New York: DWJ Books.

Foulds, H. J. 2017. High volume physical activity and cardiovascular risk. *American Journal of Hypertension.* Published online.

Francois, M. E., et al. 2017. Similar metabolic response to lower- versus upper-body interval exercise or endurance exercise. *Metabolism* 68:1–10.

Harrington, R. A., et al. 2015. More than 10 million steps in the right direction: Results from the first American Heart Association scientific sessions walking challenge. *Progress in Cardiovascular Diseases* 57(4): 296–298.

Heinrich, K. M., et al. 2014. High-intensity compared to moderate-intensity training for exercise initiation, enjoyment, adherence, and intentions: An intervention study. *BMC Public Health* 14: 789.

Hills, A. P., et al. 2015. Supporting public health priorities: Recommendations for physical education and physical activity promotion in schools. *Progress in Cardiovascular Diseases* 57(4): 368–374.

Joyner, M. J. 2017. Exercise and trainability. *Journal of Physiology.* Published online.

Kaminsky, L. A., and A. H. Montoye. 2014. Physical activity and health: What is the best dose? *Journal of the American Heart Association* 3(5): e001430.

Koohsari, M. J., et al. 2015. Public open space, physical activity, urban design and public health: Concepts, methods and research agenda. *Health & Place* 33: 75–82.

Leskinen, T., and U. M. Kujala. 2015. Health-related findings among twin pairs discordant for leisure-time physical activity for 32 years: The TWINACTIVE Study synopsis. *Twin Research in Human Genetics* 18(3): 266–272.

Lyden, K., et al. 2015. Discrete features of sedentary behaviors impact cardiometabolic risk factors. *Medicine and Science in Sports and Exercise* 47(5): 1079–1086.

Mabire, L., et al. 2017. The influence of age, sex and body mass index on the effectiveness of brisk walking for obesity management in adults. A systematic review and meta-analysis. *Journal of Physical Activity and Health* 7: 1–46.

Malina, R. M. 2015. Physical activity, health and nutrition. *World Review of Nutrition and Dietetics* 113: 68–71.

Marques, A., et al. 2015. Do students know the physical activity recommendations for health promotion? *Journal of Physical Activity and Health* 12(2): 253–256.

Marzetti, E., et al. 2017. Physical activity and exercise as countermeasures to physical frailty and sarcopenia. *Aging Clinical and Experimental Research* 29(1): 35–42.

Melanson, E. L. 2017. The effect of exercise on non-exercise physical activity and sedentary behavior in adults. *Obesity Reviews* 18(Suppl. 1): 40–49.

Moholdt, T., et al. 2014. Current physical activity guidelines for health are insufficient to mitigate long-term weight gain: More data in the fitness versus fatness debate (the HUNT Study, Norway). *British Journal of Sports Medicine* 48(20): 1489–1496.

Myers, J., et al. 2015. Physical activity and cardiorespiratory fitness as major markers of cardiovascular risk: Their independent and interwoven importance to health status. *Progress in Cardiovascular Diseases* 57(4): 306–314.

Petersen, B. A., et al. 2017. Low load, high repetition resistance training program increases bone mineral density in untrained adults. *Journal of Sports Medicine and Physical Fitness* 57(1–2): 70–76.

Picorelli, A. M., et al. 2014. Adherence to exercise programs for older people is influenced by program characteristics and personal factors: A systematic review. *Journal of Physiotherapy* 60(3): 151–156.

Puett, R., et al. 2014. Physical activity: Does environment make a difference for tension, stress, emotional outlook, and perceptions of health status? *Journal of Physical Activity and Health* 11(8): 1503–1511.

Romieu, I. 2017. Energy balance and obesity. *Cancer Causes and Control* 28(3): 247–258.

Rowlands, A. V. 2015. Physical activity, inactivity, and health. *Pediatric Exercise Science* 27(1): 21–25.

Sjogren, P., et al. 2014. Stand up for health—Avoiding sedentary behaviour might lengthen your telomeres: Secondary outcomes from a physical activity RCT in older people. *British Journal of Sports Medicine* 48(19): 1407–1409.

Soares-Miranda, L., et al. 2014. Physical activity and heart rate variability in older adults: The Cardiovascular Health Study. *Circulation* 129(21): 2100–2110.

U.S. Department of Health and Human Services. 2008. *Physical Activity Guidelines for Americans.* Washington, DC: U.S. Department of Health and Human Services.

Valle, C. G., et al. 2015. Physical activity in young adults: A signal detection analysis of Health Information National Trends Survey (HINTS) 2007 data. *Journal of Health Communication* 20(2): 134–146.

White, D. K., et al. 2015. Do short spurts of physical activity benefit cardiovascular health? The CARDIA Study. *Medicine and Science in Sports and Exercise* 47(11): 2353–2358.

SAMPLE PROGRAMS FOR POPULAR ACTIVITIES

The following sections present four sample programs based on different types of cardiorespiratory activities—walking/jogging, bicycling, swimming, and rowing. Each sample program includes regular cardiorespiratory endurance exercise, resistance training, and stretching. Read the descriptions of the programs you're considering, and decide which will work best for you based on your present routine, the potential for enjoyment, and adaptability to your lifestyle. If you choose one of these programs, complete the personal fitness program plan in Lab 7.1, just as if you had created a program from scratch.

No program will produce enormous changes in your fitness level in the first few weeks. Follow the specifics of the program for three to four weeks. Then, if the exercise program doesn't seem suitable, make adjustments to adapt it to your particular needs. But retain the basic elements of the program that make it effective for developing fitness.

GENERAL GUIDELINES

The following guidelines can help make the activity programs more effective for you:

- *Frequency and time.* To improve physical fitness, exercise for 20–60 minutes at least three times a week.

- *Intensity.* To work effectively for cardiorespiratory endurance training or to improve body composition, raise your heart rate into its target zone. Monitor your pulse or use rates of perceived exertion to monitor your intensity. If you've been sedentary, begin very slowly. Give your muscles a chance to adjust to their increased workload. It's probably best to keep your heart rate below target until your body has had time to adjust to new demands. At first you may not need to work very hard to keep your heart rate in its target zone, but as your cardiorespiratory endurance improves, you will probably need to increase intensity.

- *Interval training.* Some of the sample programs involve continuous activity. Others rely on interval training, which calls for alternating a relief interval with exercise (walking after jogging, for example, or coasting after biking uphill). Interval training is an effective method of progressive overload and improves fitness rapidly (see Chapter 3).

- *Resistance training and stretching guidelines.* For the resistance training and stretching parts of the program, remember the general guidelines for safe and effective exercise. See the summary of guidelines in Figure 7.2

- *Warm-up and cool-down.* Begin each exercise session with a 10-minute warm-up. Begin your activity at a slow pace, and work up gradually to your target heart rate. Always slow down gradually at the end of your exercise session to bring your system back to its normal state. It's a good idea to do stretching exercises to increase your flexibility *after* cardiorespiratory exercise or strength training because your muscles will be warm and ready to stretch.

Follow the guidelines presented in Chapter 3 for exercising in hot or cold weather. Drink enough liquids to stay adequately hydrated, particularly in hot weather.

- *Record keeping.* After each exercise session, record your daily distance or time on a progress chart.

WALKING/JOGGING SAMPLE PROGRAM

Walking is the perfect exercise. It increases longevity; builds fitness; expends calories; prevents weight gain; and protects against heart disease, stroke, and back pain. You don't need to join a gym, and you can walk almost anywhere. People who walk 30 minutes five times per week will lose an average of 5 pounds in 6–12 months—without dieting, watching what they eat, or exercising intensely.

Jogging takes walking to the next level. Jogging only 75 minutes per week will increase fitness, promote weight control, and provide health benefits that will prevent disease and increase longevity. Your ultimate goal for promoting wellness is to walk at a moderate intensity for 150–300 minutes per week or jog at 70% effort or more for 75–150 minutes per week.

It isn't always easy to distinguish among walking, jogging, and running. For clarity and consistency, we'll consider walking to be any on-foot exercise of less than 5 miles per hour, jogging any pace between 5 and 7.5 miles per hour, and running any pace faster than that. The faster your pace or the longer you exercise, the more calories you burn (Table 1). The greater the number of calories burned, the higher the potential training effects of these activities. Table 2 contains a sample walking/jogging program.

Equipment and Technique

These activities require no special skills, expensive equipment, or unusual facilities. Comfortable clothing, well-fitted walking or running shoes (see Chapter 3), and a stopwatch or ordinary watch with a second hand are all you need.

When you advance to jogging, use proper technique:

- Run with your back straight and your head up. Look straight ahead, not at your feet. Shift your pelvis forward and tuck your buttocks in.

- Hold your arms slightly away from your body. Your elbows should be bent so that your forearms are parallel to the ground. You may cup your hands, but do not clench your fists. Allow your arms to swing loosely and rhythmically with each stride.

- Let your heel hit the ground first in each stride. Then roll forward onto the ball of your foot and push off for the next stride. If you find this difficult, you can try a more flat-footed style, but don't land on the balls of your feet. More of a forefoot landing is recommended in barefoot running or with minimal footwear.

Table 1	Estimated Calories Expended by a 165-Pound Adult at Different Intensities of Walking and Jogging for 150 and 300 Minutes per Week (min/wk)			
	SPEED (MILES PER HOUR)	SPEED (MINUTES PER MILE)	CALORIES EXPENDED EXERCISING 150 MIN/WK	CALORIES EXPENDED EXERCISING 300 MIN/WK
	Rest	—	190	380
Walking	2.5	24	565	1,130
	3.0	20	620	1,240
	4.0	15	940	1,880
	4.3	14	1,125	2,250
Jogging	5.0	12	1,500	3,000
	6.0	10	1,875	3,750
	7.0	8.6	2,155	4,310
Running	8.0	6.7	2,530	5,060
	10.0	6	3,000	6,000

NOTE: Heavier people will expend slightly more calories, while lighter people will expend slightly fewer.

SOURCE: Adapted from Physical Activity Guidelines Advisory Committee. 2008. *Physical Activity Guidelines Advisory Committee Report.* Washington, D.C.: U.S. Department of Health and Human Services

Table 2	Sample Walking/Jogging Fitness Program

DAY	ACTIVITIES
Monday	• **Walking/jogging:** Walk briskly for 30 minutes or jog for 25 minutes. • **Stretching:** Stretch major muscle groups for 10 minutes after exercise. Do each exercise two times; hold stretch for 10–30 seconds.

Tuesday	• **Resistance workout:** Using body weight for resistance, perform the following exercises:
	  • Push-ups: 2 sets, 20 reps per set
	  • Pull-ups: 2 sets, 5 reps per set
	  • Unloaded squats: 2 sets, 10 reps per set
	  • Curl-ups: 2 sets, 20 reps per set
	  • Side bridges: 3 sets, 10-second hold (left and right sides)
	  • Spine extensions: 3 sets, 10-second hold (left and right sides)

Wednesday	• Repeat Monday activities.
Thursday	• Repeat Tuesday activities.
Friday	• Repeat Monday activities.
Saturday	• **Rest.**
Sunday	• **Rest.**

• Keep your steps short by allowing your foot to strike the ground in line with your knee. Keep your knees bent at all times.

• Breathe deeply through your mouth. Try to use your abdominal muscles rather than just your chest muscles to take deep breaths.

• Stay relaxed.

Find a safe, convenient place to walk or jog. Exercise on a trail, path, or sidewalk to stay clear of bicycles and cars. Make sure your clothes are brightly colored so that others can see you easily.

Beginning a Walking/Jogging Program

Start slowly if you have not been exercising, are overweight, or are recovering from an illness or surgery. At first, walk for 15 minutes at a slow pace, below your target heart rate zone. Gradually increase to 30-minute sessions. You will probably cover 1–2 miles. At the beginning, walk every other day.

You can gradually increase to walking five days per week or more if you want to expend more calories (which is helpful if you want to change body composition). Depending on your weight, you will expend ("burn") 90–135 calories during each 30-minute walking session. To increase the calories that you expend, walk for a longer time or for a longer distance instead of sharply increasing speed.

Start at the level of effort that is most comfortable for you. Maintain a normal, easy pace and stop to rest as often as you need to. Never prolong a walk past the point of comfort. When walking with a friend (a good motivator), let a comfortable conversation be your guide to pace. If you find that you cannot carry on a conversation without getting out of breath, you are walking too quickly.

Once your muscles have become adjusted to the exercise program, increase the duration of your sessions by no more than 10% each week. Keep your heart rate just below your target zone. Don't be discouraged by a lack of immediate progress, and don't try to speed things up by overdoing it. Remember that pace and heart rate can vary with the terrain, the weather, and other factors.

Advanced Walking

Advanced walking involves walking more quickly for longer times. You should feel an increased perception of effort, but the exercise intensity should not be too stressful. Vary your pace to allow for intervals of slow, medium, and fast walking. Keep your heart rate toward the lower end of your target zone with brief periods in the upper levels. At first, walk for 30 minutes and increase your walking time gradually until eventually you reach 60 minutes at a brisk pace and can walk 2–4 miles. Try to walk at least five days per week. Vary your program by changing the pace and distance or by walking routes with different terrains and views. You can expect to burn 200–350 calories or more during each advanced walking session.

Making the Transition to Jogging

Increase the intensity of exercise by gradually introducing jogging into your walking program. During a 2-mile walk, for example, periodically jog for 100 yards and then resume walking. Increase the number and distance of your jogging segments until you can jog continuously for the entire distance. More physically fit people may be capable of jogging without walking first. However, people unaccustomed to jogging should initially combine walking with short bouts of jogging.

A good strategy is to exercise on a 400-meter track at a local high school or college. Begin by covering 800 meters—jogging the straightaways and walking the turns. Progress to walking 200 meters (half lap) and jogging 200 meters; jogging 400 meters and walking 200 meters; jogging 800 meters, walking 200 meters; and jogging 1200 meters, walking 200 meters. Continue until you can jog 2 miles without stopping.

During the transition to jogging, adjust the ratio of walking to jogging to keep within your target heart rate zone as much as possible. Most people who sustain a continuous jogging or running program will find that they can stay within their target heart rate zone with a speed of 5.5–7.5 miles per hour (8–11 minutes per mile). Exercise at least every other day. Increasing frequency by doing other activities on alternate days will place less stress on the weight-bearing parts of your lower body than will a daily program of walking/jogging.

Developing Muscular Strength and Endurance and Flexibility

Walking, jogging, and running provide muscular endurance workouts for your lower body; they also develop muscular strength of the lower body to a lesser degree. If you'd like to increase your speed and performance, you might want to focus your program on lower-body exercises. (Don't neglect upper-body strength. It is important for overall wellness.) For flexibility, pay special attention to the hamstrings and quadriceps, which are not worked through their complete range of motion during walking or jogging. Strength training, particularly bodybuilding, can sometimes decrease flexibility, so stretching is particularly important for people who lift weights.

Staying with Your Walking/Jogging Program

Health experts have found that simple motivators such as using a pedometer, walking a dog, parking farther from the office or grocery store, or training for a fun run help people stay with their programs. Use a pedometer or GPS exercise device to track your progress and help motivate you to increase distance and speed. Accurate pedometers for walking, such as those made by Omron, Yamax, and New-Lifestyles, cost $20–$40 and are accurate to about 5%. Sophisticated GPS-based devices and apps made by Polar, Garmin, and Nike keep track of your exercise speed and distance via satellite, monitor heart rate, and store data that can be downloaded wirelessly to your computer or their own websites. Several of these units can be plugged in to programs such as Google Earth, which give you a satellite view of your walking or jogging route.

A pedometer can also help you increase the number of steps you walk each day. Most sedentary people take only 2,000 to 3,000 steps per day. Adding 1,000 steps per day and increasing gradually until you reach 10,000 steps can increase fitness and help you manage your weight.

BICYCLING SAMPLE PROGRAM

Bicycling can also lead to large gains in physical fitness. For many people, cycling is a pleasant and economical alternative to driving and a convenient way to build fitness.

Equipment and Technique

Cycling has its own special array of equipment, including helmets, lights, safety gear, and biking shoes. The bike is the most expensive item, ranging from about $100 to $1,000 or more. Avoid making a large investment until you're sure you'll use your bike regularly. While investigating what the marketplace has to offer, rent or borrow a bike. Consider your intended use of the bike. Most cyclists who are interested primarily in fitness are best served by a sturdy road bike rather than a mountain bike or sport bike. Stationary cycles are good for rainy days and areas that have harsh winters.

Clothing for bike riding shouldn't be restrictive or binding; nor should it be so loose that it catches the wind and slows you down. Shirts that wick moisture away from your skin and padded biking shorts make a ride more comfortable. Wear glasses or goggles to protect your eyes from dirt, small objects, and irritation from wind. Wear a pair of well-padded gloves if your hands tend to become numb while riding or if you begin to develop blisters or calluses.

To avoid saddle soreness and injury, choose a soft or padded saddle, and adjust it to a height that allows your legs to almost reach full extension while pedaling. To prevent backache and neck strain, warm up thoroughly and periodically shift the position of your hands on the handlebars and your body in the saddle. Keep your arms relaxed and don't lock your elbows. To protect your knees from strain, pedal with your feet pointed straight ahead or very slightly inward, and don't pedal in high gear for long periods.

Bike riding requires a number of precise skills that practice makes automatic. If you've never ridden before, consider taking a course. In fact, many courses are not just for beginners. They'll help you develop skills in braking, shifting, and handling emergencies, as well as teach you ways of caring for and repairing your bike. An **e-bike** is a good choice for people who commute to work or want some help climbing hills or riding long distances. For safe cycling, follow these rules:

- Always wear a helmet.
- Keep on the correct side of the road. Bicycling against traffic is usually illegal and always dangerous.
- Obey all the same traffic signs and signals that apply to autos.
- On public roads, ride in single file, except in low-traffic areas (if the law permits). Ride in a straight line; don't swerve or weave in traffic.
- Be alert; anticipate the movements of other traffic and pedestrians. Listen for approaching traffic that is out of your line of vision.
- Slow down at street crossings. Check both ways before crossing.
- Use hand signals—the same as for automobile drivers—if you intend to stop or turn. Use audible signals to warn those in your path.
- Maintain full control. Avoid anything that interferes with your vision. Don't jeopardize your ability to steer by carrying anything (including people) on the handlebars.
- Keep your bicycle in good shape. Brakes, gears, saddle, wheels, and tires should always be in good condition.
- See and be seen. Use a headlight at night and equip your bike with rear reflectors. Use side reflectors on pedals, front and rear. Wear light-colored clothing or use reflective tape at night; wear bright colors or use fluorescent tape by day.
- Be courteous to other road users. Anticipate the worst and practice preventive cycling.
- Use a rear-view mirror.

Developing Cardiorespiratory Endurance

Cycling is an excellent way to develop and maintain cardiorespiratory endurance and a healthy body composition.

| **e-bike** | electrically assisted bike | TERMS |

FIT-VP—frequency, intensity, time, volume, progression:

If you've been inactive for a long time, begin your cycling program at a heart rate that is 10–20% below your target zone. Beginning cyclists should pedal at about 80–100 revolutions per minute; adjust the gear so that you can pedal at that rate easily. You can equip your bicycle with a cycling computer that displays different types of useful information, such as speed, distance traveled, heart rate, altitude, and revolutions per minute.

Once you feel at home on your bike, try cycling 1 mile at a comfortable speed, and then stop and check your heart rate. Increase your speed gradually until you can cycle at 12–15 miles per hour (4–5 minutes per mile), a speed fast enough to bring most new cyclists' heart rate into their target zone. Allow your pulse rate to be your guide: More highly fit individuals may need to ride faster to achieve their target heart rate. Cycling for at least 20 minutes three days per week will improve your fitness.

At the beginning:

It may require several outings to get the muscles and joints of your legs and hips adjusted to this new activity. Begin each outing with a 10-minute warm-up. When your muscles are warm, stretch your hamstrings and your back and neck muscles. Until you become a skilled cyclist, select routes with the fewest hazards and avoid heavy automobile traffic.

As you progress:

Interval training is also effective with bicycling. Simply increase your speed to near maximum intensity for periods of 30 seconds to 2 minutes. Then ride more slowly for 2–3 minutes. Alternate the speed intervals and slow intervals for a total of 20–60 minutes, depending on your level of fitness. Biking over hilly terrain is also a form of interval training. Progress through a combination of increased speed or increased distance until you reach your fitness goals.

Developing Muscular Strength and Endurance and Flexibility

Bicycling develops a high level of endurance and a moderate level of strength in the muscles of the lower body. If one of your goals is to increase your cycling speed and performance, be sure to include exercises for the quadriceps, hamstrings, and buttocks muscles in your strength training program. For flexibility, pay special attention to the hamstrings and quadriceps, which are not worked through their complete range of motion during bike riding, and to the muscles in your lower back, shoulders, and neck.

SWIMMING SAMPLE PROGRAM

Swimming works every major muscle group in the body. It increases upper-and lower-body strength, promotes cardiovascular fitness, and is excellent for rehabilitating athletic injuries and preventing day-to-day aches and pains. It promotes weight control; builds powerful lungs, heart, and blood vessels; and promotes metabolic health. People weigh only 6–10 pounds in the water, so swimming places less stress on the knees, hips, and back than do jogging, hiking, volleyball, or basketball.

Swimming is one of the most popular recreational and competitive sports in the world. More than 120 million Americans swim regularly. More than 165,000 of these are competitive age-group swimmers (ages 5–18), and more than 30,000 competitors are over 19 years of age. You don't need a backyard pool to swim. Almost every town and city in America has a public pool. Pools are standard in many health clubs, YMCAs, and schools. Ocean and lake swimming may be options in the summer. High-tech wet suits make it possible to swim outdoors even in the middle of winter in many parts of the country.

Training Methods

Improved fitness from swimming depends on the quantity, quality, and frequency of training. Most swimmers use interval training to increase swimming fitness, speed, and endurance. Interval training calls for repeated fast swims at fixed distances followed by rest. Continuous distance or endurance training builds stamina and mental toughness. Interval and distance training each play important and different roles in improving fitness for swimming. Interval training improves overall swimming speed and the ability to swim fast at the beginning of a swim. Endurance training helps to maintain a faster average pace during a swim without becoming overly fatigued. Endurance training becomes more important when you want to compete in long, open-water swims or triathlons.

In swimming workouts, however, quality is better than quantity. Thirty years ago, elite swimmers from East Germany sometimes swam as much as 20,000 meters in a single workout (more than 12 miles). Recent studies found that competitive athletes who swam 4,000–6,000 meters per workout produced results similar to those who swam much farther. Likewise, recreational swimmers can improve fitness, strength, and power by swimming 1,000–2,000 meters (approximately 1,100–2,200 yards) per workout. Swim fast to get maximum benefits, but maintain good technique to maximize efficiency and minimize the risk of injury.

Interval training:

Interval training increases sprinting speed so that you can accelerate faster at the beginning of a swim. It also helps the body cope with metabolic waste products so that you can maintain your speed during the workout. To increase speed, swim intervals between 25 and 200 meters (or yards) at 80–90% effort. An example of a beginning program might be to swim 4 sets of 50 meters using the sidestroke at 70% of maximum effort, with a 1-minute rest between sets. A more advanced program would be to swim 10 sets of 100 meters using the freestyle stroke at 85–95% maximum effort with 30 seconds of rest between sets.

Endurance training:

Include longer swims—1,000 meters or more at a time—to build general stamina for swimming. Endurance training will improve aerobic capacity and help your cells use fuels and clear metabolic wastes. This will allow you to swim faster and longer. Longer swims promote metabolic health and build physical fitness.

Cross-training:

Cross-training combines more than one type of endurance exercise, such as swimming and jogging, in your program at a time. It also includes exercises that build strength, power, and skill. It is a good training method for people who prefer swimming but don't have daily access to a swimming pool or open water. Including multiple exercises, such as swimming and running, stair stepping, cycling, weight training exercises, and calisthenics, adds variety to the program. It also prepares you for a greater variety of physical challenges. See Chapter 3 for a discussion of cross-training and a description of typical workouts.

Technique: The Basic Swimming Strokes for General Conditioning

The best strokes for conditioning are the freestyle and sidestroke. Competitive athletes also swim the breaststroke, butterfly, and backstroke (but not the sidestroke). Learning efficient swimming strokes helps increase enjoyment and results in better workouts. Take a class from the Red Cross, local recreation department, or private coach if you are not a strong swimmer or need help with the basic strokes.

Freestyle:

While freestyle technically includes any unregulated stroke (such as the sidestroke), it generally refers to the front (Australian) crawl or overhand stroke. Freestyle is the fastest stroke and is best for general conditioning. Swim this stroke in a prone (face-down) position with arms stretched out in front and legs extended to the back. Move through the water by pulling first with the right arm and then with the left, while performing a kicking motion generated from the hips. During the stroke, rotate the thumb and palm 45 degrees toward the bottom of the pool. Pull in a semicircle downward toward the center of the body with the elbow higher than the hand. When the hand reaches the beginning of the ribcage, push the palm backward underneath the body as far as possible. Don't begin to stroke with the other hand until the first stroke is completed. Maximize the distance with each stroke by pulling fully and maintaining good posture.

The crawl uses a flutter kick, which involves moving the legs alternately with the force generated from the hips and a slight bend of the knees. Maintain a neutral spine during the stroke. A strong kick is important to minimize body roll during the stroke. For this reason, some of your training should include kicking without using the arms.

Breathing is almost always a problem for novice swimmers. Don't hold your breath! You will fatigue rapidly if you have poor air exchange during swimming. Breathe by turning the head to the side of a recovering stroke. Do not lift the head out of the water. Exhale continuously through the nose and mouth between breaths. Beginners should breathe on the same side following each stroke cycle (left and right arm strokes).

Sidestroke:

Even novices can get a good workout with minimal skill using the sidestroke. This is a good choice for beginners because you keep your head out of water and can swim great distances without fatigue. Lie in the water on your right side and stretch your right arm and hand in front of you in the direction you want to swim and place your left hand across your chest. Draw your right arm toward you, pulling at the water until your hand reaches your waist. At the same time, make a scissors kick with your legs. Repeat the stroke as your forward speed slows. Swim half the distance on your right side and the rest on your left side.

Beginning Swim Program

Take swimming lessons from a certified teacher or coach if you are a nonswimmer or have not used swimming as your primary form of exercise. A swim teacher can help you develop good technique, make more rapid progress, and avoid injuries.

To assess your starting fitness, take the 12-minute swim test described in Lab 3.1. Use the swim test table to help you measure progress in your program. Take the test every one or two months to help establish short-term goals.

Start your program by swimming one length (one-half lap) at a time, using either freestyle or sidestroke. If you can't swim the length of a standard pool (25 meters or yards), begin by swimming the width. As soon as you can, swim one length of the pool, rest for 30 seconds, and then repeat. Build up your capacity until you can swim 20 lengths with a short rest interval between each length. If you start your program with the sidestroke, try to switch to the freestyle stroke as quickly as you can.

Increase the distance of each swim to a full lap (50 meters or yards) with 30–60 seconds of rest between laps. Build up until you can swim 20 sets of 50-meter swims with 30 seconds of rest between sets. Gradually increase the distance of each set to 100-meter swims. You are ready for the next level when you can swim 10 sets of 100 meters with 30 seconds of rest between sets.

Swimming Program for Higher Levels of Fitness

This program includes a warm-up, specific conditioning drills for strokes and kicking, and a cool-down. It involves interval training three days a week and distance training two days per week.

Warm up before each workout by swimming 2–4 laps at an easy pace. It is also a good idea to warm up your legs and hips by holding on to the side of the pool and gently moving your legs using a flutter-kick motion. At the end of the workout, cool down by swimming 100–200 meters at a slow pace.

On Monday, Wednesday, and Friday, do interval training. Your goal is to swim intervals totaling 2,000 meters per workout (20 sets of 100 meters each) at a fast pace with 30 seconds of rest between each set, or interval (i.e., swim 100 meters, rest, swim 100 meters, rest, etc.). Every fifth interval, swim 25 meters using your legs alone, with your arms extended in front of you. Have someone watch you during the legs-only swims to make sure you are kicking mainly from the hips and maintaining a neutral spine. Add variety to your interval training workouts by using gloves, swim paddles, or fins.

If you are unable to do the interval workout at first, modify it by increasing rest intervals, decreasing speed, or decreasing the number of sets as you gradually increase the volume and intensity.

On Tuesday and Thursday, do distance training. Swim 1,000–2,000 meters continuously at a comfortable pace. Although distance days will help develop endurance, they are used mainly to help you recover from intense interval training days.

Rest on Saturday and Sunday. Rest is very important to help your muscles and metabolism recover and build fitness. Rest will also prevent overtraining and overuse injuries. Include two rest days per week. Rest days can be consecutive (such as Saturday and Sunday) or interspersed during the normal workout schedule.

Integrating Swimming into a Total Fitness Program

You will develop fitness best and maintain interest in continuing your exercise program by varying the structure of your workouts. Incorporate kick boards, pull-buoys, hand paddles, and fins into some of your training sessions. Cross-training is a good option for developing well-rounded fitness. Swimming results in moderate gains in strength and large gains in endurance.

Because swimming is not a weight-bearing activity and is not done in an upright position, it elicits a lower heart rate per minute. Therefore, swimmers need to adjust their target heart rate zone. To calculate your target heart rate for swimming, use this formula:

Maximum swimming heart rate (MSHR) = 205 − age

Target heart rate zone = 65−90% of MSHR

For example, a 19-year-old swimmer would calculate his or her target heart rate zone for swimming as follows:

MSHR: 205 − 19 = 186 bpm

65% intensity: 0.65 × 186 = 121 bpm

90% intensity: 0.90 × 186 = 167 bpm

Swimming does not preserve bone density as you age, so swimmers are advised to include weight training in their exercise program. Perform at least one set of 10 repetitions for 8–10 exercises that use the major muscle groups in the body. To improve swimming performance, include exercises that work key muscles. For example, if you primarily swim the freestyle stroke, include exercises to increase strength in your shoulders, arms, upper back, and hips. Training the muscles you use during swimming can also help prevent injuries. In your flexibility training, pay special attention to the muscles you use during swimming, particularly the shoulders, hips, and back. Table 3 shows a basic sample swimming program that incorporates all these types of exercises.

ROWING MACHINE SAMPLE PROGRAM

Rowing is a whole-body exercise that overloads the cardio-respiratory system and strengthens the major muscles of the body. The beauty and serenity of rowing on flat water in the

Table 3	Sample Swimming Program

DAY	ACTIVITIES
Monday	• **Warm-up:** Swim 100–200 meters (2–4 laps of a standard pool) at an easy pace. • **Intervals:** Swim 10–20 sets of 100-meter swims at 90% effort, with 30 seconds of rest between sets. After every 5 sets, swim 25 meters using your legs alone. • **Cool-down:** Swim 100–200 meters at a slow pace. • **Weight training:** Do at least 1 set of 10 repetitions of 8–10 exercises that work the body's major muscle groups. • **Flexibility:** Do standard stretching exercises for the shoulders, chest, back, hips, and thighs.
Tuesday	• **Distance:** Swim 1,000–2,000 meters continuously at a comfortable pace.
Wednesday	• Repeat Monday activities.
Thursday	• Repeat Tuesday activities.
Friday	• Repeat Monday activities.
Saturday	• **Rest.**
Sunday	• **Rest.**

morning is indescribable, but few people have access to a lake and rowing shell. Fortunately, sophisticated rowing machines simulate the rowing motion and make it possible to do this exercise at the fitness center or at a health club.

Modern rowing machines are very much like the real thing. They provide resistance with hydraulic pistons, magnets, air, or water. The best machines are solid and comfortable, provide a steady stroke, and allow you to maintain a neutral spine so that you don't injure your back. Many rowing machines come with LCD displays that show heart rate, stroke rate, power output, and estimated caloric expenditure. They are also preprogrammed with workouts for interval training, cardiovascular conditioning, and moderate-intensity physical activity. Good rowing mechanics are essential because, if done incorrectly, rowing can cause severe overuse injuries that can damage the back, hips, knees, elbows, and shoulders.

Technique: Basic Rowing Movement

Most of the power for rowing comes from the thigh and hip muscles and finishes with a pulling motion with the upper body. Maintain a neutral spine (that is, with normal curves) during the movement. Hinge at the hips and not at the back during the rowing motion.

The rowing movement includes the following phases:

• *The catch.* The catch involves sliding the seat forward on the track with arms straight as far as you can while keeping the spine neutral.

• *The drive.* The drive begins by pushing with the legs and keeping your arms straight.

• *The finish.* Finish by leaning back slightly (still maintaining a neutral spine) and pulling the handle to your abdomen.

• *The recovery.* Recover by extending your arms forward, hinging forward at the hips with a neutral spine, and sliding forward again on the seat for another "catch."

Training Methods

Your rowing program should include both continuous training and interval training. Continuous training calls for rowing for a specific amount of time—typically 20–90 minutes without stopping. Most people enjoy rowing at about 70% of maximum heart rate.

Interval training involves a series of exercise bouts followed by rest. The method manipulates distance, intensity, repetitions, and rest. An example of an interval workout would be to row for 8 sets of 4-minute exercise bouts at 85% effort with 2 minutes of rest between intervals, or sets. During interval training, changing one factor affects the others. For example, if you increase the intensity of exercise, you will need more rest between intervals and won't be able to do as many repetitions. High-intensity exercise builds fitness best but also increases the risk of injury and loss of motivation. Make intervals challenging but not so difficult that you get injured or discouraged.

Beginning Rowing Program

During the first few workouts, start conservatively by rowing for 10 minutes at a rate of about 20 strokes per minute with a moderate resistance. Exercise at about 60% effort. Do this workout three times during the first week. The movement is deceptively easy and invigorating. You are, however, using all the major muscle groups in the body and are probably not ready for a more intense exercise program.

After the first workout, do a series of 5-minute intervals during the first few weeks of training. For example, row for 5 minutes, rest 3 minutes, row 5 minutes, then rest 3 minutes. Build up until you can do 4–6 repetitions of 5-minute exercise intervals, resting only 1 minute between sets. Gradually, increase the time for each interval to 15 minutes and vary the rowing cadence from 20 to 25 strokes per minute. Your first short-term goal is to complete 30 minutes of continuous rowing without stopping.

Rowing Program for Higher Levels of Fitness

Vary your training methods after you can row continuously for 30 minutes, gain some fitness, and are used to the technique. Alternate between interval training and distance training. Doing both will help you develop fitness rapidly and improve rowing efficiency. A good strategy is to row continuously at about 70% effort for 30–60 minutes three days per week and practice interval training at 80–90% effort for two days per week. Do resistance and flexibility training two or three days per week. A basic but complete rowing machine program that includes continuous and interval training as well as resistance and flexibility exercises is shown in Table 4.

Table 4	Sample Rowing Machine Fitness Program

DAY	ACTIVITIES
Monday	• **Warm-up:** Row at low intensity for 2 minutes. • **Continuous rowing:** Row for 30 minutes at 70% effort (20–22 strokes per minute). • **Weight training (1–2 sets of 10 repetitions):** Squats, leg curls, bench press, lat pulls, raises, biceps curls, triceps extensions, curl-ups, side bridge (10 seconds per side), spine extensions (10 seconds per side). • **Stretching:** Do static stretching exercises for the shoulders, chest, back, hips, and thighs. Hold each stretch for 10–30 seconds.
Tuesday	• **Warm-up:** Row at low intensity for 2 minutes. • **Continuous rowing:** Row at 60–70% of maximum effort for 5 minutes. Rest for 3 minutes. • **Interval rowing:** Row 6 sets, for 5 minutes per set, at 25 strokes per minute (90% effort) Rest for 3 minutes between intervals.
Wednesday	• **Warm-up:** Row at low intensity for 2 minutes. • **Continuous rowing:** Row for 45 minutes at 70% effort (20–22 strokes per minute). • **Stretching:** Repeat Monday stretches.
Thursday	• **Warm-up:** Row at low intensity for 2 minutes. • **Continuous rowing:** Row for 30 minutes at 70% effort (20–22 strokes per minute). • **Weight training (1–2 sets of 10 repetitions):** Repeat Monday weight training exercises.
Friday	• **Warm-up:** Row at low intensity for 2 minutes. • **Continuous rowing:** Row for 30 minutes at 70% effort (20–22 strokes per minute). • **Stretching:** Repeat Monday stretches.
Saturday	• **Rest.**
Sunday	• **Rest.**

Name _____ Section _____ Date _____

LAB 7.1   A Personal Fitness Program Plan and Agreement

A. I, _____, am making an agreement with myself to follow a physical fitness program to work
                                         (name)

toward the following goals:

Specific or short-term goals (include current status for each):

1. _____
2. _____
3. _____
4. _____

General or long-term goals:

1. _____
2. _____
3. _____
4. _____

B. My program plan is as follows:

Activities	Components (Check ✓)					Frequency (Check ✓)							Intensity*	Time (duration)
	CRE	MS	ME	F	BC	M	Tu	W	Th	F	Sa	Su		

*Conduct activities for achieving CRE goals in your target range for heart rate or RPE.

C. My program will begin on _____. My program includes the following schedule of mini-goals. For each step in my program,
                                (date)

   I will give myself the reward listed.

_____   _____   _____
           (mini-goal 1)   (date)   (reward)

_____   _____   _____
           (mini-goal 2)   (date)   (reward)

_____   _____   _____
           (mini-goal 3)   (date)   (reward)

_____   _____   _____
           (mini-goal 4)   (date)   (reward)

_____   _____   _____
           (mini-goal 5)   (date)   (reward)

LABORATORY ACTIVITIES

D. My program will include the addition of physical activity to my daily routine (such as climbing stairs or walking to class):

1. _____
2. _____
3. _____
4. _____

E. My program will include the following strategies for reducing sedentary time:

1. _____
2. _____
3. _____
4. _____

F. I will use the following tools to monitor my program and my progress toward my goals (list any charts, graphs, or journals you plan to use):

_____
_____
_____

I sign this agreement as an indication of my personal commitment to reach my goal.

_____   _____
(your signature)   (date)

I have recruited a helper who will witness my agreement and _____

_____
(list any way your helper will participate in your program)

_____

_____   _____
(witness's signature)   (date)

Name _____ **Section** _____ **Date** _____

LAB 7.2 Getting to Know Your Fitness Facility

To help create a successful training program, take time to learn more about the fitness facility you plan to use.

Basic Information

Name and location of facility:_____

Hours of operation:_____

Times available for general use:_____

Times most convenient for your schedule:_____

Can you obtain an initial session or consultation with a trainer to help you create a program? _____ yes _____ no

If so, what does the initial planning session involve?_____
_____

Are any of the staff certified? Do any have special training? If yes, list/describe:_____
_____

What types of equipment are available for the development of cardiorespiratory endurance? Briefly list/describe:_____
_____
_____
_____

Are any group activities or classes available? If so, briefly describe:_____
_____
_____

What types of weight training equipment are available for use?_____
_____

Yes	No	
_____	_____	Is there a fee for using the facility? If so, how much? $ _____
_____	_____	Is a student ID required for access to the facility?
_____	_____	Do you need to sign up in advance to use the facility or any of the equipment?
_____	_____	Is there typically a line or wait to use the equipment during the times you use the facility?
_____	_____	Is there a separate area with mats for stretching and/or cool-down?
_____	_____	Do you need to bring your own towel?
_____	_____	Are lockers available? If so, do you need to bring your own lock?_____yes_____no
_____	_____	Are showers available? If so, do you need to bring your own soap and shampoo?_____yes_____no
_____	_____	Is drinking water available? (If not, be sure to bring your own bottle of water.)

LABORATORY ACTIVITIES

What other amenities, such as vending machines or saunas, are available at the facility? Briefly list/describe:_____

_____

_____

Information about Equipment

Fill in the specific equipment and exercise(s) that you can use to develop cardiorespiratory endurance and each of the major muscle groups. For cardiorespiratory endurance, list the type(s) of equipment and a sample starting workout: frequency, intensity, time, and other pertinent information (such as a setting for resistance or speed). For muscular strength and endurance, list the equipment and exercises, and indicate the order in which you'll complete them during a workout session. You can also combine aerobics and strength exercises by performing high-repetition kettlebell swings. Remember, you don't have to use equipment—you can use body weight or elastic bands as resistance.

Cardiorespiratory Endurance Equipment

Equipment	Sample Starting Workout

Muscular Strength and Endurance Equipment

Order	Muscle Groups	Equipment	Exercise(s)
	Neck		
	Chest		
	Shoulders		
	Upper back		
	Front of arms		
	Back of arms		
	Buttocks		
	Abdomen		
	Lower back		
	Front of thighs		
	Back of thighs		
	Calves		
	Whole body		
	Other:		

8 Nutrition

LOOKING AHEAD...

After reading this chapter, you should be able to

- List the essential nutrients and describe their functions.

- Describe the U.S. government dietary guidelines and the benefits of following them.

- Describe guidelines for vegetarians and special population groups.

- Explain how to use food labels and other consumer tools to make informed choices about foods.

- Create a personal food plan that will promote wellness.

TEST YOUR KNOWLEDGE

1. All adults should consume one serving each of fruits and vegetables every day. True or false?

2. Candy is the leading source of added sugars in the American diet. True or false?

3. Which of the following is not a whole grain?
   a. brown rice
   b. wheat flour
   c. popcorn

See answers on the next page.

©Franek Strzeszewski/Cultura/Getty Images RF

What you eat affects your energy level, well-being, and overall health. Your nutritional habits help determine your risk for major chronic diseases, including heart disease, cancer, stroke, and diabetes. Choosing a dietary pattern that provides the nutrients you need while limiting the substances linked to risk factors for disease should be an important part of your daily life.

Choosing a healthy diet is a two-part process. First, learn which nutrients you need and in what amounts. Second, translate those requirements into a diet consisting of foods you like that are available, affordable, and fit into your lifestyle. After you know what constitutes a healthy diet for you, you can adjust your current diet to bring it into line with your goals.

This chapter explains the basic principles of **nutrition**. It introduces the six classes of essential nutrients and discusses their role in the functioning of the body. You'll also find guidelines that you can use to design a healthy eating plan, and practical tools and advice to help you apply the guidelines to your life.

NUTRITIONAL REQUIREMENTS: COMPONENTS OF A HEALTHY DIET

You probably think about your diet in terms of the foods you like to eat. But more important for your health are the nutrients contained in those foods. The **essential nutrients** your body requires are proteins, fats, carbohydrates, vitamins, minerals, and water. The word *essential* means that you must get these substances from food because your body is unable to manufacture them, or at least not fast enough or in sufficient amounts to meet your physiological needs. The six classes of nutrients, along with their functions and major sources, are listed in Table 8.1.

The body needs some essential nutrients in relatively large amounts; these **macronutrients** include proteins, fats, carbohydrates, and water. **Micronutrients**, such as vitamins and minerals, are required in much smaller amounts. Your body obtains nutrients through the process of **digestion**, which breaks down food into compounds that can be absorbed and the body can use (Figure 8.1). A diet that provides enough essential nutrients is vital because they provide energy, help build and maintain body tissues, and help regulate body functions.

Food is partially broken down by being chewed and mixed with saliva in the mouth. After traveling to the stomach via the esophagus, food is broken down further by stomach acids and other secretions. As food moves through the digestive tract, it is mixed by muscular contractions and broken down by chemicals. Most absorption of nutrients occurs in the small intestine, aided by secretions from the pancreas, gallbladder, and intestinal lining. Bacteria in the digestive tract, called gut flora, also help with digestion. The large intestine reabsorbs excess water; the remaining solid wastes are collected in the rectum and excreted through the anus.

Answers (Test Your Knowledge)

1. **False.** For someone consuming 2,000 calories per day, about three servings each (2½ cups of vegetables and 2 cups of fruit) are recommended daily.
2. **False.** Regular (nondiet) sodas are the leading source of added sugars. Together with other beverages, they account for 47% of the added sugars in the American diet, and added sugars contribute an average of 13% of the total calories in American diets (more for children and teens). Each 12-ounce soda supplies about 10 teaspoons of sugar, or nearly 10% of the calories in a 2,000-calorie diet.
3. **b.** Unless labeled "whole wheat," wheat flour is processed to remove the bran and germ and is not a whole grain.

Calories

The energy in foods is expressed as **kilocalories**. One kilocalorie represents the amount of heat it takes to raise the temperature of one liter of water 1°C. A person needs about 2,000 kilocalories a day to meet his or her energy needs. Although technically inaccurate, people refer to kilocalories as *calories,* which is a much smaller energy unit: 1 kilocalorie contains 1,000 calories. This text uses the familiar word *calorie* to stand for the larger energy unit; you'll also find *calorie* used on food labels.

Table 8.1	The Six Classes of Essential Nutrients	
NUTRIENT	FUNCTION	MAJOR SOURCES
Proteins	Form important parts of muscles, bone, blood, enzymes, some hormones, and cell membranes; repair tissue; regulate water and acid-base balance; help in growth; supply energy	Meat, fish, poultry, eggs, milk, legumes, nuts
Carbohydrates	Supply energy to cells in brain, nervous system, and blood; supply energy to muscles during exercise	Grains (breads and cereals), fruits, vegetables, milk
Fats	Supply energy; insulate, support, and cushion organs; provide medium for absorption of fat-soluble vitamins	Animal foods, grains, nuts, seeds, fish, vegetables
Vitamins	Promote (initiate or speed up) specific chemical reactions within cells	Abundant in fruits, vegetables, and grains; also found in meat and dairy products
Minerals	Help regulate body functions; aid in growth and maintenance of body tissues; act as catalysts for release of energy	Found in most food groups
Water	Provides medium for chemical reactions; transports chemicals; regulates temperature; removes waste products	Fruits, vegetables, liquids

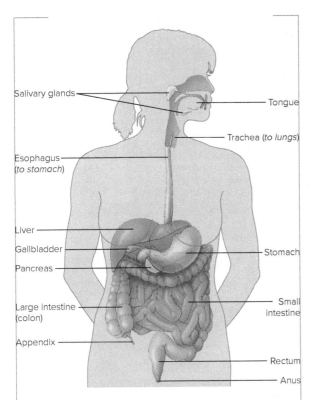

Salivary glands

Tongue

Trachea (*to lungs*)

Esophagus
(*to stomach*)

Liver

Gallbladder

Pancreas

Stomach

Large intestine
(colon)

Small
intestine

Appendix

Rectum

Anus

FIGURE 8.1   The digestive system.

Of the six classes of essential nutrients, three supply energy:

- Fat = 9 calories per gram
- Protein = 4 calories per gram
- Carbohydrate = 4 calories per gram

Alcohol, though not an essential nutrient, also supplies energy, providing 7 calories per gram.

Just meeting energy needs is not enough. Our bodies need enough of the essential nutrients to function properly. Many Americans consume sufficient or excess calories but not enough of all essential nutrients. Practically all foods contain combinations of nutrients, although foods are sometimes classified according to their predominant nutrients. For example, spaghetti contains small amounts of other nutrients, but is considered a carbohydrate food. The following sections discuss the functions and sources of each class of nutrients.

Nutrient density is an important concept related to food energy: Nutrient-dense foods are those that are high in essential nutrients but may be relatively low in calories. You can think of your daily calorie intake as a budget—you need to spend your calories wisely on nutrient-dense foods to obtain all essential nutrients while staying within your budget.

Proteins—The Basis of Body Structure

Proteins form important parts of the body's main structural components: muscles and bones. Proteins also form important parts of blood, enzymes, cell membranes, and some hormones.

When consumed, proteins also provide energy for the body (4 calories per gram).

Amino Acids   The building blocks of proteins are called **amino acids**. Twenty common amino acids are found in food. Nine of these are essential (sometimes called indispensable). As long as foods supply certain nutrients, the body can produce the other 11 amino acids.

Complete and Incomplete Proteins   Individual protein sources are considered "complete" if they supply all the essential amino acids in adequate amounts and "incomplete" if they do not. Meat, fish, poultry, eggs, milk, cheese, and soy provide complete proteins. Incomplete proteins, which come from plant sources such as nuts and **legumes** (dried beans and peas), are good sources of most essential amino acids but are usually low in one or more.

Certain combinations of vegetable proteins, such as wheat and peanuts in a peanut butter sandwich or rice and beans, allow each vegetable protein to make up for the amino acids missing in the other protein. The combination yields a complete protein. It was once believed that vegetarians had to complement their proteins at each meal in order to receive the benefit of a complete protein. Now we know that proteins consumed throughout the course of the day can complement each other as part of a pool of amino acids the body can draw from to produce proteins. Vegetarians should include a variety of vegetable protein sources in their diets to make sure they get all the essential amino acids in adequate amounts. (Healthy vegetarian diets are discussed later in the chapter.)

Recommended Protein Intake The Food and Nutrition Board of the Institute of Medicine has established goals to help ensure adequate intake of protein as well as the other macronutrients (Table 8.2). For protein, adequate intake is set at 0.8 gram per kilogram (0.36 gram per pound) of body weight. So, if you weigh 125 pounds, you should consume at least 45 grams of protein per day, and if you weigh 180 pounds, adequate intake will be 65 grams. Table 8.3 lists some popular food items and the amount of protein each provides; labels on packaged foods show how much protein there is in each serving.

Most Americans meet or exceed the protein intake needed for adequate nutrition. If you consume substantially more protein than your body needs, the extra energy from protein is synthesized into fat for storage or burned for energy requirements, depending on your overall energy intake.

Consuming some protein above the amount needed for adequate nutrition is not harmful; suggested daily intake limits have been set as a proportion of overall calories rather than as specific amounts. The Food and Nutrition Board recommendations of how much protein (and other energy-supplying nutrients) to consume as a percentage of total daily energy are called Acceptable Macronutrient Distribution Ranges (AMDRs). The AMDRs aim to ensure adequate intake of essential nutrients and to reduce the risk of chronic diseases. The protein AMDR for adults age 19 years and older should fall within the range of 10–35% of total daily calories (see Table 8.2). For someone consuming a 2,000-calorie diet, this percentage range corresponds to a suggested daily intake between 50 and 175 grams per day. Healthy protein-rich food choices are described later in the chapter.

Fats—Essential in Small Amounts

At 9 calories per gram, fats, also known as *lipids,* are the most concentrated source of energy. The fats stored in your body represent usable energy, help insulate your body, and support and cushion your organs. Fats in the diet help your body absorb fat-soluble vitamins, and they add flavor and texture to foods. Fats are the major fuel for the body during rest and light activity. Two fats—linoleic acid and alpha-linolenic acid—the essential fatty acids—are necessary components of the diet (see Table 8.2). They are used to make compounds that regulate body functions such as the maintenance of blood pressure, vision, and the progress of a healthy pregnancy.

Table 8.3	Protein Content of Common Food Items

ITEM	PROTEIN (GRAMS)
3 ounces lean meat, poultry, or fish	20–27
¼ cup (3 ounces) tofu	7
1 cup cooked beans (black, white, pinto)	15–17
1 cup yogurt	8–13
1 ounce cheese (cheddar, Swiss)	6-8
1/2–1 cup cereals	1–6
1 egg cooked	6
1 cup ricotta cheese	28
1 cup milk	8
1 ounce nuts	2–6

NOTE: For the specific protein content of a food, check the food label or the searchable U.S. Department of Agriculture food composition database (https://ndb.nal.usda.gov/ndb/search).

**SOURCE: U.S. Department of Agriculture, Agricultural Research Service, *USDA National Nutrient Database for Standard Reference,* Release 27, 2015. Nutrient Data Laboratory Home Page. (http://www.ars.usda.gov/ba/bhnrc/ndl retrieved June 24, 2015).

Table 8.2	Goals for Protein, Fat, and Carbohydrate Intake for Adults		
	DAILY ADEQUATE INTAKES (GRAMS)*		ACCEPTABLE MACRONUTRIENT DISTRIBUTION RANGES (AMDRs) (PERCENT OF TOTAL DAILY CALORIES)
	MEN	WOMEN	
Protein**	56 g	46 g	10–35%
Fat (total)			20–35%
Linoleic acid	17 g	12 g	
Alpha-linolenic acid	1.6 g	1.1 g	
Carbohydrate	130 g	130 g	45–65%

*To meet daily energy needs, you need to consume more than the minimally adequate amounts of the energy-providing nutrients listed here, which alone supply only 800–900 calories. Use the AMDRs to set overall daily goals.

**Protein intake goals can be calculated more specifically by multiplying your body weight in pounds by 0.36.

NOTE: Individuals can allocate total daily energy intake among the three classes of macronutrients to suit individual preferences. To translate percentage goals into daily intake goals expressed in calories and grams, multiply the appropriate percentages by total daily energy intake and then divide the results by the corresponding calories per gram. For example, a fat limit of 35% applied to a 2,200-calorie diet would be calculated as follows: 0.35 × 2,200 = 770 calories of total fat; 770 ÷ 9 calories per gram = 86 grams of total fat.

SOURCE: Recommendations from *Dietary Reference Intakes for Energy, Carbohydrate, Fiber, Fat, Fatty Acids, Cholesterol, Protein, and Amino Acids* (2002/2005). The report may be accessed via www.nap.edu.

Table 8.4	Types of Fatty Acids

TYPE OF FATTY ACID	FOUND IN*
Saturated	• Animal fats (especially fatty meats and poultry fat and skin) • Butter, cheese, and other high-fat dairy products • Palm and coconut oils
Trans	• Some frozen pizza • Some types of popcorn • Deep-fried fast foods • Stick margarines, shortening • Packaged cookies and crackers • Processed snacks and sweets
Monounsaturated	• Olive, canola, and safflower oils • Avocados, olives • Peanut butter (without added fat) • Many nuts, including almonds, cashews, pecans, and pistachios
Polyunsaturated—omega-3	• Fatty fish, including salmon, white albacore tuna, mackerel, anchovies, and sardines • Compared to fish, lesser amounts are found in walnut, flaxseed, canola, and soybean oils; tofu; walnuts; flaxseeds; and dark green leafy vegetables
Polyunsaturated—omega-6	• Corn, and cottonseed oils (often used in margarine, mayonnaise, and salad dressings)

Types and Sources of Fats Food fats are usually composed of both **saturated** and **unsaturated** fatty acids (Table 8.4). The dominant type of fatty acid determines the fat's characteristics. Saturated fats come mostly from animal products—red meats (hamburger, steak, roasts), whole milk, cheese, hot dogs, and lunchmeats—but are also found in tropical oils (coconut and palm oils). They are usually solid at room temperature. Most unsaturated fats in foods come from plant sources and are liquid at room temperature.

Depending on their structure, unsaturated fatty acids can be further divided into *monounsaturated* and *polyunsaturated* fats. Olive, canola, safflower, and peanut oils contain mostly monounsaturated fatty acids. Soybean, corn, and cottonseed oils contain mostly polyunsaturated fatty acids. You may sometimes see polyunsaturated fats described more specifically by chemical structure as either omega-3 or omega-6 fats.

Hydrogenation and Trans Fats **Trans fatty acids (trans fats)** are unsaturated fatty acids. Small amounts of trans fats occur naturally in animal fat, particularly beef, lamb, and dairy products, but the majority of trans fats in the American diet are artificial, from partially hydrogenated oils. When unsaturated vegetable oils undergo the process of **hydrogenation**, a mixture of saturated and unsaturated fatty acids is produced, creating a more solid fat from a liquid oil. Hydrogenation also changes some unsaturated fatty acids into trans fats.

Food manufacturers use hydrogenation to increase the stability of an oil so that it could be reused for deep frying, to improve the texture of certain foods (to make pie crusts flakier, for example), and to extend the shelf life of foods made with oil. Hydrogenation is also used to transform liquid oil into

margarine or vegetable shortening. In general, the more solid a hydrogenated oil is, the more saturated or trans fats it contains. For example, stick margarines typically contain more saturated and trans fats than do tub or squeeze margarines.

Fats and Health Scientists are still unraveling the complex effects that individual types of fats and overall dietary patterns have on health and the risk for specific diseases. Most health experts agree on the dangers of artificial trans fats because of their double-negative effect on heart health: They raise levels of **low-density lipoprotein (LDL)**—"bad" cholesterol—and they also lower **high-density lipoprotein (HDL)**—"good"

TERMS

saturated fats Fatty acids found mostly in animal products and tropical oils; usually solid at room temperature.

unsaturated fats Fatty acids found primarily in plant foods; usually liquid at room temperature.

trans fatty acid (trans fat) A type of unsaturated fatty acid produced during the process of hydrogenation; trans fats have an atypical shape that affects their chemical activity.

hydrogenation A process by which hydrogens are added to unsaturated fats, increasing the degree of saturation and turning liquid oils into solid fats. Hydrogenation produces a mixture of saturated fatty acids and standard and trans forms of unsaturated fatty acids.

low-density lipoprotein (LDL) A lipoprotein containing a moderate amount of protein and a large amount of cholesterol; "bad" cholesterol.

high-density lipoprotein (HDL) A lipoprotein containing relatively little cholesterol that helps transport cholesterol out of the arteries; "good" cholesterol.

cholesterol. Consuming trans fats appears to increase the risk for both cardiovascular disease and type 2 diabetes. In recent years, as awareness of these health risks has grown, cities and states have banned the use of trans fats in restaurants and food prepared for retail sale, and food manufacturers have reduced the amount of trans fats they use. And the Food and Drug Administration (FDA) has required that all food manufacturers stop using trans fats by June 2018. Even with the new law, it is important to check ingredient labels for partially hydrogenated oils: as long as a product has no more than half a gram of trans fats, the label may claim zero.

What about other types of fats? Many studies have examined the effects of dietary fat intake on blood **cholesterol** levels and the risk of heart disease. Longstanding advice has been to limit saturated fat intake for heart health; however, not all researchers agree. Federal dietary guidelines, as well as those from the American Heart Association and the American College of Cardiology, do strongly advise lowering saturated fat intake for reducing cardiovascular disease risk, especially for those people with risk factors for heart disease.

Continued research on the health risks and benefits of individual fats is ongoing. For example, do saturated fats in beef, butter, milk, and chocolate all have the same effect on heart disease risk? And what are the health effects of shifts in the intake of particular fats within the overall context of the diet? Dietary fat affects health in other ways besides heart disease risk. Diets high in fatty red meat are associated with an increased risk of certain forms of cancer, especially colon cancer.

What does all this mean for you? Although more research is needed on the precise effects of different types and amounts of fat on overall health, evidence suggests that most people benefit from keeping their saturated fat intake within recommended intake levels and avoiding all artificial trans fats. But dietary patterns are more important for health than a focus on a single nutrient. The fats in your diet are found in foods that contain other nutrients, and the foods you consume are in the context

Wellness Tip An isolated focus on reducing dietary fat intake contributed to an explosion in the availability of processed foods promoted as being low in fat, such as the reduced-fat cinnamon rolls shown here. Many of these choices, however, are high in refined grains and added sugars and are not healthy choices. Focus on your overall dietary pattern and limit your intake of saturated fats, processed grains, and added sugars. Choose unsaturated fats, whole grains, fruits, and vegetables.
©Diana Haronis/Getty Images

of your overall diet. Increased body weight, aging, and gender are more important for predicting negative health events than is eating one kind of dietary fat rather than another.

The U.S. Department of Agriculture recommends that Americans limit their intake of saturated fat to less than 10% of total calories per day—but that they do so in the context of a healthy dietary pattern that emphasizes vegetables, fruits, whole grains, low-fat or nonfat dairy, seafood, legumes, and nuts. The pattern should also be low in red and processed meats, sugar-sweetened foods and drinks, and refined grains. Healthy dietary patterns are described in detail later in the chapter.

Carbohydrates—A Key Source of Energy

Carbohydrates ("carbs") supply energy to body cells. Some cells, such as those in the brain and other parts of the nervous system and in the blood, use only the carbohydrate glucose for fuel. During high-intensity exercise, muscles use carbohydrates for fuel.

Simple and Complex Carbohydrates Carbohydrates are classified into two groups: simple and complex (Table 8.5). *Simple carbohydrates* consist of the single sugar molecules (monosaccharides) and the double sugars (disaccharides). Three important monosaccharides are glucose, fructose, and galactose. Glucose, the most common of the sugars, is used by both animals and plants for energy. Fructose is a very sweet sugar that is found in fruits, and galactose is the sugar in milk.

The disaccharides, pairs of single sugars, include sucrose (table sugar: fructose + glucose), maltose (malt sugar: glucose + glucose), and lactose (milk sugar: galactose + glucose). Simple carbohydrates add sweetness to foods. They are found naturally in fruits and milk and are added to soft drinks, fruit

TERMS

cholesterol A waxy substance found in the blood and cells and needed for synthesis of cell membranes, vitamin D, and hormones.

carbohydrate An essential nutrient; sugars, starches, and dietary fiber are all carbohydrates.

glucose A simple sugar circulating in the blood that can be used by cells to fuel adenosine triphosphate (ATP) production.

glycogen A complex carbohydrate stored principally in the liver and skeletal muscles; the major fuel source during most forms of intense exercise. Glycogen is the storage form of glucose.

whole grain The entire edible portion of a grain (such as wheat, rice, or oats), including the germ, endosperm, and bran; processing removes parts of the grain, often leaving just the endosperm.

glycemic index A measure of how a particular food affects blood glucose levels.

Table 8.5	Simple and Complex Carbohydrates in Foods

SIMPLE CARBOHYDRATES ("SUGARS")	COMPLEX CARBOHYDRATES
Single sugar molecules (monosaccharides) - glucose (common in foods) - fructose (fruits) - galactose (milk) Double sugar molecules (disaccharides; pairs of single sugars) - sucrose or table sugar (fructose + glucose) - maltose or malt sugar (glucose + glucose) - lactose or milk sugar (galactose + glucose)	Starches (long, complex chains of sugar molecules) - grains (wheat, rye, rice, oats, barley, millet) - legumes (dry beans, peas, and lentils) - tubers and other vegetables (potatoes, yams, corn) Fiber (nondigestible carbohydrates) - soluble (oats, barley, legumes, some fruits and vegetables) - insoluble (wheat bran, vegetables, whole grains)

drinks, candy, and desserts. There is no evidence that any type of simple carbohydrate is more nutritious than others.

Complex carbohydrates include starches and most types of dietary fiber. Starches are found in a variety of plants, especially grains (wheat, rye, rice, oats, barley, and millet), legumes (dried beans, peas, and lentils), and tubers (potatoes and yams). Most other vegetables contain a mix of complex and simple carbohydrates. Fiber, which is discussed later in this chapter, is found in fruits, vegetables, and grains.

During digestion, your body breaks down carbohydrates into simple sugar molecules, such as **glucose**, for absorption. When glucose is in the bloodstream, the pancreas releases the hormone insulin, which allows cells to take up glucose and use it for energy and fat storage. The liver and muscles also take up glucose and store it in the form of a starch called **glycogen**. The muscles use glucose from glycogen as fuel during endurance events or long workouts. Some people have problems controlling their blood glucose levels, a disorder called diabetes mellitus.

Refined versus Whole Grains Complex carbohydrates can be further divided into refined, or processed, carbohydrates and unrefined carbohydrates, or whole grains. Before they are processed, all grains are **whole grains**, consisting of an inner layer of germ, a middle layer called the endosperm, and an outer layer of bran (Figure 8.2). During processing, the germ and bran are often removed, leaving just the starchy endosperm. The refinement of whole grains transforms whole-wheat flour into white flour, brown rice into white rice, and so on.

Refined grains usually retain all the calories of their unrefined counterparts, but they tend to be less nutrient dense—lower in fiber, vitamins, minerals, and other beneficial compounds. Refined-grain products are often enriched or fortified with vitamins and minerals, but many of the nutrients lost in processing are not replaced.

Whole grains tend to take longer to chew and digest than refined ones; whole grains also generally enter the bloodstream more slowly. This slower digestive pace makes you feel full sooner and for a longer period. A slower rise in blood glucose levels after eating unrefined complex carbohydrates may help in the management of diabetes. Whole grains are also high in dietary fiber (discussed later).

Consumption of whole grains has been linked to a reduced risk of heart disease, diabetes, and cancer, and plays an important role in gastrointestinal health and body weight management. For all these reasons, whole grains are recommended over those that have been refined. See the box "Choosing More Whole-Grain Foods" for tips on increasing your intake of whole grains.

Glycemic Index and Glycemic Response Some foods cause a quick and dramatic rise in glucose and insulin levels, while others have a slower, more moderate effect. A food that has a rapid effect on blood glucose levels is said to have a high **glycemic index**. Insulin and glucose levels rise following a meal or snack containing any type of carbohydrate.

Basing food choices on the glycemic index is difficult, but for people with particular health concerns, such as diabetes, the glycemic index may be important. In addition to the type of carbohydrate in the food, the total amount of carbohydrate in the diet is important for diabetes management. The easiest way to moderate the effects shown by the glycemic index, therefore, is to choose an overall dietary pattern that includes a variety of whole grains and vegetables daily and limits foods that are high in refined grains and added sugars.

Added Sugars *Added sugars* are sugars that are added to foods by food manufacturers or individuals; they include white sugar, brown sugar, high-fructose corn syrup, and other

Bran
"Outer shell" protects seed
Contains fiber, B vitamins, trace minerals

Endosperm
Provides energy
Contains carbohydrates, protein

Germ
Provides nourishment for the seed
Contains antioxidants, vitamin E, B vitamins

FIGURE 8.2 The parts of a whole grain kernel.
©Brand X Pictures/ PunchStock RF

TAKE CHARGE
Choosing More Whole-Grain Foods

What Are Whole Grains?

The first step in adding more whole grains into your diet is to correctly identify them. The following are whole grains:

- whole wheat
- whole-grain corn
- whole rye
- popcorn
- whole oats
- brown rice
- oatmeal
- whole-grain barley

Other choices include bulgur (cracked wheat), farro, millet, kasha (roasted buckwheat kernels), quinoa, wheat and rye berries, amaranth, wild rice, graham flour, whole-grain kamut, whole-grain spelt, and whole-grain triticale.

Wheat flour, unbleached flour, enriched flour, and degerminated corn meal are not whole grains. Wheat germ and wheat bran are also not whole grains, but they are the constituents of wheat typically left out when wheat is processed and so are healthier choices than regular wheat flour, which typically contains just the grain's endosperm.

Checking Packages for Whole Grains

To find packaged foods—such as bread or pasta—that are rich in whole grains, read the list of ingredients and check for special health claims related to whole grains. The *first* item in the list of ingredients should be one of the whole grains in the preceding list. Product names and food color can be misleading. *When in doubt, always check the list of ingredients and make sure "whole" is the first word in the list.*

The FDA allows manufacturers to include special health claims for foods that contain 51% or more whole-grain ingredients. Such products may contain a statement such as the following on their packaging:

- "Rich in whole grain"
- "Made with 100% whole grain"
- "Diets rich in whole-grain foods may help reduce the risk of heart disease and certain cancers."

However, many whole-grain products will not carry such claims. This is one more reason to check the ingredient list to make sure you're buying a product made from one or more whole grains.

Box icon: ©VisualCommunications/Getty Images RF

---

sweeteners added to most processed foods. (Naturally occurring sugars in fruit and milk are not considered added sugars.) Foods high in added sugar are generally high in calories and low in nutrients and fiber, thus providing "empty calories." High intake of added sugars from foods and beverages is associated with dental caries ("cavities"), excess body weight, and increased risk of type 2 diabetes, and may also increase risk for hypertension, stroke, and heart disease.

Added sugars currently contribute about 250–300 calories in the typical daily American diet, representing about 13–17% of total energy intake. A limit of 10% is suggested by the U.S. Department of Agriculture (USDA) and other organizations; even lower intakes may be needed to meet all nutrient needs at a given level of calorie intake. Major sources of sugar in the U.S. diet are sugar-sweetened beverages, snacks, and sweets. Due to updated food labeling regulations, added sugars will begin to appear on food labels as manufacturers adopt the new label format.

To decrease added sugars from your diet, reduce your consumption of sugar-sweetened beverages (soft drinks, sweetened fruit drinks, sweetened sports beverages), sweet snacks, and desserts. In particular, choose water in place of sweetened beverages. Water is a readily available, low-cost, zero-calorie option. The sugars in your diet should come mainly from whole fruits, which are excellent sources of vitamins and minerals, and from low-fat or fat-free milk and other dairy products, which are high in protein and calcium.

Fiber—A Closer Look

Fiber is the term given to nondigestible carbohydrates in plants. Instead of being digested, like starch, fiber moves through the intestinal tract and provides bulk for feces in the large intestine, which in turn facilitates elimination. In the large intestine, some types of fiber are broken down by bacteria into acids and gases, which explains why eating too much fiber-rich food can lead to intestinal gas. Even though humans don't digest fiber, they need it for good health.

Types of Fiber **Dietary fiber** refers to the nondigestible carbohydrates (and the noncarbohydrate substance *lignin*) that are

Wellness Tip To reduce the risk of chronic disease and maintain intestinal health, daily fiber intake of 38 grams for men and 25 grams for women is recommended. Americans currently consume about half this amount. Fruits, vegetables, and whole grains are excellent sources of carbohydrates and fiber. Drink plenty of water to get the most health benefits from the fiber you consume.
©Smneedham/Getty Images

Table 8.6	Types, Effects, and Sources of Dietary Fiber	
	SOLUBLE FIBER	INSOLUBLE FIBER
Physiological effects	• Slows digestion and nutrient absorption • Helps prevent a rapid rise in blood glucose following a meal • Improves blood cholesterol levels	• Adds bulk to stool • Helps food pass more quickly through the digestive tract • Helps prevent constipation
Examples of food sources	Oat bran, barley, nuts, legumes, apples, berries	Whole wheat and other whole grains, wheat bran, vegetables

naturally present in plants such as grains, fruits, legumes, and vegetables. There are two general types of dietary fiber: soluble and insoluble (see Table 8.6). Both types are important for health.

- **Soluble (viscous) fiber**, such as that found in oat bran or legumes, can delay stomach emptying, which slows the movement of glucose into the blood after eating.

- **Insoluble fiber**, such as that found in wheat bran or psyllium seed, increases fecal bulk and helps prevent constipation, hemorrhoids, and other digestive disorders.

Functional fiber refers to nondigestible carbohydrates that have been either isolated from natural sources or synthesized in a laboratory and then added to a food product or dietary supplement. **Total fiber** refers to the sum of dietary and functional fiber in your diet.

A high-fiber diet can help reduce the risk of type 2 diabetes, heart disease, and pulmonary disease, as well as improve gastrointestinal health and aid in the management of metabolic syndrome and body weight. Some studies have linked high-fiber diets with a reduced risk of colon and rectal cancer. Other studies have suggested that it is the total dietary pattern—one rich in fruits, vegetables, and whole grains—that may be responsible for this reduction in risk. A high-fiber diet has also been linked to healthier gut bacteria, which in turn may reduce the risk of obesity and improve immune function.

Sources of Fiber All plant foods contain some dietary fiber. Fruits, legumes, oats (especially oat bran), and barley all contain the viscous types of fiber that help lower blood glucose and cholesterol levels. Wheat (especially wheat bran), cereals, grains, and vegetables are all good sources of cellulose and other fibers that help prevent constipation. Psyllium, which is often added to cereals or used in fiber supplements and laxatives, improves intestinal health and also helps control glucose and cholesterol levels. The processing of packaged foods can remove fiber, so it's important to depend on fresh fruits and vegetables and foods made from whole grains as your main fiber sources.

Vitamins—Organic Micronutrients

Vitamins are organic (carbon-containing) substances required in small amounts to regulate various processes within living cells (Table 8.7). Humans need 13 vitamins; of these, 4 are fat soluble (A, D, E, and K), and 9 are water soluble (C and the B vitamins, thiamin, riboflavin, niacin, vitamin B-6, folate, vitamin B-12, biotin, and pantothenic acid).

Solubility affects how a vitamin is absorbed, transported, and stored in the body. The water-soluble vitamins are absorbed directly into the bloodstream. Excess amounts of water-soluble vitamins are generally removed by the kidneys and excreted in urine. Fat-soluble vitamins require a more complex absorptive process. They are usually carried in the blood by special proteins and are stored in the liver and in fat tissues rather than excreted.

Functions of Vitamins Many vitamins help chemical reactions take place. They provide no energy to the body directly but help release the energy stored in carbohydrates, proteins, and fats. Other vitamins are critical in the production of red blood cells and the maintenance of the nervous, skeletal, and

Wellness Tip Vitamin and mineral supplements are popular, but they are not usually necessary for healthy people who eat a balanced diet.
©Richard Levine/Alamy Stock Photo

Table 8.7   Facts about Vitamins

VITAMIN AND RECOMMENDED INTAKES*	IMPORTANT DIETARY SOURCES	MAJOR FUNCTIONS	SIGNS OF PROLONGED DEFICIENCY	TOXIC EFFECTS OF MEGADOSES
FAT SOLUBLE				
Vitamin A Men: 900 µg Women: 700 µg	Liver, milk, butter, cheese, fortified margarine; carrots, spinach, and other orange and deep green vegetables and fruits	Maintenance of vision, skin, linings of the nose, mouth, digestive, and urinary tracts, immune function	Night blindness; dry, scaling skin; increased susceptibility to infection; loss of appetite; anemia; kidney stones	Liver damage, miscarriage and birth defects, headache, vomiting and diarrhea, vertigo, double vision, bone abnormalities
Vitamin D Men: 15 µg Women: 15 µg	Fortified milk and margarine, fish oils, butter, egg yolks (sunlight on skin also produces vitamin D)	Development and maintenance of bones and teeth; promotion of calcium absorption	Rickets (bone deformities) in children; bone softening, loss, fractures in adults	Kidney damage, calcium deposits in soft tissues, depression, death
Vitamin E Men: 15 mg Women: 15 mg	Vegetable oils, whole grains, nuts and seeds, green leafy vegetables, asparagus, peaches	Protection and maintenance of cellular membranes	Red blood cell breakage and anemia, weakness, neurological problems, muscle cramps	Relatively nontoxic but may cause excess bleeding or formation of blood clots
Vitamin K Men: 120 µg Women: 90 µg	Green leafy vegetables; smaller amounts widespread in other foods	Production of factors essential for blood clotting and bone metabolism	Hemorrhaging	None reported
WATER SOLUBLE				
Biotin Men: 30 µg Women: 30 µg	Cereals, yeast, egg yolks, soy flour, liver; widespread in foods	Synthesis of fat, glycogen, and amino acids	Rash, nausea, vomiting, weight loss, depression, fatigue, hair loss	None reported
Folate Men: 400 µg Women: 400 µg	Green leafy vegetables, yeast, oranges, whole grains, legumes, liver	Amino acid metabolism, synthesis of RNA and DNA, new cell synthesis	Anemia, weakness, fatigue, irritability, shortness of breath, swollen tongue	Masking of vitamin B-12 deficiency
Niacin Men: 16 mg Women: 14 mg	Eggs, poultry, fish, milk, whole grains, nuts, enriched breads and cereals, meats, legumes	Conversion of carbohydrates, fats, and proteins into usable forms of energy	Pellagra (symptoms include diarrhea, dermatitis, inflammation of mucous membranes, dementia)	Flushing of skin, nausea, vomiting, diarrhea, liver dysfunction, glucose intolerance
Pantothenic acid Men: 5 mg Women: 5 mg	Animal foods, whole grains, broccoli, potatoes; widespread in foods	Metabolism of fats, carbohydrates, and proteins	Fatigue, numbness and tingling of hands and feet, gastrointestinal disturbances	None reported
Riboflavin Men: 1.3 mg Women: 1.1 mg	Dairy products, enriched breads and cereals, lean meats, poultry, fish, green vegetables	Energy metabolism; maintenance of skin, mucous membranes, nervous system structures	Cracks at corners of mouth, sore throat, skin rash, hypersensitivity to light, purple tongue	None reported
Thiamin Men: 1.2 mg Women: 1.1 mg	Whole-grain and enriched breads and cereals, organ meats, lean pork, nuts, legumes	Conversion of carbohydrates into usable forms of energy; maintenance of appetite and nervous system function	Beriberi (symptoms include muscle wasting, mental confusion, anorexia, enlarged heart, nerve changes)	None reported
Vitamin B-6 Men: 1.3 mg Women: 1.3 mg	Eggs, poultry, fish, whole grains, nuts, soybeans, liver, kidney, pork	Metabolism of amino acids and glycogen	Anemia, convulsions, cracks at corners of mouth, dermatitis, nausea, confusion	Neurological abnormalities and damage
Vitamin B-12 Men: 2.4 µg Women: 2.4 µg	Meat, fish, poultry, fortified cereals, cheese, eggs, milk	Synthesis of blood cells; other metabolic reactions	Anemia, fatigue, nervous system damage, sore tongue	None reported
Vitamin C Men: 90 mg Women: 75 mg	Peppers, broccoli, brussels sprouts, spinach, citrus fruits, strawberries, tomatoes, potatoes, cabbage, other fruits and vegetables	Maintenance and repair of connective tissue, bones, teeth, cartilage; promotion of healing; aid in iron absorption	Scurvy, anemia, reduced resistance to infection, loosened teeth, joint pain, poor wound healing, hair loss, poor iron absorption	Urinary stones in some people, acid stomach from ingesting supplements in pill form, nausea, diarrhea, headache, fatigue

*Recommended intakes for adults ages 19–30; to calculate your personal Dietary Reference Intakes (DRIs) based on age, sex, and other factors, visit the Interactive DRI website (http://fnic.nal.usda.gov/fnic/interactiveDRI).

SOURCES: *Dietary Reference Intakes for Thiamin, Riboflavin, Niacin, Vitamin B6, Folate, Vitamin B12, Pantothenic Acid, Biotin and Choline* (1998); *Dietary Reference Intakes for Vitamin C, Vitamin E, Selenium, and Carotenoids* (2000); *Dietary Reference Intakes for Vitamin A, Vitamin K, Arsenic, Boron, Chromium, Copper, Iodine, Iron, Manganese, Molybdenum, Nickel, Silicon, Vanadium, and Zinc* (2001); and *Dietary Reference Intakes for Calcium and Vitamin D* (2011). These reports may be accessed via www.nap.edu; Ross, A. C., et al. 2012. eds. *Modern Nutrition in Health and Disease*, 11th ed. Baltimore: Lippincott Williams and Wilkins.

immune systems. Some vitamins act as **antioxidants**, which help preserve the health of cells. Key vitamin antioxidants include vitamin E, vitamin C, and the vitamin A precursor beta-carotene. (Antioxidants are described later in the chapter.)

Sources of Vitamins The human body must obtain most of the vitamins it requires from foods. Vitamins are abundant in fruits, vegetables, and grains. In addition, many processed foods, such as flour and breakfast cereals, contain added vitamins. Vitamin B-12 is found only in foods that are fortified or that come from animal sources. A few vitamins are made in the body: The skin makes vitamin D when it is exposed to sunlight, and intestinal bacteria make vitamin K. Nonetheless, you still need to get vitamin D and vitamin K from foods (see Table 8.7).

Vitamin Deficiencies and Excesses If your diet lacks a particular vitamin, characteristic symptoms of deficiency can develop (see Table 8.7). For example, vitamin A deficiency can cause night blindness, and people whose diets lack vitamin B-12 can develop anemia. Vitamin deficiency diseases are relatively rare in the United States because vitamins are readily available from our food supply. However, many Americans consume lower-than-recommended amounts of several vitamins, including vitamins A, D, E, and C, as well as folate. Nutrient intake that is consistently below recommended levels can have adverse effects on health even if it is not low enough to cause a deficiency disease. For example, low intake of folate increases a woman's chance of giving birth to a baby with a neural tube defect (a congenital malformation of the central nervous system). Low intake of folate and vitamins B-6 and B-12 has been linked to increased heart disease risk; low vitamin D intake may harm bone health.

Extra vitamins in the diet can be harmful, especially when taken as supplements. For example, vitamin A plays an important role in bone growth, but too much vitamin A can trigger bone loss and an increase in the risk of fracture. Megadoses of fat-soluble vitamins are particularly dangerous because the excess is stored in the body rather than excreted, increasing the risk of toxicity. Even when supplements are not taken in excess, relying on them for an adequate intake of vitamins can be problematic. There are many substances in foods other than vitamins and minerals that have important health effects. Later, this chapter discusses specific recommendations for vitamin intake and when a supplement is advisable. For now, keep in mind that it's best to get most of your vitamins from foods rather than supplements.

The vitamins and minerals in foods can be easily lost or destroyed during storage or cooking. To retain their value, eat or process vegetables immediately after buying them. If you can't do this, store them in a cool place, covered to retain moisture—either in the refrigerator (for a few days) or in the freezer (for a longer term). To reduce nutrient losses during food preparation, minimize the amount of water used and the total cooking time. Develop a taste for a crunchier texture in cooked vegetables. Baking, steaming, broiling, grilling, and microwaving are all good methods of preparing vegetables.

Minerals—Inorganic Micronutrients

Minerals are inorganic (non-carbon-containing) elements you need in relatively small amounts to help regulate body functions, aid in the growth and maintenance of body tissues, and help release energy (Table 8.8). There are about 17 essential minerals. The major minerals, those that the body needs in amounts exceeding 100 milligrams (mg) per day, include calcium, phosphorus, magnesium, sodium, potassium, and chloride. The essential trace minerals, which you need in minute amounts, include copper, fluoride, iodine, iron, selenium, and zinc.

Characteristic symptoms develop if an essential mineral is consumed in a quantity too small or too large for good health. For example, most Americans consume the mineral sodium in excess as part of dietary salt. The majority of sodium Americans consume comes from processed foods and restaurant meals. High sodium consumption raises blood pressure, and thus the risk for heart disease and stroke; reducing dietary salt has become an important public health initiative. The good news is that blood pressure begins to decrease within weeks of lowering sodium intake.

Minerals commonly lacking in the American diet include iron, calcium, magnesium, and potassium. Low potassium intake is considered a public health concern because it is linked to high blood pressure and heart disease; you can improve your potassium intake by choosing a dietary pattern rich in fruits, vegetables, and legumes. Iron-deficiency **anemia** is a problem in some age groups, and researchers fear poor calcium intakes in childhood are sowing the seeds for future **osteoporosis**, especially in women. See the box "Eating for Healthy Bones" to learn more.

Water—Vital but Often Ignored

Water is the major component in both foods and the human body: You are composed of about 50–60% water. Your need for other nutrients, in terms of weight, is much less than your need for water. You can live up to 50 days without food but only a few days without water.

Water is distributed all over the body, among lean and other tissues and in blood and other body fluids. Water is used in the digestion and absorption of food and is the medium in which

---

antioxidant A substance that protects against the **TERMS** breakdown of food or body constituents by free radicals; antioxidants' actions include binding oxygen, donating electrons to free radicals, and repairing damage to molecules.

minerals Inorganic compounds needed in relatively small amounts for the regulation, growth, and maintenance of body tissues and functions.

anemia A deficiency in the oxygen-carrying material in the red blood cells.

osteoporosis A condition in which the bones become extremely thin and brittle and break easily; due largely to insufficient calcium intake.

Table 8.8   Facts about Selected Minerals

MINERAL AND RECOMMENDED INTAKES*	IMPORTANT DIETARY SOURCES	MAJOR FUNCTIONS	SIGNS OF PROLONGED DEFICIENCY	TOXIC EFFECTS OF MEGADOSES
Calcium Men: 1,000 mg Women: 1,000 mg	Milk and milk products, tofu, fortified orange juice and bread, green leafy vegetables, bones in fish	Formation of bones and teeth; control of nerve impulses, muscle contraction, blood clotting	Stunted growth in children, bone mineral loss in adults; urinary stones	Kidney stones, calcium deposits in soft tissues, inhibition of mineral absorption, constipation
Fluoride Men: 4 mg Women: 3 mg	Fluoridated water, tea, marine fish eaten with bones	Maintenance of tooth and bone structure	Higher frequency of tooth decay	Increased bone density, mottling of teeth, impaired kidney function
Iodine Men: 150 µg Women: 150 µg	Iodized salt, seafood, processed foods	Essential part of thyroid hormones, regulation of body metabolism	Goiter (enlarged thyroid), cretinism (birth defect)	Depression of thyroid activity, hyperthyroidism in susceptible people
Iron Men: 8 mg Women: 18 mg	Meat and poultry, fortified grain products, dark green vegetables, dried fruit	Component of hemoglobin, myoglobin, and enzymes	Iron-deficiency anemia, weakness, impaired immune function, gastrointestinal distress	Nausea, diarrhea, liver and kidney damage, joint pains, sterility, disruption of cardiac function, death
Magnesium Men: 400 mg Women: 310 mg	Widespread in foods and water (except soft water); especially found in grains, legumes, nuts, seeds, green vegetables, milk	Transmission of nerve impulses, energy transfer, activation of many enzymes	Neurological disturbances, cardiovascular problems, kidney disorders, nausea, growth failure in children	Nausea, vomiting, diarrhea, central nervous system depression, coma; death in people with impaired kidney function
Phosphorus Men: 700 mg Women: 700 mg	Present in nearly all foods, especially milk, cereal, peas, eggs, meat	Bone growth and maintenance, energy transfer in cells	Impaired growth, weakness, kidney disorders, cardiorespiratory and nervous system dysfunction	Drop in blood calcium levels, calcium deposits in soft tissues, bone loss
Potassium Men: 4,700 mg Women: 4,700 mg	Meats, milk, fruits, vegetables, grains, legumes	Nerve function and body water balance	Muscular weakness, nausea, drowsiness, paralysis, confusion, disruption of cardiac rhythm	Cardiac arrest
Selenium Men: 55 µg Women: 55 µg	Seafood, meat, eggs, whole grains	Defense against oxidative stress; regulation of thyroid hormone action	Muscle pain and weakness, heart disorders	Hair and nail loss, nausea and vomiting, weakness, irritability
Sodium Men: 1,500 mg Women: 1,500 mg	Salt, soy sauce, fast food, processed foods, especially lunch meats, canned soups and vegetables, salty snacks, processed cheese	Body water balance, acid-base balance, nerve function	Muscle weakness, loss of appetite, nausea, vomiting; deficiency rarely seen	Edema, hypertension in sensitive people
Zinc Men: 11 mg Women: 8 mg	Whole grains, meat, eggs, liver, seafood (especially oysters)	Synthesis of proteins, RNA, and DNA; wound healing; immune response; ability to taste	Growth failure, loss of appetite, impaired taste acuity, skin rash, impaired immune function, poor wound healing	Vomiting, impaired immune function, decline in blood HDL levels, impaired copper absorption

*Recommended Intakes for adults ages 19–30; to calculate your personal DRIs based on age, sex, and other factors, visit the Interactive DRI website (http://fnic.nal.usda.gov/fnic/interactiveDRI).

SOURCES: *Dietary Reference Intakes for Calcium, Phosphorous, Magnesium, Vitamin D, and Fluoride* (1997); *Dietary Reference Intakes for Vitamin A, Vitamin K, Arsenic, Boron, Chromium, Copper, Iodine, Iron, Manganese, Molybdenum, Nickel, Silicon, Vanadium, and Zinc* (2001); *Dietary Reference Intakes for Water, Potassium, Sodium, Chloride, and Sulfate* (2005); *and Dietary Reference Intakes for Calcium and Vitamin D* (2011). These reports may be accessed via www.nap.edu.; Ross, A. C. et al. 2012. eds. *Modern Nutrition in Health and Disease*, 11th ed. Baltimore: Lippincott Williams and Wilkins.

most chemical reactions take place within the body. Some water-based fluids, such as blood, transport substances around the body; other fluids serve as lubricants or cushions. Water also helps regulate body temperature.

Water is contained in almost all foods, particularly in liquids, fruits, and vegetables. The foods and beverages you consume provide 80–90% of your daily water intake; the remainder is generated through metabolism. You lose water in urine, feces, and sweat and through evaporation from your lungs.

About 20% of daily water intake comes from food. Most people can make up the rest and maintain a healthy water balance by consuming beverages at meals and drinking fluids in response to thirst. The Food and Nutrition Board has set levels of adequate water intake to maintain hydration. Under these guidelines, men need to consume about 3.7 total liters of water,

TAKE CHARGE
Eating for Healthy Bones

Osteoporosis is a condition in which the bones become dangerously thin and fragile over time. An estimated 10 million Americans over age 50 have osteoporosis, and another 34 million are at risk. Women account for about 80% of osteoporosis cases.

Most of adult bone mass is built by age 18 in girls and 20 in boys. Bone density peaks between ages 25 and 35; after that, bone mass is lost over time. To prevent osteoporosis, the best strategy is to build as much bone as possible during your youth and do everything you can to maintain it as you age. Up to 50% of bone loss is determined by controllable lifestyle factors such as diet and exercise. Key nutrients in a healthy dietary pattern for bone health include the following:

- **Calcium.** Getting enough calcium is important throughout life to build and maintain bone mass. Milk, yogurt, and calcium-fortified orange juice, bread, and cereals are all good sources.

- **Vitamin D.** Vitamin D is necessary for bones to absorb calcium; a daily intake of 600 IU (15 µg) is recommended for individuals ages 1–70. Vitamin D can be obtained from foods and is manufactured by the skin when exposed to sunlight. Candidates for vitamin D supplements include people who eat few foods rich in vitamin D, get little sun (i.e., don't expose their face, arms, and hands to the sun for 5–15 minutes a few times each week), or live in higher latitudes where sunlight is weaker.

- **Vitamin K.** Vitamin K promotes the synthesis of proteins that help keep bones strong. Broccoli and leafy green vegetables are rich in vitamin K.

- **Other nutrients.** Other nutrients that may play an important role in bone health include vitamin C, magnesium, potassium, phosphorus, fluoride, manganese, zinc, copper, and boron.

Several dietary substances may have a *negative* effect on bone health, especially if consumed in excess. These include alcohol, sodium, caffeine, and retinol (a form of vitamin A). Drinking lots of soda, which often replaces milk in the diet, has been shown to increase the risk of bone fracture in teenage girls.

The effect of protein intake on bone mass depends on other nutrients: Protein helps build bone as long as calcium and vitamin D intake are adequate. But if intake of calcium and vitamin D is low, high protein intake can lead to bone loss.

Weight-bearing aerobic exercise helps maintain bone mass throughout life, and strength training improves bone density, muscle mass, strength, and balance. Drinking alcohol only in moderation, refraining from smoking, and managing depression and stress are also important for maintaining strong bones. For people who develop osteoporosis, a variety of medications are available to treat the condition.

SOURCES: Movassagh, E. Z., and H. Vatanparast, 2017. "Current evidence on the association of dietary patterns and bone health: A scoping review," *Advances in Nutrition* 8(1), 2017, 1–16; Institute of Medicine of the National Academies. 2010. *Dietary Reference Intakes for calcium and vitamin D* (http://www.iom.edu/~/media/Files/Report%20Files/2010/Dietary-Reference-Intakes-for-Calcium-and-Vitamin-D/Vitamin%20D%20and%20Calcium%202010%20Report%20Brief.pdf).

with 3.0 liters (about 13 cups) coming from beverages; women need 2.7 total liters, with 2.2 liters (about 9 cups) coming from beverages. If you exercise vigorously or live in a hot climate, you need to consume additional fluids to maintain a balance between water consumed and water lost. Severe dehydration causes weakness and can lead to death.

Other Substances in Food

Many substances in food are not essential nutrients but may influence health.

Antioxidants When the body uses oxygen or breaks down certain fats or proteins as a normal part of metabolism, substances called **free radicals** are produced. A free radical is a chemically unstable molecule that reacts with fats, proteins, and DNA, damaging cell membranes and mutating genes. Free radicals have been implicated in aging, cancer, cardiovascular disease, and other degenerative diseases like arthritis. Environmental factors such as cigarette smoke, exhaust fumes, radiation, excessive sunlight, certain drugs, and stress can increase free radical production.

Antioxidants found in foods can block the formation and action of free radicals and repair the damage they cause. Some antioxidants, such as vitamin C, vitamin E, and selenium, are also essential nutrients. Others—such as carotenoids, found in

yellow, orange, and dark green leafy vegetables—are not. In general, fruits and vegetables have a high antioxidant value, as do herbs, spices, berries, nuts, and chocolate.

Phytochemicals Antioxidants fall into the broader category of **phytochemicals**, substances found in plant foods that may help prevent chronic disease. For example, certain substances found in soy foods may help lower cholesterol levels. Sulforaphane, a compound isolated from broccoli and other **cruciferous vegetables**, may render some carcinogenic compounds harmless. Allyl sulfides, a group of chemicals found

---

free radical An electron-seeking compound that can react with fats, proteins, and DNA, damaging cell membranes and mutating genes in its search for electrons; produced through chemical reactions in the body and by exposure to environmental factors such as sunlight and tobacco smoke.

phytochemical A naturally occurring substance found in plant foods that may help prevent and treat chronic diseases such as heart disease and cancer; *phyto* means "plant."

cruciferous vegetables Vegetables of the cabbage family, including cabbage, broccoli, brussels sprouts, kale, and cauliflower; the flower petals of these plants form the shape of a cross, hence the name.

TERMS

in garlic and onions, appear to boost the activity of immune cells. Phytochemicals found in whole grains are associated with a reduced risk of cardiovascular disease, diabetes, and cancer. Carotenoids found in green vegetables may help preserve eyesight with age. Further research on phytochemicals may extend the role of nutrition to the prevention and treatment of many chronic diseases.

To get phytochemicals, eat a variety of fruits, vegetables, and unprocessed grains rather than relying on supplements. Like many vitamins and minerals, isolated phytochemicals may be harmful if taken in high doses. Another reason to get your phytochemicals from food is that their health benefits may be the result of chemical substances working in combination. The role of phytochemicals in disease prevention is discussed further in Chapters 11 and 12.

NUTRITIONAL GUIDELINES: PLANNING YOUR DIET

Scientific and government groups have created a number of useful tools to help people design healthy diets (see Table 8.9):

- The **Dietary Reference Intakes (DRIs)** set standards for nutrient intakes designed to prevent nutritional deficiencies and reduce the risk of chronic diseases.

- The **Daily Values** is a simplified version of the DRIs used on food labels.

- The **Dietary Guidelines for Americans** were established to promote health and reduce the risk of major chronic diseases through diet and physical activity.

- **MyPlate** is the U.S. Department of Agriculture (USDA) food guidance system developed to help Americans make healthy food choices consistent with the Dietary Guidelines for Americans.

Dietary Reference Intakes (DRIs)

The Food and Nutrition Board establishes dietary standards, or recommended intake levels, for Americans of all ages. The current set of standards, called Dietary Reference Intakes (DRIs), was introduced in 1997. The DRIs are frequently reviewed and are updated as substantial new nutrition-related information becomes available. The DRIs have a broad focus: They are based on research that looks not just at the prevention of nutrient deficiencies but also at the role of nutrients in promoting health and preventing chronic diseases such as cancer, osteoporosis, and heart disease.

DRI Standards The DRIs include a set of four reference values used as standards for both recommended intakes and maximum safe intakes. The recommended intake of each nutrient is expressed as either a *Recommended Dietary Allowance* (RDA) or as an *Adequate Intake* (AI). An AI is set when there is not enough information available to set an RDA value. (See Table 8.2 for examples of AIs). Regardless of the type of standard used, the DRIs represent the best available estimate of intakes for optimal health.

Used primarily in nutrition policy and research, the *Estimated Average Requirement* (EAR) is the average daily nutrient intake level estimated to meet the requirement of half the healthy individuals in a particular life stage and gender

| Table 8.9 | Agencies and their Food Guidelines |

GOVERNMENT OR SCIENTIFIC AGENCY	FOOD GUIDELINES AND TOOLS
Food and Nutrition Board of the Health and Medicine Division,* National Academy of Sciences	Dietary Reference Intakes • Recommended Dietary Allowance • Adequate Intake • Estimated Average Requirement • Tolerable Upper Intake Level
Food and Drug Administration of the U.S. Department of Health and Human Services	Daily Values
U.S. Department of Agriculture and U.S. Department of Health and Human Services	Dietary Guidelines for Americans
U.S. Department of Agriculture	MyPlate

*Formerly Institute of Medicine

SOURCE: U.S. Department of Health and Human Services and U.S. Department of Agriculture, *2015–2020 Dietary Guidelines for Americans,* 8th Edition. December 2015. Available at http://health.gov/dietaryguidelines/2015/guidelines/.

group. For example, a 2016 study shows that although most American infants under age 2 years meet their nutritional needs, 10% have an iron intake below the EAR. The *Tolerable Upper Intake Level* (UL) is the maximum daily intake that is unlikely to cause health problems in a healthy person. For example, the RDA for calcium for an 18-year-old female is 1,300 mg per day; the UL is 3,000 mg per day.

Because of a lack of data, ULs have not been set for all nutrients. This does not mean that people can tolerate long-term intakes of these vitamins and minerals above recommended levels. Like all chemical agents, nutrients can produce adverse effects if intakes are excessive. Furthermore, there is no established benefit from consuming nutrients at levels above the RDA or AI. The DRIs for many nutrients are found in Tables 8.2, 8.7, and 8.8. For a personalized DRI report for your sex and life stage, visit the Interactive DRI website (http://fnic.nal.usda.gov/fnic/interactiveDRI).

Should You Take Supplements? The aim of the DRIs, the Dietary Guidelines for Americans, and MyPlate is to guide you in meeting your nutritional needs primarily with food, rather than with vitamin and mineral supplements. Supplements lack the potentially beneficial synergistic balance of nutrients, phytochemicals, and fiber that is found only in whole foods. Most Americans can get the vitamins and minerals they need by eating a varied, nutritionally balanced diet.

Over the past two decades, high-dose supplement use has been promoted as a way to prevent or delay the onset of many diseases, including heart disease and several kinds of cancer. These claims remain controversial. According to the latest research, a balanced diet of whole foods—not high-dose supplementation—is the best way to promote health and prevent disease.

In setting the DRIs, the Food and Nutrition Board recommended supplements of particular nutrients for the following groups:

- Women who are capable of becoming pregnant should take 400 micrograms (µg) per day of folic acid (the synthetic form of the vitamin folate) from fortified foods or supplements in addition to folate from a varied diet. Research indicates that this level of folate intake reduces the risk of neural tube defects. Enriched breads, flours, corn meals, rice, noodles, and other grain products are fortified with folic acid. Folate is found naturally in green leafy vegetables, legumes, oranges, and strawberries.

- People over age 50 should eat foods fortified with vitamin B-12, take B-12 supplements, or both to meet the majority of the DRI of 2.4 µg of B-12 daily. Up to 30% of people over 50 may have problems absorbing protein-bound B-12 in foods.

- Because of the oxidative stress caused by smoking, smokers should get 35 mg *more* vitamin C per day than the RDA set for their age and sex. However, supplements are not usually needed because this extra vitamin C can easily be found in foods. For example, an 8-ounce glass of orange juice has about 100 mg of vitamin C.

Supplements may also be recommended in other cases. Women with heavy menstrual flows may need extra iron. Older people, people with dark skin, and people exposed to little sunlight may need extra vitamin D. Some vegetarians may need supplemental calcium, iron, zinc, and vitamin B-12, depending on their food choices. Other people may benefit from taking supplements based on their lifestyle, physical condition, medicines, or dietary habits.

Although dietary supplements are sold over the counter, the question of whether to take supplements is a serious one. Some vitamins and minerals are dangerous when ingested in excess, as described previously in Tables 8.7 and 8.8. Large doses of particular nutrients can also cause health problems by affecting the absorption of other vitamins and minerals or interacting with medications. For all these reasons, you should think carefully about whether to take high-dose supplements, and consult a physician or registered dietitian.

Daily Values

Because the DRIs are too cumbersome to use as a basis for food labels, the FDA developed another set of dietary standards, the Daily Values. The Daily Values are based on several different sets of guidelines and include standards for fat, cholesterol, carbohydrate, dietary fiber, and selected vitamins and minerals. The Daily Values represent appropriate intake levels for a 2,000-calorie diet. The percent Daily Value shown on a food label shows how well that food contributes to your recommended daily intake. Food labels are described in detail later in the chapter.

Dietary Guidelines for Americans

To provide general guidance for choosing a healthy diet and reducing the risk of chronic diseases, the USDA and the U.S. Department of Health and Human Services jointly issue the Dietary Guidelines for Americans, which is revised every five years. Intended for all healthy Americans age 2 years and over, the information in the Dietary Guidelines is used in developing federal food, nutrition, and health policies and programs and also serves as the basis for federal nutrition education materials.

TERMS

Dietary Reference Intakes (DRIs) An umbrella term for four types of nutrient standards: Adequate Intake (AI), Estimated Average Requirement (EAR), and Recommended Dietary Allowance (RDA) are levels of intake considered adequate to prevent nutrient deficiencies and reduce the risk of chronic disease; Tolerable Upper Intake Level (UL) is the maximum daily intake that is unlikely to cause health problems.

Daily Values A simplified version of the RDAs used on food labels; also included are values for nutrients with no established RDA.

Dietary Guidelines for Americans General principles of good nutrition intended to help prevent certain diet-related diseases.

MyPlate A food-group plan that provides practical advice to ensure a balanced intake of the essential nutrients.

Wellness Tip About half of all American adults have one or more preventable chronic diseases that are related to poor eating habits and inactivity; these include high blood pressure, type 2 diabetes, cardiovascular disease, and certain forms of cancer. The food and portion size choices you make at every meal can influence your risk for, or management of, many health conditions.
©Justin Sullivan/Getty Images

The Dietary Guidelines is designed to help Americans make healthy and informed food choices. The main objective of the *2015–2020 Dietary Guidelines* is to encourage healthy eating patterns and regular physical activity among Americans, two-thirds of whom are overweight or obese, yet undernourished in several key nutrients. The guidelines focus on the total diet and offer practical tips for how people can make shifts in their diet to integrate healthier choices. They also include findings on the broader environmental and social aspects of the American diet—that is, the "food environment."

Earlier versions of the Dietary Guidelines focused more on individual dietary components. However, people do not eat individual nutrients or single foods but rather foods in combination, to form an overall eating pattern that has cumulative effects on health. The *2015–2020 Dietary Guidelines* points out the large discrepancy between the recommendations and the actual American diet, which includes too few vegetables, fruits, high-fiber whole grains, low-fat milk and milk products, and seafood and too much added sugar, solid fat, refined grains, and sodium.

The recommendations of the Dietary Guidelines—focused on eating patterns and their food and nutrient characteristics—are based on the growing body of research that examines the relationship between overall eating patterns, health, and risk of chronic disease. Following these guidelines will promote health and reduce risk of diseases such as heart disease, cancer, diabetes, stroke, osteoporosis, and obesity. Each of the guidelines is supported by an extensive review of scientific and medical evidence.

General Recommendations The Dietary Guidelines offers five primary recommendations:

1. **Follow a healthy eating pattern across the lifespan.** All food and beverage choices matter. Choose a healthy eating pattern at an appropriate calorie level to help achieve and maintain a healthy body weight, support nutrient adequacy, and reduce the risk of chronic disease.

2. **Focus on variety, nutrient density, and amount.** To meet nutrient needs within calorie limits, choose a variety of nutrient-dense foods across and within all food groups in recommended amounts.

3. **Limit calories from added sugars and saturated fats and reduce sodium intake.** Cut back on foods and beverages higher in these components to amounts that fit within healthy eating patterns.

4. **Shift to healthier food and beverage choices.** Choose nutrient-dense foods and beverages across and within all food groups in place of less healthy choices. Consider cultural and personal preferences to make these shifts easier to accomplish and maintain.

5. **Support healthy eating patterns for all.** Everyone has a role in helping to create and support healthy eating patterns in multiple settings nationwide, from home to school to work to communities.

The Guidelines recognize the challenges that make it difficult for Americans to reach their food and fitness goals. They acknowledge that all segments of our society, from families to restaurants, food producers to policymakers, have a responsibility in supporting healthy choices. The Guidelines emphasize that a healthy eating pattern is not a rigid prescription, but rather an adaptable framework in which individuals can enjoy foods that meet their personal, cultural, and traditional preferences and fit within their budget and lifestyle. Adopting a healthy eating pattern and engaging in regular physical activity will go a long way toward improving health and reducing the risk of chronic disease in every life stage.

Building Healthy Eating Patterns A healthy eating pattern is one that meets nutrient needs while not exceeding calorie requirements, and while staying within limits for dietary components that are typically consumed in excess. The three dietary patterns developed by the *2015–2020 Dietary Guidelines* focus on healthy eating and physical activity patterns:

- **Healthy U.S.-Style Pattern.** Based on the types and proportions of foods Americans typically consume, but in nutrient-dense forms and appropriate amounts.

- **Healthy Vegetarian Pattern.** Includes more legumes, processed soy products, nuts and seeds, and whole grains; it contains no meat, poultry, or seafood, but is close to the Healthy U.S.-Style Pattern in amounts of all other food groups. Dairy and eggs are still included because the majority of vegetarians eat them; however, the plan can be vegan with plant-based substitutions.

- **Healthy Mediterranean-Style Pattern.** Reflecting a dietary pattern associated with many cultures bordering the Mediterranean Sea, which includes more fruits and seafood and less dairy than the Healthy U.S.-Style Pattern. The Mediterranean diet has been associated with positive health outcomes such as lower rates of heart disease and total mortality.

Table 8.10   USDA Food Patterns at the 2,000-Calorie Level

FOOD GROUP	HEALTHY U.S.-STYLE PATTERN	HEALTHY VEGETARIAN PATTERN	HEALTHY MEDITERRANEAN-STYLE PATTERN
Vegetables	**2½ c-eq/day**	**2½ c-eq/day**	**2½ c-eq/day**
Dark green	1½ c-eq/wk	1½ c-eq/wk	1½ c-eq/wk
Red & orange	5½ c-eq/wk	5½ c-eq/wk	5½ c-eq/wk
Legumes (beans & peas)	1½ c-eq/wk	3 c-eq/wk*	1½ c-eq/wk
Starchy	5 c-eq/wk	5 c-eq/wk	5 c-eq/wk
Other	4 c-eq/wk	4 c-eq/wk	4 c-eq/wk
Fruit	**2 c-eq/day**	**2 c-eq/day**	**2½ c-eq/day**
Grains	**6 oz-eq/day**	**6½ oz-eq/day**	**6 oz-eq/day**
Whole grains	3 oz-eq/day	3½ oz-eq/day	3 oz-eq/day
Refined grains	3 oz-eq/day	3 oz-eq/day	3 oz-eq/day
Dairy	**3 c-eq/day**	**3 c-eq per day**	**2 c-eq per day**
Protein Foods	**5½ oz-eq/day**	**3½ oz-eq/day**	**6½ oz-eq/day**
Seafood	8 oz-eq/wk	n/a	15 oz-eq/wk
Meat, poultry, eggs	26 oz-eq/wk	3 oz-eq/wk (eggs)	26 oz-eq/wk
Nuts, seeds, soy products	5 oz-eq/wk	15 oz-eq/wk	5 oz eq/wk
Oils	**27 g/day**	**27 g/day**	**27 g/day**
Limit on calories for other uses (% of total calories)**	270 cal/day (14%)	290 cal/day (15%)	260 cal/day (13%)

NOTE: c-eq = cup-equivalent, the amount of a food or beverage product that is considered equal to 1 cup from the vegetables, fruits, or dairy food groups; oz-eq = ounce-equivalent, the amount of a food product that is considered equal to 1 ounce from the grain or protein food food groups.

*For the Vegetarian Pattern, half of total legume intake counts as vegetables and half as protein foods.

** If all food choices to meet food group recommendations are in nutrient-dense forms, a small number of calories remain within the overall calorie limit of the Pattern (i.e., limit on calories for other uses). Calories up to the specified limit can be used for added sugars, added refined starches, solid fats, or alcohol, or to eat more than the recommended amount of food in a food group.

SOURCES: U.S. Department of Health and Human Services and U.S. Department of Agriculture. 2015. *2015–2020 Dietary Guidelines for Americans,* 8th ed., (http://health.gov/dietaryguidelines/2015/guidelines/); Food and Nutrition Board, Institute of Medicine, *Dietary Reference Intakes for Energy, Carbohydrate, Fiber, Fat, Fatty Acids, Cholesterol, Protein, and Amino Acids.* Washington, DC: National Academies Press, 2002.

All three patterns are based on amounts of food from different food groups (and subgroups) according to overall energy intake. They also share an emphasis on whole fruits, vegetables, whole grains, beans and peas, fat-free and low-fat milk and milk products, and healthy oils; they include less red meat and more seafood than the typical American diet. Healthy dietary patterns include oils, but they limit the amount of energy that people should consume from solid fats.

A fundamental principle of all healthy dietary patterns is that people should eat nutrient-dense foods—foods with little or no solid fats, added sugars, and added refined starches—so that they can obtain all the needed nutrients without exceeding their daily energy requirements. In addition, people should strive to get their nutrients from foods rather than from dietary supplements, although supplements or fortification may be helpful for certain populations. Following a healthy pattern allows you to meet the DRIs for essential nutrients and stay within the AMDRs established by the Food and Nutrition Board for nutrients that supply energy. Table 8.10 compares the three patterns for a 2,000-calorie diet. To see a more detailed breakdown of

the recommendations for the three healthy dietary patterns, see the Nutrition Resources section at the end of the chapter.

Although the greatest emphasis of the Dietary Guidelines is on consuming an overall healthy eating pattern, specific recommendations have been set for dietary components of particular public health concern. Sticking to these limits can help individuals stay within calorie limits while achieving a healthy eating pattern:

- Consume less than 10% of calories per day from added sugars. The current average intake among Americans is about 13–16%, with about half the total coming from sugar-sweetened beverages.

- Consume less than 10% of calories per day from saturated fats.

- Consume less than 2,300 mg per day of sodium. The current average intake among Americans is about 3,400 mg, most of it coming from processed foods.

- If you consume alcohol, do so in moderation—up to one drink per day for women and two drinks per day for men—and only if you are of legal drinking age.

In addition, all Americans should strive to meet the federal physical activity guidelines and aim to achieve and maintain a healthy body weight.

Making Shifts to Align with Healthy Eating Patterns The eating patterns of the U.S. population are low in vegetables, fruits, whole grains, dairy, seafood, and oil, while they are high in refined grains, added sugars, saturated fats, sodium, as well as meats, poultry, and eggs. Additionally, most Americans consume too many calories, and only 20% meet the physical activity guidelines. For many of us, achieving a healthy eating pattern will require changes to our current food and beverage choices. Figure 8.3 shows the lack of alignment between the typical eating patterns currently in the United States and those in the Dietary Guidelines.

Most of us would benefit from shifting food choices both within and across food groups. Some shifts can be minor and accomplished by making simple substitutions, whereas others may require greater determination. Every food choice is an opportunity to move toward a healthy eating pattern. Making small positive dietary changes over time can cumulatively support your efforts at maintaining a healthy body weight, meeting nutrient needs, and reducing your risk for chronic disease. See the box "Positive Changes to Meet the Dietary Guidelines" for some strategies to get you started.

Wellness Tip Farmers' markets are an important way to bring healthy food choices to residents of inner cities. Support the establishment of farmers' markets in your community.
©michael spring/123RF

Supporting Healthy Eating Patterns Making healthy choices can be challenging, but ultimately each person makes decisions about what, where, when, and how much to eat. Individuals are more likely to shift their eating patterns toward the guidelines if everyone makes a collaborative effort across all segments of society. By doing so, we create a culture in which healthy lifestyle choices at home, school, work, and everywhere else are easy, accessible, and affordable.

The Dietary Guidelines offer the Social-Ecological Model (SEM) as a way to understand and address these complex problems. The SEM is defined by the Centers for Disease Control and Prevention as a framework for understanding influences on health and wellness at varying levels surrounding individuals, groups, and populations. The Dietary Guidelines SEM considers how the following factors interact to influence eating and physical activity and their associated health outcomes:

- Individual factors, such as age, sex, socioeconomic status, race/ethnicity, disability, knowledge and skills, and food preferences

- Environmental settings, such as home, schools, workplaces, recreational facilities, and restaurants

- Sectors of influence, such as government, education, health care, public health and community organizations, agriculture, marketing and media, food and beverage industries, and retail

- Social and cultural norms and values, such as traditions, religion, body image, and lifestyle

How do these factors stack up in your life? Are healthy food options available and affordable at your school and worksite? How far is it from your

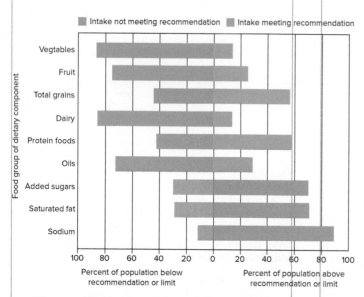

■ Intake not meeting recommendation   ■ Intake meeting recommendation

FIGURE 8.3 Dietary intakes compared to recommendations. The bars show the percentages of the U.S. population age 1 year and over who are below, at, or above each dietary goal or limit. The center (0) line is the goal or limit. For most people, meaning those represented by the orange sections of the bars, shifting toward the center line will improve eating patterns. For example, over 80% of people do not eat enough vegetables—they fall below the recommendation. Within the area of the graph demonstrating our consumption of foods we should limit—added sugars, saturated fat, and sodium—the orange bars show that over 80% of people exceed the recommended limit for sodium intake.

SOURCE: U.S. Department of Agriculture, What We Eat in America, NHANES 2007–2010, for average intakes by age-sex group. Healthy U.S.-Style Food Patterns, which vary based on age, sex, and activity level, for recommended intakes and limits (see *2015–2020 Dietary Guidelines for Americans*, https://health.gov/dietaryguidelines/2015/guidelines/chapter-2/current-eating-patterns-in-the-united-states/).

Positive Changes to Meet the Dietary Guidelines

Remember to focus on nutrient-dense options for the majority of your food choices: Use your calorie budget wisely. The tips here focus on the types of changes and swaps needed for the majority of Americans to move toward the dietary pattern recommended in the Dietary Guidelines.

Vegetables: Consume More Vegetables From All Subgroups

- Increase the vegetable content of mixed dishes while decreasing the amounts of other food components that you may overconsume—for example, cut the meat or cheese in half and double the vegetables in a soup, stew, or casserole.
- Always choose a green salad or a vegetable as a side dish. Incorporate vegetables into most meals and snacks.
- Replace foods high in calories, saturated fat, or sodium, such as some meats, poultry, cheeses, and snack foods, with vegetables.

Fruits: Increase Fruit Intake, Especially From Whole Fruits

- Choose more fruits as snacks, in salads, as side dishes, and as desserts in place of foods with added sugars such as cookies, pies, cakes, and ice cream.

Grains: Swap Whole Grains for Refined

- Shift from from white to 100% whole-wheat breads, white to whole-grain pasta, and white to brown rice (see the section on whole grains earlier in the chapter).
- Cut back on refined-grain desserts and sweet snacks that are high in added sugars, solid fats, or both. Choose smaller portions and eat them less often. For healthy swaps, try plain popcorn instead of buttered and bread instead of a croissant or biscuit, for example.

Dairy: Increase Intake

- Drink fat-free or low-fat milk (or soy beverage) with meals; choose yogurt as a snack; or use yogurt as an ingredient in salad dressings, spreads, and other prepared dishes.
- Favor milk and yogurt for additional dairy servings; cheese has more sodium and saturated fat and less potassium, vitamin A, and vitamin D than milk and yogurt.

Protein: Add Variety and Make More Nutrient-Dense Choices

- Increase seafood intake if yours is low: Try seafood as the protein choice in meals twice per week in place of meat, poultry, or eggs—for example, a tuna sandwich or a salmon steak.
- Use legumes or nuts and seeds in mixed dishes instead of some meat or poultry—for example, bean chili instead of a mixed-meat dish or almonds instead of ham on a main-dish salad.

Oils: Increase Intake As You Reduce Solid Fats

- Use vegetable oil in place of butter, stick margarine, shortening, lard, or coconut oils when cooking.

- Increase intake of foods that naturally contain oils, such as seafood and nuts, in place of some meat and poultry.
- Choose options for salad dressings and spreads made with oils instead of solid fats.

Saturated Fats: Reduce to Less Than 10% Of Calories Per Day

- Substitute foods high in unsaturated fats for foods high in saturated fats; for example, use oils rather than solid fats for food preparation.
- Read food labels to identify the types of fats in prepared foods; compare and choose lower-fat forms of foods and beverages that contain solid fats (e.g., fat-free milk instead of 2% or whole).
- Adjust proportions of ingredients in mixed dishes to increase vegetables, whole grains, lean meat, and lower-fat cheeses in place of some of the fatty meat or regular cheeses.
- Consume foods higher in solid fats less often and in smaller portions.

Added Sugars: Reduce to Less Than 10% Of Calories Per Day

- Choose beverages with no added sugars, such as water, in place of sugar-sweetened beverages.
- Reduce portion sizes of sugar-sweetened beverages, and choose them less often.
- Limit servings and decrease portion sizes of grain-based and dairy desserts and sweet snacks.
- Choose unsweetened or no-sugar-added versions of canned fruit, fruit sauces, and yogurt.

Sodium: Reduce Intake

- Read food labels to compare sodium content, choosing products with less sodium.
- Choose fresh, plain frozen, or no-salt-added canned vegetables and fresh protein sources rather than processed meat and poultry.
- Eat at home more often; cooking from scratch allows you to control the sodium content.
- Limit sauces, mixes, and "instant" flavoring packs that come with rice and noodles; use your own flavorings based on herbs and spices rather than salt.

Physical Activity: Do More!

- Increase weekly physical activity, especially during commute time and leisure activities.
- Reduce sedentary time; take frequent exercise breaks.

SOURCE: U.S. Department of Health and Human Services and U.S. Department of Agriculture. 2015. *2015–2020 Dietary Guidelines for Americans,* 8th ed. (http://health.gov/dietaryguidelines/2015/guidelines).

home to the nearest place to purchase fruits and vegetables? How many food advertisements are you exposed to daily? Factors such as these can have an enormous influence on your behavior—both positive and negative—sometimes without your awareness. The Dietary Guidelines call on all elements of society to implement strategies such as expanding access to grocery stores, farmers' markets, and other sources of healthy food; ensuring that meals and snacks served in schools are consistent with the Dietary Guidelines; encouraging physical activity in schools; developing policies to limit food and beverage marketing to children; supporting sustainable agricultural practices; and providing nutrition assistance programs.

USDA's MyPlate

To help consumers put the Dietary Guidelines for Americans into practice, the USDA also issues the food guidance system known as MyPlate. MyPlate provides a simple graphic showing how to use the five food groups to build a healthy plate at each meal (Figure 8.4). If you need to change your dietary pattern, use MyPlate to build a healthy eating style by focusing on variety, amount of food consumed, and nutrition. You can get a personalized version of MyPlate recommendations by visiting ChooseMyPlate.gov. Using the MyPlate Plan from the Online Tools menu, you can determine the amount of each food group you need based on your calorie allowance. Your plan is personalized based on your age, gender, weight, height, and level of physical activity.

FIGURE 8.4 USDA's MyPlate. illustrates the five food groups that are building blocks for a healthy diet; visit ChooseMyPlate.gov for a personalized plan.
SOURCE: U.S. Department of Agriculture. MyPlate, 2011. (http://www.ChooseMyPlate .gov; retrieved April 17, 2015).

MyPlate is available in Spanish, and it offers special recommendations for dieters, preschoolers aged 2–5, children aged 6–11, and pregnant and breastfeeding women. MyPlate On Campus is an initiative to allow students to become ambassadors of healthy eating and healthy lifestyles. MyPlate On Campus provides resources and practical guidelines for promoting health and wellness uniquely customized for students and the campus lifestyle.

Energy Intake and Portion Sizes To build a healthy eating style, base your food group goals on an appropriate level of energy intake. Table 8.11 provides guidance for determining an appropriate calorie intake for weight maintenance. Everyone is different, however, and the number of calories you need will vary depending on multiple factors. You can set a rough calorie goal by tracking your food and calorie intake for at least several days (a longer tracking period improves accuracy). Once you are comfortable with a calorie level for your eating plan, monitor your body weight over time, and adjust calorie intake and physical activity as needed to meet your personal weight goals. See Chapter 9 for much more on maintaining a healthy weight.

Most people underestimate the number of calories they consume and the size of their portions. See the box "Judging Portion Sizes" for strategies to improve the accuracy of your estimates. MyPlate doesn't use number of portions as the basis of recommendations; instead, amounts are listed in terms of cup-equivalents and ounce-equivalents. These units of measurement allow you to align servings of foods that differ—those that are concentrated versus those that are more airy or contain more water. For example, ½ cup of blueberries and ¼ cup of raisins both count as ½ cup-equivalent of fruit.

Next, let's take a look at each food group in MyPlate.

Vegetables: Vary Your Veggies Together, fruits and vegetables should make up half your plate. Vegetables contain carbohydrates, dietary fiber, vitamin C, folate, potassium, and many other nutrients, and they are naturally low in calories and fat. A 2,000-calorie diet should include 2½ cups of vegetables daily. Each of the following counts as 1 cup-equivalent from the vegetable group:

- 1 cup raw or cooked vegetables
- 2 cups raw leafy salad greens
- 1 cup vegetable juice

Because vegetables vary in the nutrients they provide, eat a variety to obtain maximum nutrition. MyPlate recommends weekly servings from the five subgroups within the vegetables group (see Table 8.10). Eat vegetables from several subgroups each day.

Table 8.11	USDA Estimated Daily Calorie Intake Levels to Maintain Energy Balance		
AGE (YEARS)	SEDENTARY*	MODERATELY ACTIVE**	ACTIVE†
FEMALE***			
16–18	1,800	2,000	2,400
19–25	2,000	2,200	2,400
26–30	1,800	2,000	2,400
31–50	1,800	2,000	2,200
51–60	1,600	1,800	2,200
61 & up	1,600	1,800	2,000
MALE			
16–18	2,400	2,800	3,200
19–20	2,600	2,800	3,000
21–25	2,400	2,800	3,000
26–35	2,400	2,600	3,000
36–40	2,400	2,600	2,800
41–45	2,200	2,600	2,800
46–55	2,200	2,400	2,800
56–60	2,200	2,400	2,600
61–65	2,000	2,400	2,600
66–75	2,000	2,200	2,600
76 & up	2,000	2,200	2,400

* A lifestyle that includes only the light physical activity associated with typical day-to-day life.

**A lifestyle that includes physical activity equivalent to walking about 1.5–3 miles per day at 3–4 miles per hour (30–60 minutes a day of moderate physical activity), in addition to the light physical activity associated with typical day-to-day life.

†Active means a lifestyle that includes physical activity equivalent to walking more than 3 miles per day at 3–4 miles per hour (60 or more minutes a day of moderate physical activity), in addition to the light physical activity associated with typical day-to-day life.

***Estimates for females do not include women who are pregnant or breastfeeding.

SOURCE: U.S. Department of Health and Human Services and U.S. Department of Agriculture. 2015. *2015–2020 Dietary Guidelines for Americans*, 8th ed. (http://health.gov/dietaryguidelines/2015/guidelines/); Food and Nutrition Board, Institute of Medicine. 2002. *Dietary Reference Intakes for Energy, Carbohydrate, Fiber, Fat, Fatty Acids, Cholesterol, Protein, and Amino Acids*. Washington, DC: National Academies Press.

- Dark-green vegetables (examples: broccoli, bok choy, romaine lettuce, spinach, collards, kale)
- Red and orange vegetables (examples: tomatoes, carrots, sweet potatoes, red peppers, winter squash)
- Beans and peas (examples: split and black-eyed peas; lentils; black, kidney, navy, pinto, white, and soybeans)
- Starchy vegetables (examples: corn, potatoes, green peas)
- Other vegetables (examples: artichokes, asparagus, beets, cauliflower, green beans, head lettuce, onions, mushrooms, zucchini)

Fruits: Focus on Whole Fruits People who eat more vegetables and fruits as part of an overall healthy diet are likely to have a reduced risk of some chronic diseases. Fruits are rich in carbohydrates, dietary fiber, and many vitamins, especially vitamin C. A 2,000-calorie diet should include 2 cups of fruits daily. Each of the following counts as 1 cup-equivalent of fruit:

- 1 cup fresh, canned, or frozen fruit
- 1 cup fruit juice (100% juice)
- 1 small whole fruit
- ½ cup dried fruit

Choose whole fruits often; they are higher in fiber and often lower in calories than fruit juices. Fruit *juices* typically contain more nutrients and less added sugar than fruit *drinks*. Choose canned fruits packed in 100% fruit juice or water rather than in syrup.

Grains: Make Half Your Grains Whole Grains Foods from this group are usually low in fat and rich in complex carbohydrates, dietary fiber (if grains are unrefined), and many vitamins and minerals. A 2,000-calorie diet should include 6-ounce-equivalent servings each day, and half of those servings should be whole grains, such as whole-grain bread, whole-wheat pasta, high-fiber cereal, or brown rice. The following count as 1 ounce-equivalents:

- 1 slice of bread
- 1 small (2½-inch diameter) muffin
- 1 cup ready-to-eat cereal flakes
- ½ cup cooked cereal, rice, grains, or pasta
- 1 6-inch tortilla

Choose foods that are typically made with little fat or added sugar (bread, rice, pasta) over those that are high in fat and added sugar (croissants, chips, cookies, doughnuts).

Dairy: Move to Low-Fat and Fat-Free Dairy This group includes all milk and milk products such as yogurt and cheeses, as well as lactose-free and lactose-reduced products. Soy milk (calcium-fortified) is also part of the dairy group. Those consuming 2,000 calories per day should include 3 cups of milk or the equivalent daily. Each of the following counts as 1 cup-equivalent:

- 1 cup milk or yogurt
- ½ cup ricotta cheese
- 1½ ounces natural cheese
- 2 ounces processed cheese

Protein Foods: Vary Your Protein Routine This group includes meat, poultry, fish, dried beans and peas, eggs, nuts, seeds, and processed soy products. A 2,000-calorie diet

TAKE CHARGE
Judging Portion Sizes

Studies have shown that most people under-estimate the size of their food portions, in many cases by as much as 50%. If you need to retrain your eye, try using measuring cups and spoons and an inexpensive kitchen scale when you eat at home. With a little practice, you'll learn the difference between 3 and 8 ounces of chicken or meat, and what a half-cup of rice really looks like. For quick estimates, use the following equivalents:

- 1 teaspoon of margarine = one die
- small cookie or cracker = a poker chip
- 2 tablespoons of peanut butter = a ping-pong ball

- ¼ cup nuts = a golf ball
- 1- to 2-ounce muffin or roll = a plum or large egg
- 1½ ounces of cheese = your thumb, four dice stacked together
- 2-ounce bagel = a hockey puck or yo-yo
- 3 ounces of chicken or meat = a deck of cards
- 1 medium potato = a computer mouse
- ½ cup of cooked rice, pasta, or potato = ½ baseball
- 1 cup of cereal flakes = a fist
- 1 medium fruit (apple or orange) = a baseball

should include 5½ ounce-equivalents daily. Each of the following counts as 1 ounce-equivalent:

- 1 ounce cooked lean meat, poultry, or fish
- ¼ cup cooked beans (legumes) or tofu
- 1 egg
- 1 tablespoon peanut butter
- ½ ounce nuts or seeds

Choose lean meats and skinless poultry, and become aware of your serving sizes. Choose at least one serving of plant proteins, such as black beans, lentils, or tofu, every day. Include at least 8 ounces of cooked seafood per week and select a variety of protein foods to improve nutrient intake and health benefits. Vegetarian options in the protein foods

group include beans and peas, processed soy products, and nuts and seeds.

Oils Oils and soft margarines include vegetable oils and soft vegetable oil table spreads that have no trans fats. Oils and fats that are liquid at room temperature and come from many plants and fish sources are included. Oils are major sources of vitamin E and unsaturated fatty acids, including the essential fatty acids, but they are not a food group. A 2,000-calorie diet should include 6 teaspoons of oils per day. One teaspoon is the equivalent of the following:

- 1 teaspoon vegetable oil or soft margarine
- 1 tablespoon salad dressing or light mayonnaise

Foods that are mostly oils include nuts, olives, avocados, and some fish. The following portions include about 1 teaspoon of oil: 8 large olives, ⅙ medium avocado, ½ tablespoon peanut butter, and ⅓ ounce roasted nuts. Food labels can help you identify the type and amount of fat in various foods.

Solid Fats and Added Sugars If you choose nutrient-dense foods from all food groups, you will have a small proportion of your daily calorie budget left to "spend." For those wanting to maintain weight, these calories may be used to increase the amount of food from a food group; to consume foods that are not in the lowest-fat form or that contain added sugars; to add oil, fat, or sugars to foods; or to consume alcohol. People who are trying to lose weight and improve their health should limit solid fats and added sugars. As described earlier, making better beverage choices is a key strategy for reducing intake of added sugars. Sodas, energy drinks, and sports drinks contribute added sugars but few nutrients to the American diet. The differences in nutrients between soda and other beverages are shown in Figure 8.5. The average American consumes

Wellness Tip Research shows that some protein-rich foods can give you a quick mental boost, which can be helpful before an exam.
©Marc Romanelli/Getty Images

Nutrient	Recommended Daily Intake* 2,000 calories		Orange Juice 168 calories		Low-Fat (1%) Milk 150 calories		Regular Cola 152 calories		Bottled Iced Tea 150 calories	
			% Daily	Nutrient value	% Daily	Nutrient value	% Daily	Nutrient value	% Daily	Nutrient value
Carbohydrate	300 g		14%	40.5 g	6%	18 g	13%	38 g	13%	37.5 g
Added sugars	32 g						119%	38 g	108%	34.5 g
Fat	65 g				6%	3.9 g				
Protein	55 g				22%	12 g				
Calcium	1,000 mg		3%	33 mg	45%	450 mg	1%	11 mg		
Potassium	4,700 mg		15%	710 mg	12%	570 mg	<1%	4 mg		
Vitamin A	700 μg		4%	30 μg	31%	216 μg				
Vitamin C	75 mg		193%	145.5 mg	5%	3.6 mg				
Vitamin D	5 μg				74%	3.7 μg				
Folate	400 μg		40%	160 μg	5%	20 μg				

Bars show percentage of recommended daily intake or limit

*Recommended intakes and limits appropriate for a 19-year-old woman consuming 2,000 calories per day.

FIGURE 8.5 Nutrient density of 12-ounce portions of selected beverages. Color bars represent percentage of recommended daily intake or limit for each nutrient.

nearly 800 calories daily from solid fats and added sugars—far higher than the recommended limits.

Physical Activity Like the Dietary Guidelines and other plans, MyPlate encourages physical activity for improving health, preventing chronic diseases, and managing weight. If you meet the U.S. Department of Health and Human Services's guidelines of 150 minutes per week of moderate physical activity, you will meet the recommendations found in MyPlate. To get the most health benefits, choose moderate physical activity such as brisk walking, cycling, and dancing, or vigorous activity such as running, swimming, basketball, or aerobics.

DASH Eating Plan

Other food-group plans have been proposed by a variety of experts and organizations, some to address the needs of special populations. One well-studied alternative is DASH, which stands for Dietary Approaches to Stop Hypertension. As its name suggests, the DASH eating plan was developed to help people lower high blood pressure and it is tailored with special attention to sodium and other nutrients of concern for managing blood pressure. Refer to Figure 4 in the Nutrition Resources at the end of the chapter for more information on DASH.

The Vegetarian Alternative

Vegetarians choose a diet with one essential difference from the diets described previously—they eliminate or restrict foods of animal origin (meat, poultry, fish, eggs, milk). Vegetarian diets tend to be lower in total calories and calories from fat, saturated fat, cholesterol, and animal protein and higher in complex carbohydrates, dietary fiber, potassium, folate, vitamins C and E, carotenoids, and phytochemicals. Individuals who follow a vegetarian diet generally have a lower body mass index than those who do not. And vegetarian-style dietary patterns are associated with lower mortality rates. Some people adopt a vegetarian diet for health reasons, whereas others do so out of concern for the environment, for financial reasons, or for reasons related to ethics or religion.

Types of Vegetarian Diets There are various vegetarian styles. The wider the variety of the diet eaten, the easier it is to meet nutritional needs.

- *Vegans* eat only plant foods.
- *Lacto-vegetarians* eat plant foods and dairy products.
- *Lacto-ovo-vegetarians* eat plant foods, dairy products, and eggs.

Others can be categorized as partial vegetarians, semi-vegetarians, or pescovegetarians. These people eat plant foods,

vegetarian Someone who follows a diet that restricts or eliminates foods of animal origin. TERMS

Wellness Tip Variety is the key to maintaining a healthy balanced vegetarian diet. Choose nutrient-dense foods rich in calcium, iron, zinc, and vitamins D and B-12.
©Nicolas McComber/Getty Images RF

dairy products, eggs, and usually a small selection of poultry, fish, and other seafood. Many other people choose vegetarian meals frequently but are not strictly vegetarian. Including some animal protein (such as dairy products) in a mostly vegetarian diet makes meal planning easier, but it is not necessary. Many Americans make dietary choices to limit their meat intake.

A Food Plan for Vegetarians Table 8.10 outlines the USDA's Healthy Vegetarian diet plan for a 2,000-calorie diet (refer to Figure 2 in the Nutrition Resources at the end of the chapter for information on other calorie levels). Adapting MyPlate for vegetarians requires only a few key modifications: For the meat and beans group, vegetarians can focus on the nonmeat choices of dry beans and peas, nuts, seeds, eggs, and soy foods like tofu. Vegans and other vegetarians who do not eat or drink any dairy products must find other rich sources of calcium. Fruits, vegetables, and whole grains are healthy choices for people following all types of vegetarian diets.

A healthy vegetarian diet, emphasizing a wide variety of plant foods, will supply all the essential amino acids. Choosing minimally processed and unrefined foods will maximize nutrient value and provide ample dietary fiber. Daily consumption of a variety of plant foods in amounts that meet total energy needs can provide all needed nutrients except vitamin B-12 and possibly vitamin D, calcium, iron, and zinc. Strategies for getting these and other nutrients include the following:

- *Vitamin B-12* is found naturally only in animal foods. If dairy products and eggs are limited or avoided, B-12 can be found in fortified foods such as ready-to-eat cereals, soy beverages, meat substitutes, special yeast products, and supplements.

- *Vitamin D* can be obtained by spending 5–15 minutes a day in the sun, by consuming vitamin D-fortified products like ready-to-eat cereals and soy or rice milk, or by taking a supplement.

- *Calcium* is found in legumes, tofu processed with calcium, dark-green leafy vegetables, nuts, tortillas made from lime-processed corn, fortified orange juice, soy milk, bread, and other foods.

- *Iron* is found in whole grains, fortified bread and breakfast cereals, dried fruits, leafy green vegetables, nuts and seeds, legumes, and soy foods. The iron in plant foods is more difficult for the body to absorb than the iron from animal sources. Eating or drinking a good source of vitamin C with most meals is helpful because vitamin C improves iron absorption.

- *Zinc* is found in whole grains, nuts, legumes, and soy foods.

If you are a vegetarian, remember that it's especially important to eat as wide a variety of foods as possible to ensure that all your nutritional needs are satisfied. Consulting with a registered dietitian will make your planning easier. Vegetarian diets for children, teens, and pregnant and lactating women warrant professional guidance.

Functional Foods

The American diet already contains numerous *functional foods*. Two of the earliest functional foods introduced in the United States were iodized salt and milk fortified with Vitamins A and D. More recently, manufacturers began fortifying breads and grains with folic acid to reduce the incidence of neural tube defects.

Although the definition of functional foods continues to evolve, this term generally refers to foods containing components that may provide positive health benefits. They include foods that are fortified, enriched, or enhanced, or that contain dietary components with additional potential to benefit health. Other examples of functional foods are calcium-fortified orange juice, margarine enriched with sterols or stanols to lower the risk of heart disease, energy bars for improved athletic performance, and vitamin B-12-enriched soy milk for vegetarians.

Dietary Challenges for Various Population Groups

MyPlate and the Dietary Guidelines for Americans provide a basis that nearly everyone can use to create a healthy diet. However, different population groups should be aware of special dietary challenges.

Children and Teenagers The best approach for parents with young children is to provide a variety of healthy food options. For example, parents can add vegetables to casseroles and fruit to cereal, or offer fruit and vegetable juices or homemade yogurt or fruit shakes instead of sugary drinks. Many children and teenagers enjoy eating at fast-food restaurants, but they should be encouraged to select the healthiest menu choices and to balance the day's diet with low-fat, nutrient-rich foods. Allowing children to help prepare meals is another good way to encourage good eating habits.

College Students Foods that are convenient for college students are not always the healthiest choices. Students who eat in buffet-style dining halls, cafeterias, and snack bars can easily overeat, and the foods offered are not necessarily high in nutrients or low in fat. The same is true of meals at fast-food restaurants. However, it is possible to make healthy eating

TAKE CHARGE
Eating Strategies for College Students

Eating Wherever

- Eat a colorful, varied diet. The more colorful your diet is, the more varied and rich in fruits and vegetables it will be. Fruits and vegetables are typically inexpensive, delicious, nutritious, and nutrient-dense.

- Eat breakfast. You'll have more energy in the morning and be less likely to grab an unhealthy snack later on.

- Choose healthy snacks—fruits, vegetables, whole grains, and cereals.

- Drink low- or nonfat milk, water, mineral water, or 100% fruit juice more often than soft drinks or sweetened beverages.

- Pay attention to portion sizes. Enjoy your food, but eat less.

- Combine physical activity with healthy eating.

- Plan to eat meals with friends and family members who choose healthy foods and can provide support and inspiration.

Eating in the Dining Hall

- Choose a meal plan that includes breakfast.

- Decide what you want to eat before you get in line, and stick to your choices.

- Build your meals around whole grains and vegetables. Ask for small servings of meat and high-fat main dishes.

- Choose leaner poultry, fish, or bean dishes rather than high-fat meats and fried entrees.

- Ask that gravies and sauces be served on the side; limit your intake.

- Choose broth-based or vegetable soups rather than cream soups.

- At the salad bar, load up on leafy greens, beans, and fresh vegetables. Avoid mayonnaise-coated salads, bacon, croutons, and high-fat dressings. Put dressing on the side; dip your fork into it rather than pouring it over the salad.

- Choose fruit for dessert rather than cookies or cakes.

Eating in Fast-Food Restaurants

- Most fast-food chains can provide a brochure with the nutritional content of their menu items. Ask for it, or check the restaurant's website for nutritional information. Order small single burgers with no cheese instead of double burgers with many toppings. If possible, get them broiled instead of fried.

- Ask for items to be prepared without mayonnaise, tartar sauce, sour cream, or other high-fat sauces. Ketchup, mustard, and fat-free mayonnaise or sour cream are better choices and are available at many fast-food restaurants.

- Choose whole-grain buns or bread for sandwiches.

- Choose chicken items made from chicken breast, not processed chicken.

- Order vegetable pizzas without extra cheese.

- If you order french fries or onion rings, get the smallest size and/or share them with a friend. Better yet, get a salad or a fruit cup instead.

- For food truck meals, use the same strategies suggested for fast-food restaurants—choose lean proteins and ask for condiments on the side. If your favorite food truck doesn't have healthy options, ask that they be added to the menu.

Eating on the Run

- When you need to eat in a hurry, remember that you can carry healthy foods in your backpack or a small insulated lunch sack (with a frozen gel pack to keep fresh food from spoiling).

- Carry items that are small and convenient but nutritious, such as fresh fruits or vegetables, whole-wheat buns or muffins, snack-size cereal boxes, and water.

- Make healthy choices at vending machines such as water or 100% fruit juice for beverages and whole-grain crackers or pretzels, nuts, seeds, baked chips, low-fat popcorn, and low-fat granola bars as snacks.

---

both convenient and affordable. See the tips in the box "Eating Strategies for College Students."

Pregnant and Breastfeeding Women Good nutrition is essential to a healthy pregnancy. Nutrition counseling before conception can help women establish a balanced eating plan and healthy body weights for a healthy pregnancy. During pregnancy and while breastfeeding, women have special nutritional needs. Pregnant or breastfeeding women are often advised to take a nutrient supplement in addition to following a special diet, as recommended by MyPlate's Daily Checklist for Moms.

To reduce the risk of neural tube defects in the fetus, the U.S. Public Health Service recommends that all women of childbearing age get 400 µg of folic acid daily from fortified foods or supplements.

Ask Yourself

QUESTIONS FOR CRITICAL THINKING AND REFLECTION

What factors influence your food choices—convenience, cost, availability, habit? Do you ever consider nutritional content or nutritional recommendations like those found in MyPlate? If not, how big a change would it be for you to think of nutritional content first when choosing food? Is it something you could do easily?

Older Adults Nutrient needs change as people age. Older adults tend to become less active and may not need as many calories to maintain body weight. At the same time, the absorption of some nutrients tends to be lower in older adults because of age-related changes in the digestive tract. For these reasons, older adults should focus on eating nutrient-dense foods. For example, foods fortified with vitamin B-12 and/or B-12 supplements are recommended for people over age 50. Calcium and vitamin D intake can be inadequate; therefore, physicians may suggest supplementation to reduce bone loss and risk of osteoporosis. Antioxidants from fruits and vegetables are important in older adults to reduce age-related changes in vision and cognitive functioning. Because constipation is a common problem, consuming foods high in dietary fiber and drinking enough fluids are important goals.

Athletes Key dietary concerns for athletes are meeting increased energy and fluid requirements for training and making healthy food choices throughout the day. For more on this topic, see the box "Do Athletes Need a Different Diet?"

People with Special Health Concerns Many Americans have special health concerns that affect their dietary needs. For example, people with diabetes benefit from a well-balanced diet that is low in simple sugars, high in complex carbohydrates, and relatively rich in monounsaturated fats. People with high blood pressure need to limit their sodium consumption and control their weight. If you have a health problem or concern that may require a special diet, discuss your situation with a physician or registered dietitian.

NUTRITIONAL PLANNING: MAKING INFORMED CHOICES ABOUT FOOD

Knowing about nutrition is a good start to making sound choices about food. It also helps if you can interpret food labels, make wise choices about dietary supplements, understand food additives, and avoid foodborne illnesses and environmental contaminants.

Food Labels

All processed foods regulated by either the FDA or the USDA include standardized nutrition information on their labels. Every food label shows serving sizes and the amount of many nutrients in each serving, including saturated fat, protein, dietary fiber, and sodium. To make informed choices about food, learn to read and understand food labels (see the box "Using Food Labels").

Food label regulations also require that foods meet strict definitions if their packaging includes terms such as *light, low-fat,* or *high-fiber* (Table 8.12). Health claims such as "good

Table 8.12	Food Package Nutrient Claims

CLAIM	WHAT IT MEANS
Healthy*	A food that is low in total fat or has predominantly mono- and/or polyunsaturated fats; has no more than 360–480 mg of sodium and 60 mg of cholesterol; and provides 10% or more of the Daily Value for vitamin A, vitamin C, vitamin D, protein, calcium, iron, potassium, or dietary fiber
Light or lite	33% fewer calories or 50% less fat than a similar product
Reduced or fewer	At least 25% less of a nutrient than a similar product; can be applied to fat ("reduced fat"), saturated fat, cholesterol, sodium, and calories
Extra or added	10% or more of the Daily Value per serving when compared to what a similar product has
Good source	10–19% of the Daily Value for a particular nutrient per serving
High, rich in, or excellent source of	20% or more of the Daily Value for a particular nutrient per serving
Low calorie	40 calories or less per serving
High fiber	5 grams or more of fiber per serving
Good source of fiber	2.5–4.9 grams of fiber per serving
Fat-free	Less than 0.5 gram of fat per serving
Low-fat	3 grams of fat or less per serving
Saturated or trans fat-free	Less than 0.5 gram of saturated fat and 0.5 gram of trans fatty acids per serving
Low saturated fat	1 gram or less of saturated fat per serving and no more than 15% of total calories
Low sodium	140 mg or less of sodium per serving
Very low sodium	35 mg or less of sodium per serving
Lean	Cooked seafood, meat, or poultry with less than 10 grams of fat, 4.5 grams or less of saturated fat, and less than 95 mg of cholesterol per serving
Extra lean	Cooked seafood, meat, or poultry with less than 5 grams of fat, 2 grams of saturated fat, and 95 mg of cholesterol per serving

*To reflect current scientific understanding and public health concerns, in 2016, the FDA updated the criteria for the "healthy" claim to also allow it for foods that are not low in total fat but instead have a fat profile makeup of predominantly unsaturated fats; the FDA also added potassium and vitamin D to the list of nutrients covered by the claim. Additional changes to the "healthy" claim are being considered.

NOTE: The FDA has not yet defined nutrient claims relating to carbohydrates, so foods labeled low- or reduced-carbohydrate do not conform to any approved standard.

THE EVIDENCE FOR EXERCISE
Do Athletes Need a Different Diet?

If you exercise vigorously and frequently or if you are an athlete in training, you likely have increased energy and fluid requirements. Research supports the following recommendations for athletes:

- **Energy intake.** Someone engaged in a vigorous training program may have energy needs as high as 6,000 calories per day—far greater than the energy needs of a moderately active person. For athletes, the Academy of Nutrition and Dietetics (formerly the American Dietetic Association) recommends a diet with 60–65% of calories coming from carbohydrates, 10–15% from protein, and no more than 30% from fat. Carbohydrates are the principal fuels used during exercise at intensities above 65% of maximum effort.

Athletes who need to maintain low body weight and fat (such as gymnasts, skaters, and wrestlers) need to get enough calories and nutrients while avoiding unhealthy eating patterns such as bulimia. The combination of low body fat, high physical activity, and disordered eating habits—and, in women, amenorrhea—is associated with osteoporosis, stress fractures, and other injuries. If keeping your weight and body fat low for athletic reasons is important to you, seek dietary advice from a qualified dietitian and make sure your physician is aware of your eating habits.

- **Carbohydrates.** Endurance athletes involved in competitive events lasting longer than 90 minutes may benefit from increasing carbohydrate intake to 65–70% of their total calories. Specifically, the American College of Sports Medicine

(ACSM) recommends that athletes consume 2.7–4.5 grams per pound of body weight daily, depending on their weight, sport, and other nutritional needs. This increase should come in the form of complex carbohydrates.

High carbohydrate intake builds and maintains glycogen stores in the muscles, resulting in greater endurance and delayed fatigue during competitive events. The ACSM recommends that before exercise an active adult or athlete eat a meal or snack that is relatively high in carbohydrates, moderate in protein, and low in fat and fiber. Eating carbohydrates 30 minutes, two hours, and four hours after exercise can help replenish glycogen stores in the liver and muscles.

- **Fat.** The ACSM recommends that all athletes get 20–35% of calories from fat in their diets. This is in line with the daily intake suggested by the Food and Nutrition Board. Reducing fat intake to less than 20% of daily calories can negatively affect performance and be harmful to health.

- **Protein.** For endurance and strength-trained athletes, the ACSM recommends eating 0.5–0.8 gram of protein per pound of body weight each day, which is considerably higher than the standard DRI of 0.36 gram per pound. This level of protein is easily obtainable from foods; in fact, most Americans eat more protein than they need every day. A balanced diet can provide the protein most athletes need.

There is no evidence that consuming supplements containing vitamins, minerals, protein, or specific amino acids builds muscle or improves sports performance. Strength and muscle are built with exercise, not extra protein, and carbohydrates provide the fuel needed for muscle-building exercise. Some research suggests spreading your protein intake across the day, every three or four hours (for example, breakfast, lunch, afternoon snack, and dinner).

- **Fluids.** If you exercise heavily or live in a hot climate, you should drink extra fluids to maximize performance and prevent heat illness. For a strenuous endurance event, prepare yourself the day before by drinking plenty of fluids. The ACSM recommends drinking 2–3 milliliters (~½ a teaspoon) of fluid per pound of body weight about four hours before the event. During the event, take in enough fluids to compensate for fluid loss due to sweating; the amount required depends on the individual and his or her sweat rate. Afterward, drink enough to replace lost fluids—about 16–24 ounces for every pound of weight lost.

Water is a good choice for fluid replacement for events lasting 60–90 minutes. For longer workouts or events, a sports drink can be a good choice. These contain water, electrolytes, and carbohydrates and can provide some extra energy as well as replace electrolytes like sodium lost in sweat.

SOURCES: Thomas, D.T., et al. 2016. "American College of Sports Medicine joint position statement. Nutrition and athletic performance," *Medicine and Science in Sports and Exercise* 48(3), 543–568; Clark, N. 2016. *Weight and protein: Hot topics at the ACSM annual meeting.* http://www.acsm.org/public-information/acsm-blog/2016/06/10/weight-and-protein-hot-topics-at-the-acsm-annual-meeting.

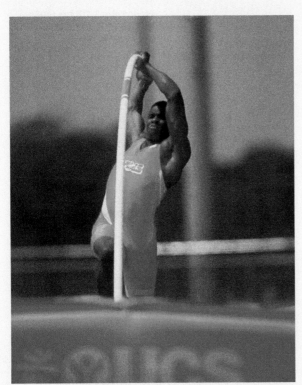

©Patrick Murphy-Racey/Sports Illustrated/Getty Images

Box icon: Vstock LLC/Getty Images

CRITICAL CONSUMER
Using Food Labels

The "Nutrition Facts" section of a food label is designed to help consumers make food choices based on the nutrients that are most important to good health. In addition to listing nutrient content by weight, the label puts the information in the context of a daily diet of 2,000 calories, with the understanding that your calorie needs may be higher or lower depending on your age, gender, height, weight, and physical activity level.

Food labels use uniform serving sizes. This means that if you look at different brands of salad dressing, for example, you can compare calories and fat content based on the serving amount. Food label serving sizes, however, may be larger or smaller than MyPlate serving size equivalents.

The Nutrition Facts label had been in use without major changes since the 1990s. Based on research into how consumers use food labels as well as changes to the nutrients of most concern to Americans, the FDA announced changes to the look and content of the label in 2016. Some new features include:

- Adding added sugars, vitamin D, and potassium to all labels; Vitamins A and C will no longer be required because deficiencies in these vitamins are rare today

- Removing the listing for "Calories from Fat" because research shows the type of fat is more important than the amount

- Revising Daily Values for certain nutrients to reflect the latest recommendations

- Updating serving size labeling for certain packages to be more realistic and to reflect amounts typically eaten at one time

- Refreshing the design to highlight calorie content and serving size and to make other parts of the label easier to read

During the transition period, you will see either the current or the new label on products. The new labels began to appear on foods in 2017, but the compliance date for all products was pushed out from the original 2018 deadline. For more on the new Nutrition Facts label, visit http://go.usa.gov/xkHru.

SOURCE: U.S. Food and Drug Administration, *New and Improved Nutrition Facts Label*, 2017. https://www.fda.gov/Food/IngredientsPackagingLabeling/LabelingNutrition/ucm537159.htm.

Box icon: ©sam74100/Getty Images RF

Previous Label

1. Serving size and calories: Based on the amount of food expected to be eaten at one time.

2. Daily Values: Generally based on a 2,000-calorie diet, Daily Value percentages tell you whether the nutrients in a serving contribute much to your total daily diet.

　　5% or less is low
　　20% or more is high

3. Limit these nutrients: Look for foods low in saturated fat, trans fat, and sodium.

4. Get enough of these nutrients: Look for foods high in dietary fiber, vitamin A, vitamin C, calcium, and iron.

Footnote: This section shows recommended daily intake for two levels of calorie consumption and values for dietary calculations.

Nutrition Facts

Serving Size 1-1/2 cup (208g)
Servings per container 2

Amount per Serving

Calories 240 Calories from Fat 36

	% Daily Value*
Total Fat 4g	**5%**
Saturated Fat 1.5g	**8%**
Trans Fat 0g	
Cholesterol 5mg	**2%**
Sodium 430mg	**19%**
Total Carbohydrate 46g	**17%**
Dietary Fiber 7g	**25%**
Sugars 4g	
Protein 11g	
Vitamin A	10%
Vitamin C	2%
Calcium	20%
Iron	35%

*Percent Daily Values are based on a 2,000 calorie diet. Your daily values may be higher or lower depending on your calorie needs:

	Calories	2,000	2,500
Total Fat	Less than	65g	80g
Sat Fat	Less than	20g	25g
Cholesterol	Less than	300mg	300mg
Sodium	Less than	2,400mg	2,400mg
Total Carbohydrate		300g	375g
Dietary Fiber	25g	30g	

Ingredients: Bulgur Wheat, Sauce (Water, Half and Half [Milk, Cream], Parmesan Cheese [Pasteurized Skim Milk, Cultures, Salt, Enzymes], Cheddar Cheese [Pasteurized Milk, Cultures, Salt, Enzymes], Olive Oil, Spice, Butter, Sugar, Xanthan Gum], Lentils, Corn, Green Beans, Red Beans, Potatoes.

Contains: Wheat and Milk

New Label

1. Servings sizes and calories: Information larger and bolder; some serving sizes have been updated to reflect what people actually eat or drink. "Calories from Fat" has been removed because research shows the type of fat consumed is more important than the amount.

2. Daily Values: Updated based on new scientific evidence; still based on 2,000-calorie diet.

3. Nutrients to look for: Look for new information on added sugars, vitamin D, and potassium. Overall, choose foods low in added sugars, saturated and trans fats, and sodium; choose foods high in fiber, vitamin D, calcium, iron, and potassium. Actual amounts of each nutrient will be listed.

Nutrition Facts

2 servings per container
Serving size 1 1/2 cup (208g)

Amount per serving

Calories   240

	% Daily Value*
Total Fat 4g	**5%**
Saturated Fat 1.5g	**8%**
Trans Fat 0g	
Cholesterol 5mg	**2%**
Sodium 430mg	**19%**
Total Carbohydrate 46g	**17%**
Dietary Fiber 7g	**25%**
Total Sugars 4g	
Includes 2g Added Sugars	**4%**
Protein 11g	
Vitamin D 2mcg	10%
Calcium 260mg	20%
Iron 6mg	35%
Potassium 240mg	6%

*The % Daily Value (DV) tells you how much a nutrient in a serving of food contributes to a daily diet. 2,000 calories a day is used for general nutrition advice.

All Food Packages

Ingredient list: Specifies each ingredient in a food by its common or usual name in descending order by weight; potential allergens must be declared at least once on a food label, in the ingredient list and/or immediately after it.

Ingredients: Bulgur Wheat, Sauce (Water, Half and Half [Milk, Cream], Parmesan Cheese [Pasteurized Skim Milk, Cultures, Salt, Enzymes], Cheddar Cheese [Pasteurized Milk, Cultures, Salt, Enzymes], Olive Oil, Spice, Butter, Sugar, Xanthan Gum], Lentils, Corn, Green Beans, Red Beans, Potatoes.

Contains: Wheat and Milk

source of dietary fiber" or "low in saturated fat" on packages are also regulated and can be signals that a product can be wisely included in your diet. Overall, the food label is an important tool to help you choose a healthy dietary pattern.

Food labels are not required on fresh meat, poultry, fish, fruits, and vegetables (many of these products are not packaged). You can get information on the nutrient content of these items from basic nutrition books, registered dietitians, nutrient analysis computer software, the Web, and the companies that produce or distribute these foods. Also, supermarkets may have posters or pamphlets listing the nutrient contents of unpackaged foods. In Lab 8.3, you compare foods using the information on their labels.

Calorie Labeling: Restaurants and Vending Machines

In 2014, the FDA issued new regulations requiring that calorie information be provided on restaurant menus and vending machines; these new rules were required as part of the 2010 Affordable Care Act. As of May 2018, calorie information is required on menus and signs near the food in chain restaurants and similar retail food establishments (those with 20 or more locations). Chain restaurants are also required to provide more detailed nutrition information about their menu items— on posters, tray liners, signs, handouts, or another similar location—so look for it!

Calorie labels are also now required (by July 2018) for vending machine operators who own or operate 20 or more machines. Calories will be shown on a sign or digital display near the food items or selection button. Use the information to help consider your options and to monitor your calorie intake.

Dietary Supplements

Dietary supplements include vitamins, minerals, amino acids, herbs, enzymes, and other compounds. Although dietary supplements are sold over the counter and are often thought of as safe and natural, they may contain powerful bioactive chemicals that can have toxic effects if consumed in excess.

In the United States, dietary supplements are not legally considered drugs and are not regulated like drugs. Before they are approved by the FDA and put on the market, drugs undergo clinical studies to determine safety, effectiveness, side effects and risks, possible interactions with other substances, and appropriate dosages. The FDA does not authorize or test dietary supplements, and manufacturers are not required to demonstrate either safety or effectiveness before these products are marketed. Although dosage guidelines exist for some of the compounds in dietary supplements, dosages for many are not well established.

Large doses of some dietary supplements can cause health problems by affecting the absorption of certain vitamins or minerals or interacting with medications. Garlic supplements, for example, can cause bleeding if taken with anticoagulant (blood-thinning) medications. Some supplements can have side effects. St. John's wort, for example, increases the skin's sensitivity to sunlight and may decrease the effectiveness of oral contraceptives, drugs used to treat HIV infection, and many other medications. For this reason, ask your doctor or a dietitian before taking any high-dosage supplement.

Drugs and supplements are also manufactured quite differently: FDA-approved medications are standardized for potency, and they require quality control and proof of purity. Dietary supplement manufacturing is not as closely regulated, and there is no guarantee that a product contains a given ingredient at all, let alone in the appropriate amount. The potency of herbal supplements can vary widely due to differences in growing and harvesting conditions, preparation methods, and storage. Contamination and misidentification of plant compounds are also potential problems.

In an effort to provide consumers with more reliable and consistent information about supplements, the FDA has developed labeling regulations. Labels similar to those found on foods are now required for dietary supplements. For more information, see the box "Using Dietary Supplement Labels."

Food Additives

Have you ever read the ingredients of your favorite processed or packaged food? Today, approximately 3,000 substances are intentionally added to foods to maintain or improve nutritional quality, to maintain freshness, to help in processing or preparation, or to alter taste or appearance. The most widely used additives in foods are sugar, salt, and corn syrup; these three, plus citric acid, baking soda, vegetable colors, mustard, and pepper, account for 98% by weight of all food additives used in the United States.

Food additives pose no significant health hazard to most people because the levels used are well below any that could produce toxic effects. Two additives of potential concern for some people are sulfites, used to keep vegetables from turning brown, and monosodium glutamate (MSG), used as a flavor enhancer. Sulfites can cause severe reactions in some people, and the FDA strictly limits their use and requires clear labeling on any food containing them. MSG may cause some people to experience episodes of sweating and increased blood pressure. If you have any sensitivity to an additive, check food labels when you shop and ask questions when you eat out.

Foodborne Illness

Many people worry about additives or pesticide residues in their food, but a greater threat comes from microorganisms that cause foodborne illnesses. Raw or undercooked animal products, such as chicken, hamburger, and oysters, pose the greatest risk, although in recent years contaminated fruits and vegetables have been catching up.

The Centers for Disease Control and Prevention (CDC) estimates that 48 million illnesses, 128,000 hospitalizations, and 3,000 deaths occur each year in the United States due to foodborne contaminants. One out of six people contract a foodborne disease each year. Symptoms include diarrhea, vomiting, fever, pain, headache, and weakness. Although the effects of foodborne

CRITICAL CONSUMER
Using Dietary Supplement Labels

Since 1999, specific types of information have been required on the labels of dietary supplements. In addition to basic information about the product, labels include a "Supplement Facts" panel, modeled after the Nutrition Facts panel used on food labels (see the sample label below).

Under the Dietary Supplement Health and Education Act (DSHEA) and food labeling laws, supplement labels can make three types of health-related claims:

● *Nutrient-content claims, such as* "high in calcium," "excellent source of vitamin C," or "high potency." The claims "high in" and "excellent source of" mean the same as they do on food labels. A "high potency" single-ingredient supplement must contain 100% of its Daily Value; a "high potency" multi-ingredient product must contain 100% or more of the Daily Value of at least two-thirds of the nutrients present for which Daily Values have been established.

● *Health claims,* if they have been authorized by the FDA or another authoritative scientific body. The association between adequate calcium intake and lower risk of osteoporosis is an example of an approved health claim. The FDA also allows so-called qualified health claims for situations in which there is emerging but as yet inconclusive evidence for a particular claim. Such claims must include qualifying language such as "scientific evidence suggests but does not prove" the claim.

● *Structure-function claims,* such as "antioxidants maintain cellular integrity" or "this product enhances energy levels." Because these claims are not reviewed by the FDA, they must carry a disclaimer (see the sample label).

Tips for Choosing and Using Dietary Supplements

● Check with your physician before taking a supplement. Many are not meant for children, older people, women who are pregnant or breastfeeding, people with chronic illnesses or upcoming surgery, or people taking prescription or over-the-counter medications. When you visit your doctor, bring a list of all dietary supplements you are taking. Do not take mega-doses (more than double DRI levels) without your doctor's approval.

● Follow the cautions, instructions for use, and dosage given on the label.

● Look for the U.S. Pharmacopeial Convention (USP) verification mark on the label, indicating that the product meets minimum safety and purity standards developed under the Dietary Supplement Verification Program by the USP. The USP mark means that the product (1) contains the ingredients stated on the label, (2) has the declared amount and strength of ingredients, (3) will dissolve effectively, (4) has been screened for harmful contaminants, and (5) has been manufactured using safe, sanitary, and well-controlled procedures. The Natural Products Association has a self-regulatory testing program for its members; other, smaller associations and labs, including consumerlab.com, also test and rate dietary supplements.

● Choose brands made by nationally known food and drug manufacturers or "house brands" from large retail chains. Due to their size and visibility, such sources are likely to have high manufacturing standards.

● If you experience side effects, stop using the product and contact your physician. Report any serious reactions to the FDA's MedWatch monitoring program (1-800-FDA-1088 or online at http://www.fda.gov/Safety/MedWatch/default.htm).

For More Information about Dietary Supplements

FDA: http://www.fda.gov/Food/DietarySupplements/
NIH Office of Dietary Supplements: http://ods.od.nih.gov
USDA: https://www.nal.usda.gov/fnic/dietary-supplements
U.S. Pharmacopeial Convention: http://www.quality--supplements.org/

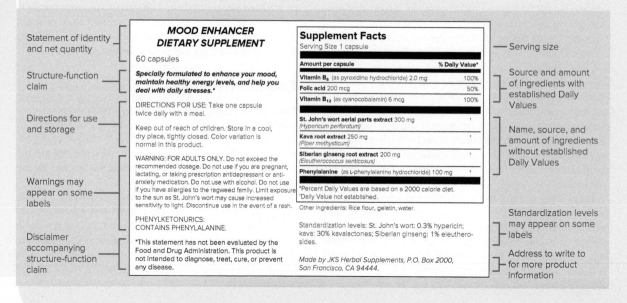

illness are usually not serious, children, pregnant women, and elderly people are more at risk for severe complications such as rheumatic diseases, seizures, blood poisoning, and death. Young children and older adults are more likely to have severe complications or to die from foodborne illnesses. In all, 13% of infections, 24% of hospitalizations, and 57% of deaths due to foodborne illnesses occurred among adults age 65 and over.

Causes of Foodborne Illnesses Most cases of foodborne illness are caused by **pathogens**, disease-causing microorganisms that contaminate food, usually from improper handling. According to the CDC, eight known pathogens contribute to the vast majority of illnesses, hospitalizations, and deaths related to foodborne illness, most notably *Salmonella* (most often found in eggs, on vegetables, and on poultry); norovirus (most often found in salad ingredients and shellfish); *Campylobacter jejuni* (most often found in meat and poultry); *Toxoplasma* (most often found in meat); *Escherichia coli* (*E. coli*) O157:H7 (most often found in meat and water); *Listeria monocytogenes* (most often found in lunch meats, sausages, and hot dogs); and *Clostridium perfringens* (most often found in meat and gravy). The most frequent causes of infection and hospitalizations are norovirus and *Salmonella*.

Although pathogens are usually destroyed during cooking, the U.S. government is taking steps to bring down levels of contamination by improving national testing and surveillance. Raw meat and poultry products are now sold with safe-handling and cooking instructions, and all packaged, unpasteurized fresh fruit and vegetable juices carry warnings about potential contamination. To ensure that the U.S. food supply is safe, the FDA Food Safety Modernization Act (FSMA) was signed into law in 2011 to reform the food safety system. The FSMA enables the FDA to focus more on preventing food safety problems rather than on reacting to problems after they occur.

Although foodborne illness outbreaks associated with food-processing plants make headlines, most cases of illness trace back to poor food handling in the home or in restaurants. The FDA encourages people to follow four basic food safety principles:

- *Clean* hands, food contact surfaces, and vegetables and fruits.
- *Separate* raw, cooked, and ready-to-eat foods while shopping, storing, and preparing foods.
- *Cook* foods to a safe temperature.
- *Chill* (refrigerate) perishable foods promptly.

The FDA also advises people to avoid certain high-risk foods, including raw (unpasteurized) milk, cheeses, and juices; raw or undercooked seafood, meat, poultry, and eggs; and raw sprouts. These precautions are especially important for pregnant women, young children, older adults, and people with weakened immune systems or certain chronic diseases. For more information on food safety, see the box "Safe Food Handling."

Treating Foodborne Illness If you think you may be having a bout of foodborne illness, drink plenty of clear fluids to prevent dehydration, and rest to speed recovery. To prevent further contamination, wash your hands often and always before

handling food until you recover. A fever higher than 102°F, blood in the stool, or dehydration deserves a physician's evaluation or a trip to your school's health clinic, especially if the symptoms persist for more than two or three days. In cases of suspected botulism—characterized by symptoms such as double vision, paralysis, dizziness, and vomiting—consult a physician immediately.

Irradiated Foods

Food irradiation is the treatment of foods with gamma rays, X-rays, or high-voltage electrons to kill potentially harmful pathogens, including bacteria, parasites, insects, and fungi that cause foodborne illness. It also reduces spoilage and extends shelf life. For example, irradiated strawberries stay unspoiled in the refrigerator up to three weeks, versus only three to five days for untreated berries. Even though irradiation has been generally endorsed by agencies such as the World Health Organization, the CDC, and the American Medical Association, few irradiated foods are currently on the market due to consumer resistance and skepticism. Studies indicate that when consumers are given information about the process of irradiation and the benefits of irradiated foods, most want to purchase them.

 All primary irradiated foods (meat, vegetables, and so on) are labeled with the flowerlike radura symbol and a brief information label; spices and foods that are merely ingredients do not have to be labeled. Proper handling of irradiated foods is still critical for preventing foodborne illness.

Environmental Contaminants and Organic Foods

Contaminants are present in the food-growing environment. Environmental contaminants include various minerals, antibiotics, hormones, pesticides, and industrial chemicals. Safety regulations attempt to keep our exposure to contaminants at safe levels, but monitoring is difficult, and many substances (such as pesticides) persist in the environment long after being banned from use.

Organic Foods Some people who are concerned about pesticides and other environmental contaminants choose to buy foods that are **organic**. To be certified as organic, foods must meet strict production, processing, handling, and labeling

---

pathogen A microorganism that causes disease. TERMS

food irradiation The treatment of foods with gamma rays, X-rays, or high-voltage electrons to kill potentially harmful pathogens and increase shelf life.

organic A designation applied to foods grown and produced according to strict guidelines limiting the use of pesticides, nonorganic ingredients, hormones, antibiotics, genetic engineering, irradiation, and other practices.

TAKE CHARGE
Safe Food Handling

Shopping

- Don't buy food in containers that leak, bulge, or are severely dented. Refrigerated foods should be cold, and frozen foods should be solid.

- Check the food label for an expiration date and for safe-handling instructions.

- Place meat, poultry, and seafood in plastic bags, and separate foods in grocery cart.

- Select cold and frozen foods last to ensure they stay refrigerated until just before checkout.

Storing Food

- Store raw meat, poultry, fish, and shellfish in containers in the refrigerator so that the juices don't drip onto other foods. Keep these items away from other foods, surfaces, utensils, and serving dishes to prevent cross-contamination.

- Store eggs in the coldest part of the refrigerator, not in the door, and use them within three to five weeks.

- Keep hot foods hot (140°F or above) and cold foods cold (40°F or below); harmful bacteria can grow rapidly between these two temperatures. Refrigerate foods within two hours of purchase or preparation and within one hour if the air temperature is above 90°F. Freeze foods at or below 0°F. Use or freeze fresh meats within three to five days and fresh poultry, fish, and ground meat within one to two days. Use refrigerated leftovers within three to four days.

Preparing Food

- Thoroughly wash your hands with warm soapy water for 20 seconds before and after handling food, especially raw meat, fish, shellfish, poultry, or eggs.

- Make sure counters, cutting boards, dishes, utensils, and other equipment are thoroughly cleaned with hot soapy water before and after use. Wash dishcloths and kitchen towels frequently.

- Use separate cutting boards for meat, poultry, and seafood and for foods that will be eaten raw, such as fruits and vegetables. Replace cutting boards once they become worn or develop hard-to-clean grooves.

- Thoroughly rinse and scrub fruits and vegetables with a brush (but not with soap or detergent), or peel off the skin.

- Don't eat raw animal products, including raw eggs in homemade hollandaise sauce, eggnog, or cookie dough.

- Thaw frozen food in the refrigerator, in cold water, or in the microwave, not on the kitchen counter. Cook foods immediately after thawing.

Cooking

- Cook foods thoroughly, especially beef, poultry, fish, pork, and eggs; cooking kills most microorganisms. Use a food thermometer to ensure that foods are cooked to a safe temperature. Hamburgers should be cooked to 160°F. Turn or stir microwaved food to make sure it is heated evenly throughout.

- Cook stuffing separately from poultry; or wash poultry thoroughly, stuff immediately before cooking, and transfer the stuffing to a clean bowl immediately after cooking. The temperature of cooked stuffing should reach 165°F.

- Cook eggs until they're firm, and fully cook foods containing eggs.

- To protect against *Listeria*, reheat ready-to-eat foods like hot dogs until steaming hot.

- Because of possible contamination with *E. coli* 0157:H7 and *Salmonella*, avoid raw sprouts.

According to the USDA, "When in doubt, throw it out." Even if a food looks and smells fine, it may not be safe. If you aren't sure that a food has been prepared, served, and stored safely, don't eat it. For more information, visit Foodsafety.gov.

©Dave King/Dorling Kindersley/Getty Images

criteria. Organic crops are grown without the use of conventional pesticides and must meet limits on pesticide residues. The use of synthetic fertilizers, genetic engineering, ionizing radiation, and sewage sludge is prohibited. For meat, milk, eggs, and other animal products to be certified organic, animals must be given organic feed and access to the outdoors and may not be given antibiotics or growth hormones. Products can be labeled "100% organic" if they contain all organic ingredients and "organic" if they contain at least 95% organic ingredients; all such products may carry the USDA organic seal. A product with at least 70% organic ingredients can be labeled "made with organic ingredients" but cannot use the USDA seal.

Organic foods, however, are not necessarily free of chemicals. They may be contaminated with pesticides used on neighboring lands or on foods transported in the same train or truck. However, they tend to have lower levels of pesticide residues than conventionally grown crops. Some experts recommend that consumers who want to buy organic fruits and vegetables spend their money on those that carry lower pesticide residues than their conventional counterparts (the "dirty dozen"): apples, bell peppers, celery, cherries, imported grapes, nectarines, peaches, pears, potatoes, red raspberries, spinach, and strawberries. Experts also recommend buying organic beef, poultry, eggs, dairy products, and baby food. Fruits and vegetables that carry little pesticide residue, whether grown conventionally or organically, include asparagus, avocados, bananas, broccoli, cauliflower, corn, kiwi, mangoes, onions, papaya, pineapples, and peas. All foods are subject to strict pesticide limits; the debate about the health effects of small amounts of residue is ongoing.

Whether organic foods are better for your health cannot be said for certain, but organic farming is better for the environment. Benefits include sustainable farming practices, preservation of biodiversity, healthier soil, protection of water supplies, reduced use of fossil fuels, improved animal welfare, protection of ecosystems, and safer conditions for farmworkers. Buying organic food, buying locally grown foods, and participating in a community garden are ways to support food production that benefits and sustains the environment.

Guidelines for Fish Consumption You may have heard reports of possible mercury contamination in fish. Overall, however, fish and shellfish are healthy sources of protein, omega-3 fats, and other nutrients, and experts continue to encourage consumption of both wild-caught and farmed fish. Prudent choices can minimize the risk of any possible negative health effects. High mercury concentrations are most likely to be found in predator fish—large fish that eat smaller fish. Mercury can cause brain damage to fetuses and young children. According to FDA and Environmental Protection Agency (EPA) guidelines, women who are or who may become pregnant and nursing mothers should follow these guidelines to minimize their exposure to mercury:

- Do not eat shark, swordfish, king mackerel, or tilefish.
- Eat 8–12 ounces each week of a variety of fish and shellfish that are lower in mercury, such as shrimp, canned light tuna, salmon, pollock, and catfish. Limit consumption of albacore tuna to 6 ounces per week.
- Check advisories about the safety of recreationally caught fish from local lakes, rivers, and coastal areas. If no information is available, limit consumption to 6 ounces per week.

The same guidelines apply to children, although they should consume smaller servings.

A PERSONAL PLAN

No single type of diet provides optimal health for everyone. Many cultural dietary patterns can meet people's nutritional requirements (see the box "Ethnic Foods"). Customize your food plan based on your age, gender, weight, activity level, medical risk factors, and personal tastes.

Assessing and Changing Your Diet

The first step in planning a healthy diet is to examine what you currently eat. Labs 8.1 and 8.2 help you analyze your current diet and compare it with optimal dietary goals. (This analysis can be completed using a nutritional analysis software program or one of several websites.)

To put your plan into action, use the behavioral self-management techniques and tips described in Chapter 1. If you identify several changes you want to make, focus on one at a time. You might start, for example, by substituting water for sugar-sweetened beverages. When you become used to that, you can try substituting whole-wheat bread for white bread. The information on eating behavior in Lab 8.1 will help you identify and change unhealthy patterns of eating.

Staying Committed to a Healthy Diet

Beyond knowledge and information, you also need support in difficult situations. Keeping to your plan is easiest when you choose and prepare your own food at home. Advance planning is the key: mapping out meals and shopping appropriately, cooking in advance when possible, and preparing enough food for leftovers. A tight budget does not necessarily make it difficult to eat healthy meals. When you are eating out, consider your food choices and portion sizes carefully.

Strategies like these are helpful, but small changes cannot transform a fundamentally high-sugar, high-calorie meal into a moderate, healthful one. Often, the best advice is to bypass a cinnamon roll with thick white icing for a flavorful but low-sugar option. Many selections offered in ethnic restaurants are healthy choices (refer to the "Ethnic Foods" box for suggestions).

DIVERSITY MATTERS
Ethnic Foods

Over the past decades, as people have come to the United States from many countries, Thai, Vietnamese, Afghani, Ethiopian, and Moroccan eateries, to name a few, have sprung up in cities and towns and near universities. For many of us, trying new foods is a fun, social, and usually delicious experience. Each cuisine arises from its local geography and the plants and animals available there. Each also evolves from cultural beliefs regarding food and health, as well as from historical events like trade, war, and immigration. For example, the cuisine of the United States began with English dishes that settlers brought to the colonies, and it was influenced later by foods and recipes of American Indians, African slaves, and immigrants from other countries in Europe as well as from Asia, Mexico, and Central America. These influences continue to shape American cuisine today.

By exploring world cuisines, you can learn about new cultures, new foods, and new flavor combinations. As you experiment, you will also want to keep healthy eating in mind, and you can do so by choosing dishes that are steamed, poached, boiled, roasted, grilled, broiled, stewed, lightly stir-fried, or broth-based—and by minimizing those that are fried, deep-fried, breaded, or cooked in butter, cream, or cheese sauces. The table below points you to healthy choices from a variety of ethnic cuisines.

Choose More Often	Choose Less Often
Chinese Hoisin sauce, oyster sauce, wine sauce, plum sauce, velvet sauce, or hot mustard Fresh fish and seafood, skinless chicken, tofu Mixed vegetables, Chinese greens	Crab rangoon Crispy (Peking) duck or chicken Sweet-and-sour dishes made with breaded and deep-fried meat, poultry, or fish
Greek Shish kabobs (souvlaki) Dolmas (grape leaves) stuffed with rice Tzatziki (yogurt, cucumbers, and garlic) Tabouli (bulgur-based salad)	Saganaki (fried cheese) Pies such as spanakopita and tyropita Deep-fried falafel (chickpea patties)
Indian Dishes prepared masala (curry), tandoori (roasted in a clay oven), or tikke (pan roasted); kebabs Raita (yogurt and cucumber salad) and other yogurt-based dishes and sauces Dal (lentils), pullao or pilau (basmati rice)	Ghee (clarified butter) Korma (meat in cream sauce) Samosas, pakoras (fried dishes) Poori, bhatura, or paratha (fried breads) Molee and other coconut milk-based dishes
Italian Pasta primavera or pasta, polenta, risotto, or gnocchi with marinara, red or white wine, white or red clam, or light mushroom sauce Dishes that are grilled or prepared cacciatore (tomato-based sauce) or piccata (lemon sauce) Cioppino (seafood stew) Vegetable soup, minestrone or fagioli (beans)	Antipasto (smoked meats) Dishes that are prepared alfredo, frito (fried), crema (creamed), alla panna (with cream), or carbonara (egg, cheese, and bacon)
Japanese Dishes prepared nabemono (boiled), shabu-shabu (in boiling broth), mushimono (steamed), nimono (simmered), yaki (broiled), or yakimono (grilled) Sushi or domburi (mixed rice dish)	Tempura (battered and fried) Agemono (deep fried) Katsu (fried pork cutlet) Sukiyaki Fried tofu
Mexican Soft corn or wheat tortillas Refried beans, nonfat or low-fat; rice and beans Ceviche (fish marinated in lime juice) Gazpacho, menudo, or black bean soup	Crispy, fried tortillas Refried beans made with lard Fried ice cream
Moroccan Couscous, harira (tomatoes, lentils, chickpeas and lamb), Zaalouk (cooked eggplant and tomatoes with olive oil), B'ssara (bean soup made with olive oil)	Makouda (deep-fried), Chebakia (deep-fried), Sfinge (doughnuts)
Thai Satay (skewered and grilled meats) Fish sauce, basil sauce, chili or hot sauces Bean thread noodles, Thai salad	Coconut milk soup Mee-krob (crispy noodles)

TIPS FOR TODAY AND THE FUTURE

Opportunities to improve your diet present themselves every day, and small changes add up.

RIGHT NOW YOU CAN

- Substitute a healthy snack for an unhealthy one.
- Drink a glass of water and put a bottle of water in your backpack for tomorrow.
- Plan to make healthy selections when you eat out, such as choosing steamed vegetables instead of french fries, or salmon instead of steak.

IN THE FUTURE YOU CAN

- Visit the MyPlate website at ChooseMyPlate.gov and use the online tools to create a personalized nutrition plan.
- Learn to cook healthier meals. There are hundreds of free websites and low-cost cookbooks that provide recipes for healthy dishes.

SUMMARY

- The six classes of nutrients are proteins, fats, carbohydrates, vitamins, minerals, and water.

- Nutrients are essential to humans when the body cannot produce them and must be gotten through food. Nutrients in foods provide energy, measured in kilocalories (commonly called calories); build and maintain body tissues; and regulate body functions.

- Protein, an important component of body tissue, is composed of amino acids; nine are essential to good health. Foods from animal sources provide complete proteins. Plants provide incomplete proteins.

- Fats, a major source of energy, also insulate the body and cushion the organs. Just 3–4 teaspoons of vegetable oil per day supply the essential fats. Unsaturated fats should be favored over saturated fats. Trans fats should be avoided.

- Carbohydrates provide energy to the brain, nervous system, and blood and to muscles during high-intensity exercise. Naturally occurring simple carbohydrates and unrefined complex carbohydrates should be favored over added sugars and refined carbohydrates.

- Fiber includes plant substances that are impossible for the human body to digest. It helps reduce cholesterol levels and promotes the passage of wastes through the intestines.

- The 13 essential vitamins are organic substances that promote specific chemical and cell processes and act as antioxidants. The 17 known essential minerals are inorganic substances that regulate body functions, aid in growth and tissue maintenance, and help in the release of energy from food. Deficiencies in vitamins and minerals can cause severe symptoms over time, but excess doses are also dangerous.

- Water aids in digestion and food absorption, allows chemical reactions to take place, serves as a lubricant or cushion, and helps regulate body temperature.

- Foods contain other substances, such as phytochemicals, that may not be essential nutrients but that may protect against chronic diseases.

- The Dietary Reference Intakes, Daily Values, Dietary Guidelines for Americans, and MyPlate food guidance system provide standards and recommendations for getting all essential nutrients from a varied, balanced diet and for eating in ways that protect against chronic disease.

- The *2015–2020 Dietary Guidelines for Americans* presents five guidelines: (1) Follow a healthy eating pattern across the lifespan; (2) focus on variety, nutrient density, and amount; (3) limit calories from added sugars and saturated fats and reduce sodium intake; (4) shift to healthier food and beverage choices; and (5) support healthy eating patterns for all.

- Choosing the right amount of foods from each group in MyPlate every day helps ensure the appropriate amounts of calories and necessary nutrients.

- A vegan diet requires special planning but can meet all human nutritional needs.

- Different population groups, such as college students and athletes, face special dietary challenges and should plan their diets to meet their particular needs.

- Consumers can get help applying nutritional principles by reading the standardized labels that appear on all packaged foods and on dietary supplements.

- Although nutritional basics are well established, no single diet provides wellness for everyone. Individuals should focus on their particular needs and adapt general dietary principles to meet them.

FOR FURTHER EXPLORATION

Academy of Nutrition and Dietetics. Provides a wide variety of educational materials on nutrition.

http://www.eatright.org

American Heart Association: Delicious Decisions. Provides basic information about nutrition, tips for shopping and eating out, and heart-healthy recipes.

https://recipes.heart.org/categories/31/delicious-decisions.

FDA: Food. Offers information and interactive tools about topics such as food labeling, food additives, dietary supplements, and foodborne illness.

http://www.fda.gov/food/default.htm

Food Safety Hotlines. Provide information on the safe purchase, handling, cooking, and storage of food.

1-888-723-3366

Forks over Knives. Shares articles by doctors from Cleveland Clinic and Cornell University on plant-based diets; also includes recipe ideas.

http://www.forksoverknives.com

Fruits and Veggies—More Matters. Hosted by the Produce for Better Health Foundation; promotes the consumption of fruits and vegetables every day.

http://www.fruitsandveggiesmorematters.org/

COMMON QUESTIONS ANSWERED

Q MyPlate recommends such large amounts of vegetables and fruit. How can I possibly eat that many servings without gaining weight?

A First, consider your typical portion sizes; you may be closer to meeting the recommendations than you think. Many people consume large servings of foods and underestimate the size of their portions. For example, a large banana may contain the equivalent of a cup of fruit. Likewise, a small salad may easily contain one cup of leafy greens and count as one-half cup of vegetables. Use a measuring cup or a food scale for a few days to train your eye to accurately estimate food portion sizes. The ChooseMyPlate. gov website includes charts of portion-size equivalents for each food group.

If you need to increase your overall intake of fruits and vegetables, look for healthy substitutions. If you are like most Americans, you are consuming more than the recommended number of calories from added sugars and solid fats; trim some of these calories to make room for additional servings of fruits and vegetables. Your beverage choices may be a good place to start. Do you routinely consume regular sodas, sweetened

energy or fruit drinks, or whole milk? One regular 12-ounce soda contains the equivalent of about 150 calories of added sugars; an 8-ounce glass of whole milk provides about 75 calories as discretionary fats. Substituting water or low-fat milk would free up calories for additional servings of fruits and vegetables. A half-cup of carrots, tomatoes, apples, or melon has only about 25 calories; you could consume six cups of these foods for the calories in one can of regular soda. Substituting lower-fat condiments for full-fat butter, mayonnaise, and salad dressing is another good way to trim calories to make room for additional servings of nutrient-rich fruits and vegetables.

Also consider your portion sizes and/ or the frequency with which you consume foods high in discretionary calories: You may not need to eliminate a favorite food— instead, just cut back. For example, cut your consumption of fast-food fries from four times a week to once a week, or reduce the size of your ice cream dessert from a cup to one-half cup. High-sugar treats should be consumed infrequently and in small amounts.

For additional help on improving food choices to meet dietary recommendations, visit ChooseMyPlate.gov and the family-friendly chart of "We Can! Go, Slow, and Whoa" foods at the site for the National Heart, Lung, and Blood Institute (http://

www.nhlbi.nih.gov/health/public/heart /obesity/wecan/downloads/gswtips.pdf).

Q What exactly are genetically modified foods? Are they safe? How can I recognize them on the shelf, and how can I know when I'm eating them?

A Genetic engineering involves altering the characteristics of a plant, animal, or microorganism by adding, rearranging, or replacing genes in its DNA; the result is a genetically modified (GM) organism. New DNA may come from related species of organisms or from entirely different types of organisms. Many GM crops are already grown in the United States. For example, more than 90% of U.S. soybean crops have been genetically modified; some GM corn crops have also been modified to carry genes for herbicide or pest resistance. Products made with GM organisms include juice, soda, nuts, tuna, frozen pizza, spaghetti sauce, canola oil, chips, salad dressing, and soup.

The potential benefits of GM foods cited by supporters include improved yields overall and in difficult growing conditions,

Gateways to Government Nutrition Information. Provides access to government resources relating to food safety, including consumer advice and information on specific pathogens.

>   http://www.foodsafety.gov
>   http://www.nutrition.gov

Harvard School of Public Health: The Nutrition Source. Provides knowledge for healthy eating, including advice on interpreting news on nutrition, and suggestions for building a healthy diet.

>   http://www.hsph.harvard.edu/nutritionsource

International Food Information Council. Food Insight. Provides information on food safety and nutrition for consumers, journalists, and educators.

>   http://www.foodinsight.org/

MedlinePlus: Nutrition. Provides links to information from government agencies and major medical associations on a variety of nutrition topics.

>   http://www.nlm.nih.gov/medlineplus/nutrition.html

MyPlate. Provides personalized dietary plans and many tips for developing a healthy eating style.

>   http://www.ChooseMyPlate.gov

National Academies' Food and Nutrition Board. Provides information about the Dietary Reference Intakes and related guidelines.

>   http://nationalacademies.org/hmd/about-hmd/leadership-staff/
>   hmd-staff-leadership-boards/food-and-nutrition-board.aspx

National Institutes of Health: Osteoporosis and Related Bone Diseases National Resource Center. Provides information about osteoporosis prevention and treatment; includes a special section on men and osteoporosis.

>   http://www.niams.nih.gov/Health_Info/Bone/

National Osteoporosis Foundation. Provides information on the causes, prevention, detection, and treatment of osteoporosis.

>   http://www.nof.org

USDA Center for Nutrition Policy and Promotion. Includes information on the Dietary Guidelines and MyPlate.

>   http://www.cnpp.usda.gov

USDA Food and Nutrition Information Center. Provides a variety of materials relating to the Dietary Guidelines, food labels, MyPlate, and many other topics.

>   http://www.nal.usda.gov/fnic

increased disease resistance, improved nutritional content, lower prices, and less use of pesticides. Critics of biotechnology argue that unexpected effects may occur: Gene manipulation could elevate levels of naturally occurring toxins or allergens, permanently change the gene pool and reduce biodiversity, and produce pesticide-resistant insects through the transfer of genes. In 2000, a form of GM corn approved for use only in animal feed was found to have commingled with other varieties of corn and to have been used in human foods; this mistake sparked fears of allergic reactions and led to recalls. Opposition to GM foods is strong in Europe; in many developing nations that face food shortages, responses to GM crops are more positive.

In 2016, the National Academy of Sciences released a report stating that there is no proof that GM food on the market is unsafe but that changes are needed to better regulate these foods and assess potential problems, especially as the related technologies and techniques change. Labeling has been another major concern. Surveys indicate that the majority of Americans want to know if their foods contain GM organisms. However, under current rules, the FDA requires special labeling only when a food's composition is changed significantly or when a known allergen is introduced. For example,

soybeans that contain a gene from a peanut would have to be labeled because peanuts are a common allergen. The only foods guaranteed not to contain GM ingredients are those certified as organic.

Q How can I tell if I'm allergic to a food?

A A true food allergy is a reaction of the body's immune system to a food or food ingredient, often a protein. This immune reaction can occur within minutes of ingesting the food, resulting in symptoms such as hives, diarrhea, difficulty breathing, or swelling of the lips or tongue. The most severe response is a systemic reaction called anaphylaxis, which involves a potentially life-threatening drop in blood pressure. Food allergies affect only about 2% of the adult population and approximately 5% of infants and young children. People with food allergies, especially children, are more likely to have asthma or other allergic conditions.

Just eight foods account for more than 90% of the food allergies in the United States: cow's milk, eggs, peanuts, tree nuts (walnuts, cashews, and others), soy, wheat, fish, and shellfish. Food manufacturers are now required to state the presence of these

eight allergens in plain language in the list of ingredients on food labels.

Many people who believe they have food allergies may actually suffer from a food intolerance, a much more common source of adverse food reactions that typically involves problems with metabolism rather than with the immune system. The body may not be able to adequately digest a food or the body may react to a particular food compound. Food intolerances have been attributed to lactose (milk sugar), gluten (a protein in some grains), tartrazine (yellow food coloring), sulfites, MSG, and the sweetener aspartame. Although symptoms of a food intolerance may be similar to those of a food allergy, they are typically more localized and not life threatening. Many people with food intolerance can safely and comfortably consume small amounts of the food that affects them.

If you suspect you have a food allergy or intolerance, a good first step is to keep a food diary. Note everything you eat or drink, any symptoms you develop, and how long after eating that the symptoms appear. Then make an appointment with your physician to go over your diary and determine if any additional tests are needed. People at risk for severe allergic reactions must diligently avoid trigger foods and carry medications to treat anaphylaxis.

USDA Hotline. Use this hotline for questions about meat and poultry.

800-535-4555

Vegetarian Resource Group. Provides information and links for vegetarians and people interested in learning more about vegetarian diets.

http://www.vrg.org

USDA Nutrient Data Laboratory Provides nutrient breakdowns of individual food items.

http://www.ars.usda.gov/ba/bhnrc/ndl

See also the resources listed in Chapters 9, 11, and 12.

SELECTED BIBLIOGRAPHY

Academy of Nutrition and Dietetics. 2015. Position of the Academy of Nutrition and Dietetics: Vegetarian diets. *Journal of the Academy of Nutrition and Dietetics* 115: 801–810.

Adebamowo, S. N., et al. 2015. Association between intakes of magnesium, potassium, and calcium and risk of stroke: 2 cohorts of US women and updated meta-analyses. *American Journal of Clinical Nutrition* 101(6): 1269–1277.

Afshin, A., et al. 2017. The prospective impact of food pricing on improving dietary consumption: A systematic review and meta-analysis. *PLoS One* 12(3): e0172277.

Ahluwalia, N., et al. 2016. Usual nutrient intakes of US infants and toddlers generally meet or exceed Dietary Reference Intakes: Findings from NHANES 2009–2012. *American Journal of Clinical Nutrition* 104(4): 1167–1174.

American Diabetes Association. 2013. *Glycemic Index and Diabetes* (http://www.diabetes.org/food-and-fitness/food/planning-meals/glycemic-index-and-diabetes.html?keymatch=glycemic-index).

American Heart Association. 2014. *Science Advisory: Omega-6 Fatty Acids* (http://www.heart.org/heartorg/gettinghealthy/fatsandoils/fats101/Omega-6-fatty-acids—science-advisory_ucm_306808_article.jsp).

American Heart Association. 2015. *Diet and Lifestyle Recommendations* (http://www.heart.org/heartorg/gettinghealthy/diet-and-lifestyle-recommendations_ucm_305855_article.jsp).

Centers for Disease Control and Prevention. 2015. *Food Safety* (http://www.cdc.gov/foodsafety/).

Centers for Disease Control and Prevention. 2016. *Burden of Foodborne Illness: Findings* (https://www.cdc.gov/foodborneburden/2011-foodborne-estimates.html).

Centers for Disease Control and Prevention. 2016. *Sodium: The Facts* (http://www.cdc.gov/salt/pdfs/Sodium_Fact_Sheet.pdf).

Centers for Disease Control and Prevention. 2017. *Know Your Limit for Added Sugars* (https://www.cdc.gov/nutrition/data-statistics/know-your-limit-for-added-sugars.html).

Chowdhury, R., et al. 2014. Association of dietary, circulating, and supplement fatty acids with coronary risk: A systematic review and metaanalysis. *Annals of Internal Medicine* 160(6): 398–406.

Denny. S. 2016. Get the Facts on Dietary Guidelines, MyPlate, and Food Labels. Academy of Nutrition and Dietetics (http://www.eatright.org/resource/food/nutrition/dietary-guidelines-and-myplate/get-the-facts).

Eckel, R. H., et al. 2013. AHA/ACC Guideline on Lifestyle Management to Reduce Cardiovascular Risk: A report of the American College of Cardiology/American Heart Association Task Force on Practice Guidelines. *Journal of the American College of Cardiology* 63(25_PA).

Estruch, R., et al. 2013. Primary prevention of cardiovascular disease with a Mediterranean diet. *New England Journal of Medicine* 368(14): 1279–1290.

Fitch, C., and K. S. Keim; Academy of Nutrition and Dietetics. 2012. Position of the Academy of Nutrition and Dietetics: Use of nutritive and nonnutritive sweeteners. *Journal of the Academy of Nutrition and Dietetics* 112(5): 739–758.

Food and Nutrition Board, Institute of Medicine. 2005. *Dietary Reference Intakes for Energy, Carbohydrate, Fiber, Fat, Fatty Acids, Cholesterol, Protein, and Amino Acids.* Washington, DC: National Academies Press.

Food and Nutrition Board, Institute of Medicine. 2005. *Dietary Reference Intakes for Water, Potassium, Sodium, Chloride, and Sulfate.* Washington, DC: National Academies Press.

Harvard Medical School. 2015. *The Truth about Fats: The Good, the Bad, and the In-Between* (http://www.health.harvard.edu/staying-healthy/the-truth-about-fats-bad-and-good).

Hedrick, V. E., et al. 2017. Dietary quality changes in response to a sugar-sweetened beverage-reduction intervention: Results from the Talking Health randomized controlled clinical trial. *American Journal of Clinical Nutrition.* doi:10.3945/ajcn.116.144543

Hooper, L., et al. 2015. Reduction in saturated fat intake for cardiovascular disease. *Cochrane Database of Systematic Reviews* 6:CD011737.

Insel, P., et al. 2016. *Nutrition,* 6th ed. Burlington, MA: Jones & Bartlett.

Jackson, S. L., et al. 2016. Prevalence of excess sodium intake in the United States—NHANES, 2009–2012. *MMWR* 64(52): 1393–1397.

Jalonick, M. C. 2015. Major shift in new federal dietary guidelines proposed. *Huffington Post,* February 19 (http://www.huffingtonpost.com/2015/02/19/federal-dietary-guidelines_n_6716130.html).

Jessri, M., W. Y. Lou, and M. R. L'Abbé. 2016. 2015 Dietary Guidelines for Americans is associated with a more nutrient-dense diet and lower risk of obesity. *American Journal of Clinical Nutrition* 104(5): 1378–1392.

Katz, D. L., and S. Meller. 2014. Can we say what diet is best for health? *Annual Review of Public Health* 35: 83–103.

Kiage, J. N., et al. 2013. Trans fat intake and all-cause mortality in the Reasons for Geographical and Racial Differences in Stroke (REGARDS) cohort. *American Journal of Clinical Nutrition* 97: 1121–1128.

Kirwan, J. P., et al. 2016. A whole-grain diet reduces cardiovascular risk factors in overweight and obese adults: A randomized controlled trial. *Journal of Nutrition* 146(11): 2244–2251.

Li, W., et al. 2016. Dietary phytochemical and cancer chemoprevention: A perspective on oxidative stress, inflammation, and epigenetics. *Chemical Research in Toxicology* 29(12): 2071–2095.

Liu, R., et al. 2012. Caffeine intake, smoking, and risk of Parkinson disease in men and women. *American Journal of Epidemiology* 175(11): 1200–1207.

Micha, R., et al. 2017. Association between dietary factors and mortality from heart disease, stroke, and type 2 diabetes in the United States. *Journal of the American Medical Association* 317(9): 912–924.

National Academy of Sciences. 2016. *Genetically Engineered Crops: Experience and Prospects* (http://nas-sites.org/ge-crops).

National Institutes of Health. Osteoporosis and Related Bone Diseases. National Resource Center. 2015. Vitamin A and Bone Health (http://www.niams.nih.gov/Health_Info/Bone/Bone_Health/Nutrition/vitamin_a.asp).

Orlich, M. J., et al. 2015. Vegetarian dietary patterns and the risk of colorectal cancers. *JAMA Internal Medicine* 175(5): 767–776.

Remig, V., et al. 2010. Trans fats in America: A review of their use, consumption, health implications, and regulation. *Journal of the American Dietetic Association* 110(4): 585–592.

Rodriguez, L. A., et al. 2016. Added sugar intake and metabolic syndrome in U.S. adolescents. *Public Health Nutrition* 19(13): 2424–2434.

Rosinger, A., et al. 2017. Sugar-sweetened beverage consumption among U.S. adults, 2011–2014. *National Center for Health Statistics Data Brief* No. 270.

Ross, S. M. 2015. Cardiovascular disease mortality: The deleterious effects of excess dietary sugar intake. *Holistic Nursing Practice* 29(1): 53–57.

Sacks, F. M., et al. 2017. Dietary fats and cardiovascular disease: A presidential advisory from the American Heart Association. *Circulation* 135 doi: 10.1161/CIR.0000000000000510.

Satya, S. J., et al. 2011. Putting the whole grain puzzle together: Health benefits associated with whole grains—Summary of American Society for Nutrition 2010 Satellite Symposium. *Journal of Nutrition* 141(5): 1011S–1022S.

Sirsikar, S., and A. Sirsikar. 2015. Prevention and management of postmenopausal osteoporosis. *International Journal of Innovative and Applied Research* 3(6): 5–26.

Slavin, J. L., and B. Lloyd. 2012. Health benefits of fruits and vegetables. *Advances in Nutrition* 3(4): 506–516.

Sofi, F., et al. 2010. Accruing evidence on benefits of adherence to the Mediterranean diet on health: An updated systematic review and meta-analysis. *American Journal of Clinical Nutrition* 92(5): 1189–1196.

Sonnenburg, E. D., et al. 2016. Diet-induced extinctions in the gut microbiota compound over generations. *Nature* 529(7585): 212–215.

Strate, L. L., et al. 2017. Western dietary pattern increases, whereas prudent dietary pattern decreases, risk of incident diverticulitis in a prospective cohort study. *Gastroenterology* S0016-5085(17)30006-9. doi:10.1053/j.gastro.2016.12.038

U.S. Department of Agriculture. 2015. *Biotechnology Frequently Asked Questions (FAQs)* (http://www.usda.gov/wps/portal/usda/usdahome?contentid=BiotechnologyFAQs.xml&navid=AGRICULTURE).

U.S. Department of Agriculture. 2015. *Scientific Report of the 2015 Dietary Guidelines Advisory Committee* (http://www.health.gov/dietaryguidelines/2015-scientific-report).

U.S. Department of Agriculture. 2016. *Adoption of Genetically Engineered Crops in the U.S.* (https://www.ers.usda.gov/data-products/adoption-of-genetically-engineered-crops-in-the-us.aspx).

U.S. Department of Agriculture and U.S. Department of Health and Human Services. 2010. *Dietary Guidelines for Americans, 2010,* 7th ed. Washington, DC: U.S. Government Printing Office.

U.S. Department of Health and Human Services and U.S. Department of Agriculture. 2015. *2015–2020 Dietary Guidelines for Americans,* 8th ed. (http://health.gov/dietaryguidelines/2015/guidelines/).

U.S. Food and Drug Administration. 2014. *Food Allergies: What You Need to Know* (http://www.fda.gov/Food/IngredientsPackagingLabeling/FoodAllergens/ucm079311.htm).

U.S. Food and Drug Administration. 2015. *Calorie Labeling on Restaurant Menus and Vending Machines: What You Need to Know* (http://www.fda.gov/Food/IngredientsPackagingLabeling/LabelingNutrition/ucm436722.htm).

U.S. Food and Drug Administration. 2015. FDA Cuts Trans Fats in Processed Foods (http://www.fda.gov/ForConsumers/ConsumerUpdates/ucm372915.htm).

U.S. Food and Drug Administration. 2016. *"Healthy" on Food Labeling* (http://www.fda.gov/Food/GuidanceRegulation/GuidanceDocuments-RegulatoryInformation/LabelingNutrition/ucm520695.htm).

U.S. Food and Drug Administration. 2016. *Use of the Term "Healthy" in the Labeling of Human Food Products: Guidance for Industry* (https://www.fda.gov/downloads/Food/GuidanceRegulation/GuidanceDocumentsRegulatoryInformation/UCM521692.pdf).

U.S. Food and Drug Administration. 2017. *Changes to the Nutrition Facts Label* (https://www.fda.gov/Food/GuidanceRegulation/GuidanceDocumentsRegulatoryInformation/LabelingNutrition/ucm385663.htm).

Vos, M. S., et al. 2016. Added sugars and cardiovascular risk in children: A scientific statement from the American Heart Association. *Circulation,* 22. doi:10.1161/CIR.0000000000000439

Wang, D. D., et al. 2016. Association of specific dietary fats with total and cause-specific mortality. *JAMA Internal Medicine* 176(8): 1134–1145.

Wang, X., et al. 2014. Fruit and vegetable consumption and mortality from all causes, cardiovascular disease, and cancer: Systematic review and dose-response meta-analysis of prospective cohort studies. *BMJ* 349: g4490.

Wu, L., and D. Sun. 2017. Adherence to Mediterranean diet and risk of developing cognitive disorders: An updated systematic review and meta-analysis of prospective cohort studies. *Scientific Reports* 7: 41317. doi:10.1038/srep41317

Zong, G., et al. 2016. Intake of individual saturated fatty acids and risk of coronary heart disease in US men and women: Two prospective longitudinal cohort studies. *BMJ* 355: i5796. doi:10.1136/bmj.i5796

NUTRITION RESOURCES

Calorie level of pattern	1,600	1,800	2,000	2,200	2,400	2,600	2,800	3,000
Food Group	**Daily amount** of food from each group (vegetable and protein foods subgroup amounts are per week)							
Fruits	1.5 c	1.5 c	2 c	2 c	2 c	2 c	2.5 c	2.5 c
Vegetables	2 c	2.5 c	2.5 c	3 c	3 c	3.5 c	3.5 c	4 c
Dark-green veg	1.5 c/wk	1.5 c/wk	1.5 c/wk	2 c/wk	2 c/wk	2.5 c/wk	2.5 c/wk	2.5 c/wk
Red/Orange veg	4 c/wk	5.5 c/wk	5.5 c/wk	6 c/wk	6 c/wk	7 c/wk	7 c/wk	7.5 c/wk
Beans and peas	1 c/wk	1.5 c/wk	1.5 c/wk	2 c/wk	2 c/wk	2.5 c/wk	2.5 c/wk	3 c/wk
Starchy veg	4 c/wk	5 c/wk	5 c/wk	6 c/wk	6 c/wk	7 c/wk	7 c/wk	8 c/wk
Other veg	3.5 c/wk	4 c/wk	4 c/wk	5 c/wk	5 c/wk	5.5 c/wk	5.5 c/wk	7 c/wk
Grains	5 oz eq	6 oz eq	6 oz eq	7 oz eq	8 oz eq	9 oz eq	10 oz eq	10 oz eq
Whole grains	3 oz eq	3 oz eq	3 oz eq	3.5 oz eq	4 oz eq	4.5 oz eq	5 oz eq	5 oz eq
Other grains	2 oz eq	3 oz eq	3 oz eq	3.5 oz eq	4 oz eq	4.5 oz eq	5 oz eq	5 oz eq
Protein foods	5 oz eq	5 oz eq	5.5 oz eq	6 oz eq	6.5 oz eq	6.5 oz eq	7 oz eq	7 oz eq
Meat poultry, eggs	23 oz eq/wk	23 oz eq/wk	26 oz eq/wk	28 oz eq/wk	31 oz eq/wk	31 oz eq/wk	33 oz eq/wk	33 oz eq/wk
Seafood	8 oz eq/wk	8 oz eq/wk	8 oz eq/wk	9 oz eq/wk	10 oz eq/wk	10 oz eq/wk	10 oz eq/wk	10 oz eq/wk
Nuts, seeds, soy	4 oz eq/wk	4 oz eq/wk	5 oz eq/wk	5 oz eq/wk	5 oz eq/wk	5 oz eq/wk	6 oz eq/wk	6 oz eq/wk
Dairy	3 c	3 c	3 c	3 c	3 c	3 c	3 c	3 c
Oils	22 g	24 g	27 g	29 g	31 g	34 g	36 g	44 g
Limit on calories for other uses (calories and % of calories)*	130 cal (8%)	170 cal (9%)	270 cal (14%)	280 cal (13%)	350 cal (15%)	380 cal (15%)	400 cal (14%)	470 cal (16%)

Food group amounts shown in cup (c) or ounce equivalents (oz eq). Oils, solid fats, and added sugars are shown in grams (g).
Quantity equivalents for each food group are:
- Grains, 1 ounce equivalent is: ½ cup cooked rice, pasta, or cooked cereal; 1 ounce dry pasta or rice; 1 slice bread; 1 cup ready-to-eat cereal flakes.
- Fruits and vegetables, 1 cup equivalent is: 1 cup raw or cooked fruit or vegetable, 1 cup fruit or vegetable juice, 2 cups leafy salad greens.
- Protein Foods, 1 ounce equivalent is: 1 ounce lean meat, poultry, or seafood; 1 egg; ¼ cup cooked beans or tofu; 1 Tbsp peanut butter; ½ ounce nuts/seeds.
- Dairy, 1 cup equivalent is: 1 cup milk or yogurt, 1½ ounces natural cheese such as cheddar cheese or 2 ounces of processed cheese.

*All foods are assumed to be in nutrient-dense forms, lean or low-fat, and prepared without added fats, sugars, refined starches, or salt. If all food choices to meet food group recommendations are in nutrient-dense forms, a small number of calories remain within the overall calorie limit of the Pattern. Calories up to the specified limit can be used for added sugars, added refined starches, solid fats, alcohol, or to eat more than the recommended amount of food in a food group. The overall eating Pattern also should not exceed the limits of less than 10% of calories from added sugars and less than 10% of calories from saturated fats. At most calorie levels, amounts that can be accommodated are less than these limits. For adults of legal drinking age who choose to drink alcohol, a limit of up to one drink per day for women and up to two drinks per day for men within limits on calories for other uses applies; and calories from protein, carbohydrate, and total fats should be within the Acceptable Macronutrient Distribution Ranges (AMDRs).

FIGURE 1. Healthy U.S.-Style Food Patterns
SOURCE: U.S. Department of Health and Human Services and U.S. Department of Agriculture, *2015–2020 Dietary Guidelines for Americans,* 8th Edition. December 2015. Available at http://health.gov/dietaryguidelines/2015/guidelines.

NUTRITION RESOURCES

Calorie level of pattern	1,600	1,800	2,000	2,200	2,400	2,600	2,800	3,000
Food Group	**Daily amount**[a] of food from each group (vegetable and protein foods subgroup amounts are per week)							
Fruits	1.5 c	1.5 c	2 c	2 c	2 c	2 c	2.5 c	2.5 c
Vegetables	2 c	2.5 c	2.5 c	3 c	3 c	3.5 c	3.5 c	4 c
Dark-green veg	1.5 c/wk	1.5 c/wk	1.5 c/wk	2 c/wk	2 c/wk	2.5 c/wk	2.5 c/wk	2.5 c/wk
Red/Orange veg	4 c/wk	5.5 c/wk	5.5 c/wk	6 c/wk	6 c/wk	7 c/wk	7 c/wk	7.5 c/wk
Beans and peas[b]	1 c/wk	1.5 c/wk	1.5 c/wk	2 c/wk	2 c/wk	2.5 c/wk	2.5 c/wk	3 c/wk
Starchy veg	4 c/wk	5 c/wk	5 c/wk	6 c/wk	6 c/wk	7 c/wk	7 c/wk	8 c/wk
Other veg	3.5 c/wk	4 c/wk	4 c/wk	5 c/wk	5 c/wk	5.5 c/wk	5.5 c/wk	7 c/wk
Grains	5.5 oz eq	6.5 oz eq	6.5 oz eq	7.5 oz eq	8.5 oz eq	9.5 oz eq	10.5 oz eq	10.5 oz eq
Whole grains	3.5 oz eq	3.5 oz eq	3.5 oz eq	4 oz eq	4.5 oz eq	5 oz eq	5.5 oz eq	5.5 oz eq
Other grains	2 oz eq	3 oz eq	3 oz eq	3.5 oz eq	4 oz eq	4.5 oz eq	5 oz eq	5 oz eq
Protein foods	2.5 oz eq	3 oz eq	3.5 oz eq	4 oz eq	4 oz eq	5 oz eq	5 oz eq	5.5 oz eq
Beans and peas[b]	4 oz eq/wk	6 oz eq/wk	6 oz eq/wk	8 oz eq/wk	8 oz eq/wk	10 oz eq/wk	10 oz eq/wk	12 oz eq/wk
Eggs	3 oz eq/wk	3 oz eq/wk	3 oz eq/wk	3 oz eq/wk	3 oz eq/wk	3 oz eq/wk	4 oz eq/wk	4 oz eq/wk
Nuts and seeds	5 oz eq/wk	6 oz eq/wk	7 oz eq/wk	8 oz eq/wk	9 oz eq/wk	10 oz eq/wk	11 oz eq/wk	12 oz eq/wk
Tofu/processed soy	5 oz eq/wk	6 oz eq/wk	7 oz eq/wk	8 oz eq/wk	9 oz eq/wk	10 oz eq/wk	11 oz eq/wk	12 oz eq/wk
Dairy	3 c	3 c	3 c	3 c	3 c	3 c	3 c	3 c
Oils	22 g	24 g	27 g	29 g	31 g	34 g	36 g	44 g
Limit on calories for other uses (calories and % of calories)c	180 cal (11%)	190 cal (11%)	290 cal (15%)	330 cal (15%)	390 cal (16%)	390 cal (15%)	400 cal (14%)	440 cal (15%)

[a]Food group amounts shown in cup (c) or ounce equivalents (oz eq). Oils, solid fats, and added sugars are shown in grams (g).
Quantity equivalents for each food group are:
- Grains, 1 ounce equivalent is: ½ cup cooked rice, pasta, or cooked cereal; 1 ounce dry pasta or rice; 1 slice bread; 1 cup ready-to-eat cereal flakes.
- Fruits and vegetables, 1 cup equivalent is: 1 cup raw or cooked fruit or vegetable, 1 cup fruit or vegetable juice, 2 cups leafy salad greens.
- Protein Foods, 1 ounce equivalent is: 1 ounce lean meat, poultry, or seafood; 1 egg; ¼ cup cooked beans or tofu; 1 tbsp peanut butter; ½ ounce nuts/seeds.
- Dairy, 1 cup equivalent is: 1 cup milk or yogurt, 1½ ounces natural cheese (e.g. cheddar cheese) or 2 ounces of processed cheese.

[b]About half of total beans and peas are shown as vegetables, in cup eqs, and half as protein foods, in ounce eqs. To determine total weekly beans and peas in cup eq, add the amount in vegetables plus the amount in protein food (in ounce eqs) divided by four. (For example, for 2,000-calorie level, 1.5 c/wk + (6 oz eq/wk ÷ 4) = 3 c eq/wk.)

[c]All foods are assumed to be in nutrient-dense forms, lean or low-fat, and prepared without added fats, sugars, refined starches, or salt. If all food choices to meet food group recommendations are in nutrient-dense forms, a small number of calories remain within the overall calorie limit of the Pattern. Calories up to the specified limit can be used for added sugars, added refined starches, solid fats, alcohol, or to eat more than the recommended amount of food in a food group. The overall eating Pattern also should not exceed the limits of less than 10% of calories from added sugars and less than 10% of calories from saturated fats. At most calorie levels, amounts that can be accommodated are less than these limits. For adults of legal drinking age who choose to drink alcohol, a limit of up to one drink per day for women and up to two drinks per day for men within limits on calories for other uses applies; and calories from protein, carbohydrate, and total fats should be within the Acceptable Macronutrient Distribution Ranges (AMDRs).

	1,600	1,800	2,000	2,200	2,400	2,600	2,800	3,000
Total beans/peas	2 c eq/wk	3 c eq/wk	3 c eq/wk	4 c eq/wk	4 c eq/wk	5 c eq/wk	5 c eq/wk	6 c eq/wk

FIGURE 2. Healthy Vegetarian Patterns.

SOURCE: U.S. Department of Health and Human Services and U.S. Department of Agriculture, *2015-2020 Dietary Guidelines for Americans*, 8th Edition. December 2015. Available at http://health.gov/dietaryguidelines/2015/guidelines.

NUTRITION RESOURCES

Calorie level of pattern	1,600	1,800	2,000	2,200	2,400	2,600	2,800	3,000
Food Group	Daily amount of food from each group (vegetable and protein foods subgroup amounts are per week)							
Fruits	1.5 c	2 c	2.5 c	2.5 c	2.5 c	2.5 c	3 c	3 c
Vegetables	2 c	2.5 c	2.5 c	3 c	3 c	3.5 c	3.5 c	4 c
Dark-green veg	1.5 c/wk	1.5 c/wk	1.5 c/wk	2 c/wk	2 c/wk	2.5 c/wk	2.5 c/wk	2.5 c/wk
Red/Orange veg	4 c/wk	5.5 c/wk	5.5 c/wk	6 c/wk	6 c/wk	7 c/wk	7 c/wk	7.5 c/wk
Beans and peas	1 c/wk	1.5 c/wk	1.5 c/wk	2 c/wk	2 c/wk	2.5 c/wk	2.5 c/wk	3 c/wk
Starchy veg	4 c/wk	5 c/wk	5 c/wk	6 c/wk	6 c/wk	7 c/wk	7 c/wk	8 c/wk
Other veg	3.5 c/wk	4 c/wk	4 c/wk	5 c/wk	5 c/wk	5.5 c/wk	5.5 c/wk	7 c/wk
Grains	5 oz eq	6 oz eq	6 oz eq	7 oz eq	8 oz eq	9 oz eq	10 oz eq	10 oz eq
Whole grains	3 oz eq	3 oz eq	3 oz eq	3.5 oz eq	4 oz eq	4.5 oz eq	5 oz eq	5 oz eq
Other grains	2 oz eq	3 oz eq	3 oz eq	3.5 oz eq	4 oz eq	4.5 oz eq	5 oz eq	5 oz eq
Protein foods	5.5 oz eq	6 oz eq	6.5 oz eq	7 oz eq	7.5 oz eq	7.5 oz eq	8 oz eq	8 oz eq
Meat, poultry, eggs	23 oz eq/wk	23 oz eq/wk	26 oz eq/wk	28 oz eq/wk	31 oz eq/wk	31 oz eq/wk	33 oz eq/wk	33 oz eq/wk
Seafood	11 oz eq/wk	15 oz eq/wk	15 oz eq/wk	16 oz eq/wk	16 oz eq/wk	17 oz eq/wk	17 oz eq/wk	17 oz eq/wk
Nut seeds, soy	4 oz eq/wk	4 oz eq/wk	5 oz eq/wk	5 oz eq/wk	5 oz eq/wk	5 oz eq/wk	6 oz eq/wk	6 oz eq/wk
Dairy	2 c	2 c	2 c	2 c	2 c	2.5 c	2.5 c	2.5 c
Oils	22 g	24 g	27 g	29 g	31 g	34 g	36 g	44 g
Limit on calories for other uses (calories and % of calories)*	140 cal (9%)	160 cal (9%)	260 cal (13%)	270 cal (12%)	300 cal (13%)	330 cal (13%)	350 cal (13%)	430 cal (14%)

Food group amounts shown in cup (c) or ounce equivalents (oz eq). Oils, solid fats, and added sugars are shown in grams (g).
Quantity equivalents for each food group are:
- Grains, 1 ounce equivalent is: ½ cup cooked rice, pasta, or cooked cereal; 1 ounce dry pasta or rice; 1 slice bread; 1 cup ready-to-eat cereal flakes.
- Fruits and vegetables, 1 cup equivalent is: 1 cup raw or cooked fruit or vegetable, 1 cup fruit or vegetable juice, 2 cups leafy salad greens.
- Protein Foods, 1 ounce equivalent is: 1 ounce lean meat, poultry, or seafood; 1 egg; ¼ cup cooked beans or tofu; 1 Tbsp peanut butter; ½ ounce nuts/seeds.
- Dairy, 1 cup equivalent is: 1 cup milk or yogurt, 1½ ounces natural cheese such as cheddar cheese or 2 ounces of processed cheese.

*All foods are assumed to be in nutrient-dense forms, lean or low-fat, and prepared without added fats, sugars, refined starches, or salt. If all food choices to meet food group recommendations are in nutrient-dense forms, a small number of calories remain within the overall calorie limit of the Pattern. Calories up to the specified limit can be used for added sugars, added refined starches, solid fats, alcohol, or to eat more than the recommended amount of food in a food group. The overall eating Pattern also should not exceed the limits of less than 10% of calories from added sugars and less than 10% of calories from saturated fats. At most calorie levels, amounts that can be accommodated are less than these limits. For adults of legal drinking age who choose to drink alcohol, a limit of up to one drink per day for women and up to two drinks per day for men within limits on calories for other uses applies; and calories from protein, carbohydrate, and total fats should be within the Acceptable Macronutrient Distribution Ranges (AMDRs).

FIGURE 3. Healthy Mediterranean-Style Patterns.

SOURCE: U.S. Department of Health and Human Services and U.S. Department of Agriculture, *2015–2020 Dietary Guidelines for Americans*, 8th Edition. December 2015. Available at http://health.gov/dietaryguidelines/2015/guidelines.

NUTRITION RESOURCES

Food groups	Number of servings per day (or per week, as noted)				Serving sizes and notes
	1,600 calories	2,000 calories	2,600 calories	3,100 calories	
Grains	6	6–8	10–11	12–13	1 slice bread, 1 oz dry cereal, ½ cup cooked rice, pasta, or cereal; choose whole grains
Vegetables	3–4	4–5	5–6	6	1 cup raw leafy vegetables, ½ cup cooked vegetables, ½ cup vegetable juice
Fruits	4	4–5	5–6	6	½ cup fruit juice, 1 medium fruit, ¼ cup dried fruit, ½ cup fresh, frozen, or canned fruit
Low-fat or fat-free dairy foods	2–3	2–3	3	3–4	1 cup milk; 1 cup yogurt, 1 ½ oz cheese; choose fat-free or low-fat types
Meat, poultry, fish	3–6	6 or less	6	6–9	1 oz cooked meats, poultry, or fish: select only lean; trim away visible fats; broil, roast, or boil instead of frying; remove skin from poultry
Nuts, seeds, legumes	3 servings per week	4–5 servings per week	1	1	⅓ cup or 1 ½ oz nuts, 2 Tbsp or ½ oz seeds, ½ cup cooked dry beans/peas, 2 Tbsp peanut butter
Fats and oils	2	2–3	3	4	1 tsp soft margarine, 1 Tbsp low-fat mayonnaise, 2 Tbsp light salad dressing, 1 tsp vegetable oil; DASH has 27% of calories as fat (low in saturated fat)
Sweets	0	5 servings/ week or less	2	2	1 Tbsp sugar, 1 Tbsp jelly or jam, ½ cup sorbet, 1 cup lemonade; sweets should be low in fat

FIGURE 4.   The DASH Eating Plan.

SOURCE: National Institutes of Health, National Heart, Lung, and Blood Institute, *Your Guide to Lowering Your Blood Pressure with DASH*, 2006. (http://www.nhlbi.nih.gov/health/public/heart/hbp/dash/new_dash.pdf).

Name _____ Section _____ Date _____

LAB 8.1   Your Daily Diet versus MyPlate

Make three photocopies of the worksheet in this lab and use them to keep track of everything you eat for three consecutive days. Break down each food item into its component parts, and list them separately in the column labeled "Food." Then enter the portion size you consumed in the correct food-group column. For example, a turkey sandwich might be listed as follows: whole-wheat bread, 2 oz-equiv of whole grains; turkey, 2 oz-equiv of meat/beans; tomato, ⅓ cup other vegetables; romaine lettuce, ¼ cup dark-green vegetables; 1 tablespoon mayonnaise dressing, 1 teaspoon (4.5 g) oils. It can be challenging to track values for added sugars and oils and fats, but use food labels to be as accurate as you can. Additional guidelines for counting discretionary calories can be found at ChooseMyPlate.gov.

For vegetables, enter your portion sizes in both the "Total" column and the column corresponding to the correct subgroup; for example, the spinach in a spinach salad would be entered under "Dark Green" and carrots would be entered under "Red & Orange." For the purpose of this three-day activity, you will compare only your total vegetable consumption against MyPlate guidelines; as described in the chapter, vegetable subgroup recommendations are based on weekly consumption. However, it is important to note which vegetable subgroups are represented in your diet; over a three-day period, you should consume several servings from each of the subgroups.

Date: _____

Food	Grains (oz-eq)		Vegetable (cups)						Fruits (cups)	Milk (cups)	Meat/ Beans (oz-eq)	Oils (g)	Discretionary Calories	
	Whole	Other	Total	Dark Green	Red & Orange	Beans & Peas	Starchy	Other					Solid Fats (g)	Added Sugars (g)
Daily Total														

LABORATORY ACTIVITIES

Next, average your daily intake totals for the three days and enter them in the chart below. For example, if your three daily totals for the fruit group were 1 cup, 1½ cups, and 2 cups, your average daily intake would be 1½ cups. Fill in the recommended intake totals that apply to you from ChooseMyPlate.gov or your chosen dietary pattern from the Nutrition Resources section.

MyPlate Food Group	Recommended Daily Amounts or Limits	Your Actual Average Daily Intake
Grains (total)	oz-eq	oz-eq
Whole grains	oz-eq	oz-eq
Other grains	oz-eq	oz-eq
Vegetables (total)	cups	cups
Fruits	cups	cups
Milk	cups	cups
Meat and beans	oz-eq	oz-eq
Oils	tsp	tsp
Solid fats	g	g
Added sugars	g/tsp	g/tsp

Using Your Results

How did you score? How close is your diet to that recommended by MyPlate? Are you surprised by the amount of food you are consuming from each food group or from added sugars and solid fats?

What should you do next? If the results of the assessment indicate that you could boost your level of wellness by improving your diet, set realistic goals for change. Do you need to increase or decrease your consumption of any food groups? List any areas of concern below, along with a goal for change and strategies for achieving the goal you've set. If you see that you are falling short in one food group, such as fruits or vegetables, but have many foods that are rich in discretionary calories from solid fats and added sugars, try decreasing those items in favor of an apple, a bunch of grapes, or some baby carrots. Think carefully about the reasons behind your food choices. For example, if you eat doughnuts for breakfast every morning because you feel rushed, make a list of ways to save time to allow for a healthier breakfast.

Problem: _____

Goal: _____

Strategies for change: _____

_____

_____

Problem: _____

Goal: _____

Strategies for change: _____

_____

_____

Problem: _____

Goal: _____

Strategies for change: _____

_____

_____

Enter the results of this lab in the Preprogram Assessment column in Appendix B. If you've set goals and identified strategies for change, begin putting your plan into action. After several weeks of your program, complete this lab again and enter the results in the Postprogram Assessment column of Appendix B. How do the results compare?

LABORATORY ACTIVITIES

Name _____ Section _____ Date _____

LAB 8.2 Dietary Analysis

You can complete this activity using either a nutrition analysis software program or information about the nutrient content of foods available online; see the For Further Exploration section and Nutritional Content of Popular Items from Fast-Food Restaurants for recommended websites. Connect users can track and analyze their food intake using the dietary analysis tool NutritionCalc Plus; launch it by clicking on the NutritionCalc Plus link on the Resources list from your Connect class home page. (This lab asks you to analyze one day's diet. For a more complete and accurate assessment of your diet, analyze the results from several different days, including a weekday and a weekend day.)

DATE _____ DAY: M Tu W Th F Sa Su

Food	Amount	Calories	Protein (g)	Carbohydrate (g)	Dietary fiber (g)	Fat, total (g)	Saturated fat (g)	Sodium (mg)	Vitamin A (RE)	Vitamin C (mg)	Calcium (mg)	Iron (mg)
Recommended totals*			10–35%	45–65%	25–38 g	20–35%	<10%	≤2300 mg	RE	mg	mg	mg
Actual totals**		cal	g / %	g / %	g	g / %	g / %	mg	RE	mg	mg	mg

*Fill in the appropriate DRI values for vitamin A, vitamin C, calcium, and iron from Tables 8.7 and 8.8 or by visiting the Interactive DRI website (http://fnic.nal.usda.gov/fnic/interactiveDRI).

**Total the values in each column. Protein and carbohydrate provide 4 calories per gram; fat provides 9 calories per gram. For example, if your day's total energy intake was 2,000 calories, including 270 grams of carbohydrate, you would calculate your percentage of total calories from carbohydrate as follows: (270 g X 4 cal/g) ÷ 2,000 = 54%. Percentages may not total 100% due to rounding.

LABORATORY ACTIVITIES

Using Your Results

How did you score? How close is your diet to that recommended in this chapter? Are you surprised by any of the results of this assessment?

What should you do next? Enter the results of this lab in the Preprogram Assessment column in Appendix B. If your daily diet meets all the recommended intakes, congratulations—and keep up the good work. If the results of the assessment pinpoint areas of concern, then work with your food record to determine what changes you could make to meet all the guidelines. Make changes, additions, and deletions until it conforms to all or most of the guidelines. Or, if you prefer, start from scratch to create a day's diet that meets the guidelines. Use the chart below to experiment and record your final, healthy sample diet for one day. Then put what you learned from this exercise into practice in your daily life. After several weeks of your program, complete this lab again and enter the results in the Postprogram Assessment column of Appendix B. How do the results compare?

DATE _____							DAY:	M	Tu	W	Th	F	Sa	Su
Food	Amount	Calories	Protein (g)	Carbohydrate (g)	Dietary fiber (g)	Fat, total (g)	Saturated fat (g)	Sodium (mg)	Vitamin A (RE)	Vitamin C (mg)	Calcium (mg)	Iron (mg)		
Recommended totals*			10–35%	45–65%	25–38 g	20–35%	<10%	≤2300 mg	RE	mg	mg	mg		
Actual totals**			g / cal	g / %	g / %	g / g	g / %	g / %	mg	RE	mg	mg		

Name _____   Section _____   Date _____

LAB 8.3   Informed Food Choices

Part I Using Food Labels

Choose three food items to evaluate. You might want to select three similar items, such as regular, low-fat, and nonfat salad dressing, or three very different items. Record the information from their food labels in the table below. Include all available values; items marked with an asterisk (*) may not appear on a label, depending on which version of the label is in use on the foods you evaluate.

Food Items			
Serving size			
Total calories	cal	cal	cal
Total fat—grams	g	g	g
—% Daily Value	%	%	%
Saturated fat—grams	g	g	g
—% Daily Value	%	%	%
Trans fat—grams	g	g	g
Cholesterol	mg	mg	mg
Sodium—milligrams	mg	mg	mg
—% Daily Value	%	%	%
Total carbohydrate—grams	g	g	g
—% Daily Value	%	%	%
Dietary fiber—grams	g	g	g
—% Daily Value	%	%	%
Total sugars—grams	g	g	g
*Added sugars—grams	g	g	g
—% Daily Value	%	%	%
Protein—grams	g	g	g
*Vitamin A—% Daily Value	%	%	%
*Vitamin C—% Daily Value	%	%	%
*Vitamin D—% Daily Value	%	%	%
Calcium—% Daily Value	%	%	%
Iron—% Daily Value	%	%	%
*Potassium—% Daily Value	%	%	%

How do the items you chose compare? You can do a quick nutrient check by totaling the Daily Value percentages for nutrients you should limit (saturated fat, sodium, added sugars) and the nutrients you should favor (dietary fiber, vitamins, minerals) for each food. Which food has the largest percent Daily Value sum for nutrients to limit? For nutrients to favor?

Food Items				
Calories		cal	cal	cal
% Daily Value total for nutrients to limit (saturated fat, sodium, added sugars)		%	%	%
% Daily Value total for nutrients to favor (fiber, vitamins, minerals)		%	%	%

LABORATORY ACTIVITIES

Part II Evaluating Fast Food

Use the nutritional information available from fast-food restaurants to complete the chart on this page for the last fast-food meal you ate. Add up your totals for the meal. Compare the values for fat, protein, carbohydrate, and sodium content for each food item and for the meal as a whole with the levels suggested by the Dietary Guidelines for Americans. Calculate the percent of total calories derived from fat, saturated fat, protein, and carbohydrate using the formulas given.

To get fast-food nutritional information, ask for a nutrition information brochure when you visit the restaurant, or visit restaurant websites:

- Arby's (http://www.arbysrestaurant.com)
- Burger King (http://www.burgerking.com)
- Domino's Pizza (http://www.dominos.com)
- Jack in the Box (http://www. jackinthebox.com)
- KFC (http://www.kfc.com)
- McDonald's (http://www.mcdonalds.com)
- Subway (http://www.subway.com)
- Taco Bell (http://www.tacobell.com)
- Wendy's (http://www.wendys.com).

If you haven't recently been to a fast-food restaurant, fill in the chart for any sample meal you might eat.

FOOD ITEMS								
	Dietary Guidelines							**Total****
Serving size (g)		g	g	g	g	g	g	g
Calories		cal	cal	cal	cal	cal	cal	cal
Total fat—grams		g	g	g	g	g	g	g
—% calories*	20–35%	%	%	%	%	%	%	%
Saturated fat—grams		g	g	g	g	g	g	g
—% calories*	<10%	%	%	%	%	%	%	%
Protein—grams		g	g	g	g	g	g	g
—% calories*	10–35%	%	%	%	%	%	%	%
Carbohydrate—grams		g	g	g	g	g	g	g
—% calories*	45–65%	%	%	%	%	%	%	%
Sodium†	800 mg	mg	mg	mg	mg	mg	mg	mg

*To calculate the percent of total calories from each food energy source (fat, carbohydrate, protein), use the following formula:

$$\frac{\text{(number of grams of energy source)} \times \text{(number of calories per gram of energy source)}}{\text{(total calories in serving of food item)}}$$

(NOTE: Fat and saturated fat provide 9 calories per gram; protein and carbohydrate provide 4 calories per gram.) For example, the percent of total calories from protein in a 150-calorie dish containing 10 grams of protein is

$$\frac{\text{(10 grams of protein)} \times \text{(4 calories per gram)}}{\text{(150 calories)}} = \frac{40}{150} = 0.27, \text{ or 27\% of total calories from protein}$$

**For the Total column, add up the total grams of fat, carbohydrate, and protein contained in your sample meal and calculate the percentages based on the total calories in the meal. (Percentages may not total 100% due to rounding.) For cholesterol and sodium values, add up the total number of milligrams.

†Recommended daily limit of sodium is divided by 3 here to give an approximate recommended limit for a single meal.

SOURCE: Insel, P. M., W. T. Roth, C. E. Insel. 2016. "Wellness Worksheet 66," *Core Concepts in Health,* 14th ed. New York: McGraw-Hill.

9 Weight Management

LOOKING AHEAD...

After reading this chapter, you should be able to

- Explain the health risks associated with overweight and obesity.
- Explain the factors that may contribute to a weight problem.
- Describe lifestyle factors that contribute to weight gain and loss.
- Identify and describe the symptoms and health risks of eating disorders.
- Design a personal plan for successfully managing body weight.

TEST YOUR KNOWLEDGE

1. About what percentage of American adults are overweight?
   a. 20%
   b. 40%
   c. 70%

2. The consumption of low-calorie sweeteners has helped Americans control their weight. True or false?

3. Approximately what percentage of female high school and college students have either anorexia or bulimia?
   a. <1%
   b. 2–4%
   c. 7–10%

See answers on the next page.

©altrendo images/Stockbyte/Getty Images RF

eredith is a college sophomore. She has been trying to manage her weight since high school with little success. At 5 feet 4 inches, she finds that her weight fluctuates from 120 to 160 pounds, depending on which popular diet she tries. "Eventually I just end up going back to my white bread, soda, and frozen pizza," she tells her friend Leroy. He too is starting to notice extra fat around his midsection. "It's our stressful schedules," he says. "We don't have time to figure out the food thing!"

Meredith and Leroy are not alone. Many Americans struggle with weight management. Over two-thirds of American adults are overweight, and about half of overweight adults fall into the higher-risk category of obese. This is a serious public health problem because being overweight or obese is linked to heart disease, type 2 diabetes, chronic liver disease, stroke, and other chronic diseases that can be fatal. Nor is the problem confined to the United States: The World Health Organization estimates that 2.2 billion people worldwide are overweight or obese.

Although this chapter uses the common terms *weight management* and *weight loss,* the goal for wellness is not to conform to rigid standards of total body weight. Rather, it is to adopt healthful behaviors that achieve an appropriate body composition. Body composition refers to the relative amounts of body fat and fat-free mass (muscle, bone, and fluids) in the body. Adopting a wellness lifestyle that includes regular exercise and a healthy dietary pattern can help you achieve and maintain a healthy body composition.

Body composition is influenced by a complex interplay of personal factors, including heredity, sex, metabolic rate, hormones, age, psychological well-being, and dietary and activity habits. But many outside forces—social and economic—shape our behavior, and some experts view obesity as a public health problem that requires an urgent and coordinated public health response. This chapter explores the factors that contribute to the development of overweight and obesity as well as to eating disorders. It also takes a close look at weight management through lifestyle and suggests specific strategies for reaching and maintaining a healthy weight.

HEALTH IMPLICATIONS OF OVERWEIGHT AND OBESITY

All U.S. population groups are affected by overweight and obesity, no matter race, ethnicity, gender, or age. Table 9.1 shows the percentage of American adults who are overweight or obese, but rates are also high among children and

Table 9.1	Weight of Americans Age 20 and Older: 2011–2014	
	OVERWEIGHT (BMI ≥ 25)	OBESE (BMI ≥ 30)
	% of population	
Both sexes	69.5	36.4
Males	73.0	34.5
Females	66.2	38.1
Not Hispanic or Latino		
White males	73.7	34.0
White females	63.5	35.3
Black males	69.6	37.9
Black females	82.0	56.5
Asian males	46.9	11.3
Asian females	34.4	11.9
Hispanic or Latino males	79.6	39.1
Hispanic or Latino females	77.1	45.6

SOURCE: National Center for Health Statistics, *Health, United States, 2015: With Special Feature on Racial and Ethnic Health Disparities.* Hyattsville. 2016. MD: National Center for Health Statistics.

adolescents: According to standards developed by the National Institutes of Health, 17% of youth, ages 6–11, and 20.5% of adolescents, ages 12–19, are obese.

As rates of overweight and obesity have risen in the United States, so has the incidence of health conditions associated with excess weight, such as type 2 diabetes. Obesity doubles mortality rates and can reduce life expectancy by 10–20 years. A response in health care technology such as gastric bypass surgery, medications, and early screening for obesity-related diseases has helped reduce the health impact of obesity, but if obesity trends persist, especially among children, average life spans may begin to decrease.

Assessing Weight

As described in Chapter 6, **overweight** is defined as total body weight above the recommended range for good health. **Obesity** is defined as a more serious degree of overweight that carries multiple health risks. Both terms, as determined by large-scale population surveys, are used to identify weight ranges that are associated with increased risk of certain diseases and health problems. But the most important thing to consider for health is the proportion of the body's total weight that is fat—the percent body fat. For example, two men of the same height and weight may differ widely in

overweight   Body weight above the recommended range for good health; sometimes defined as a body mass index between 25 and 29.9, a measure of the proportion of weight to height.

obesity   Severely overweight, characterized by an excessive accumulation of body fat; may also be defined in terms of some measure of total body weight or a body mass index of 30 or more.

TERMS

Answers (Test Your Knowledge)

1. **c.** About 70% of American adults are overweight, including 36% who are obese.
2. **False.** Studies fail to show that low-calorie sweeteners help weight loss.
3. **b.** About 2–4% of female students suffer from bulimia or anorexia, and many more occasionally engage in behaviors associated with these eating disorders.

percent body fat. If one has 12% body fat, and the other 22% body fat, only the second man's body composition will be considered unhealthy. A higher than healthy proportion of body fat is called **overfat**. Assessment methods based on body weight alone are less accurate than those based on body fat, but they are commonly used because body weight is easier to measure than body fat.

Body mass index (BMI) is a measure of body weight that is useful for estimating a person's weight status (e.g., underweight, normal, or overweight) and for classifying the health risks of body weight. This measure is helpful when more sophisticated methods aren't available. BMI is often used in surveys and studies, and it is the basis for the population statistics presented in this chapter. BMI is a fairly accurate measure of the health risks of body weight for most average people. It is less accurate for muscular athletes, people under 5 feet tall, older adults with little muscle mass, and certain other groups. BMI is calculated by dividing body weight (in kilograms) by the square of body height (in meters); an alternative equation based on pounds and inches is the following:

$$BMI = (weight \div [height \times height]) \times 703$$

(Space for calculations and a complete BMI chart appear in Labs 6.1 and 6.2.)

BMI is combined with waist measurement to more accurately assess health risks. Waist measurement helps provide an assessment of body fat distribution. **Visceral fat**, fat stored around the internal organs, is more harmful to health than **subcutaneous fat**, fat stored under the skin. For classifying your health risks, use the combination of BMI and waist measurement in Table 9.2, or complete one of the more sophisticated body composition assessment methods presented in Chapter 6.

Overweight, Obesity, and Specific Health Risks

Many studies have confirmed that obesity and—to a lesser extent—overweight can shorten lives (Figure 9.1). Obesity is one of six major controllable risk factors for heart disease, and

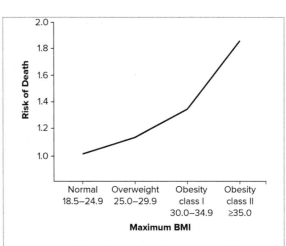

FIGURE 9.1   Weight history and all-cause mortality.
Researchers followed more than 200,000 adults for 16 years and examined the relationship between an individual's maximum BMI over the period and subsequent mortality. A maximum BMI above the normal category was associated with an excess risk of death that increased with increasing BMI.

SOURCE: Yu, E., et al. 2017. "Weight history and all-cause and cause-specific mortality in three prospective cohort studies," *Annals of Internal Medicine* DOI: 10.7326/M16-1390.

it also increases the risk for other forms of cardiovascular disease (CVD), hypertension, certain forms of cancer, gallbladder disease, kidney disease, respiratory problems, joint diseases, skin problems, impaired immune function, and sleep disorders. Obesity is strongly linked to the development of insulin resistance and type 2 diabetes; nearly 90% of people with type 2 diabetes are overweight when diagnosed.

TERMS

visceral fat   Fat located around major organs; also called *intra-abdominal fat*.

subcutaneous fat   Fat located under the skin.

Table 9.2	Body Mass Index, Waist Circumference, and Disease Risk

	BMI (KG/M²)	OBESITY CLASS	DISEASE RISK* RELATIVE TO NORMAL WEIGHT AND WAIST CIRCUMFERENCE	
			MEN: WAIST 40 IN (102 CM) OR LESS WOMEN: WAIST 35 IN (88 CM) OR LESS	MEN: WAIST >40 IN (102 CM) WOMEN: WAIST >35 IN (88 CM)
Underweight	<18.5		–	–
Normal	18.5–24.9		–	–
Overweight	25.0–29.9	I	Increased	High
Obesity	30.0–34.9	II	High	Very high
	35.0–39.9	II+	Very high	Very high
Extreme Obesity	40.0+	III	Extremely high	Extremely high

*Disease risk for type 2 diabetes, hypertension, and cardiovascular disease.

NOTE: Increased waist circumference also can be a marker for increased risk, even in persons of normal weight.

SOURCE: Adapted from National Heart, Lung, and Blood Institute. 1998. *Clinical Guidelines on the Identification, Evaluation, and Treatment of Overweight and Obesity in Adults: The Evidence Report.* Bethesda, Md.: National Institutes of Health ; De Lorenzo, A. 2016. "New obesity classification criteria as a tool for bariatric surgery indication," *World Journal of Gastroenterology* 22(2), 681–703.

Like an invasive weed slowly taking over your garden, weight gain over time can seriously affect your health. A recent study showed that women who gained more than 22 pounds since they were 18 years old had a sevenfold increase in the risk of heart disease. Gaining weight, especially as a young adult, is also strongly linked to increased risk for type 2 diabetes.

Weight loss can have a significant positive impact on health. Even modest weight loss improves blood levels of good cholesterol (HDL), triglycerides, and glucose, as well as blood pressure. A weight loss of just 5–10% in obese individuals can reduce the risk of weight-related health conditions and increase life expectancy.

FACTORS CONTRIBUTING TO EXCESS BODY FAT

Body weight and body composition are determined by multiple factors that vary with each individual, as discussed in this section.

Energy Balance

The key to achieving a healthy body weight and maintaining a healthy ratio of fat to fat-free mass is energy balance (Figure 9.2). **Energy balance** is the relationship between the amount of energy (calories) taken into the body through food and drink (energy in), and the amount of calories expended through metabolic and physical activity (energy out). If you burn the same amount of energy as you take in (a *neutral* energy balance), your weight can remain constant. The energy balance equation for many Americans today is tipped toward the energy-in side—a *positive energy balance* that promotes weight gain. This means that many people take in more calories than they expend. The opposite condition is a *negative energy balance,* which occurs when energy intake is less than energy use. To create a negative energy balance, you can burn more energy by increasing your level of physical activity and/or decrease the amount of energy you take in by consuming fewer calories.

This relatively simple equation, however, doesn't reflect the many factors that influence what and how much we eat, how much physical activity we engage in, and how our bodies process energy and respond to changes in diet and exercise patterns. These influences are grouped into genetic, physiological, lifestyle, psychosocial, and environmental factors. Although some of these factors are unchangeable, the good news is that you can control key aspects of the energy balance equation through choices you make every day. Specific strategies for altering energy balance are discussed throughout this chapter.

energy balance A condition that occurs when energy intake equals energy expenditure; the key to achieving and maintaining a healthy body weight.

TERMS

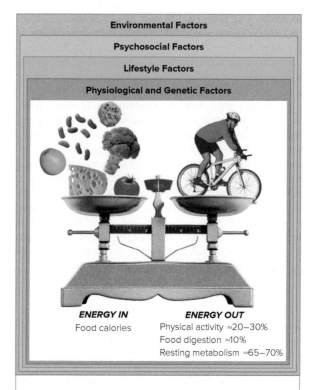

FIGURE 9.2 The energy-balance equation. Body weight remains constant if the number of calories consumed equals the number of calories expended. Many factors influence components of the energy-balance equation, some of which are out of an individual's control.

(weight scale): ©destinacigdem/123RF; (orange): ©Stockdisc/PunchStock RF; (cheese): ©Photodisc/PunchStock RF; (beans): ©C Squared Studios/Getty Images RF; (cookie): ©Brand X Pictures/PunchStock RF; (broccoli): ©Stockdisc/PunchStock RF; (tomato): ©Comstock/Jupiter Images/Getty Images RF; (biker): ©Royalty Free/Corbis RF;

Genetic Factors

Estimates of the genetic contribution to obesity vary widely, about 25–40% of an individual's body fat. More than 600 genes have been linked to obesity, but their actions are still under study. Genes influence body size and shape, body fat distribution, and metabolic rate. Genetic factors also affect the ease with which weight is gained as a result of overeating and where on the body extra weight is added.

If both parents are obese, their children have an 80% risk of being obese; children with one obese parent face a 50% risk of becoming obese. In studies that compared adoptees and their biological parents, the weights of the adoptees were found to be more like those of the biological parents than the adoptive parents, suggesting a strong genetic link.

Hereditary influences, however, must be balanced against the contribution of environmental factors. Not all children of obese parents become obese, and normal-weight parents can have overweight and obese children. Environmental factors like diet and exercise are probably responsible for such differences.

Thus, the *tendency* to develop obesity may be inherited, but the expression of this tendency can be affected by environmental influences.

Physiological Factors

Metabolism is a key physiological factor in the regulation of body fat and body weight. Hormones, fat cells, and possibly gut flora also play roles.

Metabolism   Metabolism is the sum of all the vital processes by which food energy and nutrients are made available to and used by the body. The largest component of metabolism, **resting metabolic rate (RMR)**, is the energy required to maintain vital body functions while the body is at rest, including respiration, heart rate, body temperature, and blood pressure. As shown in Figure 9.2, resting metabolism (RMR) accounts for about 65–70% of daily energy expenditure. The energy required to digest food accounts for up to an additional 10% of daily energy expenditure. The remaining 20–30% is expended during physical activity.

Both genetics and behavior affect metabolic rate. Men, who have a higher proportion of muscle mass than women, have a higher RMR because muscle tissue is more metabolically active than fat, requiring more energy to support its activities. Also, some individuals inherit a higher or lower RMR than others; RMR may vary by as much as 25% among same-weight individuals. A higher RMR means that a person burns more calories while at rest and can therefore take in more calories without gaining weight.

A number of factors reduce metabolic rate, making weight management challenging. Low-calorie intake and weight loss reduce RMR. When energy intake declines and weight is lost, the body responds by trying to conserve energy, reducing both RMR and the energy required to perform physical tasks. In essence, the body "defends" the original starting weight. Consider two people of the same size and activity level who both currently weigh 150 pounds, but one of whom used to weigh 170 pounds; the individual who lost weight will need to consume fewer calories to maintain the 150-pound weight than the person who had always been at that weight. This physiological response of the body points to the importance of preventing weight gain in the first place.

Exercise has a positive effect on metabolism. When people exercise, they slightly increase their RMR—the number of calories their bodies burn at rest. In fact, a 2011 study of college-age men showed that following 45 minutes of vigorous exercise, the participants' resting metabolic rate remained elevated for 14 hours—during which the men burned an additional 200 calories while at rest or performing normal, everyday activities. Regular exercise also increases muscle mass, which is associated with a higher metabolic rate. The exercise itself also burns calories, raising total energy expenditure. The higher the energy expenditure, the more a person can eat without gaining weight. RMR also tends to decline with age, possibly the result of a decline in lean body mass; exercise can help maintain muscle mass and metabolic rate over time.

Hormones   Hormones clearly play a role in the accumulation of body fat, especially for women. Hormonal changes at puberty, during pregnancy, and at menopause contribute to the amount and location of fat accumulation. For example, during puberty, hormones cause the development of secondary sex characteristics such as larger breasts, wider hips, and added fat under the skin. This addition of body fat at puberty is normal and healthy.

One hormone thought to be linked to obesity is *leptin*. Secreted by the body's fat cells, leptin is carried to the brain, where it appears to let the brain know how big or small the body's fat stores are. With this information, the brain can regulate appetite and metabolic rate. Leptin levels are higher in people who are obese, but obesity may cause the body to be less responsive to leptin's signals.

Insulin is another hormone that may affect weight management, possibly through regulation of appetite and fat storage. Some studies have found that when people eat foods that cause large swings in insulin levels—a rapid increase followed by a rapid decline—they feel hungrier and consume more calories. The foods most likely to cause a rapid rise in insulin are those with a high glycemic index, including foods high in added sugars and processed grains and low in fiber. Researchers are also investigating whether limiting high-glycemic-index foods might help reduce the decline in RMR that occurs with weight loss. Research is ongoing, but you can reduce the potential negative impact of insulin on weight management by limiting foods high in added sugars and highly processed grains.

Researchers hope to use leptin and other hormones to develop treatments for obesity based on appetite control. As most of us will admit, however, feelings of hunger may often *not* be the primary reason we overeat.

Fat Cells   The amount of fat (adipose tissue) the body can store is a function of the number and size of fat (adipose) cells. Some people are born with an above-average number of fat cells and thus have the potential for storing more energy as body fat. Overeating at critical times, such as in childhood, can cause the body to create more fat cells. If a person loses weight, fat cell content is depleted, but the number of fat cells may not decrease. Fat tissue is not a passive form of energy storage; rather, fat cells send out chemical signals in order to be replenished. These signals affect multiple organs and systems, including those controlling appetite, metabolism, and immunity. In many cases insulin is required to store fat.

Gut Microbiota   The human intestine houses millions of bacteria that form the intestinal flora (gut flora). These bacteria help digest the foods you eat, and they produce some vitamins, such as vitamin K. Studies show that lean people differ from

> **resting metabolic rate (RMR)**   The energy required (in calories) to maintain vital body functions while the body is at rest, including respiration, heart rate, body temperature, and blood pressure.   **TERMS**

overweight people in the composition of their intestinal flora, suggesting that intestinal flora may be involved in the development of obesity. Diets high in processed foods have been linked to less diverse intestinal microbiota. Such diets have also been linked to a higher proportion of bacteria types associated with increased energy absorption and hormonal changes that increase appetite—both factors that can contribute to obesity. More research is needed into the precise impact of gut microbiota and on how changes to the bacterial balance might help people lose weight and maintain weight loss.

Lifestyle Factors

Genetic and physiological factors may increase the risk for excess body fat, but they are not sufficient to explain the increasingly high rate of obesity in the United States. The gene pool has not changed dramatically in the past 60 years, but the rate of obesity among Americans has more than doubled. Clearly, other factors are at work—particularly lifestyle factors such as increased energy intake, especially in the form of processed carbohydrates, and decreased physical activity.

Energy Intake and Dietary Patterns Americans today consume more calories than in the past—up nearly 20% since 1983—and more of those calories come from low-quality foods. Americans eat out more often and rely more heavily on fast food and packaged convenience foods. Restaurant and convenience-food portion sizes tend to be large, and the foods are likely to be low in essential nutrients and high in empty calories from added sugars, processed carbohydrates, and solid fats.

Physical Activity Fewer than half of all adults meet the current Physical Activity Guidelines for Americans. Activity levels among Americans are declining, beginning in childhood and continuing throughout life. Many schools have cut back on physical education classes and even recess. Most adults drive to work, sit all day, and then relax in front of the TV (or continue working) at night. Incidence of overweight is consistently linked to excessive screen time—whether time spent watching TV, playing video games, or using computers.

Sleep Short sleep duration and sleep debt are associated with increased BMI and abdominal obesity, but researchers are still investigating this link. One possibility is that lack of sleep may affect hormone levels, appetite regulation, and metabolism. Short sleep duration is also associated with increased snacking and overall energy intake. Another factor is that use of multimedia devices may contribute to sleep deprivation and increase both energy intake and sedentary time. Getting adequate sleep is critical for overall wellness.

binge eating A pattern of eating in which normal food consumption is interrupted by episodes of high consumption.

TERMS

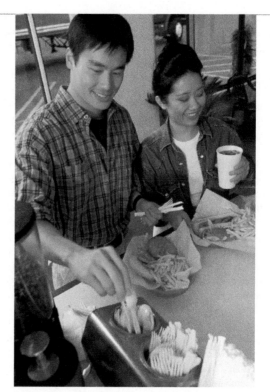

Wellness Tip If you think of fast food as your only available food option, you may find it difficult to make healthy lifestyle changes. When you do eat at a fast-food restaurant, pay special attention to your choices and your portion sizes. Choosing small instead of large fries can save 250 calories; water instead of a 12-ounce regular soda can save 150 calories. Over time, these kinds of calorie savings can add up!
©Photodisc/Alamy Stock Photo RF

Ask Yourself

QUESTIONS FOR CRITICAL THINKING AND REFLECTION

Is anyone in your family overweight? If so, can you identify factors that may contribute to this weight problem, such as heredity, eating patterns, or psychosocial factors? Has the person tried to address the problem? How is the issue handled in your family? Do family members help the situation or make it worse?

Psychosocial Factors

Many people have learned to use food as a means of coping with stress and negative emotions. Eating can provide a powerful distraction from difficult feelings—loneliness, anger, boredom, anxiety, shame, sadness, inadequacy. It can be used to combat low moods, low energy levels, and low self-esteem. When eating becomes the primary means of regulating emotions, **binge eating** or other unhealthy eating patterns can develop.

Obesity is strongly associated with socioeconomic status. The prevalence of obesity goes down as family income level goes up, especially among women and children. These differences may reflect greater access to unprocessed and low-calorie foods, to information about nutrition, and to physical activity among upper-income women. Upper-income women also may have acquired greater sensitivity and concern for a slim physical appearance. In contrast, the prevalence of obesity may reflect the greater acceptance of larger body types among certain ethnic groups, as well as different cultural values related to food choices.

In some families and cultures, food is used as a symbol of love and caring. It is an integral part of social gatherings and celebrations. In such cases, it may be difficult to change established eating patterns because they are linked to cultural and family values.

Environmental Factors

The environment in which many Americans live and work can be "obesogenic"—meaning it encourages overconsumption of calories and discourages physical activity. This combination promotes weight gain rather than weight maintenance or loss. Food marketing and pricing, food production and distribution systems, and national agricultural policies all impact individual food choices.

The food industry promotes the sale of high-calorie processed foods at every turn. For example, vending machines offer mainly chocolate bars and unhealthy snacks, airlines offer complimentary soft drinks, and restaurants provide all-you-can-eat fried food buffets. Children are especially vulnerable to marketing that pushes ultra-processed foods high in sugar, salt, fat, and additives. Because they have a stronger preference for sweets than adults do, children are targeted from a young age and encouraged to make unhealthy choices.

Many experts observe that U.S. agricultural policy encourages farmers to produce corn and its by-product, high fructose corn syrup, at the expense of fruits and vegetables. As a result, over the past 30 years, the price of fruits and vegetables has risen much faster than the prices of other consumer goods, while the price of sugar, sweets, and carbonated drinks declined. Issues of price and availability of healthy food can have a profound effect on food choices. Low-income neighborhoods often have only fast-food venues offering high-calorie, highly processed foods.

Public policies can also have a positive influence. For example, the updated food labels and new regulations requiring chain restaurants and vending machine operators to post calorie information should help consumers make more informed choices. Other public health responses recommended by experts to support positive lifestyle choices for weight management include the following:

- Change food pricing to promote healthful options. For example, tax sugary beverages and offer incentives to farmers and food manufacturers to produce and market affordable healthy choices and smaller portion sizes.

- Limit advertising of unhealthy foods targeting children.

- Fund strategies to promote physical activity by creating more walkable communities, parks, and recreational facilities.

Rather than leaving all discussion to policy makers, public health experts are encouraging people to mobilize grassroots campaigns against the way food is currently distributed and

Wellness Tip Environmental factors can have a positive or negative influence on weight management. Identify key influences in your own environment. Develop strategies to take advantage of positive opportunities and to combat negative influences.
©Photodisc/Getty Images RF

marketed. Look around your community, school, and workplace: What aspects of the environment make it easier or more difficult to make healthy choices? What foods are available for purchase—and where and at what cost? Does the community environment and transportation system support walking or cycling, or is driving the only practical way to get around?

ADOPTING A HEALTHY LIFESTYLE FOR SUCCESSFUL WEIGHT MANAGEMENT

Are most weight problems lifestyle problems? Despite the growing prevalence of obesity in children and adolescents, many young adults get away with very unhealthy eating and exercise habits and don't develop a weight problem. But as the rapid growth of adolescence slows and family and career obligations increase, maintaining a healthy weight becomes a greater challenge. Slow weight gain is a major cause of overweight and obesity, so weight management is important for everyone, not just for people who are currently overweight. A good time to develop a lifestyle for successful weight management is during early adulthood, when healthy behavior patterns have a better chance of taking hold.

Adopt healthy behaviors you can maintain throughout your life. These behaviors include good eating habits, regular physical activity and exercise, strategies that help you think positively and manage your emotions effectively, and coping strategies for the stresses and challenges in your life.

Dietary Patterns and Eating Habits

In contrast to dieting, which involves some form of food restriction, the term *diet* refers to your daily food choices. Everyone has a diet, but not everyone is dieting. It's important to develop a diet that you enjoy and that enables you to maintain a healthy body composition. Use MyPlate, DASH, or another healthy dietary pattern discussed in Chapter 8, and choose the healthiest options within each food group. For weight management, pay special attention to total calories, portion sizes, energy and nutrient density, and eating habits.

Total Calories MyPlate suggests approximate daily energy intakes based on gender, age, and activity level. However, the precise number of calories needed to maintain weight will vary from one person to another based on heredity, fitness status, level of physical activity, and other factors. Focus more on your individual energy balance than on a general recommendation for daily calorie intake. To calculate your approximate daily caloric needs, complete Lab 9.1. If you choose to track calories, keep in mind that most people underestimate their energy intake and that energy needs change as body weight changes.

If weight loss is your goal, most experts recommend an increase in physical activity with moderate calorie reduction targeting added sugars, refined carbohydrates and other processed foods, and solid fats. This way you can burn more calories than you eat (see the box, "Are All Calories and Dietary Patterns Equal for Weight Loss?"). Just as important as tracking total energy intake for successful weight loss is choosing good sources of calories from fruits, vegetables, proteins, and complex carbohydrates. To maintain weight loss, you will probably have to continue some of the calorie restriction you used to lose the weight. Therefore, adopt a level of food intake that you can live with over the long term. For most people, maintaining weight loss is more difficult than losing the weight in the first place. To identify weight-loss goals and ways to meet them, complete Lab 9.2.

Portion Sizes Overconsumption of total calories is closely tied to portion sizes. Many Americans are unaware that the portion sizes of packaged foods and of foods served at restaurants have increased, and most of us significantly underestimate the amount of food we eat (Figure 9.3). Studies have consistently found that people underestimate portion sizes by as much as 25%. When participants in one study were asked to report their food intake over the previous 24 hours, the majority underestimated their intake by about 600 calories. Another study showed that when people ordered from a restaurant menu that included calorie labels, they ate less. Limiting portion sizes is critical for weight management. For many people, concentrating on portion sizes is easier than counting calories. See Chapter 8 for more information and hints on choosing appropriate portion sizes.

Quality of Food Choices: Energy (Calorie) Density and Nutrient Density Experts also recommend that you pay attention to **energy density**—the number of calories per ounce or gram of weight in a food. Studies suggest that

energy density Number of calories per ounce or gram of food; foods with low energy density have high volume or bulk with few calories, whereas those with high energy density provide many calories in a very small portion.

FIGURE 9.3   The new (ab)normal. Portion sizes have been growing. So have we. The average restaurant meal today is more than four times larger than in the 1950s. Adults today are, on average, 26 pounds heavier. To eat healthy, there are things we can do for ourselves and our community. Order the smaller meals on the menu, split a meal with a friend, or eat half and take the rest home. Ask the managers at favorite restaurants to offer smaller meals.
SOURCE: Centers for Disease Control and Prevention; for more information, visit http://MakingHealthEasier.org/TimeToScaleBack.

it isn't consumption of a certain amount of fat or calories in food that reduces hunger and leads to feelings of fullness and satisfaction. Rather, it is consumption of a certain weight of food. Foods that are low in energy density have more volume and bulk; that is, they are relatively heavy but have few calories (Table 9.3). For example, for the same 100 calories, you could eat 20 baby carrots or four pretzel twists. You are more likely to feel fuller after eating the serving of carrots because it weighs ten times as much as the serving of pretzels (10 ounces versus 1 ounce). Fresh fruits and vegetables, with their high water and fiber content, are low in energy density, as are whole-grain foods. Fresh fruits contain fewer calories and more fiber than fruit juices or drinks. Meat, ice cream, potato chips, croissants, crackers, and cakes and cookies are examples of foods high in energy density.

Table 9.3	Examples of Foods Low in Energy Density	
FOOD	AMOUNT	CALORIES
Carrot, raw	1 medium	25
Popcorn, air popped	2 cups	62
Apple	1 medium	72
Vegetable soup	1 cup	72
Plain oatmeal	½ cup	80
Fresh blueberries	1 cup	80
Corn on the cob (plain)	1 ear	80
Cantaloupe	½ melon	95
Light (fat-free) yogurt with fruit	6 oz.	100
Unsweetened applesauce	1 cup	100
Pear	1 medium	100
Sweet potato, baked	1 medium	120

CRITICAL CONSUMER
Are All Calories and Dietary Patterns Equal for Weight Loss?

Many popular diets are promoted as the weight loss answer for all, but researchers continue to investigate the complex web of factors that influence the success or failure of efforts to lose weight and maintain that loss over time. Most researchers agree that total calorie intake is important, but preliminary evidence suggests some specific foods and eating patterns may help improve the odds for people trying to manage their weight.

Evaluating Dietary Composition: Balance of Protein, Carbohydrates, and Fats

Scientists are investigating whether particular patterns of macronutrient intake (e.g., higher protein, lower fat, or lower carbohydrate) are better for weight loss, for weight loss maintenance, and/or for improving health markers such as blood fat levels. How might macronutrient balance impact weight management? Two possible areas of influence are appetite and resting metabolic rate (RMR). Eating foods high in protein tends to make people feel fuller than eating foods high in fat or carbohydrate. This increase in satiety may help people refrain from overeating, thereby managing overall energy intake. On the flip side, foods high in simple sugars and refined carbohydrates may cause increased appetite (and eating) due to swings in the level of insulin.

One key challenge for weight-loss maintenance is the drop in RMR that follows weight loss. In some small, short-term studies, researchers compared the three dietary patterns—low fat, low glycemic index, and low carbohydrate—and the effect each had on RMR following weight loss. On average, the low-carbohydrate dietary pattern was associated with the smallest reduction in RMR. However, additional studies are needed to confirm the findings and determine their importance over a longer time period. An additional challenge is that extreme shifts in macronutrient balance are difficult for people to maintain over time.

How do various diets measure up over months and years? Researchers have not found significant differences. A study comparing weight loss among adults assigned to one of four reduced-calorie diets differing in percentages of protein, carbohydrate, and fat found that weight loss at two years was similar for all four diets (about nine pounds). However, weight loss was strongly associated with attendance at group sessions. Other studies have also found little difference in weight loss among popular reduced-calorie diets; most resulted in modest weight loss and reduced heart disease risk factors. The more closely people adhered to each diet, however, the more weight they lost. The American Heart Association notes that many dietary patterns can produce weight loss, and their latest guidelines list more than 15 approaches that can lead to weight loss if calories are reduced.

An interesting finding of multiple weight-loss and weight-maintenance studies is that people respond differently to different diets. So, for example, on a diet with a given balance of protein, carbohydrates, and fats, some people experience much greater weight loss than others. Similarly, changes in RMR after weight loss on different diets also vary. These findings point to individual differences in the factors affecting weight management—genetics, metabolism, hormones, and intestinal flora. Thus, there is no single diet that is for everyone. Researchers are trying to identify methods of matching people to an approach likely to be effective, but in the meantime, people can experiment with different dietary patterns to see what works best for them.

Making Quality Food Choices in Healthy Dietary Patterns

The typical American dietary pattern—high in sugary beverages, refined carbohydrates, red meat, and solid fats—is associated with obesity. For weight loss, choose high-quality calorie sources in a healthier dietary pattern; refer back to the patterns and food choices recommended in Chapter 8. Remember that there is more to foods than energy. Consume high-quality calorie sources, whatever dietary composition you choose. Nutrient-dense foods can help with both weight management and chronic disease prevention.

Maintaining Energy Balance Counts: The National Weight Control Registry

Important lessons can be drawn from the National Weight Control Registry—an ongoing study of people who have lost significant amounts of weight and kept it off. The participants (80% women, 20% men) in the registry lost 66 pounds and kept the weight off for more than five years. Nearly all participants use a combination of diet and exercise to manage their weight. Fifty-five percent of the participants chose a diet program to lose weight. Forty-five percent manage their weight on their own. Common strategies include eating breakfast, self-monitoring weight and food intake, and getting exercise of about one hour per day. The most common dietary pattern used by registry participants is low-fat/high-carbohydrate. Greater weight regain in this group of individuals came as a result of decreases in physical activity, fewer dietary restraints, less individual monitoring of body weight, and increased percentage of energy intake from fat. This study illustrates that to lose weight and keep it off, you must decrease daily calorie intake and increase daily physical activity—and continue to do so over your lifetime. Whatever dietary pattern you choose, make sure it contains high-quality, nutrient-dense foods and that it is a pattern you can maintain over the long term.

SOURCES: Hall, K. D., et al. 2016. "Energy expenditure and body composition changes after an isocaloric ketogenic diet in overweight and obese men," *American Journal of Clinical Nutrition* 104(2), 324–333; Ebeling, C. B., et al. 2012. "Effects of dietary composition on energy expenditure during weight-loss maintenance," *Journal of the American Medical Association* 307(24), 2627–2634; M. D. Jensen, et al. 2014. "AHA/ACC/TOC guideline for the management of overweight and obesity in adults: A report of the American College of Cardiology/American Heart Association Task Force on Practice Guidelines and the Obesity Society," *Circulation* 129(25 Suppl. 2), S102–S138; Thomas, J. G., et al. 2014. "Weight-loss maintenance for 10 years in the National Weight Control Registry," *American Journal of Preventive Medicine* 46(1), 17–23; Sacks, F. M., et al. 2009. "Comparison of weight loss diets with different compositions of fat, protein, and carbohydrates," *New England Journal of Medicine* 360, 859–873.

Box icon: ©sam74100/Getty Images RF

As you decrease consumption of foods high in energy density, choose those that are also high in nutrient density—foods that are relatively low in calories but high in nutrients. Strategies for lowering the energy density of your diet while also increasing its nutrient density include the following:

- Eat fruit with breakfast and for dessert.

- Add extra vegetables to sandwiches, casseroles, stir-fry dishes, pizza, pasta dishes, and fajitas

- Start meals with a bowl of broth-based soup; include a green salad or fruit salad.

- Snack on fresh fruits and vegetables rather than crackers, chips, or other energy-dense snack foods.

- Limit serving sizes of energy-dense foods such as butter, mayonnaise, cheese, chocolate, fatty meats, croissants, and snack foods that are fried, are high in added sugars (including reduced-fat products), or contain trans fat.

- Pay special attention to your beverage choices. Many sweetened drinks are low in nutrients and high in calories from added sugar.

- Limit processed foods, especially those high in added sugars and refined carbohydrates; these are usually energy dense, nutrient poor, and also high on the glycemic index, which may increase rather than reduce your appetite.

Eating Habits Equally important to weight management is eating small, frequent meals—including breakfast and snacks—on a regular schedule. Eating every 3–4 hours can help fuel healthy metabolism, maintain muscle mass, and prevent between-meal hunger that often leads to unhealthy snacking. Skipping meals leads to excessive hunger, feelings of deprivation, and increased vulnerability to binge eating or snacking. Establish a regular pattern of eating; it is better to consume the majority of calories during the day rather than in the evening. Set some rules governing food choices. Breakfast rules might include choosing a high-fiber cereal that is low in added sugar with low-fat milk on most days, and saving pancakes and waffles for special occasions unless they are whole grain. A good goal is to eat in moderation; no foods need to be entirely off-limits, though some should be eaten judiciously.

Physical Activity and Exercise

Making significant cuts in food intake in order to lose weight is a difficult strategy to maintain; increasing your physical activity is a much better approach. Physical activity and exercise burn calories and keep the metabolism geared to using food for energy instead of storing it as fat. Regular physical activity protects against weight gain and is essential for maintaining weight loss.

Physical Activity All physical activity will help you manage your weight. The first step in becoming more active is to incorporate more physical activity into your daily life. If you are currently sedentary, start by accumulating short bouts of moderate-intensity physical activity—walking, gardening, doing housework, and so on—for a total of 150 minutes or more

per week. If you are overweight and want to lose weight, or if you are trying to maintain a lower weight following weight loss, a greater amount of physical activity can help. Researchers have found that people who lose weight and don't regain it typically burn about 2,800 calories per week in physical activity—the equivalent of about one hour of brisk walking per day.

As shown in the energy balance equation in Figure 9.2, your daily physical activity accounts for about 20–30% of your total energy expenditure. This total includes purposeful exercise like a cycling workout but also includes what's called non-exercise activity thermogenesis (NEAT), which is the energy you use for daily activities like walking to class, completing homework, cooking, and cleaning. Even a small increase in activity level can help you maintain your current weight or lose a modest amount of weight. In fact, research suggests that fidgeting—stretching, squirming, standing up, and so on—may prevent weight gain in some people. Moreover, short bouts of activity spread throughout the day can produce many of the same health benefits as continuous physical activity. See the box "Be More Active During Screen Time" for strategies for adding more NEAT to your life even while you are engaged in fairly sedentary activities.

Exercise After you become more active every day, begin a formal exercise program that includes cardiorespiratory endurance exercise, resistance training, and stretching exercises (see the box "What Is the Best Way to Exercise for Weight Loss?"). Moderate-intensity endurance exercise, if performed frequently for a relatively long duration, can burn a significant number of calories. Endurance training also increases the rate at which your body uses calories after your exercise session is over—burning an additional 5–180 extra calories, depending on the intensity and duration of exercise. Resistance training builds muscle mass, and more muscle translates into a higher metabolic rate. Resistance training can also help you maintain your muscle mass during a period of weight reduction, helping you avoid the significant drop in RMR associated with weight loss.

Regular physical activity, maintained throughout life, makes weight management easier. The sooner you establish good habits, the better. The key to success is making exercise an integral part of a lifestyle you can enjoy now and will enjoy in the future.

Thoughts and Emotions

The way you think about yourself and your world influences, and is influenced by, how you feel and how you act. In fact, research on people who struggle with their weight indicates that many suffer from low self-esteem, and the negative emotions that accompany it are significant problems. Often, people with low self-esteem compare the actual self to an internally held picture of the "ideal self," an image based on perfectionist goals and beliefs about how they and others should look. The more these two pictures differ, the larger the negative impact on self-esteem and the more likely the presence of negative emotions.

Besides the internal picture we hold of ourselves, all of us carry on an internal dialogue about events happening to us and around us. This *self-talk* can be either deprecating or positively motivating, depending on our beliefs and attitudes. Having

TAKE CHARGE
Be More Active During Screen Time

Ten and a half: That's the number of hours per day a 2016 Nielsen report says average Americans spend with smartphones, computers, tablets, televisions, video games, and radios. And that's up one hour from 2015. Because much of our time spent with technology asks little of our bodies, excessive hours sitting in front of a screen, whether for work, study, or pleasure, contributes to the health risks of a sedentary lifestyle—and makes weight management more challenging. (See Chapters 2 and 7 for more on the dangers of sedentary time and suggestions for reducing it.)

You'll benefit from limiting the amount of time you spend sitting, but you can also incorporate some physical activity and boost NEAT even when engaged in screen time. Try some of the following suggestions.

Your working position and posture:

- If you can, alternate between a chair and a standing desk and/or a stability ball to avoid spending an extended period in the same position. Balancing on a stability ball works your back and core muscles; be sure to use good form at all times.

- When you do sit in a chair, tap your feet, fidget, wiggle, bounce, and dance in your chair. Any extra movements keep you more physically active.

- Follow the suggestions for posture in Chapter 5 to prevent stress on your joints.

Strength training in place—try some of the following or develop your own screen-time workout:

- *Leg extensions:* Extend one leg and rest the heel on the floor; lift your leg off the ground three inches or higher while keeping your back straight, and hold 5–10 seconds. Repeat with the other leg.

- *Air or chair squats:* Perform air squats as described in Chapter 4, or use a sturdy chair (without wheels) to indicate the bottom position of the squat. Don't lean forward or put your full weight on the chair as you lower into the squat position.

- *Desk, chair, or wall push-ups:* Place your hands on a sturdy surface and perform push-ups while keeping your body in a straight line; the lower the surface, the more difficult the exercise.

- *Press-ups:* Sit in a sturdy chair with armrests. Lean slightly forward and use your arms to push your body slowly off the seat; hold for a few seconds and release. Repeat.

- *Seated toe press:* Start with your feet flat on the floor and then push down with your toes as you raise your heels; hold the contraction of the calf muscles for several seconds, and then return to the starting position. Repeat.

- *Isometric chest press:* With elbows out to the side and palms together in front of your chest, press your hands and hold the position; relax and repeat. Be sure to breath throughout the contraction.

- *Isometric abdominals:* Use your abdominal muscles to pull your belly button toward your spine; hold the position, relax, and repeat. You can also do isometric contractions of your gluteals and many other muscle groups. Squeeze a tennis ball to develop grip strength.

- Add exercises that use a resistance band or small hand weights, such as arm curls; seated rows; front, side, and overhead arm raises; side and back leg raises; and knee curls.

Stretch and breathe:

- Try the upper-body stretches from Chapter 5 from a seated position: head turns and tilts, towel stretch, across-the-body and overhead stretch, upper-back stretch, and lateral stretch.

- Stretch your calves by extending your legs, one at a time, and pulling your toes back.

- Pull your shoulders back to open your chest; expand your abdomen as you breathe deeply.

SOURCES: *The Total Audience Report Q1 2016.* Nielsen Company, 2016. http://www.nielsen.com/us/en/insights/reports/2016/the-total-audience-report-q1-2016.html; Villablanca, P. A., et al. 2015. "Nonexercise activity thermogenesis in obesity management," *Mayo Clinic Proceedings* 90(4), 509–519; *Exercise and Physical Activity: Your Everyday Guide—Sample Exercises—Strength,* NIH National Institute on Aging, 2016. https://www.nia.nih.gov/health/publication/exercise-physical-activity/sample-exercises-strength

Box Icon: ©VisualCommunications/Getty Images RF

---

realistic beliefs and goals and engaging in positive self-talk and problem solving support a healthy lifestyle. (Chapter 10 and Activity 11 in the Behavior Change Workbook at the end of the text include strategies for developing realistic self-talk.)

Coping Strategies

Appropriate coping strategies help you deal with the stresses of life; they are also an important lifestyle factor in weight management. Many people use drugs, alcohol, smoking, or gambling as ways to cope; others use eating. Those who overeat use food to alleviate loneliness or fatigue, as an antidote to boredom, or as a distraction from problems. Some people even overeat to punish themselves for real or imagined transgressions.

An interesting phenomenon regarding weight-loss interventions among college students has recently been observed: Groups of students who shared certain characteristics did better at losing and managing weight than did groups of dissimilar students. The study grouped students according to common psychosocial factors (such as emotional eating) that contribute to weight gain. These clusters of similar students were able to lose more weight and keep more weight off than were groups of students who did not share common dietary or psychosocial characteristics. The findings of this study may help shape

THE EVIDENCE FOR EXERCISE
What Is the Best Way to Exercise for Weight Loss?

If weight loss is your primary goal, the guidelines for planning a fitness program can vary depending on your weight, body composition, and current level of fitness. If you are obese or your fitness level is very low, start with a lower-intensity workout (55% of maximum heart rate), and stick with it until your cardiorespiratory fitness level improves enough to support short bouts of higher-intensity exercise. A study of 136 obese men and women found that those who included aerobic exercise in their regimens achieved a much better outcome than those who engaged only in resistance exercises: The aerobicizers achieved more cardiopulmonary fitness, reduced more abdominal and visceral fat, and improved their insulin sensitivity. Those who added resistance training (like using resistance bands or lifting weights) lost the most weight. On top of aerobics and resistance training, balance and flexibility exercises have been shown to reduce injury for obese people as well as any mobile person.

For weight loss to occur, exercise at lower intensities has to be offset by longer and/or more frequent exercise sessions. Experts recommend 60–90 minutes of daily exercise for anyone who needs to lose weight or maintain weight loss. If you cannot fit such a large block of activity into your daily schedule, break your workouts into short segments—as little as 10–15 minutes each. This approach is probably best for someone who has been sedentary because it allows the body to become accustomed to exercise at a gradual pace while preventing injury and avoiding strain on the heart.

Many research studies have shown that walking is an ideal form of exercise for losing weight and avoiding weight gain. A landmark 15-year study by the University of North Carolina at Charlotte showed that, over time, people who did not walk gained 18 pounds more than people who walked just 30 minutes per day. Those who regularly walked farther were better able to lose or maintain weight. Other studies found that people who walked 30 minutes five times per week lost an average of five pounds in 6–12 months, without dieting, watching what they ate, or exercising intensely. You can lose even more weight if you eat sensibly and walk farther and faster.

A 165-pound adult who walks at a speed of three miles per hour for 60 minutes a day, five days a week, can lose about one-half pound of body weight per week. Regular walking is the simplest and most effective health habit for controlling body weight and promoting health. Even if you're sedentary, a few months of walking can increase your fitness level to the point where more vigorous types of exercise—and even greater health benefits—are possible.

©Ariel Skelley/Getty Images RF

SOURCES: Gordon-Larsen, P., et al. 2009. "Fifteen-year longitudinal trends in walking patterns and their impact on weight change," *American Journal of Clinical Nutrition* 89(1), 19–26; Higgins, J. P., and C. L. Higgins. 2016. "Prescribing exercise to help your patients lose weight," *Cleveland Clinic Journal of Medicine* 83(2), 141–150; Levine, J. A., et al. 2008. "The role of free-living daily walking in human weight gain and obesity," *Diabetes* 57(3), 548–554.

Box Icon: ©Vstock LLC/Getty Images RF

---

group-oriented weight-loss programs in the future and contribute to an understanding of coping strategies.

For a summary of the components of weight management through healthy lifestyle choices, see the box "Lifestyle Strategies for Successful Weight Management."

APPROACHES TO OVERCOMING A WEIGHT PROBLEM

Each year, Americans spend more than $60 billion on various weight-loss plans and products. If you are overweight, you may already be creating a plan to lose weight and keep it off. You have many options.

Doing It Yourself

If you need to lose weight, focus on adopting the healthy lifestyle described throughout this book. The "right" weight for you will evolve naturally, and you won't have to diet. Combine modest cuts in energy intake with exercise, and avoid very-low-calorie diets.

Set Reasonable Goals According to the Centers for Disease Control (CDC), reasonable weight loss for someone who is obese is 5–10% of body weight over 6 months. For example, for someone who weighs 200 pounds, a 5% weight loss would be 10 pounds. The person in this example may still be in the "overweight" or "obese" range, but this degree of weight loss can reduce the chronic-disease risks related to obesity.

Lifestyle Strategies for Successful Weight Management

Food Choices

- Focus on making good choices from each food group, eating a variety of foods, and balancing your food intake with your energy expenditure.

- Select foods with a *low energy* (calorie) density and a *high nutrient* density.

- Check labels for serving sizes, calories, and nutrients. Watch for hidden calories. Reduced-fat foods often have as many calories as their full-fat versions.

- Limit calories in the form of soda, fruit drinks, sports drinks, alcohol, and specialty coffees and teas. Water and nonfat or low-fat milk are good beverage choices.

- For very tempting high-calorie foods, eat small amounts under controlled conditions. Go out for a scoop of ice cream, for example, rather than buying half a gallon for your freezer.

Planning and Serving

- Periodically monitor your calorie intake and compare this to your calorie expenditure, noting where your energy balance is. Do you need to exercise more? Eat less?

- Don't go longer than three to four hours without eating, and consume the majority of your calories during the day rather than in the evening. Avoid late-night eating, a behavior specifically associated with weight gain among college students.

- Fix more meals yourself and eat out less often.

- Keep low-calorie snacks on hand to combat the "munchies." Fresh fruits and vegetables are good choices.

- When shopping, make a list and stick to it. Don't shop when you're hungry. Avoid aisles that contain problem foods.

- Pay attention to portion sizes. Use measuring cups and spoons and a food scale to become familiar with portion sizes.

- Serve meals on small plates and in small bowls to help you eat smaller portions without feeling deprived. (Research has shown that using a larger plate makes food portions appear smaller, so people serve themselves more food and overeat.)

- Eat only in specifically designated spots. Remove food from other areas of your home. When you eat, just eat. Don't do anything else.

- Eat slowly. It takes time for your brain to get the message that your stomach is full. Take small bites and chew food thoroughly. Pay attention to every bite, and enjoy your food.

Special Occasions

- When you eat out, choose a restaurant where you can make healthy food choices. Ask the server not to put bread and butter on the table before the meal, and request that sauces and salad dressings be served on the side. If portion sizes are large, take half your food home for a meal later in the week. Don't choose supersized meals.

- If offered food you don't want by friends or family, accept a small portion or politely decline.

Physical Activity and Stress Management

- Increase your level of daily physical activity as slowly as necessary based on your current fitness level.

- Begin an exercise program that includes cardiorespiratory endurance exercise, strength training, and stretching.

- Get six to eight hours of sleep a night.

- Develop techniques for handling stress that don't involve food. See Chapter 10 for more on stress management.

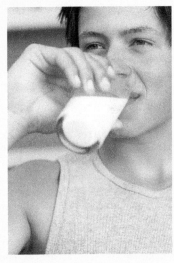

- Develop strategies for coping with non-hunger cues to eat, such as boredom, sleepiness, or anxiety. Try calling a friend, taking a walk, or reading a magazine.

- Tell family members and friends that you're changing your eating and exercise habits. Ask them to be supportive.

©Klaus Tiedge/Corbis/Getty Images RF

Modest weight loss can also be easier to maintain. American Heart Association guidelines state that an even smaller weight loss, in the 3–5% range, is beneficial if maintained. Relatively modest weight loss—and the lifestyle changes used to achieve and maintain it—is likely to improve blood pressure as well as reduce cholesterol and glucose levels and the risk for diabetes.

Some diet plans have an initiation phase of rapid weight loss, such as 6–8 pounds for the first two weeks. Then the plans transition to a reduced weight loss of 0.5–2.0 pounds per week. The rapid weight loss goal for the first two weeks can work, but if continued, it may have adverse results such as lean tissue and water loss. The reduced weight loss goal is not only more realistic but healthier.

A pound of body fat represents 3,500 calories, which means that as you strive to lose weight, you may need a negative energy balance of at least 250–1,000 calories per day.

Although this balance may help you lose weight at the start of a diet, some people need an even greater negative calorie balance as their metabolic rate slows: As described earlier in the chapter, your lower energy intake and loss of weight prompt the body to conserve energy and lower the RMR. The National Institutes of Health has a planning tool that provides individual energy-intake estimates for reaching a goal weight within a specific time period and maintaining it afterward (https://www.niddk.nih.gov/health-information/weight-management/body-weight-planner). The tool can provide a starting point for planning, as well as a reality check on your goals.

In general, a low-calorie diet provides 1,200–1,500 calories per day. Most low-calorie diets cause a rapid loss of body water at first. After this phase, weight loss declines, and dieters are often misled into believing that their efforts are not working. They give up, not realizing that the large initial fluid loss is not as significant as smaller fat losses occurring later in the diet.

Develop a Plan You Can Stick With Maintaining weight loss is usually a bigger challenge than losing weight. Without lifestyle changes, most weight lost during a period of dieting is regained. Weight management is a lifelong project. When planning a weight-management program, include strategies that you can maintain over the long term, both for food choices and for physical activity. If you want to use a digital tracking tool in your program, consider the tips in the box "Apps and Wearables for Weight Management." A registered dietitian or nutritionist can recommend a personalized plan when you want to lose weight on your own. For more strategies, refer to the section on "Adopting a Healthy Lifestyle for Successful Weight Management."

Diet Books

Many people who try to lose weight by themselves fall prey to one or more of the dozens of diet books on the market. Although some books contain useful advice and motivational tips, most make empty promises. Look for books that advocate a balanced approach to diet plus exercise and sound nutritional advice. Reject those with any of the following:

- An approach based on an unbalanced way of eating, such as a high-carbohydrate-only diet or one focused on a single food, such as cabbage or grapefruit
- A claim that it is based on a "scientific breakthrough" or that it has the "secret to success"
- Gimmicks, such as matching eating to blood type, hyping insulin resistance as the cause of obesity, or combining foods in special ways to achieve weight loss
- Promises of quick weight loss or limits placed on the selection of healthy foods

Many diets cause weight loss if maintained. The real difficulty is finding a safe and healthy pattern of food choices and physical activity that results in long-term maintenance of a healthy body weight and reduced risk of chronic disease.

Wellness Tip Many plans and supplements claim to promote weight loss, but few have any research supporting their effectiveness for long-term weight management. If you're tempted to start taking an over-the-counter weight-loss supplement, do your homework first. Ask for your doctor's opinion, and check the FDA's supplement website at http://www.fda.gov/Food/DietarySupplements.
©VStock LLC/Tanya Constantine/Getty Images RF

Dietary Supplements and Diet Aids

The number of dietary supplements and other weight-loss aids on the market has also increased in recent years. Promoted in advertisements, magazines, direct mail campaigns, infomercials and on websites, these products typically promise a quick and easy path to weight loss. Most of these products are marketed as dietary supplements and so are subject to fewer regulations than over-the-counter (OTC) medications. According to the Federal Trade Commission (FTC), more than half of advertisements for weight-loss products make representations that are likely to be false. And although the FTC will order companies to stop making baseless and bogus product claims when monitors become aware of them, consumers are urged to critically evaluate any product that sounds too good to be true.

Potentially harmful hidden and undisclosed ingredients are a growing problem in products promoted for weight loss. Consumers may take a diet product that doesn't list quantities of approved prescription drug ingredients. In some cases the products also contain untested and unstudied ingredients or controlled substances (substances whose use is strictly regulated by the government). All of these ingredients could have harmful effects. Such situations are becoming more common because the FDA cannot test for potentially harmful hidden ingredients in all products. Also, consumer advisories for tainted products identify only a small proportion of the potentially harmful products on the market.

Public notifications available on the FDA website reveal that even some products labeled "Natural and Safe" contain prescription medications, including sibutramine (a weight-loss medication sold under the brand name Meridia) and phenytoin (an antiseizure medication). In its consumer alert, the FDA noted that a number of the recalled supplements contained pharmaceuticals in amounts far exceeding FDA-recommended levels. Some of the supplements contained substances that are

WELLNESS IN THE DIGITAL AGE
Apps and Wearables for Weight Management

A wide and ever-growing range of wearable trackers and weight-loss apps are available to consumers. You can find hundreds of smartphone apps to help you keep a nutrition journal and calculate your daily intake of calories and nutrients. You can also pair such apps with wearable trackers that can monitor your physical activity and calculate the calories you burn throughout the day. The apps may also synchronize data with a website that can display your results and progress in multiple formats; some also let you share your results across your social media networks or with a group of behavior change "buddies."

Do these digital tools help with weight loss and weight maintenance? Research findings have been mixed. As with any health habit, tracking alone is unlikely to create permanent behavior change. Apps and wearables for weight management may be most effective when you pair tracking with evidence-based behavior-change techniques, such as reviewing goals, developing a specific action plan, planning for relapse prevention, and providing prompts, personalized feedback, rewards, and opportunities for motivational support. Pairing a digital tool with in-person or phone counseling from a health professional may further boost success.

If you decide to use a wearable and/or app to track diet and exercise for your weight-management program, consider the following:

- Does the app track what you want to track, and is it easy to use? Try it for a week or more: Did you stick with it?

- Does the app incorporate evidence-based behavior-change strategies? What does it offer besides tracking? Look for apps with motivation components (e.g., feedback, rewards

and challenges, and a system of points or levels).

- If you want to share your results with friends on social media, is that functionality supported? Can you join other app users in a supportive group?

- How was the app developed? Has it undergone scientific evaluation? Were behavior-change or medical experts involved in its development? If users claim the app has provided some level of effectiveness or success, what evidence is provided to back up the claim? Satisfaction or popularity ratings do not necessarily reflect effectiveness for supporting weight loss.

Even with the help of digital devices and programs, weight management is still primarily a matter of personal effort, perseverance, and a commitment to lifestyle changes that last for life.

SOURCES: Abedtash, H., and R. J. Holden. 2017. "Systematic review of the effectiveness of health-related behavioral interventions using portable activity sensing devices (PASDs)," *Journal of the American Medical Informatics Association.* doi: 10.1093/jamia/ocx006; Ross, K. M., and R. R. Wing. 2016. "Impact of newer self-monitoring technology and brief phone-based intervention on weight loss: A randomized pilot study," *Obesity* 24(8), 1653–1659; Jakicic, J. M., et al. 2016. "Effect of wearable technology combined with lifestyle intervention on long-term weight loss: The IDEA randomized clinical trial," *JAMA* 316(11), 1161–1171; Flores Mateo, G., et al. 2015. "Mobile phone apps to promote weight loss and increase physical activity: A systematic review and meta-analysis," *Journal of Medical Internet Research* 17(11), E253.

---

not approved for sale in the United States, including lorcaserin (a controlled substance), and phenolphthalein, which is thought to be a carcinogen. The use of these drugs could lead to complications such as heart attack, stroke, suicide, and cancer.

The following sections describe some commonly marketed OTC products for weight loss.

Formula Drinks and Food Bars Canned diet drinks, powders used to make shakes, and diet food bars and snacks are meal replacements. They are designed to help you lose weight by substituting for some or all of your daily food intake. Meal replacements are convenient. However, most people find it difficult to use these products for long periods, and although they sometimes result in rapid short-term weight loss, the weight is typically regained because users don't learn to change their eating and lifestyle behaviors.

Herbal Supplements As described in Chapter 8, herbs are marketed as dietary supplements, and there is little information about effectiveness, proper dosage, drug interactions, and side effects. In addition, labels may not accurately reflect the ingredients and dosages present, and safe manufacturing practices are not guaranteed. Herbal supplements on the market today are described in Table 9.4.

Other Supplements Fiber is another common ingredient in OTC diet aids, promoted for appetite control. However, dietary fiber acts as a bulking agent in the large intestine, not the stomach, so it doesn't have a pronounced effect on appetite. In addition, many diet aids contain only 3 or fewer grams of fiber, which do not contribute much toward the recommended daily intake of 25–38 grams.

Other popular dietary supplements include conjugated linoleic acid, carnitine, chromium, pyruvate, calcium, B vitamins, chitosan, and a number of products labeled "fat absorbers," "fat blockers," or "starch blockers." Research has not found these products to be effective, and many have potentially adverse side effects.

Weight-Loss Programs

Weight-loss programs come in a variety of types, including noncommercial support organizations, commercial programs, websites, and clinical programs.

Noncommercial Weight-Loss Programs Noncommercial programs such as TOPS (Take Off Pounds Sensibly) and Overeaters Anonymous (OA) mainly provide group support. They do not advocate any particular diet, but they do recommend seeking professional advice for creating an individualized

Table 9.4   Safety and Effectiveness of Common Over-the-Counter Weight-Loss Pills

INGREDIENT	PROPOSED MECHANISM OF ACTION	EVIDENCE OF EFFICACY	REPORTED ADVERSE EFFECTS
Alli (OTC form of orlistat)	Decreases absorption of dietary fat	Possible modest benefit; less effective than prescription strength form (Xenical)	Loose stools, gas with oily spotting, more frequent and hard to control bowel movements; reduced absorption of some nutrients; rare cases of liver damage
Bitter orange (synephrine)	Increased energy expenditure, mild appetite suppressant	Possible effect on resting metabolic rate; inconclusive effects on weight loss	Chest pain, anxiety, increased blood pressure and heart rate
Caffeine (as added caffeine or from guarana, kola nut, yerba mate, or other herbs)	Stimulates central nervous system, increases fat oxidation	Possible modest effect on body weight or decreased weight gain over time	Nervousness, jitteriness, vomiting, and tachycardia
Chitosan	Binds dietary fat in the digestive tract	Minimal effect on body weight	Bloating, flatulence, indigestion, constipation, nausea, heartburn
Chromium	Increases lean muscle mass; promotes fat loss; reduced hunger and fat cravings	Minimal effect on body weight and body fat	Headache, watery stools, constipation, weakness, vertigo, nausea, vomiting, hives
Conjugated linoleic acid	Promotes reduction in fat cells	Minimal effect on body weight and body fat	Abdominal pain, constipation, diarrhea, indigestion, and (possibly) adverse effects on blood lipid levels
Green tea extract	Increases energy expenditure and fat use, reduces fat absorption	Possible modest effect on body weight	Abdominal pain, constipation, nausea, increased blood pressure, liver damage
Guar gum	Acts as bulking agent in the gut, increases feelings of fullness	No effect on body weight	Abdominal pain, flatulence, diarrhea, nausea, cramps
Hoodia	Suppresses appetite, reduces food intake	Limited research, but no apparent effect on energy intake or body weight	Headache, dizziness, nausea, and vomiting
Pyruate	Increases fat burning and energy expenditure	Possible minimal effect on body weight and body fat	Diarrhea, gas, bloating, and (possibly) decreased good cholesterol (HDL)
Raspberry ketone	Alters fat metabolism	Insufficient research to draw firm conclusions	None known

SOURCE: Adapted from *Dietary Supplements for Weight Loss: Fact Sheet for Health Professionals.* National Institutes of Health: Office of Dietary Supplements, 2015. (http://ods.od.nih.gov/factsheets/WeightLoss-HealthProfessional)

diet and exercise plan. Like Alcoholics Anonymous, OA is a 12-step program with a spiritual orientation that promotes abstinence from compulsive overeating. These types of programs are generally free. Your physician or a registered dietitian can also provide information and support for weight loss.

Commercial Weight-Loss Programs Commercial weight-loss programs typically provide group support, nutrition education, physical activity recommendations, and behavior modification advice. Some also make packaged foods available to assist in following dietary advice.

A responsible and safe weight-loss program should have the following features:

- Healthy eating plans that reduce calories but do not exclude specific foods or food groups
- Tips on ways to increase moderate-intensity physical activity
- Tips on healthy habits that also keep your cultural needs in mind, such as lower-fat versions of your favorite foods
- Slow and steady weight loss

- A recommendation for medical evaluation and care if you have health problems, are taking medication, or are planning to follow a special formula diet that requires monitoring by a doctor
- A plan to keep the weight off after you have lost it
- Information on all fees and costs, including those of supplements and prepackaged foods, as well as data on risks and expected outcomes of participating in the program

You should also consider whether a program fits your lifestyle and whether you are truly ready to make a commitment to it. A strong commitment and a plan for maintenance are especially important because only 10–15% of program participants maintain their weight loss; the rest gain back all they had lost or more. One study of participants found that regular exercise was the best predictor of maintaining weight loss, and frequent television viewing was the best predictor of weight gain.

Clinical Weight-Loss Programs Medically supervised clinical programs are usually located in a hospital or other medical setting. Designed to help those who are severely obese, these programs typically involve a closely monitored very-low-calorie

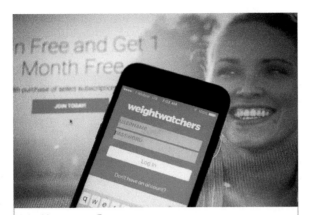

Wellness Tip Commercial weight-loss programs yield mixed results, but most provide nutritional counseling and support for people who are serious about losing weight. If the structure and support a program provides seem like something you'd like to try, be sure to evaluate the recommended dietary and activity patterns carefully.

©Bloomberg/Getty Images

diet. The cost of a clinical program is usually high, but insurance often covers part of the fee.

Prescription Drugs for Obesity

For a medicine to cause weight loss, it must (1) reduce energy consumption, (2) increase energy expenditure, and/or (3) interfere with energy absorption. The medications most often prescribed for weight loss are appetite suppressants that reduce feelings of hunger or increase feelings of fullness. Appetite suppressants usually work by increasing levels of catecholamine or serotonin, two brain chemicals that affect mood and appetite. Although some medications are approved only for short-term use, most experts agree that medications must be safe to use over the long term in order to be effective for treatment of obesity.

Appetite suppressants approved for long-term use include Belviq (lorcaserin), Qsymia (phentermine and topiramate extended-release), Contrave (bupropion and naltrexone), and Saxenda (liraglutide). All have potential side effects: Reported side effects include sleeplessness, nervousness, and euphoria, as well as increases in blood pressure and heart rate. Headaches, constipation or diarrhea, dry mouth, and insomnia are other side effects. If you are taking a prescription medication, discuss any concerns about side effects with your physician.

Orlistat lowers calorie consumption by blocking fat absorption in the intestines; it prevents about 30% of the fat in food from being digested. Similar to the fat substitute olestra, orlistat also reduces the absorption of fat-soluble vitamins and antioxidants. Therefore, a vitamin supplement is highly recommended for people taking orlistat. Side effects include severe liver injury, diarrhea, cramping, and other gastrointestinal problems if users do not follow a low-fat diet. Alli is a lower-dose version of orlistat that is sold over the counter.

Prescription medications work best in conjunction with behavior modification. Studies have generally found that appetite suppressants produce modest weight loss above the loss expected with nondrug obesity treatments. In a review published in 2016, researchers reported that people taking a prescription medication were two to three times more likely to have at least 5% weight loss than people taking a placebo. Individuals respond differently, however, and some lose more weight than others. Weight loss tends to level off or reverse after four to six months on a medication, and many people regain the weight they've lost when they stop taking the drug.

Prescription weight-loss drugs are not for people who just want to lose a few pounds. The latest federal guidelines advise people to try lifestyle modification for at least six months before trying drug therapy. Prescription drugs are recommended only for people who have been unable to lose weight with nondrug options and who have a BMI over 30 (or over 27 if an additional risk factor such as diabetes or high blood pressure is present). For severely obese people who have been unable to lose weight by other methods, prescription drugs may provide a good option.

Surgery

An estimated 6.3% of adult Americans age 20 and older have a BMI greater than 40, qualifying them as severely or morbidly obese. In 1975 in the U.S., .5% of men and 1.5% of women were severely obese. Forty years later, these percentages have jumped to 5.2% of men and 12.7% of women. Severe obesity is a serious medical condition that is often complicated by other health problems such as diabetes, sleep disorders, heart disease, and arthritis. Surgical intervention—known as *bariatric surgery*—may be necessary as a treatment of last resort. Bariatric surgery may be recommended for patients with a BMI greater than 40, or greater than 35 with obesity-related illnesses.

Due to the increasing prevalence of severe obesity, surgical treatment of obesity is becoming more common worldwide. Obesity-related health conditions, as well as risk of premature death, generally improve after surgical weight loss. Surgery, however, carries risks. Patients with poor cardiorespiratory fitness prior to surgery experience more postoperative complications, including stroke, kidney failure, and even death, than patients with higher fitness levels.

Bariatric surgery modifies the gastrointestinal tract. One method partitions the stomach with staples or a band, while another modifies the way the stomach drains (gastric bypass). The goal is to promote weight loss by reducing the amount of food the patient can eat. Potential complications from surgery include nutritional deficiencies, fat intolerance, nausea, vomiting, and reflux. As many as 10–20% of patients may require follow-up surgery to address complications.

Weight loss from surgery generally ranges between 40% and 70% of total body weight over the course of a year. The key to success is to have adequate follow-up and to stay motivated so that life behaviors and eating patterns are changed permanently.

The surgical technique of liposuction involves the removal of small amounts of fat from specific locations. Liposuction is not a method for treating obesity.

Ask Yourself

QUESTIONS FOR CRITICAL THINKING AND REFLECTION

Why do you think people like Meredith and Leroy (at the start of the chapter) continue to buy in to fad diets and weight-loss gimmicks, even though they are constantly reminded that the key to weight management is lifestyle change? Have you ever tried a fad diet or dietary supplement? If so, what were your reasons for trying it? What were the results?

Psychological Help

When concerns about body weight and shape have developed into an eating disorder, professional help is recommended. Therapists who help people with these disorders should have experience in weight management, body image issues, eating disorders, addictions, and abuse issues.

BODY IMAGE

The cultural picture of the body as seen through the mind's eye, **body image** consists of perceptions, images, thoughts, attitudes, and emotions. A negative body image is characterized by dissatisfaction with the body in general or some part of the body in particular.

Developing a positive body image is an important aspect of psychological wellness and successful weight management. Dissatisfaction with body size and shape comes from external, cultural forces as well as internal, psychological perceptions that are specific to life stages. For example, a cultural ideal of female body shape in Western society has become progressively thinner, whereas actual female body size continues to increase. How we individually perceive these norms and act on them, for example, not eating enough or refusing to appear in a bathing suit, represents our psychological response.

Severe Body Image Problems

Poor body image can cause significant psychological distress. Preoccupation with a perceived defect in appearance can damage self-esteem and interfere with relationships. Adolescents and adults who have a negative body image are more likely to diet restrictively, eat compulsively, or develop some other form of disordered eating.

When dissatisfaction becomes extreme, the condition is called *body dysmorphic disorder (BDD)*. BDD affects about 2% of Americans, males and females in equal numbers. BDD

usually begins before age 18 but can begin in adulthood. Sufferers are overly concerned with physical appearance, often focusing on slight flaws that are not obvious to others. Individuals with BDD may spend hours every day thinking about their flaws and looking at themselves in mirrors; they may desire and seek repeated cosmetic surgeries. BDD is related to obsessive-compulsive disorder and can lead to depression, social phobia, and suicide if left untreated. Medication and therapy can help people with BDD.

In some cases, body image may bear little resemblance to fact. A person with the eating disorder anorexia nervosa typically has a severely distorted body image, believing herself to be fat even when she has become emaciated (see the next section for more on anorexia). Distorted body image is also a hallmark of *muscle dysmorphia,* a disorder experienced by some bodybuilders and other active people who see themselves as small and out of shape despite being very muscular. People with muscle dysmorphia may let obsessive weight training interfere with their work and relationships. They may also use potentially dangerous muscle-building drugs.

To assess your body image, complete the body image self-test in Lab 9.3.

Acceptance and Change

There are limits to the changes that can be made to body weight and body shape, both of which are influenced by heredity. Knowing when the limits to healthy change have been reached—and learning to accept those limits—is crucial for overall wellness. Women in particular tend to measure self-worth in terms of their appearance. When they don't measure up to an unrealistic cultural ideal, they see themselves as defective, and their self-esteem falls. The result can be negative body image, disordered eating, or even a full-blown eating disorder (see the box "Gender, Ethnicity, and Body Image."

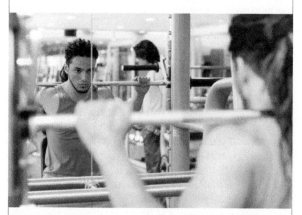

Fitness Tip   Exercise is a healthy practice, but people with eating disorders or body image problems sometimes exercise excessively, building their lives around their workouts. Compulsive exercise can lead to injuries, low body fat, and other health problems. Track your exercise habits for a week; if they seem excessive and you can't seem to cut back, talk to a professional counselor or your doctor to find out if you have a body image problem.
©PhotoAlto/Odilon Dimier/Getty Images RF

---

body image   The mental representation a person holds about her or his body is influenced by cultural models and consists of perceptions, images, thoughts, attitudes, and emotions about the body.   TERMS

DIVERSITY MATTERS
Gender, Ethnicity, and Body Image

Body Image and Gender

Women are much more likely than men to be dissatisfied with their bodies, often wanting to be thinner. Body weight perception has been found to begin in girls as young as 7 years old. Approximately 50% of girls and undergraduate women report being dissatisfied with their bodies. Girls and women are much more likely than boys and men to diet, develop eating disorders, and become obese.

The image of the ideal woman presented in the media is often unrealistic and even unhealthy. In a review of BMI data for Miss America pageant winners since 1922, researchers noted a significant decline in BMI over time, with an increasing number of recent winners having BMIs in the "underweight" category. The average fashion model is four to seven inches taller and almost 50 pounds lighter than the average American woman. Most fashion models are thinner than 98% of American women.

Our culture may be promoting an unattainable masculine ideal as well. Researchers have found that males who form their ideals from media-generated images show a preference for thinness and muscularity. Researchers studying male action figures note that they have become increasingly muscular. Such media messages can be demoralizing; boys and men also suffer from body image problems, although not as commonly as girls and women.

Body Image and Ethnicity

Although some groups espouse thinness as an ideal body type, others, like many traditional African societies, prefer full-figured women's bodies, which are

seen as symbols of health, prosperity, and fertility. African American teenage girls have a more positive body image than European American girls; in one survey, two-thirds of them defined beauty as "the right attitude," whereas European American girls were more preoccupied with weight and body shape. In another study about pressure to look like idealized images, Latina women reported the greatest pressure (over white or black women) to be physically attractive.

Nevertheless, recent evidence indicates that African American women are as likely to engage in disordered eating behavior—especially binge eating and vomiting—as their Latina, Native American, and European American counterparts. This finding underscores the complex nature of eating disorders and body image.

Avoiding Body Image Problems

To minimize your risk of developing a body image problem, keep the following strategies in mind:

- Focus on healthy habits and good physical health.

- Put concerns about physical appearance in perspective. Your worth as a human being does not depend on how you look.

- Practice body acceptance. You can influence your body size and type through lifestyle to some degree, but the fact is that some people are

©Gary Burchell/Getty Images

genetically designed to be bigger or heavier than others.

- Find things to appreciate in yourself besides an idealized body image. People who can learn to value other aspects of themselves are more accepting of the physical changes that occur naturally with age.

- View eating as a morally neutral activity—eating dessert isn't "bad" and doesn't make you a bad person.

- See the beauty and fitness industries for what they are. Realize that their goal is to prompt you to be dissatisfied with yourself so that you will buy their products.

SOURCES: Bruns, G. L, and M. M. Carter. 2015. "Ethnic differences in the effects of media on body image: The effects of priming with ethnically different or similar models," *Eating Behaviors* 17, 33–36; Haytko, D. L, et al. 2014. "Body image and ethnicity: A qualitative exploration," *Journal of Management and Marketing Research* 17; Webb, J. B., et al. 2013. "Do you see what I see: An exploration of inter-ethnic body size comparisons among college women," *Body Image* 10(3), 369–379.

Box icon: ©Rawpixel Ltd/Getty Images RF

Weight management is most successful in a positive and realistic atmosphere. For an obese person, losing as few as 10 pounds can reduce blood pressure and improve mood. The hazards of excessive dieting and overconcern about body weight need to be countered by a change in attitude. A reasonable weight must take into account a person's weight history, social circumstances, metabolic profile, and psychological well-being.

EATING DISORDERS

Problems with body weight and weight control are not limited to excessive body fat. A growing number of people, especially adolescent girls and young women, experience **eating disorders**. Eating disorders are characterized by severe disturbances in body image, eating patterns, and eating-related behavior. In the United States, it is estimated that 20 million women and 3 million men suffer from an eating disorder (anorexia nervosa, bulimia nervosa, and binge-eating disorder) some time in their lives. Many more people have abnormal eating habits and attitudes about food that disrupt their lives, even though these habits do not meet the criteria for a major eating disorder. To assess your eating habits, complete Lab 9.3.

Eating disorders are classified as mental disorders. Although many explanations for the development of eating disorders have been proposed, individuals with such disorders share one central feature: a dissatisfaction with body image and body weight. Such dissatisfaction is created by distorted thinking, including perfectionist beliefs, unreasonable demands for self-control, and excessive self-criticism. Dissatisfaction with body weight leads to dysfunctional attitudes about eating, such as fear of fat, preoccupation with food, and problematic eating behaviors.

Anorexia Nervosa

People with **anorexia nervosa** have an intense fear of gaining weight or becoming fat. Although they may express a great interest in food, they do not eat enough food to maintain a reasonable body weight. They may engage in compulsive behaviors or rituals that help them avoid eating. People with anorexia are typically introverted, emotionally reserved, and socially insecure. Their entire sense of self-esteem may be tied up in their evaluation of their body shape and weight. An estimated 0.5–3.7% of women suffer from anorexia nervosa in their lifetime. Although it can occur earlier or later, anorexia typically develops during puberty and the late teenage years, with an average onset age of about 19 years.

---

eating disorder   A serious disturbance in eating patterns or eating-related behavior, characterized by a negative body image and concerns about body weight or body fat.

anorexia nervosa   An eating disorder characterized by a refusal to maintain body weight at a minimally healthy level and an intense fear of gaining weight or becoming fat; self-starvation.

bulimia nervosa   An eating disorder characterized by recurrent episodes of binge eating and then purging to prevent weight gain.

purging   The use of vomiting, laxatives, excessive exercise, restrictive dieting, enemas, diuretics, or diet pills to compensate for food that has been eaten and that the person fears will produce weight gain.

binge-eating disorder   An eating disorder characterized by repeated episodes of eating large amounts of food in a short period of time; episodes are marked by feelings of lack of control.

TERMS

Anorexia nervosa has been linked to a variety of medical complications, including disorders of the cardiovascular, gastrointestinal, and endocrine systems. Because of extreme weight loss, females with anorexia often stop menstruating. When body fat is virtually gone and muscles are severely wasted, the body turns to its organs in a desperate search for protein. Death can occur from heart failure caused by electrolyte imbalances. About 1 in 10 women with anorexia dies of starvation, cardiac arrest, or other medical complications—one of the highest death rates for any psychiatric disorder. Depression is also a serious risk, and about half the fatalities relating to anorexia are suicides.

Bulimia Nervosa

A person with **bulimia nervosa** engages in recurrent episodes of binge eating followed by **purging**. Bulimia is often difficult to recognize because sufferers conceal their eating habits and usually maintain a normal weight, although they may experience weight fluctuations of 10–15 pounds. Although bulimia usually begins in adolescence or young adulthood, it has begun to emerge at increasingly younger (11–12 years) and older (40–60 years) ages. The average age of onset is about 20 years.

A bulimic person may rapidly consume thousands of calories by binge eating; during a binge, bulimics feel as though they have lost control and cannot stop or limit how much they eat. This is followed by an attempt to get rid of the food by purging, usually by vomiting or using laxatives or diuretics. Some binge and purge only occasionally; others do so many times every day. Binges may be triggered by a major life change or other stressful event. Binge eating and purging may become a way of dealing with difficult feelings such as anger and disappointment.

The binge-purge cycle of bulimia places a tremendous strain on the body and can have serious health effects, including tooth decay, esophageal damage and chronic hoarseness, menstrual irregularities, depression, liver and kidney damage, and cardiac arrhythmia.

Binge-Eating Disorder

Binge-eating disorder (BED) affects 3–5% of American women and 2% of men. It is characterized by uncontrollable eating without any compensatory purging behaviors. Common eating patterns are eating more rapidly than normal, eating until uncomfortably full, eating when not hungry, and preferring to eat alone. Uncontrolled eating is usually followed by weight gain and feelings of guilt, shame, and depression. Many people with binge-eating disorder mistakenly see rigid dieting as the only solution to their problem, but this usually causes feelings of deprivation and a return to overeating.

Compulsive overeaters rarely eat because of hunger. Instead, they use food to cope with stress, conflict, and other difficult emotions or to provide solace or entertainment. Binge eaters are almost always obese, so they face all the health risks associated with obesity. In addition, binge eaters may have higher-than-average rates of depression and anxiety.

Other Specified Feeding or Eating Disorders (OSFED)

Eating habits and body image run along a continuum from healthy to seriously disordered. Where an individual falls along that continuum can change depending on life stresses, illnesses, and many other factors. People with feeding or eating disorders that can cause significant distress or impairment, but do not meet the criteria for another feeding or eating disorder, may be classified as having "other specified feeding or eating disorders" (OSFED).

Formally described as *eating disorders not otherwise specified (EDNOS),* OSFED is a feeding or eating disorder that does not meet full diagnostic criteria for anorexia, bulimia, or binge-eating disorder. Examples of OSFED include atypical anorexia nervosa, a condition in which weight is not below normal; bulimia nervosa, a condition with less frequent bulimic episodes; purging disorder, a condition without binge eating; and night eating syndrome, in which the individual engages in excessive nighttime food consumption.

Ideally, our relationship to food should be a happy one. The biological urge to satisfy hunger is one of our most basic drives, and eating is associated with many pleasurable sensations. For some of us, food triggers pleasant memories of good times, family, holidays, and fun. But for too many people, food is a source of anguish rather than pleasure. In the lives of affected individuals, eating results in feelings of guilt and self-loathing rather than satisfaction, causing tremendous disruption.

How do you know if you have disordered eating habits (for example, skipping meals or avoiding vegetables) that can lead to the more serious eating disorder? When thoughts about weight and food dominate your life, you have a problem. If you're convinced that your worth as a person hinges on how you look and how much you weigh, it's time to get help. Self-induced vomiting or laxative use after meals, even if only once in a while, is reason for concern. Do you feel compelled to exercise excessively to compensate for what you've eaten? Do you routinely restrict your food intake and sometimes eat nothing

in an effort to feel more in control? These are all danger signs and could mean that you are developing a serious problem. Lab 9.3 can help you determine whether you are at risk for an eating disorder.

Treating Eating Disorders

The treatment of eating disorders must address both problematic eating behaviors and the misuse of food to manage stress and emotions. Treatment for anorexia nervosa first involves averting a medical crisis by restoring adequate body weight; similarly, the first step for treating bulimia nervosa or binge-eating disorder involves stabilizing the eating patterns. Afterward, psychological aspects of the disorders can be addressed, such as identifying and changing the patterns of thinking that lead to disordered eating. Treatment usually involves a combination of psychotherapy, medication, and medical management. Friends and family members often want to know what they can do to help; for suggestions, see the box "If Someone You Know Has an Eating Disorder."

People with milder patterns of disordered eating may benefit from getting a nutrition checkup with a registered dietitian. A professional can determine appropriate body weight and calorie intake and offer advice on how to budget calories into a balanced, healthy diet.

TIPS FOR TODAY AND THE FUTURE

Many approaches work, but the simplest formula for weight management is moderate food intake coupled with regular exercise.

RIGHT NOW YOU CAN

- Assess your weight-management needs. Do you need to gain weight, lose weight, or stay at your current weight?
- List five things you can do to add more physical activity (not exercise) to your daily routine.
- Identify the foods you regularly eat that may be sabotaging your ability to manage your weight.

IN THE FUTURE YOU CAN

- Make an honest assessment of your body image. Is it accurate and fair, or is it unduly negative and unhealthy? If your body image presents a problem, consider getting professional advice on how to view yourself realistically.
- Keep track of your energy needs to determine whether your energy-balance equation is correct. Use this information as part of your long-term weight-management efforts.

Ask Yourself

QUESTIONS FOR CRITICAL THINKING AND REFLECTION

Have you known someone you thought may be suffering from an eating disorder? How did you come to that conclusion?

TAKE CHARGE
If Someone You Know Has an Eating Disorder...

Secrecy and denial are two hallmarks of eating disorders, so it can be hard to know if someone has anorexia or bulimia. Signs that someone may have anorexia include sudden weight loss, excessive dieting or exercise, guilt or preoccupation with food or eating, frequent weighing, fear of becoming fat despite being thin, and baggy or layered clothes to conceal weight loss. Signs that someone may have bulimia include excessive eating without weight gain; secretiveness about food (stealing, hiding, or hoarding food); self-induced vomiting (bathroom visits during or after a meal); swollen glands or puffy face; erosion of tooth enamel; and use of laxatives, diuretics, or diet pills to control weight.

If you decide to approach a friend with your concerns, here are some tips to follow:

• Find out about treatment resources in your community (see the "For Further Exploration" section for suggestions). You may want to consult a professional at your school clinic or counseling center about the best way to approach the situation.

• Arrange to speak with your friend in a private place, and allow enough time to talk.

• Express your concerns, with specific observations of your friend's behavior. Expect him or her to deny or minimize the problem and possibly to become angry with you. Stay calm and nonjudgmental, and continue to express your concern.

• Avoid giving simplistic advice about eating habits. Listen if your friend wants to talk, and offer your support and understanding. Give your friend the information you found about where he or she can get help, and offer to go along.

• If the situation is an emergency—if your friend has fainted, for example, or attempted suicide—call 9-1-1 for help immediately.

• If you are upset about the situation, consider talking to someone yourself. The professionals at the clinic or counseling center are there to help you. Remember, you are not to blame for another person's eating disorder.

SUMMARY

• Excess body weight increases the risk of numerous diseases, particularly cardiovascular disease, cancer, and diabetes.

• The influence of heredity on weight can in many cases be overcome with attention to lifestyle factors.

• Physiological factors involved in the regulation of body weight and body fat include metabolic rate and hormones.

• Energy-balance components that an individual can control are calories taken in and calories expended in physical activity.

• Nutritional guidelines for weight management and wellness include controlling consumption of total calories, unhealthy fats and carbohydrates, and protein; monitoring portion sizes and calorie density; increasing consumption of whole grains, fruits, and vegetables; and developing an eating schedule based on rules for food choices.

• Activity guidelines for weight control emphasize engaging in moderate-intensity physical activity for 60–90 minutes or more per day; regular, prolonged endurance exercise and weight training can burn a significant number of calories while maintaining muscle mass.

• The sense of well-being that results from a well-balanced diet can reinforce commitment to weight control; improve self-esteem; and lead to realistic, as opposed to negative, self-talk. Those who are successfully managing their weight find strategies other than eating as means of coping with stress.

• In cases of extreme obesity, weight loss requires medical supervision; in less extreme cases, people can set up individual programs,

perhaps getting guidance from reliable books or by joining a formal weight-loss program.

• Dissatisfaction with body image and body weight can lead to physical problems and serious eating disorders, including anorexia nervosa, bulimia nervosa, binge-eating disorder, and other specified feeding or eating disorders (OSFED).

FOR FURTHER EXPLORATION

Calorie Control Council. Includes a variety of interactive calculators, including an Exercise Calculator that estimates the calories burned from various forms of physical activity.

http://www.caloriecontrol.org

Centers for Disease Control and Prevention: Healthy Weight. Provides a variety of information and tools to help people assess their weight and plan healthy lifestyle changes.

http://www.cdc.gov/healthyweight

Frontline: Fat. Information from a PBS *Frontline* special that looked at how society, genetics, and biology have influenced our relationship with food and at current problems with obesity and eating disorders.

http://www.pbs.org/wgbh/pages/frontline/shows/fat

MedlinePlus: Obesity and Weight Control. Provides reliable information from government agencies and key professional associations.

http://www.nlm.nih.gov/medlineplus/obesity.html
http://www.nlm.nih.gov/medlineplus/weightcontrol.html

National Heart, Lung, and Blood Institute (NHLBI): Aim for a Healthy Weight. Provides information and tips on diet and physical activity, as well as a BMI calculator.

http://www.nhlbi.nih.gov/health/public/heart/obesity/lose_wt

COMMON QUESTIONS ANSWERED

Q How can I safely gain weight?

A Just as for losing weight, a program for weight gain should be gradual and should include both exercise and dietary changes. The foundation of a successful and healthy program for weight gain is a combination of strength training and in most cases a high-carbohydrate, high-protein diet that also contains healthy fats. Strength training will help you add weight as muscle rather than fat.

Energy balance is also important in a program for gaining weight. You need to consume more calories than your body requires in order to gain weight, but you need to choose those extra calories wisely. Fatty, sweet, high-calorie foods may seem like an obvious choice, but consuming additional calories as empty calories from solid fats and added sugars can jeopardize your health and your weight-management program. Your body is more likely to convert excess dietary fat into fat tissue than into muscle mass.

A better strategy is to consume additional calories as protein, healthy fats, and complex carbohydrates from whole grains, fruits, and vegetables. Add healthy calories from nutrient-dense, energy-dense foods such as nuts and whole grains. A diet for weight gain should contain about 60–65% of total daily calories from carbohydrates. You probably do not need to be concerned with protein. Although protein requirements increase when you exercise, the protein consumption of most Americans is already well above the DRI.

To gain primarily muscle weight instead of fat, a gradual program of weight gain is your best bet. Try these strategies for consuming extra calories:

- Don't skip any meals. If you fill up too fast, try eating five or six smaller meals.
- Add two or three snacks to your daily eating routine. Try trail mix, smoothies, and nut butters on crackers.
- Try a sports drink or supplement that has at least 60% of calories from carbohydrates, as well as significant amounts of protein, vitamins, and minerals. (But don't use supplements to replace meals because they don't contain all of the components of food.)

Q How can I achieve a "perfect" body?

A The current cultural ideal of an ultratoned, ultrafit body is impossible for most people to achieve. A reasonable goal for body weight and body shape must take into account your heredity, weight history, social circumstances, metabolic rate, and psychological well-being. Don't set goals based on movie stars or fashion models. Modern photographic techniques can make people look much different on film or in magazines than they do in person. Many of these people are also genetically endowed with body shapes that are impossible for most of us to emulate. The best approach is to work with what you've got. Adopting a wellness lifestyle that includes regular exercise and a healthy diet will naturally result in the best possible body shape for you. Obsessively trying to achieve unreasonable goals can lead to problems such as eating disorders, overtraining, and injuries.

Weight-control Information Network (WIN). A service of the National Institute of Diabetes and Digestive and Kidney Diseases, serves as an online clearinghouse of weight-management information.

http://win.niddk.nih.gov/

WHO: Global Strategy on Diet, Physical Activity and Health. Provides information on the World Health Organization's global strategy on diet and physical activity.

http://www.who.int/dietphysicalactivity/en

There are also many resources for people concerned about body image and eating disorders:

MedlinePlus: Eating Disorders

http://www.nlm.nih.gov/medlineplus/eatingdisorders.html

National Association of Anorexia Nervosa and Associated Disorders

http://www.anad.org

National Eating Disorders Association

http://www.nationaleatingdisorders.org

Women's Body Image and Health

http://www.womenshealth.gov/body-image/

See also the listings in Chapters 1, 6, and 8.

SELECTED BIBLIOGRAPHY

American Academy of Child and Adolescent Psychiatry. 2016. *Obesity in Children and Teens* (http://www.aacap.org/cs/root/facts_for_families/obesity_in_children_and_teens).

American Psychiatric Association. 2013. *Diagnostic and Statistical Manual of Mental Disorders*, 5th ed. Washington, DC: American Psychiatric Publishing.

Andreyeva, T., A. S. Tripp, and M. B. Schwartz. 2015. Dietary quality of Americans by Supplemental Nutrition Assistance Program participation status: A systematic review. *American Journal of Preventive Medicine* 49(4): 594–604.

Arora, T., et al. 2016. The impact of sleep debt on excess adiposity and insulin sensitivity in patients with early type 2 diabetes mellitus. *Journal of Clinical Sleep Medicine* 12(5): 673–680.

Basen-Engquist, K., and M. Chang. 2011. Obesity risk and cancer: Recent review and evidence. *Current Oncology Reports* 13(1): 71–76.

Bayon, V., et al. 2014. Sleep debt and obesity. *Annals of Medicine* 46(5): 264–272.

Boulangé, C. L., et al. 2016. Impact of the gut microbiota on inflammation, obesity, and metabolic disease. *Genome Medicine* 8: 42.

Bray, M. S., et al. 2016. NIH working group report—using genomic information to guide weight management: From universal to precision treatment. *Obesity* 24(1): 14–22.

Brown, P. 2016. Carbohydrate study leaves diet researchers divided. *MedPageToday*, 11 July (http://www.medpagetoday.com/primarycare/dietnutrition/59012).

Cheung, P. C., et al. 2016. Childhood obesity incidence in the United States: A systematic review. *Childhood Obesity* 12(1): 1–11.

Donnelly, J. E., et al. 2009. American College of Sports Medicine position stand: Appropriate physical activity intervention strategies for weight loss and prevention of weight regain for adults. *Medicine and Science in Sports and Medicine* 41(2): 459–471.

Federal Trade Commission. 2011. *Facts for Consumers: Dietary Supplements* (http://www.ftc.gov/bcp/edu/pubs/consumer/health/hea11.shtm).

Federal Trade Commission. 2012. *Facts for Consumers: Weighing the Evidence in Diet Ads* (http://www.ftc.gov/bcp/edu/pubs/consumer/health/hea03.shtm).

Fothergill, E., et al. 2016. Persistent metabolic adaptation 6 years after "The Biggest Loser" competition. *Obesity* 24(8): 1612–1619.

Freedhoff, Y., and K. D. Hall. 2016. Weight loss diet studies: We need help not hype. *Lancet* 388(10047): 849–851.

Hall, K. D., et al. 2016. Energy expenditure and body composition changes after an isocaloric ketogenic diet in overweight and obese men. *American Journal of Clinical Nutrition* 104(2): 324–333.

GBD 2015 Obesity Collaborators. 2017. Health effects of overweight and obesity in 195 countries over 25 years. *New England Journal of Medicine* doi: 10.1056/NEJMoa1614362.

Global BMI Mortality Collaboration. 2016. Body-mass index and all-cause mortality: Individual-participant-data meta-analysis of 239 prospective studies in four continents. *Lancet* 388(10046): 776–786.

Grant, S. F. A., ed. 2014. *The Genetics of Obesity.* New York: Springer.

Guedes, E. P., et al. 2013. Body composition and depressive/anxiety symptoms in overweight and obese individuals with metabolic syndrome. *Diabetology & Metabolic Syndrome* 5(1): 82.

Harvard T. H. Chan School of Public Health. 2015. *Toxic Food Environment: How Our Surroundings Influence What We Eat* (http://www.hsph.harvard.edu/obesity-prevention-source/obesity-causes/food-environment-and-obesity/).

Healthy Seniors: Portal for Aging and Health in the Americas. 2015. *Sedentary Lifestyle Causes More Deaths Than Smoking, Says Study* (http://www.healthyolderpersons.org/news/sedentary-lifestyle-causes-more-deaths-smoking-says-study).

Holland, L. A., et al. 2014. Defining features of unhealthy exercise associated with disordered eating and eating disorder diagnoses. *Psychology of Sport and Exercise* 15(1): 116–123.

Huang, T. T.-K., et al. 2015. Mobilisation of public support for policy actions to prevent obesity. *Lancet* 385(9985): 2422–2431.

Jensen M. D., et al. 2014. AHA/ACC/TOS guideline for the management of overweight and obesity in adults: A report of the American College of Cardiology/American Heart Association Task Force on Practice Guidelines and the Obesity Society. *Circulation* 129: S102–138.

Karl, J. P., et al. 2015. Effects of carbohydrate quantity and glycemic index on resting metabolic rate and body composition during weight loss. *Obesity* 23(11): 2190–2198.

Kaur, J., et al. 2015. The association between food insecurity and obesity in children—the National and Nutrition Examination Survey. *Journal of the Academy of Nutrition and Dietetics* 115: 751–758.

Kenney, E. L., and S. L. Gortmaker. 2016. United States adolescents' television, computer, videogame, smartphone, and tablet use: Associations with sugary drinks, sleep, physical activity, and obesity. *Journal of Pediatrics* S0022-3476(16): 31243–31244.

Khera, R., et al. 2016. Association of pharmacological treatments for obesity with weight loss and adverse events: A systematic review and meta-analysis. *Journal of the American Medical Association* 315(22): 2424–2434.

Kiviruusu, O., et al. 2016. Self-esteem and body mass index from adolescence to mid-adulthood. A 26-year follow-up. *International Journal of Behavioral Medicine* 23(3): 355–363.

Knab, A. M., et al. 2011. A 45-minute vigorous exercise bout increases metabolic rate for 14 hours. *Medicine and Science in Sports and Exercise* 43(9): 1643–1648.

Kodama, S. et al. 2014. Quantitative relationship between body weight gain in adulthood and incident type 2 diabetes: A meta-analysis. *Obesity Research* 15(3): 202–214.

Kovesdy, C. P., et al. 2017. Obesity and kidney disease: Hidden consequences of the epidemic. *American Journal of Nephrology* 45(3): 283–291.

Lane, R. 2015. Christina Roberto: Taking a broad view on combating obesity. *Lancet* 385(9985): 2345.

Lasikiewicz, N., et al. 2014. Psychological benefits of weight loss following behavioural and/or dietary weight loss interventions. A systematic research review. *Appetite* 72: 123–137.

Levis, L. 2016. Are all calories equal? *Harvard Magazine,* May–June.

Ludwig, D. 2016. Lifespan weighed down by diet. *Journal of the American Medical Association* 315(21): 2269–2270.

MacLean, P. S., et al. 2015. NIH working group report: Innovative research to improve maintenance of weight loss. *Obesity* 23(1): 7–15.

Mayo Clinic. 2015. *Gastric Bypass Surgery* (http://mayoclinic.com/health/gastric-bypass/MY00825/DSECTION_results).

Mazidi, M., et al. 2016. Gut microbiome and metabolic syndrome. *Diabetes and Metabolic Syndrome* 10(2 Suppl 1): S150–157.

Mozzafarian, D. 2016. Dietary and policy priorities for cardiovascular disease, diabetes, and obesity: A comprehensive review. *Circulation* 133(2): 187–225.

NCD Risk Factor Collaboration. 2016. Trends in adult body-mass index in 200 countries from 1975 to 2014: a pooled analysis of 1698 population-based measurement studies with 19.2 million participants. *The Lancet* 387(10026): 1377–1396.

Ogilvie, R. P., et al. 2016. Actigraphy measured sleep indices and adiposity: The Multi-Ethnic Study of Atherosclerosis (MESA). *Sleep* 39(9): 1701–1708.

Nunez, C., et al. 2017. Obesity, physical activity and cancer risks: Results from the Cancer, Lifestyle and Evaluation of Risk Study (CLEAR). *Cancer Epidemiology* 47: 56–63.

Pellegrini, C. A., et al. 2012. The comparison of a technology-based system and an in-person behavioral weight loss intervention. *Obesity* 20(2):356–363.

Postrach, E., et al. 2013. Determinants of successful weight loss after using a commercial web-based weight reduction program for six months: Cohort study. *Journal of Medical Internet Research* 15(10).

Roberto, C. A., et al. 2015. Patchy progress on obesity prevention: Emerging examples, entrenched barriers, and new thinking. *Lancet* 385(9985): 2400–2409.

Rouhani, M. H., et al. 2016. Associations between dietary energy density and obesity: A systematic review and meta-analysis of observational studies. *Nutrition* 32(10): 1037–1047.

Schmidt, M. E., et al. 2012. Systematic review of effective strategies for reducing screen time among young children. *Obesity* 20(7): 1338–1545.

Schroder, K. E. 2011. Computer-assisted dieting: Effects of a randomized nutrition intervention. *American Journal of Health Behavior* 35(2): 175–188.

Sheikh, V. K., and H. A. Raynor. 2016. Decreases in high-fat and/or high added-sugar food group intake occur when a hypocaloric, low-fat diet is prescribed within a lifestyle intervention: a secondary cohort analysis. *Journal of the Academy of Nutrition and Dietetics* 116(10): 1599–1605.

Siegel, K. R., et al. 2016. Association of higher consumption of foods derived from subsidized commodities with adverse cardiometabolic risk among US adults. *JAMA Internal Medicine* 176(8): 1124–1132.

Slevec, J. H., and M. Tiggerman. 2011. Predictors of body dissatisfaction and disordered eating in middle-aged women. *Clinical Psychology Review* 31(4): 515–524.

U.S. Department of Health and Human Services and U.S. Department of Agriculture. 2015. *2015–2020 Dietary Guidelines for Americans,* 8th ed. (http://health.gov/dietaryguidelines/2015/guidelines).

U.S. Department of Health and Human Services. 2012. *Healthy People 2020: Nutrition and Weight Status* (http://healthypeople.gov/2020/topicsobjectives2020/overview.aspx?topicid_29).

U.S. Food and Drug Administration. 2017. *Tainted Weight Loss Products* (https://www.fda.gov/Drugs/ResourcesForYou/Consumers/BuyingUsingMedicineSafely/MedicationHealthFraud/ucm234592.htm).

Wansink, B., et al. 2006. Bottomless bowls: Why visual cues of portion size may influence intake. *Obesity Research* 13(1), 93–100.

Wing, R. R., et al. 2011. Benefits of modest weight loss in improving cardiovascular risk factors in overweight and obese individuals with type 2 diabetes. *Diabetes Care* 34(7): 1481–1486.

Wong, J. C., et al. 2016. A glucocorticoid- and diet-responsive pathway toggles adipocyte precursor cell activity in vivo. *Science Signaling* 9(451): ra103.

Yanovski, S. Z., and J. A. Yanovski. 2014. Long-term drug treatment for obesity: A systematic and clinical review. *Journal of the American Medical Association* 311(1): 74–86.

Yu, E., et al. 2017. Weight history and all-cause and cause-specific mortality in three prospective cohort studies. *Annals of Internal Medicine.* doi:10.7326/M16-1390.

Zheng, H., et al. 2013. Obesity and mortality risk: New findings from body mass index trajectories. *American Journal of Epidemiology* 178(11): 1591–1599.

Name _____ Section _____ Date _____

LAB 9.1 Calculating Daily Energy Needs

Part I Estimating Current Energy Intake from a Food Record

If your weight is stable, your current daily energy intake is the number of calories you need to consume to maintain your weight at your current activity level. For women, average calorie requirements are 1,600–2,400 calories per day; for men, 2,000–3,000. The low end of the range is for sedentary individuals, the high end for active individuals. In addition, caloric needs tend to decrease with age.

If you completed Lab 8.2, you should have a record of your current energy intake; if you didn't complete the lab, keep a careful and complete record of everything you eat for one day, and then total the calories in all the foods and beverages you consumed. Record your total energy intake below:

Current energy intake (from food record):_____**calories per day**

Part II Estimating Daily Energy Requirements Using Food and Nutrition Board Formulas

Many people underestimate the size of their food portions, and so energy goals based on estimates of current calorie intake from food records can be inaccurate. You can estimate your daily energy needs using the formulas listed below. To use the appropriate formula for your sex, you'll need to plug in the following:

- Age (in years)
- Height (in inches)

- Weight (in pounds)
- Physical activity coefficient (PA) from the table below.

To help estimate your physical activity level, consider the following guidelines: Someone who typically engages in 30 minutes of moderate-intensity activity, equivalent to walking two miles in 30 minutes, in addition to the activities involved in maintaining a sedentary lifestyle, is considered "low active";

	Physical Activity Coefficient (PA)	
Physical Activity Level	*Men*	*Women*
Sedentary	1.00	1.00
Low active	1.12	1.14
Active	1.27	1.27
Very active	1.54	1.45

someone who typically engages in the equivalent of 90 minutes of moderate-intensity activity is rated as "active." You might find it helpful to refer back to Lab 2.3 to estimate your physical activity level.

Estimated Daily Energy Requirement for Weight Maintenance in Men

$$864 - (9.72 \times age) + (PA \times [(6.39 \times weight) + (12.78 \times height)])$$

1. $9.72 \times$ _____ age (years) = _____
2. $864 -$ _____ result from step 1 = _____ [*result may be a negative number*]
3. $6.39 \times$ _____ weight (pounds) = _____
4. $12.78 \times$ _____ height (inches) = _____
5. _____ result from step 3 + _____ result from step 4 = _____
6. _____ PA (from table) × _____ result from step 5 = _____
7. _____ result from step 2 + _____ result from step 6 = _____ calories per day

LABORATORY ACTIVITIES

Estimated Daily Energy Requirement for Weight Maintenance in Women

$$387 - (7.31 \times age) + (PA \times [(4.91 \times weight) + (16.78 \times height)])$$

1. $7.31 \times$ _____ age (years) = _____

2. $387 -$ _____ result from step 1 = _____ [*result may be a negative number*]

3. $4.91 \times$ _____ weight (pounds) = _____

4. $16.78 \times$ _____ height (inches) = _____

5. _____ result from step 3 + _____ result from step 4 = _____

6. _____ PA (from table) × _____ result from step 5 = _____

7. _____ result from step 2 + _____ result from step 6 = _____ calories per day

Daily energy needs for weight maintenance (from formula): _____ **calories/day**

Part III Determining an Individual Daily Energy Goal for Weight Maintenance

If you calculated values for daily energy needs based on both methods, examine the two values. Some difference is likely—people tend to underestimate their food intake and overestimate their level of physical activity—but if the two values are very far off, check your food record and your physical activity estimate for accuracy, and make any necessary adjustments. For an individualized estimate of daily calorie needs, average the two values:

Daily energy needs = (food record result _____ **calories/day + formula result** _____ **calories/day) ÷ 2 =** _____ **calories/day**

Using Your Results

How did you score? Are you surprised by the value you calculated for your approximate daily energy needs? If so, is the value higher or lower than you expected?

What should you do next? Enter the results of this lab in the Preprogram Assessment column in Appendix B. If you want to change your energy balance to lose weight, complete Lab 9.2 to set goals and develop specific strategies for change. (If your goal is weight gain, see Common Questions Answered for basic guidelines.) One of the best ways to tip your energy balance toward weight loss is to increase your daily physical activity. If you include increases in activity as part of your program, then you can use the results of this lab to chart changes in your daily energy expenditure (and needs). Look for ways to increase the amount of time you spend in physical activity, thus increasing your physical activity coefficient. After several weeks of your program, complete this lab again, and enter the results in the Postprogram Assessment column of Appendix B. How do the results compare? Did your program for increasing physical activity show up as an increase in your daily energy expenditure and need?

SOURCE: Estimating Daily Energy Requirements Using Food and Nutrition Board Formulas Part II: Reprinted with permission from *Dietary Reference Intakes for Energy, Carbohydrate, Fiber, Fat, Fatty Acids, Cholesterol, Protein, and Amino Acids (Macronutrients)*. Reprinted with permission from the National Academies Press, Copyright 2005, National Academy of Sciences.

LABORATORY ACTIVITIES

Name _____   Section _____   Date _____

LAB 9.2   Identifying Weight-Loss Goals

Negative Calorie Balance

Complete the following calculations to determine your daily negative calorie balance goal.

Your current weight: _____ lb

Your target weight (from Lab 6.2):_____ lb

Total pounds to lose: _____ lb

Your target date for achieving your target weight: _____

    Enter your personal data (age, sex, activity level) along with your current and target weight in the National Institute of Health's Body Weight Planner (https://www.niddk.nih.gov/health-information/weight-management/body-weight-planner) to provide an estimate of the calorie level you'll need to achieve to meet your weight loss goal. Don't enter any changes in activity level at this point (leave the changes in activity level at 0%). Enter your results from the tool below; if the calorie level is not realistic, adjust your target weight and/or your target date.

Results from the Body Weight Planner:

(1) Calories to maintain current weight: _____ calories/day

(2) Calories to reach goal by target date: _____ calories/day

    Subtract value 2 from value 1 to obtain your daily negative calorie balance: _____ **calories per day**

    To keep your weight-loss program on schedule, you must achieve the daily negative calorie balance by either decreasing your calorie consumption (eating less) or increasing your calorie expenditure (being more active). Combining the two strategies may be most successful. Below, make a plan for changes in activity and diet that will allow you to achieve your daily negative calorie balance.

Changes in Activity Level

Adding a few minutes of exercise every day is a good way to expend calories. Use the calorie costs for different activities listed in the following table.

Activity	Cal/lb/min	×	Body weight	×	min	=	Total calories
Aerobic dance	.046		_____		_____		_____
Basketball (half court)	.045		_____		_____		_____
Bicycling (casual)	.049		_____		_____		_____
Bicycling (13 mph)	.071		_____		_____		_____
Elliptical exercise	.049		_____		_____		_____
Football (touch)	.049		_____		_____		_____
Hiking	.051		_____		_____		_____
Housework	.029		_____		_____		_____
Jogging	.060		_____		_____		_____
Rope skipping	.071		_____		_____		_____
Rowing	.032		_____		_____		_____
Skating	.049		_____		_____		_____
Soccer	.052		_____		_____		_____
Swimming	.032		_____		_____		_____
Walking (normal pace)	.029		_____		_____		_____
Walking (briskly)	.048		_____		_____		_____

Activity	Duration	Calories Used
_____	_____	_____
_____	_____	_____
_____	_____	_____

Total calories expended: _____

LABORATORY ACTIVITIES

Changes in Diet

Look closely at your diet from one day, as recorded in Lab 8.2. Identify ways to cut calorie consumption by eliminating certain items or substituting lower-calorie choices. Be realistic in your cuts and substitutions; you need to develop a plan you can live with.

Food Item   Substitute Food Item   Calorie Savings

_____   _____   _____

_____   _____   _____

_____   _____   _____

                                                                    Total calories cut: _____

Total calories expended _____ + total calories cut _____ = total negative calorie balance _____

Common Problem Eating Behaviors

For each group of statements that appear below, check those that are true for you. If you check several statements for a given pattern or problem, it will probably be a significant factor in your weight-management program. One possible strategy for dealing with each type of problem is given. For those eating problems you identify as important, add your own ideas to the strategies listed.

1. _____ I often skip meals.

   _____ I often eat a number of snacks in place of a meal.

   _____ I don't have a regular schedule of meal and snack times.

   _____ I make up for missed meals and snacks by eating more at the next meal.

Problem: Irregular eating habits

Possible solutions:

- Write out a plan for each day's meals in advance. Carry it with you and stick to it.
- _____
- _____

2. _____ I eat more than one sweet dessert or snack each day.

   _____ I usually snack on foods high in calories and fat (chips, cookies, ice cream).

   _____ I drink regular (not sugar-free) soft drinks.

   _____ I choose types of meat that are high in fat.

   _____ I consume more than one alcoholic beverage a day.

Problem: Poor food choices

Possible solutions:

- Keep a supply of raw fruits and vegetables handy for snacks.
- _____
- _____

3. _____ I always eat everything on my plate.

   _____ I often go back for seconds and thirds.

   _____ I take larger helpings than most people.

   _____ I eat leftovers instead of putting them away.

Problem: Portion sizes too large

Possible solutions:

- Measure all portions with a scale or measuring cup.
- _____
- _____

Name _____ Section _____ Date _____

LAB 9.3 Checking for Body Image Problems and Eating Disorders

Assessing Your Body Image

	Never	Sometimes	Often	Always
1. I dislike seeing myself in mirrors.	0	(1)	2	3
2. When I shop for clothing, I am more aware of my weight problem, and consequently I find shopping for clothes somewhat unpleasant.	0	(1)	2	3
3. I'm ashamed to be seen in public.	(0)	1	2	3
4. I prefer to avoid engaging in sports or public exercise because of my appearance.	(0)	1	2	3
5. I feel somewhat embarrassed about my body in the presence of someone of the other sex.	0	(1)	2	3
6. I think my body is ugly.	0	(1)	2	3
7. I feel that other people must think my body is unattractive.	0	1	(2)	3
8. I feel that my family or friends may be embarrassed to be seen with me.	(0)	1	2	3
9. I find myself comparing myself with other people to see if they are heavier than I am.	0	(1)	2	3
10. I find it difficult to enjoy activities because I am self-conscious about my physical appearance.	(0)	1	2	3
11. Feeling guilty about my weight problem occupies most of my thinking.	(0)	1	2	3
12. My thoughts about my body and physical appearance are negative and self-critical.	0	(1)	2	3
Now add up the number of points you have circled in each column: __6__	0	+ _6_	+ _2_	+ ____

Score Interpretation

The lowest possible score is 0, and this indicates a positive body image. The highest possible score is 36, and this indicates an unhealthy body image. A score higher than 14 suggests a need to develop a healthier body image.

SOURCE: Nash, J. D. *The New Maximize Your Body Potential*. Copyright 1997 by Bull Publishing. Reprinted with permission from Bull Publishing. All rights reserved.

Eating Attitudes Test to Evaluate Eating Disorder Risk

To help determine whether you might have an eating disorder that needs professional attention, answer the questions as accurately, honestly, and completely as possible; there are no right or wrong answers.

Part 1. Eating Attitudes Test (EAT-26)

Circle a response for each of the following statements.

	Always	Usually	Often	Some times	Rarely	Never
1. Am terrified about being overweight.	3	2	(1)	0	0	0
2. Avoid eating when I am hungry.	3	2	1	0	0	(0)
3. Find myself preoccupied with food.	3	2	(1)	0	0	0
4. Have gone on eating binges where I feel that I may not be able to stop.	3	(2)	1	(0)	0	0
5. Cut my food into small pieces.	3	2	(1)	(0)	0	0
6. Aware of the calorie content of foods that I eat.	3	2	(1)	0	0	0
7. Particularly avoid food with a high carbohydrate content (i.e. bread, rice, potatoes, etc.).	3	2	1	(0)	0	0
8. Feel that others would prefer if I ate more.	3	2	1	(0)	0	0

LABORATORY ACTIVITIES

	Always	Usually	Often	Some times	Rarely	Never
9. Vomit after I have eaten.	3	2	1	0	0	(0)
10. Feel extremely guilty after eating.	3	2	(1)	0	0	0
11. Am preoccupied with a desire to be thinner.	3	(3)	1	0	0	0
12. Think about burning up calories when I exercise.	3	(2)	1	0	0	0
13. Other people think that I am too thin.	3	2	1	(0)	0	0
14. Am preoccupied with the thought of having fat on my body.	3	(2)	1	0	0	0
15. Take longer than others to eat my meals.	3	2	1	(0)	0	0
16. Avoid foods with sugar in them.	3	2	1	(0)	0	0
17. Eat diet foods.	3	2	1	(0)	0	0
18. Feel that food controls my life.	3	2	(0)	0	0	0
19. Display self-control around food.	3	(2)	1	0	0	0
20. Feel that others pressure me to eat.	3	2	1	(0)	0	0
21. Give too much time and thought to food.	3	2	(1)	0	0	0
22. Feel uncomfortable after eating sweets.	3	2	1	(0)	0	0
23. Engage in dieting behavior.	3	2	1	(0)	0	0
24. Like my stomach to be empty.	3	2	1	(0)	0	0
25. Have the impulse to vomit after meals.	3	2	1	(0)	0	0
26. Enjoy trying new rich foods.	(0)	0	0	1	2	3

Total the points for your responses to determine your EAT-26 score: __6__

Part 2. Behavioral Questions

Answer the following questions according to your behavior in the past 6 months. Check the boxes with the most appropriate responses.

In the past 6 months have you:	Never	Once a month or less	2–3 times a month	Once a week	2–6 times a week	Once a day or more
A Gone on eating binges where you feel that you may not be able to stop?					✓	
B Ever made yourself sick (vomited) to control your weight or shape?	✓					
C Ever used laxatives, diet pills, or diuretics (water pills) to control your weight or shape?	✓					
D Exercised more than 60 minutes a day to lose or to control your weight?				✓		
E Lost 20 pounds or more in the past 6 months		Yes		No ✓		

Interpreting Your Results

If you meet one or more of the following criteria, evaluation by a qualified professional is recommended:

- A score of 20 or higher on EAT-26,
- A check in any of the gray boxes in the Behavioral Questions section, or
- A body mass index (BMI) that classifies you as underweight or very underweight using norms for sex and age (see the following table).

LABORATORY ACTIVITIES

This screening is not designed to make a diagnosis of an eating disorder or take the place of a professional consultation. A high score on the EAT-26 assessment does not mean that you have an eating disorder, but it does indicate that you should seek the advice of a qualified mental health professional who has experience with treating eating disorders. If you have a low score on the EAT-26, you still could have problems with eating behavior or body image; if you are suffering from feelings that are causing you concern or interfering with your daily functioning, seek help.

Body Mass Index (BMI) Cutoffs for Classification of Underweight

Age (years)	Females					Males			
	18	**19**	**20**	**20+**		**18**	**19**	**20**	**20+**
Very underweight	≤17.5	≤17.5	≤17.5	≤18.5		≤18.0	≤18.5	≤19.0	≤19.5
Underweight	17.6–18.0	17.6–18.0	17.6–18.5	18.6–19.0		18.1–18.5	18.6–19.0	19.1–19.5	19.6–20.0

SOURCE: Based on Garner et al. 1982. *Psychological Medicine*, 12, 871–878.

Using Your Results

How did you score? Are you surprised by your scores? Do the results of either assessment indicate that you may have a problem with body image or disordered eating?

What should you do next? If your results are borderline, consider trying some of the self-help strategies suggested in the chapter. If body image or disordered eating is a significant problem for you, get professional advice; a physician, therapist, and/or registered dietitian can help. Make an appointment today.

10 Stress Management and Sleep

LOOKING AHEAD...

After reading this chapter, you should be able to

- Explain what stress is and how people react to it.
- Describe the relationship between stress and disease.
- List common sources of stress.
- Describe techniques for preventing and managing stress.
- Put together a plan for managing the stress in your life.
- Explain the consequences of disrupted sleep and strategies for improving sleep.

TEST YOUR KNOWLEDGE

1. Which of the following events can cause stress?
   a. taking out a loan
   b. failing a test
   c. graduating from college

2. Exercise stimulates which of the following?
   a. analgesia (pain relief)
   b. birth of new brain cells
   c. relaxation

3. Which of the following can be a result of chronic stress?
   a. violence
   b. heart attack
   c. stroke

See answers on the next page.

© Caiaimage/Robert Daly/Getty Images RF

Like the term *fitness, stress* is a word many people use without understanding its precise meaning. Stress is popularly viewed as an uncomfortable response to a negative event, which probably describes *nervous tension* more than the cluster of physical and psychological responses that actually constitutes stress. In fact, stress is not limited to negative situations: It is also a response to pleasurable physical challenges and the achievement of personal goals. Whether stress is experienced as pleasant or unpleasant depends largely on the situation and the individual.

Because learning effective responses to stress can enhance psychological health and help prevent a number of serious diseases, stress management can be an important part of daily life. In this chapter we explain the physiological and psychological reactions that make up the stress response and how these reactions can be risks to good health. We also present a variety of methods of managing stress and establishing healthy sleep patterns.

WHAT IS STRESS?

In common usage, the term *stress* refers to two things: the mental states or events that trigger physical and psychological reactions *and* the reactions themselves. We use the more precise term **stressor** for a situation that triggers physical and emotional reactions and the term **stress response** for those reactions. We

use the term **stress** to describe the general physical and emotional state that accompanies the stress response.

Each person's experience of stress depends on many factors, including the nature of the stressor and how the person perceives it. Thoughts or feelings about an approaching event—a first date or a final exam—can be just as stressful as the event itself, or more so. Stressors take many forms. Like a fire in your home, some occur suddenly and neither last long nor repeat. Others, like air pollution or quarreling parents, can continue for a long time. The memory of a stressful occurrence, such as the loss of a loved one, can itself be a stressor years after the event. Responses to stressors can include a wide variety of physical, emotional, and behavioral changes. A short-term response might be an upset stomach or insomnia, whereas a long-term response might be a change in your personality or social relationships.

Physical Responses to Stressors

Imagine that you have stepped off the curb and see a car speeding toward you. With a fraction of a second to spare, you leap out of harm's way. In that split second of danger and the moments that follow, you experience a predictable series of physical reactions. Your body goes from a relaxed state to one prepared for physical action to cope with a threat to your life.

Two systems in your body are responsible for your physical response to stressors: the nervous system and the endocrine system. Through rapid chemical reactions affecting almost every part of your body, these systems allow you to act quickly and appropriately.

Actions of the Nervous System The nervous system consists of the brain, spinal cord, and nerves. Part of the nervous system is under voluntary control, as when you tell your arm to reach for an orange. What is not under conscious supervision—for example, the part that controls the digestion of the orange—is the **autonomic nervous system**. In addition to digestion, it controls your heart rate, breathing, blood pressure, and hundreds of other involuntary functions.

The autonomic nervous system consists of two divisions:

- The **parasympathetic division** is in control when you are relaxed. It aids in digesting food, storing energy, and promoting growth.

- The **sympathetic division** is activated during times of arousal, including exercise, and when you face an emergency or experience severe pain, anger, or fear.

Sympathetic nerves use the neurotransmitter **norepinephrine** (or *noradrenaline*) to affect nearly every organ, sweat gland, blood vessel, and muscle to enable your body to handle an emergency. In general, the sympathetic division commands your body to stop storing energy and to use it in response to a crisis.

Actions of the Endocrine System During stress, the sympathetic nervous system triggers the **endocrine system**. This system of glands, tissues, and cells helps control body functions by releasing **hormones** and other chemical messengers into the bloodstream to influence metabolism and other body processes.

TERMS

stressor   Any physical or psychological event or condition that produces physical and psychological reactions.

stress response   The physical and emotional reactions to a stressor.

stress   The general physical and emotional state that accompanies the stress response.

autonomic nervous system   The branch of the nervous system that controls basic body processes; consists of the sympathetic and parasympathetic divisions.

parasympathetic division   A division of the autonomic nervous system that moderates the excitatory effect of the sympathetic division, slowing metabolism and restoring energy supplies.

sympathetic division   A division of the autonomic nervous system that reacts to danger or other challenges by almost instantly accelerating body processes.

Answers (Test Your Knowledge)

1. **All three.** Stress-producing factors can be pleasant or unpleasant and can include physical challenges, goal achievements, and events that are perceived as negative.

2. **All three.** Regular exercise is linked to improvements in many dimensions of wellness.

3. **All three.** Chronic—or ongoing—stress can last for years. People who suffer from long-term stress may ultimately become violent toward themselves or others. They also run a greater-than-normal risk for certain ailments, especially cardiovascular disease.

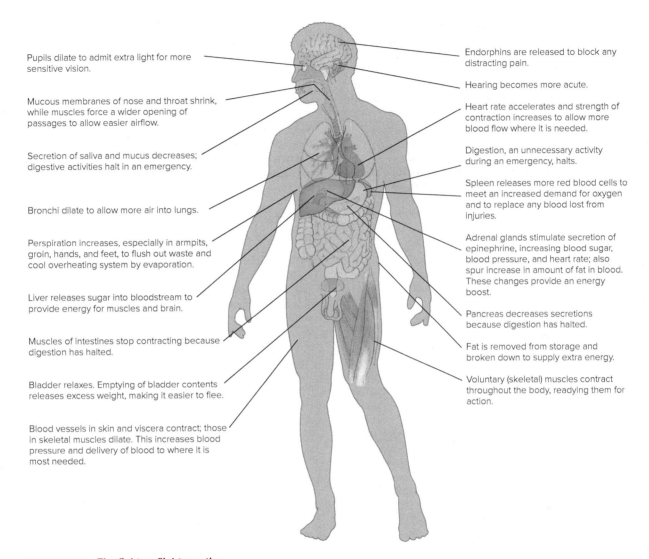

Pupils dilate to admit extra light for more sensitive vision.

Mucous membranes of nose and throat shrink, while muscles force a wider opening of passages to allow easier airflow.

Secretion of saliva and mucus decreases; digestive activities halt in an emergency.

Bronchi dilate to allow more air into lungs.

Perspiration increases, especially in armpits, groin, hands, and feet, to flush out waste and cool overheating system by evaporation.

Liver releases sugar into bloodstream to provide energy for muscles and brain.

Muscles of intestines stop contracting because digestion has halted.

Bladder relaxes. Emptying of bladder contents releases excess weight, making it easier to flee.

Blood vessels in skin and viscera contract; those in skeletal muscles dilate. This increases blood pressure and delivery of blood to where it is most needed.

Endorphins are released to block any distracting pain.

Hearing becomes more acute.

Heart rate accelerates and strength of contraction increases to allow more blood flow where it is needed.

Digestion, an unnecessary activity during an emergency, halts.

Spleen releases more red blood cells to meet an increased demand for oxygen and to replace any blood lost from injuries.

Adrenal glands stimulate secretion of epinephrine, increasing blood sugar, blood pressure, and heart rate; also spur increase in amount of fat in blood. These changes provide an energy boost.

Pancreas decreases secretions because digestion has halted.

Fat is removed from storage and broken down to supply extra energy.

Voluntary (skeletal) muscles contract throughout the body, readying them for action.

FIGURE 10.1 The fight-or-flight reaction.

The Two Systems Together How do both systems work together in an emergency? Let's go back to your near-collision with a car. Reflexes as well as higher cognitive (thinking) areas in your brain quickly determine that you are facing a threat, and your body prepares to meet the danger. The two systems activate the adrenal glands, causing the release of the hormones **cortisol** and **epinephrine** (also called *adrenaline*). These hormones trigger the physiological changes shown in Figure 10.1, including these:

- Heart and respiration rates accelerate to speed oxygen through the body.
- Hearing and vision become more acute.
- The liver releases extra sugar into the bloodstream to boost energy.
- Perspiration increases to cool the skin.
- The brain releases **endorphins**—chemicals that can inhibit or block sensations of pain—in case you are injured.

norepinephrine A neurotransmitter released by ⬤ **TERMS** the sympathetic nervous system onto specific tissues to increase their function in the face of increased activity; when released by the brain, causes arousal (increased attention, awareness, and alertness); also called *noradrenaline*.

endocrine system The system of glands, tissues, and cells that secretes hormones into the bloodstream to influence metabolism and other body processes.

hormone A chemical messenger produced in the body and transported in the bloodstream to targeted cells or organs for specific regulation of their activities.

cortisol A hormone secreted by the cortex (outer layer) of the adrenal gland; also called *hydrocortisone*.

epinephrine A hormone secreted by the medulla (inner core) of the adrenal gland that affects the functioning of organs involved in responding to a stressor; also called *adrenaline*.

endorphins Brain secretions that have pain-inhibiting effects.

and build energy reserves. When the next crisis comes, you'll be ready to respond again.

The Fight-or-Flight Reaction in Modern Life The fight-or-flight reaction is a part of our biological heritage, a survival mechanism that has served both humans and animals well. In modern life, however, it is often absurdly inappropriate. Many stressors we face in everyday life—such as an exam, a mess left by a roommate, or a stop light—do not require a physical response. The fight-or-flight reaction prepares the body for physical action regardless of whether such action is a necessary or appropriate response to a particular stressor.

Psychological and Behavioral Responses to Stressors

We all experience a similar set of physical responses to stressors (the fight-or-flight reaction). Nevertheless, these responses vary from person to person and from one situation to another. People's perceptions of potential stressors—and their responses to them—also vary greatly. You may feel confident about taking exams but nervous about talking to people you don't know, while your roommate may love challenging social situations but dread taking tests.

Your cognitive appraisal of a potential stressor—how you think about it—strongly influences how you respond to it. Two factors that can reduce the magnitude of the stress response are successful prediction and the perception of control. For instance, receiving course syllabi at the beginning of the term allows you to predict the timing of major deadlines and exams. This gives you control over your study plans and can help reduce the stress caused by exams.

The way we appraise potentially stressful situations is highly individual and strongly related to emotions. The facts of a situation—Who? What? Where? When?—are typically evaluated in the same way by each person. However, different people can evaluate the potential personal outcomes of a situation very differently: What does this mean for me? Can I do anything about it? Will it get better or worse? If you think you can't cope with a situation, you may respond negatively and with an inappropriate stress response. On the other hand, if you approach a situation as a challenge you can manage, you are likely to have a more positive and appropriate response. A moderate level of stress, if handled appropriately, can actually promote optimal performance (Figure 10.2).

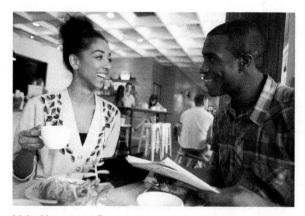

Wellness Tip Many people experience the set of almost-instantaneous physical changes that make up the stress response, such as increased heart rate and sweaty hands and feet, in reaction to positive stressors, such as a first date. Recognize the symptoms for what they are. If the physical stress response isn't appropriate for the situation, try a quick relaxation technique such as deep breathing.
©Monkeybusinessimages/Getty Images RF

Taken together, these almost-instantaneous physical changes are called the **fight-or-flight reaction**. They give you the heightened reflexes and strength you need to dodge the car or respond appropriately in the face of other stressors. Although these physical changes may vary in intensity, the same basic set of physical reactions occurs in response to any type of stressor—positive or negative, physical or psychological.

The Return to Homeostasis A short time after your near miss with the car, you begin to feel normal again. When a stressful situation ends, the parasympathetic division of your autonomic nervous system takes command and halts the stress response. It restores **homeostasis**, a state in which your body maintains blood pressure, heart rate, hormone levels, and other vital functions within a narrow range of normal. Your parasympathetic nervous system calms your body down, slowing a rapid heartbeat, drying sweaty palms, and returning breathing to normal. Gradually, your body resumes its normal "housekeeping" functions, such as digestion and temperature regulation. Some damage sustained during the fight-or-flight reaction can be repaired. The day after you narrowly dodge the car, you wake up feeling fine. In this way, your body can grow, repair itself,

Effective and Ineffective Responses Common responses to stressors include anxiety, depression, and fear. Although emotional responses are part of personality or temperament, we can learn to control them. Coping techniques are discussed later in the chapter.

Our less emotional, more mindful and behavioral responses to stressors are controlled by the **somatic nervous system**, which manages our conscious actions. Effective behavioral responses such as talking, laughing, exercising, meditating, learning time-management skills, and becoming more assertive can promote wellness and enable us to function at our best. Ineffective behavioral responses to stressors include

---

fight-or-flight reaction A defense reaction that prepares a person for conflict or escape by triggering hormonal, cardiovascular, metabolic, and other changes.

homeostasis A state of stability and consistency in a person's physiological functioning.

somatic nervous system The branch of the peripheral nervous system that governs motor functions and sensory information, largely under conscious control.

personality The sum of behavioral, cognitive, and emotional tendencies.

TERMS

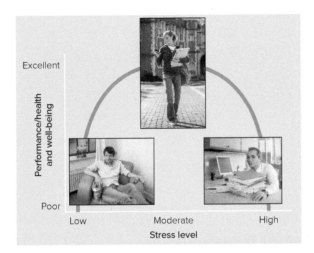

FIGURE 10.2   Stress level, performance, and well-being. A moderate level of stress challenges individuals in a way that promotes optimal performance and well-being. Too little stress, and people are not challenged enough to improve; too much stress, and the challenges become stressors that can impair physical and emotional health.
(low): ©Image Source/Getty Images RF; (moderate): ©John Fedele/Blend Images/Getty Images RF; (high): ©John Lund/Drew Kell /Blend Images LLC RF

overeating; expressing hostility; and using tobacco, alcohol, or other drugs.

Personality and Stress   You probably know some people who are nervous, irritable, and easily upset by minor annoyances, and other people who are calm and composed even in difficult situations. **Personality**—the sum of behavioral, cognitive, and emotional tendencies—clearly affects how people perceive and react to stressors. To investigate the links among personality, stress, and wellness, researchers have looked at characteristics, "personality types," and "personality traits."

PERSONALITY TYPES   Depending on the situation, most of us display some of the behaviors characteristic of one or more of the following types:

- *Type A.* People with Type A personality are described as ultracompetitive, controlling, impatient, aggressive, and even hostile. Type A people have a higher perceived stress level and more problems coping with stress. They may react explosively to stressors and are upset by events that others would consider only annoyances. Studies suggest that certain characteristics of the Type A pattern—anger, cynicism, and hostility—increase the risk of heart disease.
- *Type B.* The Type B personality is relaxed and contemplative. Type B people are less frustrated by daily events and more tolerant of the behavior of others.
- *Type C.* The Type C personality is characterized by anger suppression, difficulty expressing emotions, feelings of hopelessness and despair, and an exaggerated response to minor stressors.
- *Type D.* The Type D personality tends toward negative emotional states such as anxiety, depression, and

irritability. Type D people also avoid social interactions, worrying that others will react negatively toward them. Having this kind of personality predicts a number of poor health outcomes, including cardiovascular disease.

PERSONALITY TRAITS   Researchers have also looked for personality traits that enable people to deal more successfully with stress. One such trait is *hardiness,* a form of optimism. People with a hardy personality view potential stressors as challenges and opportunities for growth and learning, rather than as burdens. Hardy people perceive fewer situations as stressful, and their reaction to stressors tends to be less intense. They are committed to their activities, have a sense of inner purpose and an inner locus of control, and feel at least partly in control of their lives.

Personality traits related to motivation also affect how people behave. Two types of motivation have been studied that relate to stress and health. *Stressed power motivation* is associated with people who are aggressive and argumentative, and who need to have power over others. One study of college students found that persons with this personality trait tend to get sick when their need for power is blocked or threatened. In contrast, people with *unstressed affiliation motivation* are drawn to others and want to be liked as friends. The same study of college students found that students with this trait reported the fewest illnesses.

Another important personality trait—*resilience*—is especially associated with social and academic success in groups at risk for stress, such as people from low-income families and those with mental or physical disabilities. Resilient people tend to face adversity by accepting the reality of their situation, holding on to a belief that life is meaningful, and possessing a great ability to improvise.

Academic resilience helps college students flourish. Whether they need to bounce back from a poor grade or negative feedback, or master the art of juggling multiple academic pressures, students can learn techniques to stay or become resilient. One technique is to identify resources such as peers and counselors to lean on in times of crisis.

Contemporary research is repeatedly demonstrating that you can change some basic elements of your personality as well as your typical behaviors and patterns of thinking by using positive stress-management techniques like those described later in the chapter.

Gender and Stress   Your gender role—the activities, abilities, and behaviors your culture expects based on your sex—can affect your experience of stress. Some behavioral responses to stressors, such as crying or openly expressing anger, may be deemed more appropriate for one gender than another.

Strict adherence to gender roles, however, can limit your response to stress and can itself become a source of stress. Gender roles can also affect your perception of a stressor. For example, some medical situations may be more stressful for gay or bisexual men because they are often stereotyped as being HIV positive.

Since the American Psychological Association began its yearly "Stress in America" survey in 2007, women have reported a higher level of stress than men. In 2016, 12% of female college students reported "tremendous stress," as compared to 9% of male college students. In her book *Overwhelmed,* Brigid Schulte describes a continuing unequal gendered division of labor: Families are working more hours than they used to, but

American women spend even more time with their children than they did in the 1960s. How is this possible? Mothers tend to choose jobs that are flexible rather than high powered, and they spend less time cleaning (either hiring someone else or leaving their houses dirtier), sleep less, and take less time for themselves.

Cultural Background Because young adults from around the world come to the United States for a higher education, most students finish college with a greater appreciation for other cultures and worldviews. The clash of cultures, however, can be a big source of stress for many students—especially when it leads to disrespectful treatment, harassment, or violence. Everyone's reaction to stress is influenced by his or her upbringing and cultural background. Learning to accept and appreciate the cultural backgrounds of other people is both a mind-opening experience and a way to avoid stress over cultural differences.

Experience Past experiences can profoundly influence the way you evaluate a potential stressor. If you had a bad experience giving a speech in the past, you are much more likely to perceive an upcoming speech as stressful than someone who has had positive public-speaking experiences. Effective behavioral responses, such as preparing carefully and visualizing success, can help overcome the effects of negative past experiences.

PHYSICAL SYMPTOMS	EMOTIONAL SYMPTOMS	BEHAVIORAL SYMPTOMS
Dry mouth	Anxiety	Crying
Excessive perspiration	Depression	Disrupted eating habits
Frequent illnesses	Edginess	Disrupted sleeping habits
Gastrointestinal problems	Fatigue	Harsh treatment of others
Grinding of teeth	Hypervigilance	Problems communicating
Headaches	Impulsiveness	Sexual problems
High blood pressure	Inability to concentrate	Social isolation
Pounding heart	Irritability	Increased use of tobacco, alcohol, or other drugs
Stiff neck or aching lower back	Trouble remembering things	

FIGURE 10.3 Symptoms of excessive stress.
(man rubbing neck): ©Fancy Collection/SuperStock RF; (woman sitting in corner): ©Izf/Getty Images RF; (couple arguing): ©Latin Stock Collection/Corbis RF

the emotional response, the stronger the physical response. Sometimes people have such intense responses to stressors or such ineffective coping techniques that they need professional help. More often, however, people can learn to handle stressors on their own (see the section "Managing Stress" later in the chapter).

STRESS AND WELLNESS

According to the American Psychological Association's Stress in America survey, the average overall stress level among Americans rose between 2016 and 2017, the first significant increase since the survey began in 2007. Increased stress rates corresponded to higher levels of physical and emotional stress symptoms: 80% of respondents reported having at least one symptom of stress in the past month. The role of stress in health is complex, but evidence suggests that stress can increase our vulnerability to many ailments. Several theories have been proposed to explain the relationship between stress and disease.

The General Adaptation Syndrome

The concepts of homeostasis (inner balance) and adaptations to stressors came from the work of several scientists across the 20th century. The **general adaptation syndrome (GAS)**, developed by biologist Hans Selye beginning in the 1930s and 1940s, is a theory that describes a universal and predictable response pattern to all stressors. It identifies an automatic self-regulation system of the mind and body that attempts to return the body to a state of homeostasis after being subjected to stress.

Some stressors are viewed as pleasant, such as attending a party, while others are viewed as unpleasant, such as getting a bad grade. In the GAS theory, stress triggered by a positive stressor is called **eustress**; stress triggered by a negative stressor is called **distress**. The sequence of physical responses associated with GAS (Figure 10.4) is the same for both eustress and distress and occurs in three stages:

The Stress Experience as a Whole

As Figure 10.3 shows, the physical, emotional, and behavioral symptoms of excess negative stress are distinct, but you might guess that they are also intimately interrelated. The more intense

general adaptation syndrome (GAS) A pattern **TERMS** of stress responses consisting of three stages: alarm, resistance, and exhaustion.

eustress Stress resulting from a pleasant stressor.

distress Stress resulting from an unpleasant stressor.

allostatic load The long-term negative impact of the stress response on the body.

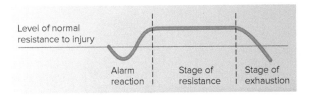

FIGURE 10.4 The general adaptation syndrome. During the alarm stage, a lower resistance to injury is evident. With continued stress, resistance to injury is actually enhanced. With prolonged exposure to repeated stressors, exhaustion sets in, with a return of low resistance levels seen during acute stress.

Ask Yourself

QUESTIONS FOR CRITICAL THINKING AND REFLECTION

Have you ever been so stressed that you felt ill in some way? If so, what were your symptoms? How did you handle them? Did the experience affect the way you reacted to other stressful events?

- *Alarm.* The alarm stage includes the complex sequence of events brought on by the fight-or-flight reaction. At this stage, the body is more susceptible to disease or injury because it is geared up to deal with a crisis. Someone in this phase may experience headaches, indigestion, anxiety, and disrupted sleeping and eating patterns.

- *Resistance.* With continued stress, the body develops a new level of homeostasis in which it is more resistant to disease and injury than normal. In this stage, a person can cope with normal life and added stress.

- *Exhaustion.* The first two stages of GAS require a great deal of energy. If a stressor persists, or if several stressors occur in succession, general exhaustion results. This is not the sort of exhaustion you feel after a long, busy day. Rather, it's a life-threatening type of physiological exhaustion.

Stress research further advanced in the 1970s and 1980s with the advent of *biofeedback techniques.* Researchers developed instruments to measure brain waves, skin conduction, heart rates, and muscle tone (see discussion of biofeedback in the section "Managing Stress"). These tools allow the study of specific immediate and long-term impacts of the stress response.

Allostatic Load

The wear and tear on the body that results from long-term exposure to repeated or chronic stress is called the **allostatic load**. A person's allostatic load depends on many factors, including genetics, life experiences, and emotional and behavioral responses to stressors. The concept of allostatic load explains how frequent activation of the body's stress response, although essential for managing acute threats, can damage the body in the long run. For example, a student who suffers from test anxiety manages a week of exams but collapses on the weekend with a severe cold. Although physical stress reactions may promote a new level of homeostasis (resistance stage of GAS), they also have negative effects on the body. The increased susceptibility to disease after repeated or prolonged stress may be due to effects of the stress response itself rather than to a depletion of resources (exhaustion stage of GAS). Over time, the student's allostatic load, along with susceptibility to disease, can increase. Allostatic load is generally measured through indicators of cumulative strain on several organs and tissues, especially on the cardiovascular system.

Stress and Specific Conditions

Although much remains to be learned, it is clear that people who have unresolved chronic stress in their lives or who handle stressors poorly are at risk for a wide range of health problems. In the short term, the problem might just be a cold or a stomachache. Over the long term, the problems can be more severe, such as reduced functioning of the immune system and cardiovascular disease.

Stress and the Immune System Studies of the stress hormones cortisol and epinephrine have provided a physical link between emotions and immune function. In general, increased levels of stress hormones are linked to a decrease in the number or functioning of immune system cells. Some of the health problems linked to stress-related changes in immune function include vulnerability to colds and other infections, asthma and allergy attacks, and flare-ups of chronic diseases such as genital herpes. Stress reactions over a prolonged length of time can have a negative impact on health.

Chronic (ongoing) stressors such as unemployment have negative effects on almost all functional measures of immunity. *Chronic stress* may cause prolonged secretion of cortisol (sometimes called the "antistress hormone" because it seeks to return the nervous system to homeostasis after a stress reaction) and may accelerate the course of diseases that involve inflammation, including multiple sclerosis, heart disease, type 2 diabetes, and clinical depression.

Mood, personality, behavior, and immune functioning are intertwined. For example, people who are generally pessimistic may neglect the basics of health care, become passive when ill, and fail to engage in health-promoting behaviors. People who are depressed may reduce physical activity and social interaction, which may in turn affect the immune system and the cognitive appraisal of a stressor. Optimism, successful coping, and positive problem solving, by contrast, may positively influence immunity.

Cardiovascular Disease The stress response profoundly affects the cardiovascular system. During the stress response, heart rate increases, blood vessels constrict, and blood pressure rises. Chronic high blood pressure is a major cause of strokes and heart attacks (Chapter 11). As a related matter, people who react to situations with anger and hostility are more likely to have heart attacks than are people with less explosive, more relaxed personalities.

Other Health Problems Many other health problems may be caused or worsened by excessive stress, including the following:

- Digestive problems such as stomachaches, diarrhea, constipation, irritable bowel syndrome, and ulcers
- Tension headaches and migraines
- Insomnia and fatigue
- Injuries, including on-the-job injuries caused by repetitive strain
- Menstrual irregularities, impotence, and pregnancy complications
- Psychological problems, including depression, anxiety, panic attacks, eating disorders, and posttraumatic stress disorder (PTSD), which afflicts people who have suffered or witnessed severe trauma

COMMON SOURCES OF STRESS

Recognizing potential sources of stress is an important step in successfully managing the stress in your life.

Major Life Changes

Any major change in your life that requires adjustment and accommodation can be a source of stress. Early adulthood and the college years are associated with many significant changes, such as moving out of the family home and into a new, unfamiliar environment. Even changes typically thought of as positive—graduation, job promotion, marriage—can be stressful.

Life changes that are traumatic, such as getting fired or divorced or experiencing the death of a loved one, may be linked to subsequent health problems in some people. Personality and coping skills, however, are important moderating influences. People with a strong support network and a stress-resistant personality are less likely to become ill in response to life changes than are people with fewer resources.

Daily Hassles

Although major life changes are undoubtedly stressful, they seldom occur regularly. Researchers have proposed that minor problems—life's daily hassles, such as losing your keys or sitting in traffic—can be an even greater source of stress because they occur much more often.

People who perceive hassles negatively are likely to experience a moderate stress response every time they are faced with one. Over time, this can take a significant toll on health. Studies indicate that for some people, daily hassles contribute to a general decrease in overall wellness.

College Stressors

College is a time of major changes and minor hassles. For many students, college means being away from home and family

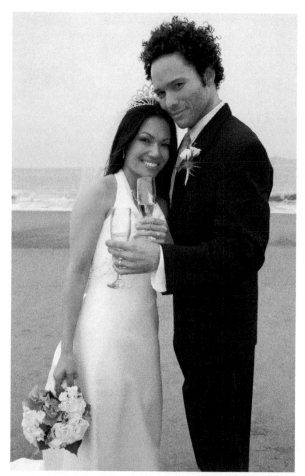

Wellness Tip Even a joyful occasion can be a source of stress, especially if it involves a major life change. To combat the stress of major life changes, develop a strong social support network and focus on the positive opportunities presented by the changes.
©VStock LLC/Tanya Constantine/VStock/Alamy Stock Photo RF

for the first time. Nearly all students share stresses like the following:

- *Academic stress.* Exams, grades, and an endless workload await every college student but can be especially troublesome for young students just out of high school.
- *Interpersonal stress.* All students are more than just students; they are also friends, sons and daughters, employees, spouses, parents, and so on. Managing relationships while juggling the rigors of college life can be daunting.
- *Time pressures.* Class schedules, assignments, and deadlines are an inescapable part of college life. But these time pressures can be compounded dramatically for students who also have a job or family responsibilities.
- *Financial concerns.* The majority of college students need financial aid not just to cover the cost of tuition but also to survive from day to day while in school. For many,

college life isn't possible without a job, and the pressure to stay afloat financially competes with academic and other stressors.

- *Worries about the future.* As college life comes to an end, students face the reality of life after college. This means thinking about a career, choosing a place to live, and leaving behind the friends and routines of school.

Job-Related Stressors

Work was the second highest reported source of stress for Americans in 2016 (money was the first), according to the Stress in America survey. Tight schedules and overtime leave less time for exercising, socializing, and other stress-proofing activities. Worries about job performance, salary, job security, and interactions with others can contribute to stress. High levels of job stress are also common for people who are left out of important decisions relating to their jobs. When workers are given the opportunity to shape their job descriptions and responsibilities, job satisfaction goes up and stress levels go down.

If job-related (or college-related) stress is severe or chronic, the result can be *burnout,* a state of physical, mental, and emotional exhaustion. Burnout occurs most often in highly motivated and driven individuals who come to feel that their work is not recognized or that they are not accomplishing their goals. People in the helping professions—teachers, social workers, caregivers, police officers, and so on—are also prone to burnout. For some people who suffer from burnout, a vacation or leave of absence may be appropriate. For others, a reduced work schedule, better communication with superiors, or a change in job goals may be necessary. Improving time-management skills can also help.

Relationships and Stress

Human beings need social relationships; we cannot thrive as solitary creatures. Simply put, people need people. Even so, our interpersonal relationships—even our deepest, most intimate ones—can be one of the most significant sources of stress in our life.

The first relationships we form outside the family are friendships. With members of either the same or the other sex, friendships give people the opportunity to share themselves and discover others. Friendships are often more stable and longer lasting than intimate partnerships. Because expectations surrounding friends differ from those surrounding romantic partners, friends are often more accepting and less critical than lovers. During times of stress, in fact, many people initially turn to their friends for comfort, rather than family members or lovers.

Intimate love relationships are among the most profound human experiences. When two people fall in love, their relationship at first is likely to be characterized by high levels of passion and rapidly increasing intimacy. In time, passion decreases as the partners become more familiar. The diminishing passion can create stress (usually affecting one partner more than the other) and can be experienced as a crisis in the relationship. If a quieter, more lasting love fails to emerge, the relationship will likely break up, and each person will search for another who will once again ignite his or her passion.

The key to developing and maintaining any type of friendship or intimate relationship is good communication. Miscommunication creates frustration and distances us from our friends and partners. (For more information, see the section "Communication" later in this chapter.)

Social Stressors

Social networks can be real or virtual. Both types can improve your ability to deal with stress, but they can also become stressors.

Real Social Networks The college years can be a time of great change in interpersonal relationships—becoming part of a new community, meeting people from different backgrounds, leaving old relationships behind. You may feel stress as you meet people of other ethnic, racial, or socioeconomic groups. You may feel torn between sticking with people who share your background versus connecting with individuals and groups you've not encountered before. If English is not your first language, you may face the added burden of interacting in a language with which you are not completely comfortable. All these pressures can become significant sources of stress. (See the box "Diverse Populations, Discrimination, and Stress.")

Virtual Social Networks Technology can connect you with people all over the world and make many tasks easier, but it can also increase stress. Being electronically connected to work, family, and friends all the time can impinge on your personal space, waste time, and distract you. The 2017 Stress in America survey looked at "constant checkers"—the 43% of Americans who report continually checking their e-mails, texts, or social media accounts. These constant checkers report higher levels of overall stress than those who do not engage with technology as frequently. They are also more likely to report feeling disconnected from their family as a result of technology and to being stressed by political and cultural discussions on social media. Many Americans feel that taking breaks from technology is important for mental health, but fewer than 30% of them actually do so.

Other Stressors

Environmental stressors are external conditions or events that cause stress and include a noisy atmosphere, unpleasant odors, pollen, industrial accidents, violence, and natural disasters. (See Appendix A for preparation and coping strategies for large-scale disasters.) Internal stressors are the pressures we put on ourselves to reach personal goals. Striving to reach goals can enhance self-esteem if the goals are reasonable, but unrealistic expectations can damage self-esteem and become a significant source of stress. Physical states such as illness and exhaustion, and emotional states such as despair or hostility, are also internal stressors.

DIVERSITY MATTERS
Diverse Populations, Discrimination, and Stress

Stress is universal, but an individual's response to stress can vary depending on gender, cultural background, prior experience, and genetic factors. In diverse multiethnic and multicultural nations such as the United States, some groups face special stressors and have higher-than-average rates of stress-related physical and emotional problems. These groups include ethnic and sexual minorities, the poor, and those with physical or mental disabilities.

Discrimination occurs when people speak or act according to their prejudices—biased, negative beliefs or attitudes toward a group. Rising to the level of hate speech and criminal activity would be painting a swastika on a Jewish community center or vandalizing a mosque. A more subtle example would be when Middle Eastern American or African American students in mostly white college towns notice that shopkeepers tend to monitor them more closely. More than 60% of U.S. adults report experiencing day-to-day discrimination, such as being treated with less courtesy or respect, receiving poorer service than others, or being harassed or threatened.

Immigrants to the United States have to learn to live in a new society.

Doing so requires a balance between assimilating to fit in with the majority culture and maintaining a connection to their own culture, language, and religion. The process of acculturation is a two-way street: Both the newcomers and the established members of the community adapt to each other. This process of adapting is generally stressful, especially when our background is radically different from that of our neighbors, or when people are suspicious or unwelcoming. The stress induced by prejudice, denial of civil rights, and social rejection in general can show up in outward symptoms of chronic stress and unhealthy coping behaviors, as well as in internal disruptions at the hormonal level.

One study using 20 years of data found that the more racial discrimination participants reported experiencing or perceiving, the more dysfunctional their cortisol rhythms were. Cortisol levels normally start high in the morning, decrease throughout the day, and lower in the evening. But constant stress can alter this rhythm, keeping cortisol levels flat during the day and high at night. Irregular cortisol rhythms are linked with weakened immunity, cardiovascular disease, mental health and cognitive problems like impaired

memory, as well as fatigue and disrupted sleep. Another study showed that while perceived discrimination produces stress in both blacks and whites, its impact on cortisol rhythms was greater for the black participants.

Many people who experience hardship and prejudice develop effective goal-directed coping skills. Some of these skills include building support networks where people share experiences; discovering and maintaining a strong cultural identity (for example, taking a class on the history of one's own cultural background, or joining campus cultural groups); and joining groups working for social action and equality.

SOURCES: Adam, E. K., et al. 2015. Developmental histories of perceived racial discrimination and diurnal cortisol profiles in adulthood. *Psychoneuroendocrinology* 62: 279–91; American Psychological Association. 2016. *Stress in America: The Impact of Discrimination.* Washington, DC: American Psychological Association; Anderson, K. F. 2013. Diagnosing discrimination: Stress from perceived racism and the mental and physical health effects. *Sociological Inquiry* 83: 55–81; Cook, S. H., et al. 2017. Cortisol profiles differ by race/ethnicity among young sexual minority men. *Psychoneuroendocrinology* 75: 1–4.

Box icon: ©Rawpixel Ltd/Getty Images RF

MANAGING STRESS

Can you do anything about all this stress? A great deal.

- Develop healthy exercise and eating habits.
- Shore up your support system.
- Improve your communication skills.
- Identify and moderate individual stressors.
- Practice relaxation and mindfulness techniques.

Adequate sleep is another key strategy for managing stress and for improving your overall wellness. See the section "Sleep" later in the chapter.

Exercise

Researchers have found that people who exercise regularly react with milder physical stress responses before, during, and after

exposure to stressors. Exercisers' overall sense of well-being increases as well (see the box "Does Exercise Improve Mental Health?"). Although even light exercise can have a beneficial effect, an integrated fitness program can have a significant impact on stress.

For some people, however, exercise can become just one more stressor in an already stressful life. People who exercise compulsively risk overtraining, a condition characterized by fatigue, irritability, depression, and diminished athletic performance. An overly strenuous exercise program can even make a person sick by compromising immune function. (For information on creating a safe and effective exercise program, refer to Chapter 7.)

Nutrition

A healthy, balanced diet can help you cope with stress. Eating wisely enhances your feelings of self-control and self-esteem.

THE EVIDENCE FOR EXERCISE
Does Exercise Improve Mental Health?

The overall conclusion from many published studies is that exercise—even modest activity such as taking a daily walk—can combat a variety of mental health problems. Overall, physically active people who exercise 2.5–7.5 hours per week are about 25–30% less likely to feel anxious or stressed than inactive people. Regardless of the number, age, or health status of the people being studied, those who were active managed stress better than their inactive counterparts. Among athletic teenagers, there is a correlation between exercise and improved social interaction, as well as between exercise and improved body image, two factors that contribute to good mental health. Physical activity has also been shown to improve conditions for people with anxiety; with affective, eating, and substance use disorders; and with schizophrenia and dementia.

A simple walk can be very effective: One study found that taking a long walk can reduce anxiety and blood pressure. Another showed that a brisk walk of as little as 10 minutes' duration can leave people feeling more relaxed and energetic for up to two hours. People who took three brisk 45-minute walks each week for three months reported that they perceived fewer daily hassles and had a greater sense of general wellness.

These findings are not surprising. The stress response mobilizes energy resources and readies the body for physical emergencies. If you experience stress and do not exert yourself physically, you are not completing the energy cycle. You may not be able to exercise while your daily stressors are occurring, but you can be active later in the day. Such activity allows you to expend the nervous energy you have built up and trains your body to return more readily to homeostasis after stressful situations. Physical activity also helps you sleep better, which is in turn critical to managing stress (see the section "Sleep" later in the chapter). Regular activity promotes better sleep and provides some protection against sleep interruptions such as insomnia and sleep apnea. Consistent, restful sleep is now regarded as a protective factor in disorders such as depression, anxiety, obesity, and heart disease.

SOURCES: Stubs, B., et al. 2017. An examination of the anxiolytic effects of exercise for people with anxiety and stress-related disorders: A meta-analysis. *Psychiatry Research* 249: 102–108; Kim, Y. S., et al. 2012. Relationship between physical activity and general mental health. *Preventive Medicine* 55(5):458–463; Zschucke, E., et al. 2013. Exercise and physical activity in mental disorders: Clinical and experimental evidence. *Journal of Preventive Medicine and Public Health* J46 (Suppl. 1): S12–S21; Eime, R. M., et al. 2013. A systematic review of the psychological and social benefits of participation in sport for children and adolescents: Informing development of a conceptual model of health through sport. *International Journal of Behavioral Nutrition and Physical Activity* 10: 98.

Box Icon: ©Vstock LLC/Getty Images RF

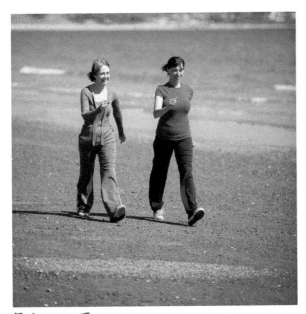

Fitness Tip Stressed out? Then walk away—literally. Walking is a proven countermeasure against stress. A brisk, 10-minute walk may be enough to help you put things in perspective and get back to your normal routine. If not, just keep walking until you feel better. As you walk, try not to think too much about anything specific; the idea is to clear your head!
©Pamplemousse/Getty Images RF

Avoiding or limiting caffeine may also be important in stress management. Caffeine, a mildly addictive stimulant, leaves some people jittery, irritable, and unable to sleep. Consuming caffeine during stressful situations can raise blood pressure and increase levels of cortisol. (For more on sound nutrition and for advice on evaluating dietary supplements, many of which are marketed for stress management, see Chapter 8.)

Social Support

Meaningful connections with others can play a key role in stress management and overall wellness. One study of college students living in overcrowded apartments, for example, found that those with a strong social support system were less distressed by their cramped quarters than those who navigated life's challenges on their own. Other studies have shown that married people live longer than single people and have lower death rates from a wide range of conditions, although some studies suggest that marriage benefits men more than women. A sense of isolation can lead to chronic stress, which in turn can increase one's susceptibility to illnesses like colds and to chronic illnesses, such as heart disease. Although the mechanism isn't clear, social isolation can be as significant to mortality rates as factors like smoking, high blood pressure, and obesity.

There is no single best pattern of social support that works for everyone. However, research suggests that having a variety of types of relationships may be important for wellness. Here are some tips for strengthening your social ties:

- *Foster friendships.* Keep in regular contact with your friends. Offer respect, trust, and acceptance, and provide help and support in times of need. Build your communication skills, and express appreciation for your friends.

- *Keep your family ties strong.* Stay in touch with the family members you feel close to. If your family doesn't function well as a support system for its members, create a second "family" of people with whom you have built meaningful ties.

- *Get involved with a group.* Do volunteer work, take a class, attend a lecture series, or join a religious group. These types of activities can give you a sense of security, a place to talk about your feelings or concerns, and a way to build new friendships. Choose activities that are meaningful to you and that include direct involvement with other people.

Communication

Good communication skills can help everyone form and maintain healthy relationships. Communicating in an assertive, confident way that respects the rights of others—as well as your own—can prevent potentially stressful situations from getting out of control. When friends or partners communicate effectively, they can reduce the stresses in their relationship and spend more time focusing on the positive aspects of being together.

Three keys to good communication in relationships are self-disclosure, listening, and feedback:

Wellness Tip Social support can be a key means of reducing stress. College offers many antidotes to loneliness in the forms of clubs, organized activities, sports, and just hanging out with friends.
©Lori Adamski Peek/Getty Images

- *Self-disclosure* involves revealing personal information that we ordinarily wouldn't reveal because of the risk involved. It usually increases feelings of closeness and moves the relationship to a deeper level of intimacy.

- *Listening* is a rare skill. Those with good listening skills focus their time and energy on fully understanding another person's "story" rather than on judging, evaluating, blaming, advising, analyzing, or trying to control. Empathy, warmth, respect, and genuineness are qualities of skillful listeners. Attentive listening encourages friends or partners to share more and, in turn, to be attentive listeners. To connect with other people and develop real emotional intimacy, listening is essential.

- *Feedback,* a constructive response to another's self-disclosure, is the third key to good communication. Giving positive feedback means acknowledging that the friend's or partner's feelings are valid—no matter how upsetting or troubling—and offering self-disclosure in response. Self-disclosure and feedback can open the door to change.

For tips on improving your communication skills, see the box "Guidelines for Effective Communication."

Some people have trouble telling others what they need or saying no to the needs of others. They may suppress their feelings of anger, frustration, and resentment, and they may end up feeling taken advantage of or suffering in unhealthy relationships. At the other extreme are people who express anger openly and directly by being verbally or physically aggressive or indirectly by making critical, hurtful comments to others. Their abusive behavior pushes other people away, so they also have problems with relationships.

If you typically suppress your feelings, you might want to take an assertiveness training course that can help you identify and change your patterns of communication. If you have trouble controlling your anger, you can benefit from learning anger-management strategies; see the box "Dealing with Anger."

Conflict Resolution

Conflict is natural in any relationship, and it can become a key source of stress for friends, coworkers, family members, and intimate partners. No matter how close two people become, they still remain separate individuals with their own needs, desires, past experiences, and ways of seeing the world. Conflict itself isn't dangerous to a relationship; it may simply indicate that the relationship is growing. But if it isn't handled in a constructive way, conflict can damage—and ultimately destroy—a relationship.

Conflict is often accompanied by anger—a universal emotion, but one that can be difficult to handle. When angry, both

TAKE CHARGE
Guidelines for Effective Communication

Getting Started

- When you want to have a serious discussion with your partner, choose an appropriate time and place. Find a private place and a time when you will not be interrupted. Avoid having important conversations via text or other media.

- Face your partner and maintain eye contact. Use nonverbal feedback (gestures and facial expressions) to show you are interested and involved in the communication process.

Managing Conflicts

- State your concern or issue as clearly as you can.

- Use "I" statements—statements about how *you* feel—rather than statements beginning with "You," which tell another person how you think he or she feels. When you use "I" statements, you are taking responsibility for your feelings. "You" statements are often blaming or accusatory and may get a defensive or resentful response. "I feel unloved," sends a clearer, less blaming message than "You don't love me."

- Focus on a specific behavior rather than on the whole person. Be specific about the behavior you like or don't like. Avoid generalizations beginning with "You always" or "You never." Such statements make people feel defensive.

- Make constructive requests. Opening your request with "I would like" keeps the focus on your needs rather than on your partner's deficiencies.

- Avoid blaming, accusing, and belittling. Even if you are right, you have little to gain by putting people down. Studies have shown that when people feel criticized or attacked, they are less able to think rationally or solve problems constructively.

- Set your partner up for success. Tell your partner what you would like to have happen in the future; don't wait for him or her to blow it and then express anger or disappointment.

Being an Effective Listener

- Provide appropriate nonverbal feedback.

- Don't interrupt.

- Develop the skill of reflective listening. Don't judge, evaluate, analyze, or offer solutions (unless asked to do so). Your partner may just need to have you there in order to sort out feelings. By jumping in right away to "fix" the problem, you may be cutting off communication.

- Don't offer unsolicited advice. Giving advice implies that you know more about what a person needs to do than he or she does; therefore, it often evokes anger or resentment.

- Clarify your understanding of what your partner is saying by restating it in your own words and asking if your understanding is correct.

- Be sure you are really listening, not off somewhere in your mind rehearsing your reply. Tune in to your partner's feelings and needs as well as the words. Accurately reflecting the other person's feelings and needs is often a more powerful way of connecting than just reframing his or her thoughts.

- Let your partner know that you value what she or he is saying and want to understand. Respect for the other person is the cornerstone of effective communication.

Box icon: ©VisualsCommunications/Getty Images RF

---

parties should back off, calm down, and then come back to the issue later to try to resolve it rationally.

Negotiation helps dissipate anger so the conflict can be resolved. Some basic strategies are useful in successfully negotiating with a friend, family member, colleague, or intimate partner:

1. *Clarify the issue.* Take responsibility for thinking through your feelings and discovering what's really bothering you. Agree that one of you will speak first and have the chance to speak fully while the other listens. Then reverse the roles. Try to understand the other person's position fully by repeating what you've heard and asking questions to clarify or elicit more information.

2. *Find out what each person wants.* Ask the other person to express her or his desires. Don't assume you already know what those desires are, and don't try to speak for your friend or partner.

3. *Determine how both of you can get what you want.* Brainstorm to generate a variety of options.

4. *Decide how to negotiate.* Work out a plan for change. For example, agree that one of you will do one task and the other will do another task or that one of you will do a task in exchange for something she or he wants.

5. *Solidify the agreements.* Go over the plan verbally and write it down, if necessary, to ensure that both of you understand and agree to it.

6. *Review and renegotiate.* Decide on a time frame for trying out the new plan and set a time to discuss how it's working. Make adjustments as needed.

TAKE CHARGE
Dealing with Anger

Anger is a universal response to something we perceive as injustice, betrayal, insult, or some other wrong—whether real or imagined. We may respond physically with faster heart and breathing rates, muscle tension, trembling, a knot in the stomach, or a red face. When anger alerts us that something is wrong, it is a useful emotion that can lead to constructive change. When anger leads to loss of control and to aggression, it causes problems.

According to current popular wisdom, it's healthy to express your feelings, including anger. However, research has shown that people who are overtly hostile are at higher risk for heart disease and heart attacks than calmer people. In addition, expressing anger in thoughtless or out-of-control ways can damage personal and professional relationships.

People who experience rage or explosive anger are particularly at risk for negative repercussions. Some of these people may have *intermittent explosive disorder,* characterized by aggressiveness that is impulsive and out of proportion to the stimulus. Explosive anger renders people temporarily unable to think straight or act in their own best interests. Counseling can help very angry people learn how to manage their anger.

In dealing with anger, distinguish between self-assertiveness and aggression. When you are *assertive,* you stand up for your own rights at the same time that you respect the rights of others. When you are *aggressive,* you may violate the rights of others.

Managing Your Own Anger

What are the best ways to handle anger? If you find yourself in a situation where you are getting angry, answer these questions:

- Is the situation important enough to get angry about?

- Are you truly justified in getting angry?

- Is expressing your anger going to make a positive difference?

If the answer to all these questions is yes, then calm, assertive communication may be appropriate. Use "I" statements to express your feelings ("I would like . . ." "I feel . . ."), and listen respectfully to the other person's point of view. Don't attack verbally or make demands; try to negotiate a constructive, mutually satisfying solution.

If you answer no to any of the questions, try to calm yourself. First, reframe the situation by thinking about it differently. Try these strategies:

- Don't take it personally. Maybe the driver who cut you off simply didn't see you.

- Look for mitigating factors. Maybe the classmate who didn't say hello was preoccupied.

- Practice empathy. See the situation from the other person's point of view.

- Ask questions. Clarify the situation by asking what the other person meant. Avoid defensiveness.

- Focus on the present. Don't let this situation trigger thoughts of past incidents that you perceive as similar.

Second, calm your body.

- Use the old trick of counting to 10 before you respond.

- Concentrate on your breathing, taking long, slow breaths.

- Imagine yourself in a beautiful, peaceful place.

- If needed, take a longer cooling-off period by leaving the situation until your anger has subsided.

Dealing with Other People's Anger

If someone you are with becomes very angry, try these strategies:

- Respond "asymmetrically" by reacting not with anger but with calm.

- Apologize if you think you are to blame. (Don't apologize if you don't think you are to blame.)

- Validate the other person by acknowledging that he or she has some reason to be angry. However, don't accept verbal abuse.

- Focus on the problem and ask what can be done to alleviate the situation.

- If the person cannot be calmed, disengage from the situation, at least temporarily. After a time-out, attempts at rational problem solving may be more successful.

Warning Signs of Violence

Violence is never acceptable. The following behaviors, feelings, or circumstances over a period of time suggest the potential for violence:

- A history of making threats and engaging in aggressive behavior

- Drug or alcohol abuse

- Gang membership

- Access to or fascination with weapons

- Feelings of rejection or aloneness; the feeling of constantly being disrespected; victimization by bullies

- Withdrawal from usual activities and friends; poor school performance

- Failure to acknowledge the rights of others

The following are immediate warning signs of violence:

- Daily loss of temper or frequent physical fighting

- Significant vandalism or property damage

- Increased risk-taking behavior; increased drug or alcohol abuse

- Threats or detailed plans to commit acts of violence

- Pleasure in hurting animals

- The presence of weapons

Avoid people who shows these warning signs of violence. Don't carry a weapon or resort to violence to protect yourself. Ask someone in authority or an experienced professional for help.

Striving for Spiritual Wellness

Spiritual wellness is associated with more effective coping skills and higher levels of overall wellness. Researchers have linked spiritual wellness to longer life expectancy, reduced risk of disease, faster recovery, and improved emotional health. Although spirituality is difficult to define and study, and researchers aren't sure how or why spirituality seems to improve health, several explanations have been offered. To develop spiritual wellness, choose activities that are meaningful to you, such as the following:

Look inward. Spend quiet time alone with your thoughts and feelings:

- Spend time in nature, experiencing continuity with the natural world.
- Notice art, architecture, or music.
- Engage in a favorite activity that allows you to express your creative side.
- Engage in a personal spiritual practice, such as prayer, meditation, or yoga.

Reach out to others:

- Share writings that inspire you.
- Practice small acts of personal kindness for people you know as well as for strangers.
- Perform community service.

Confiding in Yourself through Writing

Keeping a diary is like confiding in someone else, except that you are confiding in and becoming more attuned to yourself. This form of coping with severe stress may be especially helpful for those who find it difficult to open up to others. Although writing about traumatic and stressful events may have a short-term negative effect on mood, over the long term, stress is reduced and positive changes in health occur. A key to promoting health and well-being through journaling is to write about your emotional responses to stressful events. Set aside a special time each day or week to write down your feelings about stressful events in your life.

Time Management

Learning to manage your time can be crucial to coping with everyday stressors. Over-commitment, procrastination, and even boredom are significant stressors for many people. Try these strategies for improving your time-management skills:

- *Set priorities.* Divide your tasks into three groups: essential, important, and trivial. Focus on the first two, and ignore the third.
- *Schedule tasks for peak efficiency.* You probably know that you're most productive at certain times of the day (or night). Schedule as many of your tasks for those hours as you can, and stick to your schedule.
- *Set realistic goals and write them down.* Attainable goals spur you on. Impossible goals, by definition, cause frustration and failure. Fully commit yourself to achieving your goals by putting them in writing.
- *Budget enough time.* For each project you undertake, calculate how much time you will need to finish it. Then tack on another 10–15%, or even 25%, as a buffer.
- *Break up long-term goals into short-term ones.* Instead of waiting for large blocks of time, use short amounts of time to start a project or keep it moving.
- *Visualize achieving your goal.* By mentally rehearsing a task, you will be able to do it more smoothly.
- *Keep track of the tasks you put off.* Analyze the reasons you procrastinate. If the task is difficult or unpleasant, look for ways to make it easier or more fun. For example, if you find the readings for one of your classes particularly difficult, choose an especially nice setting for your reading, and then reward yourself each time you complete a section or chapter.
- *Consider doing your least favorite tasks first.* Once you have the most unpleasant ones out of the way, you can work on the tasks you enjoy more.
- *Consolidate tasks when possible.* For example, try walking to the store so that you run your errands and exercise in the same block of time.
- *Identify quick transitional tasks.* Keep a list of 5- to 10-minute tasks you can do while waiting or between other tasks, such as watering your plants, doing the dishes, or checking a homework assignment.
- *Delegate responsibility.* Asking for help when you have too much to do is no cop-out; it's good time management. Just don't delegate the jobs you know you should do yourself.
- *Say no when necessary.* If the demands made on you don't seem reasonable, say no—tactfully but without guilt or apology.
- *Give yourself a break.* Allow time for play—free, unstructured time when you can ignore the clock. Don't consider this a waste of time. Play renews you and enables you to work more efficiently.
- *Avoid your personal "time sinks."* You can probably identify your own time sinks—activities like watching television, surfing the Internet, or talking on the phone—that consistently use up more time than you anticipate and put you behind schedule. On particularly busy days, avoid these problematic activities altogether; for example, if you have a big paper due, don't sit down for a five-minute TV break if it is likely to turn into a two-hour break. Try a five-minute walk instead.
- *Stop thinking or talking about what you're going to do, and just do it!* Sometimes the best solution for procrastination is to stop waiting for the right moment and just get started. You will probably find that things are not as bad as you feared, and your momentum will keep you going.

For more help with time management, complete Activity 10 in the Behavior Change Workbook.

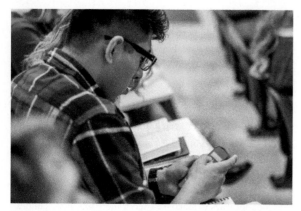

Wellness Tip Managing the many commitments of adult life—including work, school, and parenthood—can sometimes feel overwhelming and produce a great deal of stress. Time-management and problem-solving skills, including careful scheduling with a date book, smartphone, or tablet, can help you cope with busy days.
©Hill Street Studios/Tobin Rogers/Getty Images RF

Cognitive Techniques

Certain thought patterns and ways of thinking, including ideas, beliefs, and perceptions, can contribute to stress and have a negative impact on health. But other habits of mind, if practiced with patience and consistency, can help break unhealthy thought patterns. An important skill is to distinguish between types of stressors: *eustress* or "challenge stressors" create positive experiences and opportunities for growth, versus *distress* or "hindrance stressors," which can impede growth and life satisfaction levels.

Practice Affirmations and Avoid Negative Self-Talk If you tend to beat up on yourself—"Late for class again! You can't even cope with college! How do you expect to ever hold down a real job?"—try being kind to yourself instead. Monitor your self-talk and try to minimize hostile, critical, suspicious, and self-deprecating thoughts. Substituting positive self-talk for negative self-talk can help you build and maintain self-esteem and cope better with the challenges in your life (see Table 10.1).

Act Constructively and Problem Solve Focus on things you can control. Accept what you can't change, forgive others for their faults, and be flexible. Identify key stressors that you can address, and take a constructive approach to dealing with them. If you find yourself stewing over a problem, try this approach:

1. Define the problem in one or two sentences.
2. Identify the causes of the problem.
3. Consider several alternative solutions. Don't stop with the most obvious one.
4. Weigh positive and negative consequences for each alternative.
5. Make a decision—that is, choose a solution.
6. Make a list of tasks you must perform to act on your decision.
7. Carry out the tasks on your list.
8. Evaluate the outcome and revise your approach if necessary.

Modify Your Expectations and Live in the Present The fewer expectations you have, the more you can live spontaneously and joyfully in the present. Try to accept life as it comes. The more you expect from others, the more often you will feel let down. And trying to meet the expectations others have of you is often futile.

Cultivate Your Sense of Humor Cultivating your sense of humor is another key cognitive stress-management technique. Even a fleeting smile produces changes in your autonomic nervous system that can lift your spirits. Hearty laughter triggers the release of endorphins, and after a good laugh, your muscles go slack and your pulse and blood pressure dip below normal; you are relaxed.

Table 10.1	Avoiding Negative Self-Talk	
COGNITIVE DISTORTION	NEGATIVE SELF-TALK	POSITIVE SELF-TALK
Focusing on negatives	School is so discouraging—nothing but one hassle after another.	School is pretty challenging and has its difficulties, but there certainly are rewards. It's really a mixture of good and bad.
Expecting the worst	Why would my boss want to meet with me this afternoon if not to fire me?	I wonder why my boss wants to meet with me. I guess I'll just have to wait and see.
Overgeneralizing	[*After getting a poor grade on a paper*] Just as I thought—I'm incompetent at everything.	I'll start working on the next paper earlier. That way, if I run into problems I'll have time to talk to the TA.
Minimizing	I won the speech contest, but none of the other speakers was very good. I wouldn't have done as well against stiffer competition.	It may not have been the best speech I'll ever give, but it was good enough to win the contest.
Blaming others	I wouldn't have eaten so much last night if my friends hadn't insisted on going to that restaurant.	I overdid it last night. Next time I'll make different choices.
Expecting perfection	I should have scored 100% on this test. I can't believe I missed that one problem through a careless mistake.	Too bad I missed one problem through carelessness, but overall I did very well on this test. Next time I'll be more careful.

Relaxation and Body Awareness Techniques

The **relaxation response** is a physiological state characterized by a feeling of warmth and quiet mental alertness. This state is the opposite of the fight-or-flight response. When you induce the relaxation response by using a relaxation technique, your heart rate, breathing, and metabolism slow down. Blood pressure and oxygen consumption decrease. At the same time, blood flow to the brain and skin increases, and brain waves shift from an alert beta rhythm to a relaxed alpha rhythm.

The techniques described in this section are among the most popular techniques and the easiest to learn. All of them take practice, so it may be several weeks before the benefits become noticeable in everyday life.

Progressive Muscle Relaxation In this simple relaxation technique, you tense and then relax the muscles of the body one group at a time. Also known as deep muscle relaxation, this technique addresses the muscle tension that occurs when the body is experiencing stress. Consciously relaxing tensed muscles sends a message to other body systems to reduce the stress response.

To practice progressive relaxation, begin by inhaling as you contract your right fist. Then exhale as you release your fist. Repeat. Contract and relax your right bicep. Repeat. Do the same using your left arm. Then, working from forehead to feet, contract and relax other muscles. Repeat each contraction at least once, inhaling as you tense and exhaling as you relax. To speed up the process, tense and relax more muscles at one time—for example, both arms simultaneously. With practice, you'll be able to relax quickly just by clenching and releasing only your fists.

Visualization Also known as imagery, visualization is so effective in enhancing sports performance that it has become part of the curriculum at training camps for U.S. Olympic athletes. This same technique can be used to induce relaxation; to help change habits; and to improve performance on an exam, on stage, or on a playing field.

To practice visualization, imagine yourself floating on a cloud, sitting on a mountaintop, or lying in a meadow. Try to identify all the perceptible qualities of the environment—sight, sound, temperature, smell, and so on. Your body will respond as if your imagery were real.

An alternative is to close your eyes and imagine a deep purple light filling your body. Then change the color to a soothing gold. As the color lightens, so should your distress. Imagery can also enhance performance: Visualize yourself succeeding at a task that worries you.

Deep Breathing Your breathing pattern is closely tied to your stress level. Deep, slow breathing is associated with relaxation. Rapid, shallow, often irregular breathing occurs during the stress response. With practice, you can learn to slow and quiet your breathing pattern, thereby also quieting your mind and relaxing your body. Try one of the breathing techniques

described here for on-the-spot tension relief, as well as for long-term stress reduction.

BELLY BREATHING:

1. Lie on your back and relax.
2. Place one hand on your chest and the other on your abdomen. Your hands will help you gauge your breathing.
3. Take in a slow, deep breath through your nose and into your belly. Your abdomen should rise significantly (check with your hand); your chest should rise only slightly. Focus on filling your abdomen with air.
4. Exhale through your mouth, gently pushing out the air from your abdomen.

TENSION-RELEASE BREATHING:

1. Lie down or sit in a chair and get comfortable.
2. Take a slow, deep breath into your abdomen. Inhale through your nose. Try to visualize the air moving to every part of your body. As you breathe in, say to yourself, "Breathe in relaxation."
3. Exhale through your mouth. Visualize tension leaving your body. Say to yourself, "Breathe out tension."

These techniques have many variations. For example, sit in a chair and raise your arms, shoulders, and chin as you inhale; lower them as you exhale. Or slowly count to four as you inhale, then again as you exhale. Breathing in time to soothing music can work well, too. Experts suggest inhaling through the nose and exhaling through the mouth. Breathe slowly, deeply, and gently. To focus on breathing gently, imagine a candle burning a few inches in front of you. Try to exhale softly enough to make the candle's flame flicker, not hard enough to blow it out. Practice is important, too. Perform your chosen breathing exercise two or more times daily, for 5–10 minutes per session.

Body Awareness Techniques and Mindfulness
Mindfulness is both a mental state and the practices that cultivate this mental state. We cultivate mindfulness by paying attention to our mental states, physical activities, and behaviors as they happen. Practicing mindfulness promotes stronger connections between the brain's prefrontal cortex and amygdala. These connections have been demonstrated to facilitate improved problem-solving skills, emotional self-regulation, and resilience. Techniques for practicing mindfulness include forms of meditation (see the box "Mindfulness Meditation") as well as more familiar forms of neuromuscular activities.

YOGA Hatha yoga, the most common yoga style practiced in the United States, emphasizes physical balance and breath

---

relaxation response A physiological state characterized by a feeling of warmth and quiet mental alertness.

mindfulness The intentional cultivation of attention in a way that is nonjudging and nonstriving.

TERMS

TAKE CHARGE
Mindfulness Meditation

Mindful Breathing

You are always breathing, so this is a powerful and convenient way to become present wherever you go and whatever you do. After you read these instructions, close your eyes and invest 5–15 minutes in being present with your breath. Sitting comfortably where you are right now, bring your body into a posture that is upright and supported, with a sense of balance and dignity. See if you can align your head, neck, and body in a way that is neither too rigid nor too relaxed, but somewhere in between. The intention is to be wakeful and alert, yet not tense; at ease, but not sleeping.

Bring attention to your breathing, wherever you feel it most prominently and notice the sensations of your breath coming and going as it will, in its own way and with its own pace. If your mind wanders from your breath, return to it by feeling the sensations of the breath as they come and go. Use these sensations as your way to be present, here and now, in each successive moment for the time you have set aside. Research has repeatedly demonstrated that extending this practice to 30 or 45 minutes on a regular basis significantly reduces stress and stress-related illnesses and conditions.

Many cultures have developed ways of quieting the mind over the centuries. Qigong, yoga, tai chi, and meditation can all complement or supplement other stress therapies.

At its most basic level, meditation, or self-reflective thought, involves quieting or emptying the mind to achieve deep relaxation. Some practitioners of meditation view it on a deeper level as a means of focusing concentration, increasing self-awareness, and bringing enlightenment to their lives. Meditation has been integrated into the practices of several religions—Buddhism, Hinduism, Confucianism, Taoism—but it is not a religion itself, nor does its practice require any special knowledge, belief, or background.

Walking Meditation

Find a place where you can walk and be uninterrupted by other people or traffic—if possible, in natural surroundings. You can adapt this practice to fit yourself, whatever your circumstances are with mobility—for example, it can become a mindful-rolling practice if you use a wheelchair. Once you're ready, begin walking—slowly at first (as slowly as possible for about 10 minutes)—paying close attention to each step and using the sensations of each foot touching the ground as your way to be present. When you are ready, accelerate your pace, broadening your attention to take in more of your experience as you walk. In this mindful-movement practice, you may walk any distance, anywhere, at any speed that feels right for you. In the beginning, however, give yourself about 30 minutes.

The key instruction is to be fully present in each moment you are walking rather than consumed with mind chatter or destination. Be open to the experience of your environment and notice, for example, the way clouds move or how the sunlight glistens in the trees and foliage around you. Turn toward whatever calls your attention and be with it as long as you like, stopping if you want to take a close look at a bug or flowers or to listen to the rustling of leaves.

As you become more skilled in mindful awareness practice, you will be able to do this anywhere, even on a bustling college campus. If you want to pick up the speed or duration of your walk, you can make this walking practice part of a regular exercise program, and you will grow in strength and cardiovascular health as well as mindfulness.

control. It integrates components of flexibility, muscular strength, endurance, and muscle relaxation. A session of yoga typically involves a series of postures, each held for a few seconds to several minutes. With yoga, you can cultivate body awareness, ease, and flexibility. If you are interested in trying yoga, take a class with an experienced instructor.

TAI CHI This martial art (in Chinese, *taijiquan*) is a system of self-defense that incorporates philosophical concepts from Taoism and Confucianism. In addition to being a self-defense system, tai chi aims to bring the body into balance and harmony to promote health and spiritual growth. It teaches practitioners to remain calm and centered, to conserve and concentrate energy, and to manipulate force by becoming part of it—by "going with the flow." Tai chi consists of a series of slow, fluid, elegant movements that reinforce the idea of moving with rather than against the stressors of everyday life. As with yoga, it's best to start tai chi with a class led by an experienced instructor.

Listening to Music Music can relax us. It influences pulse, blood pressure, and the electrical activity of muscles. Listening to soothing, lyrical music can lessen depression, anxiety, and stress levels. To experience the stress-management benefits of music, set aside a period of at least 15 minutes to listen quietly. Choose music you enjoy and selections that make you feel relaxed.

Other Stress-Management Techniques

Techniques such as biofeedback, hypnosis and self-hypnosis, and massage require a partner or professional training or assistance. As with the relaxation techniques presented, all take practice, and it may be several weeks before the benefits are noticeable.

Biofeedback helps people reduce their response to stress by enabling them to become more aware of their level of physiological arousal. In biofeedback, some measure of stress—perspiration, heart rate, skin temperature, or muscle tension—is electronically monitored, and feedback is given using sound (a tone or music), light, or a meter or dial. With practice, people begin to exercise conscious control over their physiological stress responses. The point of biofeedback training is to develop the ability to transfer the skill to daily life without the use of electronic equipment.

Counterproductive Strategies for Coping with Stress

As we've seen, there are many effective coping techniques for dealing with stress. However, college students sometimes develop habits in response to stress that are ineffective and even unhealthy. Here are a few unhealthy coping techniques to avoid:

- *Alcohol.* A few drinks might make you feel at ease, and getting drunk may help you forget the stress in your life—but any relief alcohol provides is temporary. Binge drinking and excessive alcohol consumption are not effective ways to handle stress, and using alcohol to deal with stress puts you at risk for all the short- and long-term problems associated with alcohol abuse.

- *Tobacco.* The nicotine in cigarettes and other tobacco products can make you feel relaxed and may even increase your ability to concentrate. Tobacco, however, is highly addictive, and smoking causes cancer, heart disease, sexual problems, and many other health problems. Tobacco use is the leading preventable cause of death in the United States.

- *Other drugs.* Altering your body chemistry to cope with stress is a strategy with many pitfalls. Stimulants, such as amphetamines, can activate the stress response; they also affect the same areas of the brain that are involved in regulating the stress response. Repeated use of marijuana can elicit panic attacks. Opioids such as morphine and heroin can mimic the effects of your body's natural painkillers and reduce anxiety; however, tolerance develops quickly, and many users become dependent.

- *Binge eating.* Eating can induce relaxation, which reduces stress. Eating as a means of coping with stress, however, may lead to weight gain and to binge eating, a risky behavior associated with eating disorders.

There is one other problem with these methods of fighting stress: None of them addresses the actual cause of the stress in your life. To combat stress in a healthy way, learn some of the stress-management techniques described in this chapter.

GETTING HELP

You can use the principles of behavioral self-management described in Chapter 1 to create a stress-management program tailored specifically to your needs. The starting point of a successful program is to listen to your body. When you learn to recognize the stress response and the emotions and thoughts that accompany it, you'll be in a position to begin handling stress. Labs 10.1 and 10.2 can guide you in identifying and finding ways to cope with stress-inducing situations.

If you feel you need guidance beyond the information in this text, excellent self-help guides can be found in bookstores or the library; helpful websites are listed in "For Further Exploration" at the end of the chapter. Some people also find it helpful to express their feelings in a journal. Grappling with a painful experience in this way provides an emotional release and can help you develop more constructive ways of dealing with similar situations in the future.

Peer Counseling and Support Groups

If you still feel overwhelmed despite efforts to manage your stress, you may want to seek outside help. Peer counseling, often available through the student health center or counseling center, is usually staffed by volunteer students with special training that emphasizes maintaining confidentiality. Peer counselors can steer those seeking help to appropriate campus and community resources or just offer sympathetic listening.

Support groups are typically organized around a particular issue or problem: All group members might be entering a new school, reentering school after an interruption, struggling with single parenting, experiencing eating disorders, or coping with particular kinds of trauma. Simply voicing concerns that others share can relieve stress.

Professional Help

Psychotherapy, especially a short-term course of sessions, can also be tremendously helpful in dealing with stress-related problems. Not all therapists are right for all people, so it's a good idea to shop around for a compatible psychotherapist who has reasonable fees. (See the box "Choosing and Evaluating Mental Health Professionals.")

Wellness Tip The most important predictor of whether therapy will be helpful is how much rapport you feel with your therapist at the first session. You have to like your therapist and feel that she or he will be able to help you. If you do, there's a good chance that therapy will be helpful. If you seek professional help for stress-related problems, take the time to find someone who feels right for you.
©Africa Studio/Shutterstock.com RF

CRITICAL CONSUMER
Choosing and Evaluating Mental Health Professionals

College students are usually in a good position to find convenient, affordable mental health care. Larger schools typically have health services that employ psychiatrists and psychologists as well as counseling centers staffed by professionals and peer counselors. Resources in the community may include a school of medicine, a hospital, and a variety of professionals who work independently. It's a good idea to get recommendations from physicians, friends who have been in therapy, or community agencies, rather than to pick a counselor or therapist at random.

In choosing a mental health professional, financial considerations are also important. Find out the costs and what your health insurance will cover. If you're not adequately covered by a health plan, don't let that stop you from getting help; investigate low-cost alternatives on campus and in your community. The cost of treatment is linked to how many therapy sessions will be needed, which in turn depends on the type of therapy and the nature of the problem. Psychological therapies focusing on specific problems may require 8–24 sessions at weekly intervals. Therapies aiming for psychological awareness and personality change can last months or years.

Deciding whether a therapist is right for you requires meeting the therapist in person. Before or during your first meeting, find out about the therapist's background and training:

- Does she or he have a degree from an appropriate professional school and a state license to practice?

- Has she or he had experience treating people with problems similar to yours?

- How much will therapy cost?

You have a right to know the answers to these questions and should not hesitate to ask them. After your initial meeting, evaluate your impressions:

- Does the therapist seem like a warm, intelligent person who would be able to help you and is interested in doing so?

- Are you comfortable with the personality, values, and beliefs of the therapist?

- Is the therapist willing to talk about the techniques he or she will use? Do these techniques make sense to you?

If you answer yes to these questions, this therapist may be satisfactory for you. If you feel uncomfortable—and if you are not in need of emergency care—it's worthwhile to set up one-time consultations with one or two others before you make up your mind. Take the time to find someone who feels right for you.

Later in your treatment, evaluate your progress:

- Are you being helped by the treatment?

- If you are displeased, is it because you aren't making progress or because therapy is raising difficult, painful issues you don't want to deal with?

- Can you express dissatisfaction to your therapist? Such feedback can improve your treatment.

If you're convinced your therapy isn't working or is harmful, thank your therapist for her or his efforts and find another.

Box icon: ©sam74100/Getty Images RF

Is It Stress or Something More Serious?

Most of us have periods of feeling down when we become pessimistic, anxious, less energetic, and less able to enjoy life. Such feelings and thoughts can be normal responses to the ordinary challenges of life. Symptoms that may indicate a more serious problem include the following:

- Depression, anxiety, or other emotional problems that interfere seriously with school or work performance or in getting along with others
- Attempted or serious consideration of suicide

- Symptoms such as hallucinations, delusions, incoherent speech, or loss of memory
- Alcohol or drug use to the extent that they impair normal functioning, occupy much of the week, or result in psychological or physical withdrawal symptoms when a dosage is reduced

Depression is of particular concern because severe depression is linked to suicide, one of the leading causes of death among college students. In some cases, depression, like severe stress, is a clear-cut reaction to a specific event, such as losing a loved one or failing in school or work. In other cases, no trigger event is obvious. Depression differs from person to person but includes the following symptoms that persist most of the day and last more than two consecutive weeks:

- A feeling of sadness and hopelessness or loss of pleasure in doing usual activities (anhedonia)
- Poor appetite and weight loss, or alternatively, increased eating compared to usual
- Insomnia or disturbed sleep, including waking up and being unable to fall back to sleep or sleeping more than normal
- Decreased energy
- Restlessness or, alternatively, slowed thinking or activity

TERMS

depression A mood disorder characterized by loss of interest, sadness, hopelessness, loss of appetite, disturbed sleep, and other physical symptoms.

rapid eye movement (REM) sleep The portion of the sleep cycle during which dreaming occurs.

non–rapid eye movement (NREM) sleep The portion of the sleep cycle that involves deep sleep; NREM sleep includes four stages of successively deeper sleep.

- Thoughts of worthlessness and guilt
- Trouble concentrating or making decisions
- Thoughts of death or suicide

Not everyone who is depressed has all these symptoms, but most have depressed mood or anhedonia and at least four other symptoms. Someone who has symptoms of major depression for more than two weeks, even if it is in reaction to a specific event, should consider treatment. About 60% of people who commit suicide are depressed. The more symptoms of depression a person has, the greater the risk. Warning signs of suicide include expressing the wish to be dead, revealing contemplated suicide methods, increasing social withdrawal and isolation, and exhibiting a sudden, inexplicable lightening of mood (which can indicate the person has finally decided to commit suicide).

If you are severely depressed or know someone who is, expert help from a mental health professional is essential. Most communities and many colleges have hotlines and/or health services and counseling centers that can provide help. The National Suicide Prevention Lifeline can be reached at 1-800-273-TALK. Treatments for depression and many other psychological disorders are highly effective.

Ask Yourself

QUESTIONS FOR CRITICAL THINKING AND REFLECTION
What percentage of your daily stress is time related? How effective are your time-management skills? Identify one thing you can start doing right now to manage your time better, and describe how you can apply it to one aspect of your daily routine.

SLEEP

Don't underestimate sleep as a means of managing stress. Getting enough sleep isn't just good for you physically. Adequate sleep also improves mood, fosters feelings of competence and self-worth, enhances mental functioning, and supports emotional functioning.

How Sleep Works: The Physiology of Sleep

Sleep occurs in two phases: **rapid eye movement (REM) sleep** and **non–rapid eye movement (NREM) sleep**. A sleeper goes through several cycles of NREM and REM sleep each night.

NREM Sleep NREM sleep includes stages of successively deeper sleep (I, II, III, IV). As you move through these stages, a variety of physiological changes occur: Your blood pressure drops, respiration and heart rates slow, body temperature declines, and growth hormone is released. Each state of sleep is characterized by a different pattern of electrical brain activity. Brain waves become slow and even in NREM sleep. People in the deepest stages (III and IV) are difficult to arouse quickly, and when awakened, they may be confused. Some models of sleep group stages III and IV into a single stage of deep sleep, but the overall pattern is the same.

REM Sleep The last stage is REM sleep. During REM sleep, dreams occur. REM sleep is characterized by rapid movement of the eyes under closed eyelids, similar to when people move their eyes while awake. Blood pressure and respiration and heart rates rise, and brain activity increases to levels equal to or greater than those during waking hours. Because the body is prevented from moving during dreaming, like a form of paralysis, muscles in the limbs relax completely.

Sleep Cycles When people fall asleep, they cycle through the four stages of NREM and then REM sleep (Figure 10.5). The sequence lasts about 90 minutes, and then the cycle repeats. During one night of sleep, a person is likely to go through four or five cycles, but the cycles differ somewhat over the course of the night: The NREM periods are longer in the first part of the night, and the REM periods are longer in the last part of the night. Because of this pattern, confusional awakening and sleepwalking are more likely to occur in the earlier part of the night, whereas dreaming is more likely to occur in the last part of the night.

Natural Sleep Drives

Two main natural forces drive us toward sleep—the homeostatic sleep drive and the circadian rhythm. Understanding how these work and learning how to strengthen them can have a big impact on sleep.

Homeostatic Sleep Drive The homeostatic sleep drive gets stronger the longer you are awake. When people are awake during the day, a neurochemical called adenosine accumulates in the brain. This is a by-product of energy used by the brain, and it promotes sleep onset. The homeostatic drive is strengthened if you get up at a reasonably early time in the morning and then remain awake until your

FIGURE 10.5 Sleep stages and cycles. During one night of sleep, the sleeper typically goes through four or five cycles of NREM sleep (four stages) followed by REM sleep.
SOURCE: Adapted from Krejcar, O., Jirka, J, and Janckulik, D. 2011. "Use of mobile phones as intelligent sensors for sound input analysis and sleep state detection," *Sensors* 11(6): 6037–6055.

intended bedtime at night. Naps or dozing in the afternoon will strongly reduce this sleep drive at night, as will sleeping late in the morning. People who have problems falling asleep or staying asleep can strengthen the sleep drive by avoiding naps and setting a reasonably early wake time goal every day. This allows for enough wake time during the day for the sleep drive to accumulate. Caffeine blocks the homeostatic sleep drive by blocking adenosine receptors in the brain. If a person has problems falling asleep, reduction of caffeine can be very important.

Circadian Rhythm The circadian rhythm is the sleep and wake pattern coordinated by the brain's master internal clock, which sends signals throughout the body. You may be familiar with the sensation of jet lag—when a change of time zone causes the internal body clock to be out of sync with the new environment—but travel between time zones is not the only disrupter of circadian rhythm. Some people have habits that cause their internal body clocks to be set at a time that differs from the time zone where they live. An example is a person who stays up regularly until four in the morning and then sleeps until noon, a pattern called delayed sleep phase. If this person occasionally has to wake up earlier, the change can be difficult, and the person will feel poorly, just like a person with jet lag.

The master clock can be reset by "time-givers," or *zeitgebers*. Although there are many zeitgebers, including activity, exercise, and eating, the strongest is light. If a person is exposed to light in the morning at a certain time on a regular basis, it will indicate to the brain that it should set the internal clock to wake around that time. When light is reduced at night, as when natural dusk occurs, the internal clock triggers the production of melatonin. Melatonin signals systems involved in preparation for sleep. People who are blind often have problems with sleep because they do not have the usual light signals to help synchronize their circadian rhythms.

To strengthen the circadian rhythm, get good light exposure in the morning and daytime and reduce exposure to light at night. The challenge in the modern age is that we live with abundant sources of artificial light, which can insulate us from the natural 24-hour rhythm of the sun. For information on personal electronic devices and sleep, see the box "Digital Devices: Help or Harm for a Good Night's Sleep?"

Adequate Sleep and Your Health

Poor-quality or insufficient sleep has been associated with a number of health problems and impairments, including heart disease, high blood pressure, depression, stress, earlier death, increased risk for dementia, weight gain, poorer glucose control, increased risk for accidents, reduced motivation and attention, and increased irritability or hyperactivity. The good news is that people can improve their sleep and, in turn, their health. Along with exercise and good nutrition, good sleep is a critical pillar of good health.

Sleep and Stress Hormones Stress-hormone levels in the bloodstream vary throughout the day and are related to

sleep patterns. Stress-hormone levels are low during NREM sleep and increase during REM sleep. Peak concentrations occur in the early morning, followed by a slow decline during the day and evening. Concentrations return to peak levels during the final stages of sleep and in the early morning hours.

Even though stress hormones are released during sleep, it is the lack of sleep that has the greatest impact on stress. In someone who is suffering from sleep deprivation (not getting enough sleep over time), mental and physical processes deteriorate steadily. A sleep-deprived person experiences headaches, feels irritable, cannot concentrate, and is prone to forgetfulness. Acute sleep deprivation slows the daytime decline in stress hormones, so evening levels are higher than normal. A decrease in total sleep time also causes an increase in the level of stress hormones. Together these changes may increase stress-hormone levels throughout the day and contribute to physical and mental exhaustion. Extreme sleep deprivation can lead to hallucinations and other psychotic symptoms, as well as to a significant increase in heart attack risk.

Sleep and Driving Drowsy driving is responsible for more than 70,000 crashes, 40,000 injuries, and as many as 7,500 deaths per year. Even if you don't fall asleep completely, drowsiness slows your reaction time and lessens your ability to pay attention and make good decisions. Going 24 hours without sleep can impair a driver to the same extent as a blood alcohol level of 0.10%, which is above the legal limit.

People who are most at risk for falling asleep while driving include young adults aged 18–29, with men at slightly greater risk than women; parents with small children; shift workers; people who have accumulated sleep debt; and those who have other untreated sleep disorders such as sleep apnea or insomnia. Sleepiness is worsened when people take substances such as muscle relaxants, antihistamines, cold medicines, or alcohol.

The good news is that accidents due to sleepiness are preventable. First and foremost, if you find yourself drowsy while driving, pull over. Taking a nap or short rest can help, but if drowsiness persists, let someone else do the driving.

Sleep Disorders

Although many of us can attribute the lack of sleep to long workdays and family responsibilities, as many as 70 million Americans suffer from chronic sleep disorders—medical conditions that prevent them from sleeping well. Some of the most common ones are described in the sections that follow.

Chronic Insomnia Many people have trouble falling asleep or staying asleep—a condition called insomnia. For most people, insomnia is brief and is due to life circumstances, such as worrying about an upcoming deadline or consuming too much caffeine or alcohol on a particular day. A person is considered to have chronic insomnia if sleep disruption occurs at least three nights per week and lasts at least three months. If you experience insomnia, try the strategies described in this

WELLNESS IN THE DIGITAL AGE
Digital Devices: Help or Harm for a Good Night's Sleep?

Many apps are promoted as sleep aids and trackers. Can they really improve sleep? Or can using digital devices hurt the body's natural sleep cycles?

Digital Devices and Sleep

Before we look at sleep apps, let's consider how use of your digital devices can negatively affect your sleep. Tablets, smartphones, and computers emit blue light, which impedes the release of melatonin, a hormone that affects sleep and wake cycles. In one study, researchers compared the sleep of people who read an e-book on a digital device in the hours before bedtime with people who did so with a print book. Those who read the digital book took longer to fall asleep, had reduced melatonin release, and were less alert the next morning. In another study that compared the impact of playing smartphone games with either a standard or suppressed blue light phone, use of the blue light phone was associated with decreased sleepiness and worsened mood as well as a decline in memory performance.

Does heavy texting affect sleep? Psychologist Karla Murdock reported that texting was a direct predictor of sleep problems among first-year students in a study that examined links among interpersonal stress, text-messaging behavior, and three indicators of college students' health: burnout, sleep problems, and emotional well-being.

Murdock and other sleep experts suggest turning off your screens. Use them less during the day and also when preparing to sleep at night. If you have trouble relaxing and transitioning to sleep in the evenings, shut down all your devices an hour or more before you intend to sleep. Now that you are resting in the dark, why would you consider using a sleep app or digital tracker? Ironically, a smartphone may help you get to sleep—if you tuck it into the corner of your bed.

Digital Aids for Relaxation

Many free and low-cost apps provide aids to assist with relaxation and improve sleep. Some include music, white noise, or sounds of nature (e.g., wind, rain, waves, or songbirds). Others offer specific techniques, such as guided meditation or breathing exercises, to promote relaxation and sleep. Experiment to find the aids that work best for you.

Digital Sleep Trackers

More complicated technologies attempt to track and analyze sleep. Many are based on movement detectors in smartphones. These apps estimate the amount and type of sleep you get based on your movements during the night; they may generate detailed graphs of your sleep quality and then time your wake-up alarm to a specific sleep cycle. Some apps also include a sound recorder, which detects sleep talking, snoring, and other night noises, providing further information.

In addition to smartphone apps, specialized fitness wristbands such as those by Fitbit and Garmin include sleep trackers. Many of these are also based on movement detectors, but some incorporate heart-rate data as well; preliminary research indicates that adding heart-rate data to movement tracking may improve the accuracy of the results. Fitbit and other wearables, along with some apps, may combine sleep and fitness data into an overall picture of an individual's activity over the course of a day.

Apps and devices may be popular, but no consumer technology yet developed can equal the capability of a sleep lab at detecting sleep stages or diagnosing specific sleep disorders. If you enjoy the features of an app or wearable tracker, go ahead and use them, but don't rely on an app to diagnose the presence or absence of a serious sleep problem. One good effect of using a sleep tracker is simply the greater focus it places on sleep.

SOURCES: Heo, J. Y., et al. 2016. Effects of smartphone use with and without blue light at night in healthy adults: A randomized, double-blind, crossover, placebo-controlled comparison. *Journal of Psychiatric Research* 87: 61–70; Chang, A. M., et al. 2015. Evening use of light-emitting eReaders negatively affects sleep, circadian timing, and next-morning alertness. *Proceedings of the National Academy of Sciences* 112(4): 1232–1237; Bhat, S., et al. 2015. Is there a clinical role for smartphone sleep apps? Comparison of sleep cycle detection by a smartphone application to polysomnography. *Journal of Clinical Sleep Medicine,* February 3; Behar, J., et al. 2013. A review of current sleep screening applications for smartphones. *Physiological Measurement* 34(7): R29–R46; Lewis, J. G. 2013. Sleep cycle app: Precise, or placebo? Mind Read: Connecting Brain and Behavior (http://www.nature.com/scitable/blog/mind-read/sleep_cycle_app_precise_or); Murdock, K. K. 2013. Texting while stressed: Implications for students' burnout, sleep, and well-being. *Psychology of Popular Media Culture* 2(4): 207–221.

chapter for promoting healthy sleep patterns and in the box "Overcoming Insomnia."

Restless Leg Syndrome Restless leg syndrome (RLS) affects about 5% of the adult population and as many as 25% of pregnant women. RLS is characterized by muscle throbbing or creeping or other uncomfortable sensations in the legs, which create an uncontrollable urge to move them. Symptoms occur primarily at night or while resting.

RLS can be associated with small kicking movements during the night, can interfere with falling asleep, and can make falling back to sleep more difficult. Simple measures that help

RLS include getting more exercise during the day; avoiding all caffeine, tobacco, and alcohol; massaging the legs or using heating pads or a warm bath; maintaining a regular sleep pattern; and correcting any deficiencies in iron, folate, or magnesium. Medications are also available, but certain substances should be avoided: Diphenhydramine (Benadryl), which is a common ingredient in over-the-counter sleeping pills, paradoxically worsens RLS symptoms and can worsen sleep.

Sleep Apnea Sleep apnea occurs when a person repeatedly stops breathing for short periods while asleep. Apnea can be caused by a number of factors, but it typically results when

Most people can overcome insomnia by discovering the cause of poor sleep and taking steps to remedy it. If you're bothered by insomnia, try the following:

- Determine how much sleep you need to feel refreshed the next day, and don't sleep longer than that.

- Go to bed at the same time every night and, more important, get up at the same time every morning, seven days a week, regardless of how much sleep you got. Adjust your sleep schedule to keep your wake time consistent and early enough for the sleep drive to accumulate.

- Anchor your circadian rhythm with more light in the morning.

- Don't nap during the day if you can help it. If you fall asleep in the afternoon, make the nap short—less than 30 minutes.

- Exercise every day, but not too close to bedtime. Your metabolism takes up to six hours to slow down after exercise.

- Avoid caffeine late in the day and alcohol before bedtime (it causes disturbed, fragmented sleep). If you take any medications (prescription or not), ask your doctor or pharmacist if they are known to interfere with sleep.

- Do what you can to make your sleeping environment quiet, dark, and a comfortable temperature. Overhearing music or talking can make it hard to sleep.

- Have a light snack before bedtime; you'll sleep better if you're not hungry.

- Use your bed only for sleep. Don't eat, read, study, or watch television in bed.

- Relax before bedtime with a bath, a book, music, or relaxation exercises. Avoid bright lights and electronic activities in the hour prior to bedtime.

- If you don't fall asleep in 15–20 minutes, or if you wake up and can't fall asleep again, turn on your back and engage in a mindful breathing exercise.

If sleep problems last more than six months and interfere with daytime functioning, ask your physician for a referral to a sleep specialist. You may be a candidate for a sleep study—an overnight evaluation of your sleep pattern that can uncover many sleep-related disorders. Sleeping pills are not recommended for chronic insomnia because they can be habit-forming; they often lose their effectiveness over time.

---

the soft tissue at the back of the mouth (such as the tongue or soft palate) "collapses" during sleep, blocking the airway (Figure 10.6). When breathing is interrupted, so is sleep, because the sleeper awakens throughout the night to begin breathing again. In most cases, this occurs without the sleeper's awareness. However, the disruption to sleep can be significant, and over time, acute sleep deprivation can result.

Sleep apnea is most common among people who are overweight, but it can occur in people classified as at normal weight. Risk increases with age, and up to 50% of adults over age 65 may have some degree of sleep apnea. Untreated, sleep apnea increases the risk of high blood pressure, heart attack, stroke, obesity, and diabetes. It also increases the risk of

work-related or driving accidents. Treatments for sleep apnea include the following:

- Lifestyle changes, including weight loss, sleeping on your side, quitting smoking, and using nasal sprays or allergy medicines to keep nasal passages open at night.

- Mouthpieces (oral appliances) that are worn at night and adjust the position of the lower jaw to help keep airways open.

- Breathing devices such as the continuous positive airway pressure (CPAP) machine, which has a mask that fits over the mouth and/or nose and gently blows air into the throat.

Improving Sleep

If you're like the average American, you get less than the recommended amount of sleep each night. The Centers for Disease Control and Prevention calls sleep deprivation a national public epidemic. In adults, between seven and nine hours of sleep is generally sufficient, but sleep needs vary from person to person; some people need only six hours, while others need more than nine. Complete Lab 10.3 to learn more about your current sleep.

Support Natural Sleep Rhythms and Drives Sleep is a natural physiological process, so you can't "will" yourself to sleep—meaning, don't get frustrated if you don't fall asleep. As noted, to strengthen physiological sleep drives, keep a consistent sleep schedule throughout the week. To support circadian rhythm, set a target wake time with good light exposure, and avoid bright lights and electronic devices at night. To enhance

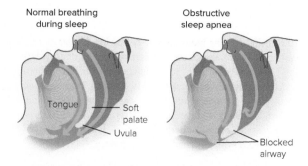

FIGURE 10.6 Sleep apnea. Sleep apnea occurs when soft tissues surrounding the airway relax, "collapsing" the airway and restricting airflow.

the homeostatic drive, make your wake time sufficiently early, avoid naps, and minimize caffeine.

Create a Good Sleep Environment Your bedroom should be cool, dark, and quiet, ideally without pets. Although you'll want to be warm when you get into bed, sleep comes more easily in cool temperatures. Therefore, you may want to take a warm shower or bath before bed, to warm the body, and wear socks if you tend to have cold extremities at night. But after that, fewer blankets and a cooler temperature setting are beneficial. Generally if you tend to awaken at night, avoid activities in the bedroom that might be stimulating, such as watching television or using electronic devices.

Avoid Substances That Disrupt Sleep People vary greatly in how they are affected by caffeine, but those with poor-quality sleep, difficulty falling asleep, or nighttime awakenings need to be especially careful. Caffeine can have physiological effects for over 24 hours in susceptible people, and even caffeine consumed in the morning can affect sleep throughout the night. Alcohol is another substance that can affect sleep. Some people think that alcohol improves sleep, but it can cause poorer sleep in the second part of the night when the effects wear off, leading to increased activation and arousal. For people with poor sleep, reducing alcohol consumption can be beneficial.

Treat Conditions That Interfere with Sleep A number of readily treated medical conditions, including nasal congestion and acid reflux, can disrupt sleep. Simple interventions, such as using medications or saline spray to treat allergies or limiting foods and fluids for several hours before bedtime, can help in some cases. If symptoms are severe and continue to interfere with sleep, consult a health care provider.

Don't Equate Sleeplessness with Job or School Performance We live in a society where people work long hours, and our culture can seem to reward people who sleep less and work more. But establishing balance between sleep and life activities is important. "Cramming" all night before an exam, or staying up all night to write a paper, is something most college students have been tempted to do, but all-nighters can interfere with learning and memory. Having a full night's sleep after studying promotes long-term memory formation.

Similarly, some job environments encourage longer working hours. But equating work ethic with long work hours and less sleep can lead to burnout and lower productivity. People who work the night shift must try especially hard to protect downtime and sleep periods and refrain from adding other daytime commitments that interfere with sleep. It can be tempting in the short term to cut back on sleep, but in the longer term this is likely to backfire, resulting in increased mood problems and the health-related issues associated with sleep loss.

Avoid Sleep Pitfalls Don't be concerned with a bout of sleeplessness. Worry can worsen sleep, and when you are having trouble sleeping, it can be easy to start worrying about the consequences for the next day. Most of the time, even if you sleep poorly, the next day's activities will be fine. The ups and down of mental and physical performance are not always correlated to the prior night's sleep. In addition, remember the value of relaxation. Quiet relaxation has restorative value. You don't have to be sound asleep to benefit from quiet time during the night; resting, relaxing, and dozing can also be beneficial. Consider the relaxation techniques presented earlier in this chapter. If you find that despite everything, you feel anxious or frustrated during the night when awake, leave the bedroom and engage in a quiet activity like reading until you feel more relaxed and sleepy again.

Wellness Tip Don't use electronic devices, especially those that emit blue light, in the hour before bed. Use of blue-light-emitting devices affects melatonin levels and is associated with problems falling asleep and greater sleepiness the following day. Take a break from your devices.
©acinquantadue/Shutterstock.com RF

TIPS FOR TODAY AND THE FUTURE

For the stress you can't avoid, develop a range of stress-management techniques and strategies.

RIGHT NOW YOU CAN
- Practice deep breathing for 5–10 minutes.
- Visualize a relaxing, peaceful place and imagine yourself experiencing it as vividly as possible. Stay there as long as you can.
- Do some stretching exercises.
- Get out your datebook and schedule what you'll be doing the rest of today and tomorrow. Plan a short walk and a conversation with a friend. Schedule a reasonable bedtime to ensure adequate sleep.

IN THE FUTURE YOU CAN
- Take a class or workshop, such as one in assertiveness training or time management, that can help you overcome a source of stress.
- Find a way to build relaxing time into every day. Just 15 minutes of meditation, stretching, or deep breathing can induce the relaxation response.
- Evaluate your sleep patterns and gradually make changes that will help you get the sleep you need to feel and do your best.

COMMON QUESTIONS ANSWERED

Q **Are there any relaxation techniques I can use in response to an immediate stressor?**

A Yes. Try the deep breathing techniques described in the chapter, and try some of the following to see which work best for you:

- Do a full-body stretch while standing or sitting. Stretch your arms out to the sides and then reach them as far as possible over your head. Rotate your body from the waist. Bend over as far as is comfortable for you.
- Do a partial session of progressive muscle relaxation. Tense and then relax some of the muscles in your body. Focus on the muscles that are stiff or tense. Shake out your arms and legs.
- Take a short, brisk walk (three to five minutes). Breathe deeply.
- Engage in realistic self-talk about the stressor. Mentally rehearse dealing successfully with the stressor. As an

alternative, focus your mind on some other activity.

- Briefly reflect on something personally meaningful. In one study of college students, researchers found that self-reflection on important personal values prior to a stressful task reduces the hormonal response to the stressor.

Q **Can stress cause headaches?**

A Stress is one possible cause of the most common type of headache, the tension headache. About 90% of headaches are tension headaches, characterized by a dull, steady pain, usually on both sides of the head. It may feel as though a band of pressure is tightening around the head, and the pain may extend to the neck and shoulders. Acute tension headaches may last from hours to days, while chronic tension headaches may occur almost every day for months or even years. Ineffective stress-management skills, poor posture, and immobility are leading causes of tension

headaches. There is no cure, but the pain can sometimes be avoided and relieved with mindfulness skills and over-the-counter painkillers; many people also try therapies such as massage, relaxation, hot or cold showers, and rest. Stress is also one possible trigger of migraine headaches, which are typically characterized by throbbing pain (often on one side of the head), heightened sensitivity to light and noise, visual disturbances such as flashing lights, nausea, and fatigue.

If your headaches are frequent, keep a journal with details about the events surrounding each one. Are your tension headaches associated with late nights, academic deadlines, or long periods spent sitting at a computer? Are migraines associated with certain foods, stress, fatigue, specific sounds or odors, or (in women) menstruation? If you can identify the stressors or other factors that are consistently associated with your headaches, you can begin to gain more control over the situation. If you suffer persistent tension or migraine headaches, consult your physician.

SUMMARY

- Stress is the collective physiological and emotional response to any stressor. Physiological responses to stressors are the same for everyone.

- The autonomic nervous system and the endocrine system are responsible for the body's physical response to stressors. The sympathetic nervous system mobilizes the body and activates key hormones of the endocrine system, causing the fight-or-flight reaction. The parasympathetic system returns the body to homeostasis.

- Behavioral responses to stress are controlled by the somatic nervous system and fall under a person's conscious control, though personality, gender, culture, and experience affect one's response to stress.

- The general adaptation syndrome model contributes to our understanding of the links between stress and disease. People who have many stressors in their lives or who handle stress poorly are at risk for cardiovascular disease, impairment of the immune system, and many other problems.

- Potential sources of stress include major life changes, daily hassles, college- and job-related stressors, and interpersonal and social stressors, both real and virtual.

- Positive ways of managing stress include regular exercise; good nutrition; support from other people; clear communication; conflict resolution; spiritual wellness; effective time management; cognitive techniques; and techniques for relaxation, body awareness, and mindfulness.

- If a personal program for stress management doesn't work, peer counseling, support groups, and psychotherapy are available.

- Getting adequate sleep is an important means of managing stress. Understanding the physiology of sleep, the basic sleep drives, and a variety of sleep disorders can be key steps in analyzing your own sleep patterns and determining strategies for getting the sleep you need to feel and do your best.

FOR FURTHER EXPLORATION

American Headache Society. Provides information for consumers and clinicians about different types of headaches, their causes, and their treatment.
   http://www.americanheadachesociety.org/

American Institute of Stress. A resource of in-depth information on stress, its causes, and its treatments.
   http://www.stress.org

American Psychiatric Association: Healthy Minds, Healthy Lives. Provides information on mental wellness, especially for college students.

http://apahealthyminds.blogspot.com/

American Psychological Association. Provides information on stress management and psychological disorders.

http://www.apa.org

http://www.apa.org/helpcenter/index.aspx

Association for Applied Psychophysiology and Biofeedback. Provides information about biofeedback and referrals to certified biofeedback practitioners.

http://www.aapb.org

Benson-Henry Institute for Mind Body Medicine. Provides information about stress management and relaxation techniques.

http://www.massgeneral.org/bhi

National Institute of Mental Health (NIMH). Publishes informative brochures about stress and stress management as well as other aspects of mental health.

http://www.nimh.nih.gov

National Sleep Foundation. Provides information about sleep and how to overcome sleep problems such as insomnia, apnea, and jet lag.

http://www.sleepfoundation.org

WebMD Stress Management Health Center. Offers a range of digestable subtopics of stress.

http://www.webmd.com/balance/stress-management/default.htm

SELECTED BIBLIOGRAPHY

American College Health Association. 2016. *American College Health Association–National College Health Assessment II Reference Group Executive Summary, Spring 2016.* Hanover, MD: American College Health Association.

American Psychological Association. 2017. *Stress in America 2017 Part 1: Coping with Change.* Washington, DC: American Psychological Association.

American Psychological Association. 2017. *Stress in America 2017 Part 2: Technology and Social Media.* Washington, DC: American Psychological Association.

American Psychological Association. 2014. *Stress in America: Paying with Our Health* (http://www.apa.org/news/press/releases/stress/2014/stress-report.pdf).

American Psychological Association. 2015. *Mind/Body Health: Stress* (http://www.apa.org/helpcenter/stress.aspx).

Butler, C. 2011. Research suggests that good friends may actually be great medicine. *Washington Post,* March 14.

Cassidy, S. 2016. The Academic Resilience Scale (ARS-30): A new multidimensional construct measure. *Frontiers in Psychology* 7: 1787.

Chen, L. J., et al. 2017. Physical activity, smoking, and the incidence of clinically diagnosed insomnia. *Sleep Medicine* 30: 189–194.

Cohen, S., and D. Janicki-Deverts. 2012. Who's stressed? Distributions of psychological stress in the United States in probability samples from 1983, 2006 and 2009. *Journal of Applied Social Psychology* 42: 1320–1334.

Dyar, C., et al. 2016. The mediating roles of rejection sensitivity and proximal stress in the association between discrimination and internalizing symptoms among sexual minority women. *Archives of Sexual Behavior.* doi:10.1007/s10508-016-0869-1.

Edes, A. N., and D. E. Crews. 2017. Allostatic load and biological anthropology. *American Journal of Physical Anthropology* 162(S63): 44–70.

Flinchbaugh, C., et al. 2015. A challenge or a hindrance? Understanding the effects of stressors and thriving on life satisfaction. *International Journal of Stress Management* 22(4): 323.

Greenberg, J. 2016. *Comprehensive Stress Management,* 14th ed. New York: McGraw-Hill.

Javaheri, S., et al. 2017. Sleep apnea: Types, mechanisms, and clinical cardiovascular consequences. *Journal of the American College of Cardiology* 69(7): 841–858.

Kabat-Zinn, J. 2011. *Mindfulness for Beginners: Reclaiming the Present Moment—and Your Life.* Louisville, CO: Sounds True.

Knutson, K. 2015. Sleep and pain: Summary of the 2015 Sleep in America Poll. *Sleep Health: Journal of the National Sleep Foundation* 1(2): 85.

Kurek, S. J., Jr. 2016. EAST 2016 presidential address: Resilience. *Journal of Trauma and Acute Care Surgery* 81(1): 1–87.

Leppink, E. W., et al. 2016. The young and the stressed: Stress, impulse control, and health in college students. *Journal of Nervous and Mental Disease* 204(12): 931–938.

Max Planck Institute for Demographic Research. 2011. Marriage and life expectancy [press release]. May 11.

Manzoni, G. C., et al. 2016. Age of onset of episodic and chronic cluster headache—a review of a large case series from a single headache centre. *Journal of Headache Pain* 17: 44.

Mayo Foundation for Medical Education and Research. 2015. *Stress: Constant Stress Puts You Health at Risk* (http://www.mayoclinic.com/health/stress/SR00001).

McGonigal, K. 2015. *The Upside of Stress: Why Stress Is Good for You, and How to Get Good At It.* New York: Avery.

National Institute of Neurological Disorders and Stroke. 2015. Restless Legs Syndrome Fact Sheet (http://www.ninds.nih.gov/disorders/restless_egs/detail_restless_legs.htm).

National Sleep Foundation. 2013. *National Sleep Foundation Poll Finds Exercise Key to Good Sleep.* Arlington, VA: National Sleep Foundation.

National Sleep Foundation. 2017. Insomnia (http://sleepfoundation.org/insomnia/content/symptoms).

O'Driscoll, M., et al. 2017. The effects of mindfulness-based interventions for health and social care undergraduate students: A systematic review of the literature. *Psychology, Health, and Medicine.* doi:10.1080/13548506.2017.1280178.

Pascoe, M. C., and I. E. Bauer. 2015. A systematic review of randomised control trials on the effects of yoga on stress measures and mood. *Journal of Psychiatric Research* 68: 270–282.

Pennebaker, J. W., and J. Evans. 2014. *Expressive Writing: Words That Heal.* Enumclaw, WA: Idyll Arbor.

Pew Research Center. 2013. Modern parenthood: How mothers and fathers spend their time (http://www.pewsocialtrends.org/2013/03/14/chapter-5-americans-time-at-paid-work-housework-child-care-1965-to-2011).

Ramikie, T. S., et al. 2014. Multiple mechanistically distinct modes of endocannabinoid mobilization at central amygdala glutamatergic synapses. *Neuron* 81(5): 1111–1125.

Schulte, B. 2014. *Overwhelmed.* New York: Sarah Crichton Books.

Seaward, B. L. 2015. *Managing Stress: Principles and Strategies for Health and Well-Being,* 8th ed. Boston: Jones and Bartlett.

Torpy, J. M., et al. 2007. Chronic stress and the heart. *Journal of the American Medical Association* 298(14): 1722.

Turner, J. B. and R. J. Turner. 2013. Social relations, social integration, and social support. In *Handbook of the Sociology of Mental Health,* ed. C. S. Aneshensel, J. C. Phelan, and A. Bierman, pp. 341–456. Dordrecht, Netherlands: Springer.

U.S. Department of Health and Human Services, National Institutes of Health. 2015. *Stress* (http://www.nlm.nih.gov/medlineplus/stress.html).

Vaccarino, V., et al. 2016. Sex differences in mental stress-induced myocardial ischemia in patients with coronary heart disease. *Journal of the American Heart Association* 5(9): e003630.

Van der Zwan, J. E., et al. 2015. Physical activity, mindfulness meditation, or heart rate variability biofeedback for stress reduction: A randomized controlled trial. *Applied Psychophysiology and Biofeedback* 40(4):257–268.

Wang C.-W., et al. 2014. Managing stress and anxiety through qigong exercise in healthy adults: A systematic review and meta-analysis of randomized controlled trials. *BMC Complementary and Alternative Medicine* 14: 8.

White, R. L., et al. 2017. Domain-specific physical activity and mental health: A meta-analysis. *American Journal of Preventive Medicine.* doi:10.1016/j.amepre.2016.12.008.

Yano, Y., et al. 2016. Blood pressure reactivity to psychological stress in young adults and cognition in midlife: The Coronary Artery Risk Development in Young Adults (CARDIA) study. *Journal of the American Heart Association* 5(1): e002718.

Name _____   **Section** _____   **Date** _____

LAB 10.1   Identifying Your Stress Level and Key Stressors

How Stressed Are You?

To help determine how much stress you experience on a daily basis, answer the following questions.
How many of the symptoms of excessive stress in the list below do you experience frequently?

Symptoms of Excessive Stress

Physical Symptoms	*Emotional Symptoms*	*Behavioral Symptoms*
Dry mouth	Anxiety	Crying
Excessive perspiration	Depression	Disrupted eating habits
Frequent illnesses	Edginess	Disrupted sleeping habits
Gastrointestinal problems	Fatigue	Harsh treatment of others
Grinding of teeth	Hypervigilance	Increased use of tobacco, alcohol, or other drugs
Headaches	Impulsiveness	Problems communicating
High blood pressure	Inability to concentrate	Sexual problems
Pounding heart	Irritability	Social isolation
Stiff neck or aching lower back	Trouble remembering things	

Yes   No

_____   _____   1. Are you easily startled or irritated?

_____   _____   2. Are you increasingly forgetful?

_____   _____   3. Do you have trouble falling or staying asleep?

_____   _____   4. Do you continually worry about events in your future?

_____   _____   5. Do you feel as if you are constantly under pressure to produce?

_____   _____   6. Do you frequently use tobacco, alcohol, or other drugs to help you relax?

_____   _____   7. Do you often feel as if you have less energy than you need to finish the day?

_____   _____   8. Do you have recurrent stomachaches or headaches?

_____   _____   9. Is it difficult for you to find satisfaction in simple life pleasures?

_____   _____   10. Are you often disappointed in yourself and others?

_____   _____   11. Are you overly concerned with being liked or accepted by others?

_____   _____   12. Have you lost interest in intimacy or sex?

_____   _____   13. Are you concerned that you do not have enough money?

Experiencing some stress-related symptoms or answering yes to a few questions is normal. However, if you experience a large number of stress symptoms or you answered yes to a majority of the questions, you may be experiencing a high level of stress. Take time out to develop effective stress-management techniques. Many coping strategies that can aid you in dealing with college stressors are described in this chapter. In addition, your school's counseling center can provide valuable support.

LABORATORY ACTIVITIES

Weekly Stress Log

Now that you are familiar with the signals of stress, complete the weekly stress log to map patterns in your stress levels and identify sources of stress. Enter a score for each hour of each day according to the ratings listed below.

	A.M.							P.M.												
	6	7	8	9	10	11	12	1	2	3	4	5	6	7	8	9	10	11	12	*Average*
Monday																				
Tuesday																				
Wednesday																				
Thursday																				
Friday																				
Saturday																				
Sunday																				
Average																				

Ratings: 0 = Asleep

1 = No anxiety; general feeling of well-being

2 = Mild anxiety; no interference with activity

3 = Moderate anxiety; specific signal(s) of stress present

4 = High anxiety; interference with activity

5 = Very high anxiety and panic reactions; general inability to engage in activity

To identify daily or weekly patterns in your stress level, average your stress rating for each hour and each day. For example, if your scores for 10:00 a.m. are 4, 3, 4, 3, 4, 3, and 4, your 10:00 a.m. rating would be 25 ÷ 7 , or 3.6 (moderate to high anxiety). Then calculate an average weekly stress score by averaging your daily average stress scores. Your weekly average will give you a sense of your overall level of stress.

Using Your Results

How did you score? How high are your daily and weekly stress scores? Are you satisfied with your stress rating? If not, set a specific goal:

What should you do next? Enter the results of this lab in the Preprogram Assessment column in Appendix B. If you've set a goal for improvement, begin by using your log to look for patterns and significant time periods in order to identify key stressors in your life. Below, list any stressors that caused you a significant amount of discomfort this week; these can be people, places, events, or recurring thoughts or worries. For each, enter one strategy that would help you deal more successfully with the stressor. Examples of strategies might include practicing an oral presentation in front of a friend or engaging in positive self-talk.

Next, begin to put your strategies into action. In addition, complete Lab 10.2 to help you incorporate lifestyle stress-management techniques into your daily routine.

Name _____ Section _____ Date _____

LAB 10.2   Stress-Management Techniques

Part I Lifestyle Stress Management

For each of the areas listed in the table below, describe your current lifestyle as it relates to stress management. For example, do you have enough social support? How are your exercise and nutrition habits? Is time management a problem for you? For each area, list two ways that you could change your current habits to help you manage your stress. Sample strategies might include calling a friend before a challenging class, taking a short walk before lunch, and buying and using a datebook to track your time.

	CURRENT LIFESTYLE	LIFESTYLE CHANGE #1	LIFESTYLE CHANGE #2
Social support system			
Exercise habits			
Nutrition habits			
Time-management techniques			
Self-talk patterns			
Sleep habits			

LABORATORY ACTIVITIES

Part II Relaxation Techniques

Choose two relaxation techniques described in this chapter (progressive relaxation, visualization, deep breathing, meditation, listening to music). If a recording is available for progressive relaxation or visualization, these techniques can be performed by your entire class as a group.

List the techniques you tried.

1. _____

2. _____

How did you feel before you tried these techniques?

_____

_____

_____

What did you think or how did you feel during each of the techniques you tried?

1. _____

_____

_____

2. _____

_____

_____

How did you feel after you tried these techniques?

_____

_____

_____

Name _____ Section _____ Date _____

LAB 10.3 Evaluating and Improving Sleep

Adequate sleep helps you stay healthy and function at your best. However, chronic sleep loss and sleep disorders affect many Americans and contribute to lost productivity as well as health care expenses. Complete the checklists, log, and analysis below to evaluate and improve your sleep habits.

Do You Get Enough Sleep?

To determine whether you get enough high-quality sleep, review the following list of statements and check any that are true for you.

_____ 1. I feel very tired during the day.

_____ 2. I do not feel refreshed and alert when I wake up.

_____ 3. I often feel I could doze off while

_____ sitting and reading or watching media.

_____ sitting in a public place, such as a classroom, meeting, or movie theater.

_____ riding in a car for an hour without stopping.

_____ sitting and talking to someone.

_____ sitting quietly after lunch.

_____ sitting in traffic for a few minutes.

_____ 4. I often have trouble focusing, making decisions, solving problems, remembering things, and coping with change.

The more items you check, the more likely it is that you are not getting enough sleep. Insufficient or poor sleep can be due to a sleep disorder (see next section) or to not allotting enough time for sleep.

Do You Have Signs of a Sleep Disorder?

Review this list of common signs of a sleep disorder and check any that are true for you on three or more nights per week.

_____ 1. It takes me more than 30 minutes to fall asleep at night.

_____ 2. I awaken frequently in the night and then have trouble falling back to sleep again.

_____ 3. I awaken too early in the morning.

_____ 4. I often don't feel well rested despite spending seven to eight hours or more asleep at night.

_____ 5. I feel sleepy during the day and fall asleep within five minutes if I have an opportunity to nap, or I fall asleep unexpectedly or at inappropriate times during the day.

_____ 6. My bed partner claims that I snore loudly, snort, gasp, or make choking sounds while I sleep, or that my breathing stops for short periods.

_____ 7. I have creeping, tingling, or crawling feelings in my legs that are relieved by moving or massaging them, especially in the evening and when I try to fall asleep.

_____ 8. I have vivid, dreamlike experiences while falling asleep or dozing.

_____ 9. I have episodes of sudden muscle weakness when I am angry or fearful, or when I laugh.

_____ 10. I feel as though I cannot move when I first wake up.

_____ 11. My bed partner notes that my legs or arms jerk often during sleep.

_____ 12. I regularly need to use stimulants to stay awake during the day.

LABORATORY ACTIVITIES

If you checked any of these items, get an evaluation by a health care provider. Some items on the list can be symptoms of multiple types of sleep disorders, but some are characteristic of specific disorders:

- *Chronic insomnia:* Difficulty falling asleep or staying asleep on at least three nights per week for more than one month
- *Sleep apnea:* Intermittent blocking of the upper airway, causing pauses in breathing and sleep; often characterized by loud and frequent snoring, with periodic gasping or snorting noises
- *Restless leg syndrome:* Unpleasant prickling or tingling in the legs that is relieved by moving or massaging them; may also be characterized by brief and abrupt limb movements during sleep that can awaken the sleeper
- *Narcolepsy:* Overwhelming daytime sleepiness, sudden muscle weakness, sleep paralysis, and vivid dreams

Tracking Your Sleep

One of the best ways to determine if you are getting enough high-quality sleep, or if you have signs of a sleep disorder, is to keep a sleep log. Your log will give you an idea of how much uninterrupted sleep you need to avoid daytime sleepiness. You can also use the log to identify patterns or practices that may keep you from getting a good night's sleep.

Complete the log for at least a week to capture your typical pattern, which may vary between weekdays and weekends. You don't need to be exact; your best estimate is good enough. You may use a sleep app to inform your estimates, but don't keep checking the time, as that may negatively affect your sleep.

Date							
Complete in the morning:							
Time I went to bed last night							
Time I got up this morning							
How long I took to fall asleep last night							
Number of awakenings							
Total time awake last night							
Number of hours of sleep last night							
Medications taken last night							
How awake did I feel this morning 1 = wide awake 2 = awake but a little tired 3 = sleepy							
Complete in the evening:							
Number of caffeinated drinks and time when I had them today							
Number of alcoholic drinks and time when I had them today							
Naptimes and lengths today							
Exercise times and lengths today							
How sleepy did I feel today? 1 = so sleepy I had to struggle to stay awake 2 = somewhat tired 3 = fairly alert 4 = wide awake							

Analyzing Your Sleep Log

What is your current sleep schedule during the week? On the weekends?

How many hours of sleep do you currently average per night? How much sleep do you need to function well? How do the numbers compare? Remember, the amount of sleep time varies by individual; if you get eight hours of sleep a night and are still sleepy during the day, you may naturally require more sleep and should plan accordingly.

What would be your ideal sleep period if you could sleep anytime you wanted? What would be the best sleep period for you to get adequate sleep, considering your obligations and preferences? Why?

Could your consumption of caffeine or alcohol be affecting your sleep? What about your pattern of exercise? Do you have any medical conditions like nasal allergies or acid reflux that could interfere with sleep? Do you take any medications that can affect sleep?

Using Your Results

How did you score? Do you have signs of insufficient sleep or a sleep disorder? What did you learn from your sleep log?

What should you do next? Based on your analysis, identify at least one problem with your sleep pattern or with possible blockers of quality sleep. Set an appropriate SMART goal to address the problem, and then identify at least two concrete strategies to try. Your goal and strategies can focus on a specific sleep problem or on a time-management issue that limits your ability to schedule enough time for sleep.

SOURCES: Centers for Disease Control and Prevention. 2014. *Key Sleep Disorders* (https://www.cdc.gov/sleep/about_sleep/key_disorders.html); U.S. Department of Health and Human Services, National Institutes of Health, National Heart Lung and Blood Institute. 2011. *Your Guide to Healthy Sleep*. NIH Publication No. 11-5271.

11 Cardiovascular Health and Diabetes

LOOKING AHEAD...

After reading this chapter, you should be able to

- Describe the risk factors associated with cardiovascular disease.
- Discuss the major forms of cardiovascular disease and how they develop.
- List the steps you can take to protect yourself against cardiovascular disease.
- Describe types, risk factors, and prevention strategies for diabetes.

TEST YOUR KNOWLEDGE

1. Women are less likely to die of cardiovascular disease than they are to die of breast cancer. True or false?

2. On average, how much earlier does heart disease develop in people who don't exercise regularly than in people who do?
   a. 6 months
   b. 2 years
   c. 6 years

3. Which of the following foods would be a good choice for promoting heart health?
   a. whole grains
   b. salmon
   c. bananas

See answers on the next page.

©Hero Images/Getty Images

Cardiovascular disease (CVD) includes the diseases that affect the heart and blood vessels: heart disease, heart attack (blockage of the coronary artery), stroke (blockage of the cerebral artery), and angina (chest pain), as well as blood vessel diseases, arrhythmias (heart rhythm problems), congenital heart defects, and other conditions affecting the heart's muscle, valves, or rhythms.

As the country's leading cause of death, CVD claims more than 2,200 American lives every day. About 92 million American adults have one or more types of CVD, and of these, 46.7 million are estimated to be 60 years of age or younger. Heart disease, one form of CVD, is the leading cause of death for both U.S. men and women. Among the life-threatening manifestations of CVD, heart disease and strokes rank first and second on the list of the leading causes of death among Americans. High blood pressure, which is both a form of CVD and a risk factor for other types of disease, affects nearly 1 in every 3 adults, or about 86 million Americans. Although CVD may seem like a disease that affects only adults, evidence has been mounting that atherosclerosis, the underlying cause of CVD, begins in childhood.

CVD is largely due to our way of life. Millions of Americans are overweight and sedentary; we smoke, manage stress ineffectively, have uncontrolled high blood pressure or high cholesterol levels, and don't know the signs of CVD. Not all risk factors for CVD are controllable—for example, some people have an inherited tendency toward high cholesterol levels—but many risk factors are within your control.

In this chapter you'll learn about the major forms of CVD, including hypertension, atherosclerosis, and stroke, and also the factors that put people at risk for CVD. We'll also talk about diabetes because it is a key CVD risk factor and one of the leading causes of death among Americans. Most important, you'll learn the steps you can take to protect your heart and promote cardiovascular health throughout your life.

MAJOR FORMS OF CARDIOVASCULAR DISEASE

Although deaths from CVD have declined dramatically over the past 60 years, it remains the leading cause of death in the United States. Together, heart disease and stroke kill about 750,000 Americans per year. The financial burden of CVD, including the costs of medical treatments and lost productivity, exceeds $315 billion annually. Although the main forms of CVD are interrelated and have elements in common, we treat them separately here for the sake of clarity.

Atherosclerosis

Atherosclerosis, a form of arteriosclerosis, is a thickening and hardening of the arteries. In atherosclerosis, arteries narrow from deposits of fat, cholesterol, and other substances (Figure 11.1). The process begins when the cells lining the arteries (endothelial cells) become damaged, most likely through a combination of factors such as smoking, high blood pressure, high insulin or glucose levels, and deposits of oxidized LDL particles. The body's response to this damage results in inflammation and changes in the artery lining. Deposits, called **plaques**, accumulate on artery walls, and the arteries lose their elasticity and their ability to expand and contract, restricting blood flow. Once narrowed by a plaque, an artery is vulnerable to blockage by blood clots. The risk of life-threatening clots and heart attacks increases if the fibrous cap covering a plaque ruptures.

Inflammation deprives the heart, brain, or other organs of blood and oxygen, and can be deadly. Coronary arteries, which supply the heart with blood, are particularly susceptible to plaque buildup, a condition called **coronary heart disease (CHD)**, or *coronary artery disease* (*CAD*). The blockage of a coronary artery causes a heart attack. If a cerebral artery (leading to the brain) is blocked, the result is a stroke. The main risk factors for atherosclerosis are cigarette smoking, physical inactivity, high levels of blood cholesterol, high blood pressure, and diabetes.

Heart Disease and Heart Attacks

The American Heart Association estimates that 580,000 Americans have a first heart attack each year, and 210,000 suffer a recurrent attack. About 165,000 people suffer a symptomless, or "silent," heart attack each year. Although a **heart attack**, also called *myocardial infarction* (*MI*), may come without warning, it is usually the end result of a long-term disease process. The heart requires a steady supply of oxygen-rich blood to function properly (Figure 11.2). If one

---

TERMS

cardiovascular disease (CVD)   A collective term for various diseases of the heart and blood vessels.

atherosclerosis   A form of CVD in which the inner layers of artery walls are made thick and irregular by plaque deposits; arteries become narrowed, and blood supply is reduced.

plaque   A deposit of fatty (and other) substances on the inner wall of an artery.

coronary heart disease (CHD)   Heart disease caused by atherosclerosis in the arteries that supply blood to the heart muscle; also called *coronary artery disease (CAD)*.

heart attack   Damage to, or death of, heart muscle, resulting from a failure of the coronary arteries to deliver enough blood to the heart; also known as *myocardial infarction (MI)*.

Answers (Test Your Knowledge)

1. **False.** Cardiovascular disease kills far more. Among American women, nearly 1 in 4 die of cardiovascular disease, taking more lives than all forms of cancer combined.

2. **C, 6 years.** Both aerobic exercise and strength training significantly improve cardiovascular health.

3. **All three.** Whole grains (whole wheat, oatmeal, rye, barley, and brown rice), foods with omega-3 fatty acids (salmon), and foods high in potassium and low in sodium (bananas) all improve cardiovascular health.

1. A healthy artery allows blood to flow through freely.

2. Plaque buildup begins when endothelial cells lining the arteries are damaged by smoking, high blood pressure, oxidized LDL cholesterol, and other causes. Excess cholesterol particles collect beneath these cells.

3. In response to the damage, platelets and other types of cells collect at the site. A fibrous cap forms, isolating the plaque within the artery wall. An early-stage plaque is called a fatty streak.

4. Chemicals released by cells in and around the plaque cause further inflammation and buildup. An advanced plaque contains LDL cholesterol, white blood cells, connective tissue, smooth muscle cells, platelets, and other compounds.

5. The narrowed artery is vulnerable to blockage by blood clots. The risk of blockage and heart attack or stroke rises if the fibrous cap cracks, probably due to the action of destructive enzymes released by white blood cells within the plaque.

6. If a clot is traveling through the bloodstream, it may become trapped in the narrowed artery at the site of the plaque buildup, cutting off blood supply and oxygen to tissue.

FIGURE 11.1 Atherosclerosis: The process of cardiovascular disease.

coronary artery that supplies blood to the heart becomes blocked, a heart attack results. A heart attack caused by a blood clot is called *coronary thrombosis.* During a heart attack, part of the heart muscle (myocardium) may die from lack of blood flow.

Chest pain, called **angina pectoris**, is a signal that the heart isn't getting enough oxygen to supply its needs. Although not actually a heart attack, angina—felt as an extreme tightness in the chest and heavy pressure behind the breastbone or in the shoulder, neck, arm, hand, or back—is a warning that the heart is overloaded.

If the electrical impulses that control heartbeat are disrupted, the heart may beat too quickly, too slowly, or in an irregular fashion, a condition known as **arrhythmia**. The symptoms of arrhythmia range from imperceptible to severe and even fatal. **Sudden cardiac death**, also called *cardiac arrest,* is most often caused by an arrhythmia called *ventricular fibrillation,* a kind of "quivering" of the ventricle that makes it ineffective in pumping blood. If ventricular fibrillation continues for more than a few minutes, it is generally fatal. Cardiac defibrillation, in which an electrical shock is delivered to the heart, can jolt the heart into a more efficient rhythm. This shock can be administered with an automated external defibrillator (AED), a first-aid device that is available in many public places in case someone experiences a heart attack.

Heart attack symptoms may include pain or pressure in the chest; pain in the arm, neck, or jaw; difficulty breathing; excessive sweating; nausea and vomiting; and loss of

angina pectoris A condition in which the heart muscle does not receive enough blood, causing severe pain in the chest and often in the arm and shoulder.

arrhythmia A change in the normal pattern of the heartbeat.

sudden cardiac death A nontraumatic, unexpected death from sudden cardiac arrest, most often due to arrhythmia; in most instances, victims have underlying heart disease.

TERMS

FIGURE 11.2 Blood supply to the heart. Blood is supplied to the heart from the right and left coronary arteries, which branch off the aorta. If a coronary artery becomes blocked by plaque buildup or a blood clot, a heart attack occurs; part of the heart muscle may die due to lack of oxygen.

consciousness. But not all heart attacks involve sharp chest pain. Women, in particular, are more likely to have different symptoms—shortness of breath, weakness, unusual fatigue, cold sweat, and dizziness.

If symptoms of heart trouble occur, contact an emergency medical service or go immediately to the nearest hospital or clinic (see the box "Warning Signs of Heart Attack, Stroke, and Cardiac Arrest"). Many experts also suggest that the heart attack victim chew and swallow one adult aspirin tablet (325 mg); aspirin has an immediate anticlotting effect. If someone having a heart attack gets to the emergency department quickly enough, an injection can be used to dissolve a clot in the coronary artery, reducing the amount of damage to the heart muscle.

Physicians have a variety of diagnostic tools and treatments for heart disease. Patients may undergo a stress or exercise test, in which they run on a treadmill or pedal a stationary cycle while being monitored with an electrocardiogram (ECG or EKG). Characteristic changes in the heart's electrical activity during the test can reveal particular heart problems, such as restricted blood flow to the heart muscle. Tools that allow the physician to visualize a patient's heart and arteries include a special type of X-ray known as an angiogram, magnetic resonance imaging (MRI), electron-beam computed tomography (EBCT), echocardiograms, and others.

If tests indicate a cardiovascular problem, or if a person has already had a heart attack, several treatments are possible. Along with a low-fat diet, regular exercise, and smoking

cessation, many patients are also advised to take a low-dose aspirin tablet (81 mg) daily. Aspirin has an anticlotting effect, keeping platelets in the blood from sticking to arterial plaques and forming clots; it also reduces inflammation. Low-dose aspirin therapy may help prevent first heart attacks in men, second heart attacks in men and women, and strokes in women over age 65. In addition to aspirin, prescription drugs can also help reduce the strain on the heart.

Several surgical treatments exist for certain forms of heart disease. *Balloon angioplasty* threads a catheter with an inflatable balloon tip through a coronary artery until it reaches the area of blockage; as the balloon is inflated, it flattens the plaque, widening the arterial opening. Many surgeons implant permanent coronary *stents*—flexible stainless steel tubes—to prop open the artery and prevent reclogging after angioplasty. In coronary bypass surgery, healthy blood vessels are grafted to coronary arteries to bypass blockages.

Stroke

A **stroke**, called a *cerebrovascular accident* (*CVA*), occurs when the blood supply to the brain is cut off. If brain cells are deprived of blood for more than a few minutes, they die. Once brain cells die, about two million cells are lost every minute that blood flow is not restored. Nerve cells control sensation and most body movements; depending on the area of the brain affected, a stroke may cause paralysis, walking disability, speech impairment, memory loss, and changes in behavior. Prompt treatment of stroke can greatly decrease the risk of permanent disability. The American Heart Association estimates that 795,000 Americans suffer a stroke each year.

There are two major types of strokes: ischemic and hemorrhagic. Ischemic strokes are the more common type and account for 87% of all strokes. They are caused by a blockage in a blood vessel. There are two types of ischemic strokes:

- A *thrombotic stroke* is caused by a blood clot that forms in a cerebral or carotid artery that has been narrowed or damaged by atherosclerosis.

- An *embolic stroke* is caused by an embolus, a wandering blood clot that is carried in the bloodstream and may become wedged in a cerebral artery.

A *hemorrhagic stroke* occurs when a blood vessel in the brain bursts, spilling blood into the surrounding tissue. Cells normally nourished by the vessel are deprived of blood and cannot function. In addition, accumulated blood from the burst vessel may put pressure on surrounding brain tissue, causing damage and even death.

Hemorrhages can be caused by head injuries, by a malformed blood vessel bursting, or by an *aneurysm*, which is a blood-filled pocket that bulges out from a weak spot in the artery wall. Aneurysms in the brain may remain stable and never break, but when they do, the result is a hemorrhagic stroke. Aneurysms may be caused or worsened by hypertension.

Many people have strokes without knowing it. Because silent strokes do not cause symptoms while they are occurring, many people do not realize they need evaluation or treatment

Warning Signs of Heart Attack, Stroke, and Cardiac Arrest

Heart Attack Warning Signs

The most common warning symptoms of a heart attack for both men and women are the following:

- *Chest pain or discomfort (angina)* in the center or left side of the chest that usually lasts for more than a few minutes or goes away and comes back. It can feel like pressure, squeezing, fullness, or pain. It can also feel like heartburn or indigestion and can be mild or severe.

- *Upper body discomfort* in one or both arms, the back, shoulders, neck, jaw, or upper part of the stomach (above the navel).

- *Shortness of breath* may be the only symptom, or it may occur before or along with chest pain or discomfort. It can occur when you are resting or doing mild physical activity.

But remember these additional facts:

- Heart attacks can start slowly and cause only mild pain or discomfort. Symptoms can be mild or more intense and sudden. Symptoms also may come and go over several hours.

- People who have high blood sugar (diabetes) may have no symptoms or very mild ones. Heart attacks without symptoms or with very mild symptoms are called silent heart attacks.

- The most common symptom, in both men and women, is chest pain or discomfort.

- Women are somewhat more likely to have shortness of breath; nausea and vomiting; unusual tiredness (sometimes for days); and pain in the back, shoulders, and jaw.

- Other possible symptoms include breaking out in a cold sweat, light-headedness or sudden dizziness, or a change in the pattern of usual symptoms.

The signs and symptoms of a heart attack can develop suddenly or slowly—within hours, days, or weeks of a heart attack. If you think you or someone you know might be having heart attack symptoms or a heart attack, don't ignore it or feel embarrassed to call for help. **Call 9-1-1 right away.** Here's why:

- Acting fast can be life saving. Every minute matters. Never delay calling 9-1-1 to do anything you think might help.

- An ambulance is the best and safest way to get to the hospital. Emergency medical services (EMS) personnel start life-saving treatments right away. People who arrive by ambulance often receive faster treatment at the hospital.

- The 9-1-1 operator or EMS technician can give you advice. You might be told to crush or chew an aspirin if you're not allergic, unless there is a medical reason for you not to take one.

Stroke Warning Signs

The symptoms of stroke are distinctive because they happen quickly:

- Sudden numbness or weakness of the face, arm, or leg (especially on one side of the body)

- Sudden confusion, trouble speaking or understanding speech

- Sudden trouble seeing from one or both eyes

- Sudden trouble walking, dizziness, loss of balance or coordination

- Sudden severe headache with no known cause

An acronym to help you remember the signs of stroke and what to do is FAST. This stands for Facial drooping, Arm weakness, Speech difficulties, and Time to call 9-1-1. If you believe someone is having a stroke, call 9-1-1 immediately. Ischemic strokes, the most common type, can be treated with a drug called t-PA, which dissolves blood clots. The drug must be administered within three hours, but to be evaluated and treated in time, patients must get to the hospital within 60 minutes.

A transient ischemic attack (TIA) occurs when blood to the brain is briefly blocked. TIAs have the same signs and symptoms as a stroke but usually last less than 1–2 hours (although they may last up to 24 hours). A TIA, which may occur only once in a person's lifetime or more often, can be a warning sign for future strokes.

Sudden Cardiac Arrest Signs

In sudden cardiac arrest (SCA), the heart suddenly and unexpectedly stops beating. As a result, blood stops flowing to the brain and other vital organs. The person suddenly becomes unresponsive and stops breathing, and if not treated within minutes, death can occur. Some people may have a racing heartbeat or feel dizzy or light-headed just before they lose consciousness (faint). Within an hour before SCA, some people have chest pain, shortness of breath, nausea, or vomiting. Usually, however, the first sign of SCA is loss of consciousness. At the same time, no heartbeat (or pulse) can be felt.

If you are with someone who suddenly experiences these symptoms, begin CPR (see Appendix A) and call 9-1-1 immediately. Rapid treatment of SCA with a defibrillator can save a life. A defibrillator is a device that sends an electric shock to the heart to restore its normal rhythm. Automated external defibrillators (AEDs) can be used by bystanders to save the lives of people who are having SCA. (See how to use one at the National Heart, Blood, and Lung Institute website: https://www.nhlbi.nih.gov/health/health-topics/topics/aed/howtouse.) These portable devices are often found in public places, such as shopping malls, golf courses, businesses, airports, airplanes, convention centers, hotels, sports venues, and schools.

©Robert Alexander/Getty Images

SOURCES: National Heart, Lung, and Blood Institute. 2013. *What Are the Symptoms of a Heart Attack?* (http://www.nhlbi.nih.gov/health/health-topics/topics/heartattack/signs); National Institute of Neurological disorders and Stroke. 2013. *Know Stroke. Know the Signs. Act in Time.* (http://www.ninds.nih.gov/disorders/stroke/knowstroke.htm); National Heart, Lung, and Blood Institute. 2011. *What Is Sudden Cardiac Arrest?* (http://www.nhlbi.nih.gov/health/health-topics/topics/scda).

Box icon: ©VisualCommunications/Getty Images RF

for the risk of a full-blown stroke in the future. Although they may be mild, silent strokes leave their victims at a higher risk for subsequent and more serious strokes later in life. They also contribute to loss of mental and cognitive skills.

Some stroke victims have a transient ischemic attack (TIA), or "ministroke," days, weeks, or months before they have a full-blown stroke (see the box "Warning Signs of Heart Attack, Stroke, and Cardiac Arrest"). A TIA produces temporary stroke-like symptoms, such as weakness or numbness in an arm or a leg, speech difficulty, or dizziness. These symptoms are brief, often lasting just a few minutes, and do not cause permanent damage. Still, anyone with a suspected TIA should get immediate medical attention.

Congestive Heart Failure

The heart's pumping mechanism can be damaged by a number of conditions, including high blood pressure, heart attack, atherosclerosis, viral infections, rheumatic fever, and birth defects. When the heart cannot maintain its regular pumping rate and force, fluids begin to back up. When extra fluid seeps through capillary walls, edema (swelling) results, usually in the legs and ankles, but sometimes in other parts of the body as well. Fluid can collect in the lungs and interfere with breathing, particularly when a person is lying down. This condition is called *pulmonary edema,* and the entire process is known as **congestive heart failure**. Treatment includes reducing the workload on the heart, modifying salt intake, and using drugs that help the body eliminate excess fluid.

RISK FACTORS FOR CARDIOVASCULAR DISEASE

Researchers have identified a variety of factors associated with an increased risk of developing CVD. They have categorized them as major risk factors and contributing risk factors. Some are linked to controllable aspects of lifestyle and can therefore be changed. Others are beyond your control. (You can evaluate your personal CVD risk factors in Part I of Lab 11.1.)

Major Risk Factors That Can Be Changed

The American Heart Association (AHA) has identified six major risk factors for CVD that can be changed: tobacco smoke, high blood pressure, unhealthy cholesterol levels, physical

---

congestive heart failure A condition resulting from the heart's inability to pump out all the blood that returns to it; blood backs up in the veins leading to the heart, causing an accumulation of fluid in various parts of the body.

platelets Cell fragments in the blood that are necessary for the formation of blood clots.

hypertension Sustained abnormally high blood pressure.

TERMS

---

inactivity, obesity, and diabetes. Most Americans, including young adults, have at least one major risk factor for CVD that they can control.

Tobacco Smoke Annually, nearly 1 in 5 deaths is attributable to smoking, equivalent to 1,300 deaths per day. More than 16% of adult men and 13% of adult women smoke. Among young adults aged 18–24, 13.0% are current smokers. Smoking remains the leading preventable causes of CVD in the United States. People who smoke a pack of cigarettes a day have twice the risk of heart attack that nonsmokers do; smoking two or more packs a day triples the risk. When smokers have heart attacks, they are two to three times more likely than nonsmokers to die from them. Cigarette smoking also doubles the risk of stroke. Exposure to other people's smoke also increases the risk of heart disease even for nonsmokers.

Smoking harms the cardiovascular system in several ways:

- It damages the lining of arteries.
- It reduces the level of *high-density lipoproteins (HDL),* or "good" cholesterol.
- It raises the levels of triglycerides and *low-density lipoproteins (LDL),* or "bad" cholesterol.
- Nicotine increases blood pressure and heart rate.
- The carbon monoxide in cigarette smoke displaces oxygen in the blood, reducing the oxygen available to the body, and decreases exercise tolerance.
- Smoking causes **platelets** to stick together in the bloodstream, leading to clotting.
- Smoking speeds the development of fatty deposits in the arteries.

You don't have to smoke to be affected. The risk of developing heart disease increases up to 30% among people exposed to environmental tobacco smoke (ETS)—also known as "secondhand smoke." As of 2016, researchers estimate that about 69,000 nonsmokers die from heart disease each year as a result of exposure to ETS.

Recently, electronic cigarettes (or e-cigarettes) have become popular, especially among teenagers and young adults. As of 2016, approximately 13% of high school seniors were current (past 30-day) users of electronic cigarettes. Notably, e-cigarettes contain nicotine, which causes addiction, may harm brain development, affects cardiovascular function, and could lead to continued tobacco product use among youth. The Centers for Disease Control and Prevention (CDC) has identified electronic cigarettes as an area of concern due to the potential harm to public health in the United States.

High Blood Pressure In addition to being a form of CVD in itself, high blood pressure, or **hypertension**, is a risk factor for other forms of cardiovascular disease, including heart attacks and strokes.

Created by the pumping action of the heart, blood pressure is the force exerted by the blood on the vessel walls. High blood pressure occurs when too much force is exerted against the walls of the arteries, thereby increasing the heart's workload and decreasing its efficiency. Short periods of high blood pressure—such as in response to excitement or exertion—are normal, but chronic high blood pressure is a health risk.

Blood pressure is expressed as two numbers—for example, 120 over 80—and measured in millimeters of mercury (mmHg). The first number measures systolic blood pressure, the greatest pressure your blood exerts against artery walls as your heart beats, pushing blood around the body. The second measures diastolic blood pressure, the lowest pressure, which occurs when your heart relaxes between beats (see Chapter 3). A normal blood pressure reading for a healthy adult is below 120 systolic and below 80 diastolic. Blood pressure readings above this level indicate an increased risk for CVD and are classified as prehypertension or hypertension. High blood pressure (hypertension) in adults is defined as equal to or greater than 140 over 90 (Table 11.1). Health care professionals measure blood pressure with a stethoscope and an instrument called a *sphygmomanometer*. Professional measurement is needed for a diagnosis of hypertension, but you can track your own blood pressure at a drugstore or at home with an inexpensive monitor, and some new technologies measure blood pressure with wearable devices.

High blood pressure results from the heart's increased output of blood or from the arteries' increased resistance to blood flow. Arterial resistance can be caused by the constriction of smooth muscle surrounding the arteries or by atherosclerosis, a disease process that causes arteries to clog and narrow. High blood pressure also scars and hardens arteries, making them less elastic and further increasing blood pressure. When a person has high blood pressure, the heart must work harder than normal to force blood through the narrowed and stiffened arteries, straining both the heart and the arteries. Eventually, the strained heart weakens and tends to enlarge, which weakens it even more.

High blood pressure is often called a silent killer, because it usually has no symptoms. A person may have high blood pressure for years without realizing it. But during that time, it damages vital organs and increases the risk of heart attack, congestive heart failure, stroke, kidney failure, and blindness.

Recent research has shed new light on the importance of lowering blood pressure to improve cardiovascular health. The risk of death from heart attack or stroke begins to rise even within the "normal" range when blood pressure is above 115 over 75, well below the traditional 140 over 90 cutoff for hypertension. People with blood pressures in the prehypertension range (defined as systolic pressure of 120–139 and diastolic pressure of 80–89) are at increased risk of heart attack and stroke as well as at significant risk of developing full-blown hypertension.

About 53% of American adults age 20 and older have hypertension or prehypertension. The incidence of high blood pressure rises dramatically with age, but it can occur among children and young adults. In most cases, hypertension cannot be cured, but it can be controlled. The key to avoiding complications is to have your blood pressure tested at least once every two years (or if you have other CVD risk factors, at least once every year).

Lifestyle changes are recommended for everyone with high "normal" range blood pressure, prehypertension, and hypertension. These changes include weight reduction, regular physical activity, a healthy diet, and moderation of alcohol use. The DASH diet (see Chapter 8) is recommended specifically for people with high blood pressure; it emphasizes fruits, vegetables, and whole grains—foods that are rich in potassium and fiber, both of which may reduce blood pressure. Sodium restriction is also helpful. The *2015–2020 Dietary Guidelines for Americans* recommends restricting sodium consumption to less than 2,300 mg (equivalent to a teaspoon of salt) per day for adults and children age 14 and older. This recommendation applies to all people but is particularly important for those with hypertension or prehypertension, African Americans, and middle-aged and older adults. For these groups, further reduction in sodium intake to 1,500 mg per day can result in even greater blood pressure reduction. Adequate potassium intake is also important. New blood pressure drug treatments are available, as well as particular combinations for the elderly and people with diabetes, chronic kidney disease, and cardiovascular diseases. People who fall into the category of prehypertension or the high normal blood pressure range may not benefit from drug therapy.

Unhealthy Cholesterol Levels *Cholesterol* is a fatty, waxlike substance that circulates through the bloodstream and is an important component of cell membranes, sex hormones, vitamin D, the fluid that coats the lungs, and the protective sheaths around nerves. Adequate cholesterol is essential for the proper functioning of the body. Excess cholesterol, however, can clog arteries and increase the risk of CVD (Figure 11.3). Your liver manufactures cholesterol; foods can also increase the cholesterol level.

Table 11.1	Blood Pressure Classification for Healthy Adults		
CATEGORY*	SYSTOLIC (mm Hg)		DIASTOLIC (mm Hg)
Normal**	below 120	and	below 80
Prehypertension	120–139	or	80–89
Hypertension[1]			
Stage 1	140–159	or	90–99
Stage 2	160 and above	or	100 and above

*When systolic and diastolic pressure fall into different categories, the higher category should be used to classify blood pressure status.

**Blood pressure 120/80 and above carries risk of heart attack and stroke.

[1]Based on the average of three or more readings taken at different times. In persons over age 50, systolic blood pressure greater than 140 is a much more significant CVD risk factor than elevated diastolic blood pressure.

SOURCE: Benjamin, E. J. et al. 2017. "Heart disease and stroke statistics—2017 update," *Circulation* 135:00—00; James, P. A., et al. 2014. "2014 Evidence-based guideline for the management of high blood pressure in adults," Report from the panel members appointed to the Eighth Joint National Committee (JNC 8), *JAMA* 311(5): 507—520.

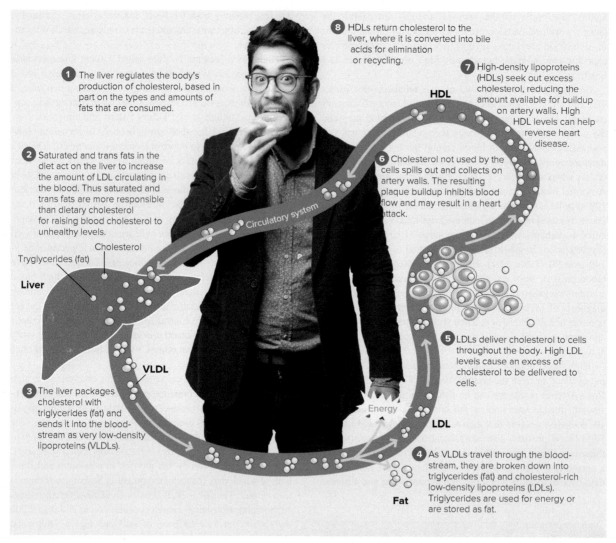

1. The liver regulates the body's production of cholesterol, based in part on the types and amounts of fats that are consumed.

2. Saturated and trans fats in the diet act on the liver to increase the amount of LDL circulating in the blood. Thus saturated and trans fats are more responsible than dietary cholesterol for raising blood cholesterol to unhealthy levels.

Tryglycerides (fat)

Cholesterol

Liver

3. The liver packages cholesterol with triglycerides (fat) and sends it into the blood-stream as very low-density lipoproteins (VLDLs).

VLDL

Circulatory system

8. HDLs return cholesterol to the liver, where it is converted into bile acids for elimination or recycling.

7. High-density lipoproteins (HDLs) seek out excess cholesterol, reducing the amount available for buildup on artery walls. High HDL levels can help reverse heart disease.

HDL

6. Cholesterol not used by the cells spills out and collects on artery walls. The resulting plaque buildup inhibits blood flow and may result in a heart attack.

5. LDLs deliver cholesterol to cells throughout the body. High LDL levels cause an excess of cholesterol to be delivered to cells.

Energy

LDL

4. As VLDLs travel through the blood-stream, they are broken down into triglycerides (fat) and cholesterol-rich low-density lipoproteins (LDLs). Triglycerides are used for energy or are stored as fat.

Fat

FIGURE 11.3 **Travels with cholesterol.**

©Asier Romero/Shutterstock.com RF

GOOD VERSUS BAD CHOLESTEROL   Cholesterol is carried in the blood by protein-lipid packages called **lipoproteins**. **Low-density lipoproteins (LDLs)** shuttle cholesterol from the liver to the organs and tissues that require it. LDL is known as "bad" cholesterol because if there is more than the body can use, the excess can be deposited in the blood vessels. The accumulated LDL becomes encased in artery walls and may be oxidized by free radicals, speeding inflammation and damage to artery walls and increasing the likelihood that an artery will become blocked, causing a heart attack or stroke. **High-density lipoproteins (HDLs)**, or "good" cholesterol, act as scavengers and are transported in a protein package that takes LDL choles-terol back to the liver for recycling. By removing cholesterol from blood vessels, HDLs help protect against atherosclerosis.

RECOMMENDED BLOOD CHOLESTEROL LEVELS   Screening for cholesterol provides one part of the assessment of the risk of cardiovascular disease. This risk for CVD increases with higher LDL cholesterol levels. The National Cholesterol Education Program recommends testing at least once every five years for all adults, beginning at age 20. The recommended test is a fasting lipoprotein profile that measures total cholesterol, LDL cholesterol, HDL cholesterol, and triglycerides (a type of blood

TERMS

lipoproteins   Protein-and-lipid substances in the blood that carry fats and cholesterol; classified according to size, density, and chemical composition.

low-density lipoprotein (LDL)   A lipoprotein containing a moderate amount of protein and a large amount of cholesterol; "bad" cholesterol.

high-density lipoprotein (HDL)   A lipoprotein containing relatively little cholesterol that helps transport cholesterol out of the arteries; "good" cholesterol.

fat). In general, high LDL, total cholesterol, and triglyceride levels, combined with low HDL levels, are associated with a higher risk for CVD. You can reduce this risk by lowering LDL, total cholesterol, and triglycerides. Raising HDL is important because a high HDL level seems to offer some protection from CVD even in cases where total cholesterol is high. This appears to be especially true for women.

In 2013 the American College of Cardiology (ACC) and the AHA updated their guidelines for the treatment of elevated blood cholesterol levels. The new guidelines focus on lifestyle change as well as therapy with *statins,* a group of medications that lower LDL. Although the previous guidelines set specific targets for LDL and HDL, the new guidelines do not; instead, they focus on identifying the groups of people for whom medical treatment has the greatest chance of preventing heart attacks and strokes. For these at-risk groups, treatment with statin therapy is recommended (Table 11.2). Experts hope that the new recommendations will mean that more people who would benefit from statin therapy will get it, while those who would not benefit will avoid unnecessary treatment.

Subjects can review their specific risk factors and the pros and cons of therapy with their health care providers. Lifestyle choices to help improve cholesterol levels include exercising regularly, limiting saturated and trans fat intake, and choosing a healthy dietary pattern. To lower LDL, the ACC and AHA recommend a dietary pattern that is rich in fruits, vegetables, and whole grains; includes low-fat dairy, poultry, fish, legumes, nontropical vegetable oils, and nuts; and limits sweets, sugar-sweetened beverages, and red meats.

Physical Inactivity At risk for CVD, about 1 in every 3 Americans is sedentary during leisure time. Exercise is thought to be the closest thing we have to a magic bullet against heart disease. It lowers CVD risk by helping to decrease blood pressure and resting heart rate, increase HDL levels, maintain desirable weight, improve the condition of the blood vessels, and prevent or control diabetes. One study found that women who got in at least three hours of brisk walking each week cut their risk of heart attack and stroke by more than half. (See Chapter 3 for more information on the benefits of cardiorespiratory exercise.)

Obesity The risk of death from CVD is two to three times higher in obese people (BMI $\geq$ 30) than it is in lean people (BMI 18.5–24.9), and for every five-unit increment of BMI, a person's risk of death from coronary heart disease increases by 30%. Excess weight increases the strain on the heart by contributing to high blood pressure and high cholesterol. It can also lead to diabetes, another CVD risk factor (see the next section). As discussed in Chapter 6, distribution of body fat is also significant: Fat that collects in the abdomen is more dangerous than fat that collects around the hips. Obesity in general, and abdominal obesity in particular, is significantly associated with narrowing of the coronary arteries, even in young adults in their 20s.

A sensible diet and regular exercise are the best ways to achieve and maintain a healthy body weight (see Chapter 9 for an extensive discussion of weight control). For someone who is overweight, even modest weight reduction can reduce CVD risk by lowering blood pressure, improving cholesterol levels, and reducing diabetes risk.

Diabetes **Diabetes mellitus** is a disorder in which the metabolism of glucose is disrupted, causing a buildup of glucose in the bloodstream. People with diabetes are at increased risk for CVD, partly because elevated blood glucose levels can damage

> **diabetes mellitus** A disease that disrupts normal metabolism, interfering with cells' ability to take in glucose for energy production. **TERMS**

Table 11.2	Groups Who Benefit from Treatment of Elevated Cholesterol
GROUP	TREATMENT RECOMMENDATION
1. People age 75 or younger with known CVD*	High-intensity statin therapy unless contraindicated; no recommendation for people with heart failure or those on dialysis for kidney disease
2. People age 21 and older with high LDL levels, 190 mg/dL or greater	High-intensity statin therapy unless contraindicated, or maximum tolerated intensity of therapy
3. People ages 40–75 *with* diabetes *and* an LDL level 70–189 mg/dL who do *not* have a history of cardiovascular disease	Moderate-intensity statin therapy, with high-intensity therapy considered for those with a 7.5% or greater estimated risk of developing CVD over the next 10 years**
4. People ages 40–75 *without* diabetes or known cardiovascular disease but *with* a high risk of developing CVD over the next 10 years *and* an LDL level 70–189 mg/d	Moderate- to high-intensity therapy for those with an estimated 10-year risk of CVD of 7.5% or greater; moderate-intensity therapy considered for those with an estimated 10-year risk of CVD of 5% to less than 7.5%**

*Atherosclerotic cardiovascular disease types include previous heart attacks, chest pain due to partially clogged arteries, history of invasive treatment for clogged arteries, previous stroke, or previous clogged arteries in the limbs.

**10-year cardiovascular risk is calculated using a new tool available on the AHA website (https://professional.heart.org/professional/GuidelinesStatements/PreventionGuidelines/UCM_457698_Prevention-Guidelines.jsp).

SOURCE: Stone, N. J., et al. 2014. "2013 ACC/AHA guideline on the treatment of blood cholesterol to reduce atherosclerotic cardiovascular risk in adults. A report of the American College of Cardiology/American Heart Association Task Force on Practice Guidelines," *Journal of the American College of Cardiology* 63(25_PA).

the lining of arteries, making them more vulnerable to atherosclerosis. Diabetics also often have other risk factors, including hypertension, obesity, unhealthy cholesterol and triglyceride levels, and platelet and blood coagulation abnormalities. Even people whose diabetes is under control face an increased risk of CVD. Therefore, careful control of other risk factors is critical for people with diabetes. Diabetes is described in detail later in the chapter.

Contributing Risk Factors That Can Be Changed

As with the major risk factors, some contributing CVD risk factors can be changed, including triglyceride levels, psychological and social factors, and drug use.

High Triglyceride Levels *Triglycerides* are blood fats that are absorbed from food and manufactured by the body. High triglyceride levels are a reliable predictor of heart disease, especially if associated with other risk factors, such as low HDL levels, obesity, and diabetes. Factors contributing to elevated triglyceride levels include excess body fat, physical inactivity, cigarette smoking, type 2 diabetes, excessive alcohol intake, very-high-carbohydrate diets, and certain diseases and medications. A full lipid profile should include testing and evaluation of triglyceride levels.

For people with high triglyceride levels, lifestyle changes can bring levels down into the healthy range: losing weight, reducing intake of added sugars while increasing intake of unsaturated fats, and increasing physical activity. Limiting alcohol use is also helpful. For some people with very high triglyceride levels, drug therapy may be prescribed.

Insulin Resistance and Metabolic Syndrome As people gain weight and become less active, their muscles, fat, and liver become less sensitive to the effect of insulin—a condition known as *insulin resistance* (or prediabetes). As the body becomes increasingly insulin resistant, the pancreas must secrete more and more insulin (hyperinsulinemia) to keep glucose levels within a normal range. Eventually even high levels of insulin may become insufficient, and blood glucose levels start to rise (hyperglycemia), resulting in type 2 diabetes.

Those who have insulin resistance tend to have several other related risk factors. This cluster of abnormalities is called *metabolic syndrome* or *insulin resistance syndrome* (Table 11.3). Metabolic syndrome significantly increases the risk of CVD—more so in women than in men. It is estimated that about 34% of the adult U.S. population has metabolic syndrome.

To reduce your risk of developing metabolic syndrome, choose a healthy dietary pattern and get plenty of aerobic exercise. Reducing calorie intake to prevent weight gain, or losing weight if needed, also reduces insulin resistance. Eating more protein, vegetables, and fiber while limiting fat, added sugars, and starches may be beneficial.

Table 11.3	Characteristics of Metabolic Syndrome*
FACTOR	CRITERIA
Large waistline	35 or more inches for women
	40 or more inches for men
High triglyceride level	150 mg/dL or higher
	Or taking medication to treat high triglycerides
Low HDL level	Less than 50 mg/dL for women
	Less than 40 mg/dL for men or taking medication to treat low HDL
High blood pressure	130/85 mmHg
	Or higher (one or both numbers)
	Or taking medication to treat high blood pressure
High fasting blood sugar	100 mg/dL or higher
	Or taking medication to treat high blood sugar

*A person having three or more factors listed here is diagnosed with metabolic syndrome.

SOURCE: Adapted from National Heart, Lung, and Blood Institute. 2011. *How Is Metabolic Syndrome Diagnosed?* (http://www.nhlbi.nih.gov/health/health-topics/topics/ms/diagnosis).

Inflammation Inflammation plays a key role in the development of CVD. When an artery is injured by hypertension, smoking, cholesterol, or other factors, the body's response is to produce inflammation. A substance called C-reactive protein (CRP) is released into the bloodstream during the inflammatory response, and high levels of CRP indicate a substantially elevated risk of heart attack and stroke. CRP may also be harmful to the coronary arteries themselves. Gum disease involves another type of inflammation that may moderately influence the progress of coronary heart disease.

Lifestyle changes and certain drugs can reduce CRP levels. Statin drugs, widely prescribed to lower cholesterol, also decrease inflammation; this may be one reason that statin drugs seem to lower CVD risk even in people with normal blood lipid levels.

Psychological and Social Factors Many of the psychological and social factors that influence other areas of wellness are also important risk factors for CVD. They include chronic stress, chronic hostility and anger, lack of social support, and others. The cardiovascular system is affected by both sudden, acute episodes of mental stress and the more chronic, underlying emotions of anger, anxiety, and depression. See Chapter 10 for more information on stress, its effects, and ways to combat these effects.

Alcohol and Drugs Drinking too much alcohol raises blood pressure and can increase the risk of stroke and heart failure. Stimulant drugs, particularly cocaine and methamphetamines—and associated stimulants, such as designer drugs like ecstasy (MDMA)—can also cause serious cardiac problems, including heart attack, stroke, and sudden cardiac death. Injection drug use can cause heart infections and stroke.

Wellness Tip Stress and social isolation increase the risk of cardiovascular disease, whereas social support buffers risk and may prevent or delay the onset of CVD. A strong social support network improves both heart health and overall wellness and can provide opportunities for exercise and relaxation. Take time out to develop and nurture friendships and family ties.

©David Buffington/Blend Images/Getty Images RF

Major Risk Factors That Can't Be Changed

A number of major risk factors for CVD cannot be changed. They include genetics, aging, being male, and ethnicity.

Genetics Multiple genes contribute to the development of CVD and its risk factors. Having an unfavorable set of genes increases your risk, but risk is modifiable by lifestyle factors such as whether you smoke, exercise, or eat a healthy diet. People who inherit a tendency for CVD are not destined to develop it, but they may have to work harder than other people to prevent it.

Age About 70% of all heart attack victims are age 65 or older, and about 75% who suffer fatal heart attacks are over 65. For people over 55, the incidence of stroke more than doubles in each successive decade. However, even people in their 30s and 40s, especially men, can have heart attacks.

Gender Although CVD is the leading killer of both men and women in the United States, men face a greater risk of heart attack than women, especially earlier in life. Until age 55, men

also have a greater risk of hypertension than women. The incidence of stroke is higher for males than females until age 65. Estrogen production, which is highest during the child-bearing years, may protect premenopausal women against CVD (see the box "Gender, Race/Ethnicity, and CVD"). By age 75, the gender gap nearly disappears.

Race/Ethnicity Rates of heart disease and CVD risk factors vary among racial and ethnic groups in the United States. African Americans have much higher rates of hypertension, heart disease, and stroke than other groups do. Figure 11.4 shows how rates of CVD compare among non-Hispanic whites, non-Hispanic blacks, and Hispanics in the United States. American Indians and Alaska Natives have higher rates of hypertension than non-Hispanic whites; Hispanic women have higher rates of angina (a warning sign of heart disease) than other racial/ethnic groups. Asian Americans historically have had far lower rates of CVD than white Americans.

Possible Risk Factors Currently Being Studied

In recent years, several other possible risk factors for cardiovascular disease have been identified.

Elevated blood levels of homocysteine, an amino acid that may damage the lining of blood vessels, are associated with an increased risk of CVD. Men generally have higher homocysteine levels than women, as do individuals with diets low in folic acid, vitamin B-12, and vitamin B-6. Most people can lower homocysteine levels easily by adopting a healthy diet rich in fruits, vegetables, and grains. Severe vitamin D deficiency has also been associated with heart dysfunction, independent of homocysteine levels.

Several infectious agents, including *Chlamydia pneumoniae*, cytomegalovirus, and *Helicobacter pylori*, have also been identified as possible risk factors for cardiovascular disease. *Chlamydia pneumoniae*, a common cause of flulike respiratory

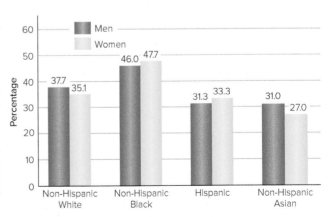

FIGURE 11.4 Percentage of adult Americans with cardiovascular disease.

SOURCE: Benjamin, E. J. et al. 2017. "Heart disease and stroke statistics—2017 update," *Circulation* 135:00—00

DIVERSITY MATTERS
Gender, Race/Ethnicity, and CVD

CVD is the leading cause of death for all Americans, but significant differences exist between men and women and among racial/ethnic groups in the incidence, diagnosis, and treatment of this deadly disease.

CVD in Women

CVD has been thought of as a "man's disease," but it actually kills more women than men. Polls indicate that women vastly underestimate their risk of dying of a heart attack and overestimate their risk of dying of breast cancer. In reality, nearly 1 in 3 women dies of CVD, whereas 1 in 31 dies of breast cancer. And although CVD typically does not develop in women younger than age 50, recent research suggests that the number of CVD deaths in women aged 35–45 may be increasing.

The hormone estrogen, produced naturally by a woman's ovaries until menopause, improves blood lipid concentrations and reduces other CVD risk factors. For several decades, many physicians encouraged menopausal women to take hormone replacement therapy (HRT), which includes estrogen, to relieve menopause symptoms and presumably to reduce their risk of CVD. However, some studies found that HRT may actually *increase* a woman's risk for heart disease and other health problems, including breast cancer. Some newer studies have found that the increased risk of CVD in women who start HRT may be age dependent; women in the early stages of menopause or ages 50–59 did not appear to have excess risk. This suggests that outcomes may depend on several factors, including the timing of hormone use. The U.S. Preventive Services Task Force and the American Heart Association recommend that HRT not be used to protect against CVD.

When women have heart attacks, they are more likely than men to die within a year. One reason is that because they develop heart disease at older ages, women are more likely to have other health problems that complicate treatment. Women with CVD are less likely than men to report the usual symptoms of a heart attack, such as chest pain, and more likely to report less-specific symptoms; this

pattern may obscure the diagnosis. These less-specific symptoms include fatigue, weakness, shortness of breath, nausea, vomiting, and pain in the abdomen, neck, jaw, and back. Women are also more likely than men to have pain at rest, during sleep, or accompanying mental stress. A woman who experiences these symptoms should be persistent in seeking accurate diagnosis and appropriate treatment.

Careful diagnosis of cardiac symptoms is also key in avoiding unnecessary invasive procedures in cases of stress cardiomyopathy ("broken heart syndrome"), which occurs much more commonly in women than in men. In this condition, hormones and neurotransmitters associated with a severe stress response stun the heart, producing heart-attack-like symptoms and decreased pumping function of the heart, but no damage to the heart muscle. Typically, the condition reverses quickly.

Women should be aware of their CVD risk factors and consult with a physician to assess their risk and determine the best way to prevent CVD.

CVD in African Americans and Other Racial/Ethnic Groups

Although cardiovascular disease is the leading cause of death for all Americans, there is a higher prevalence of CVD in adult African Americans, and a higher prevalence of many associated risk factors in Mexican Americans, than in non-Hispanic whites and Asian Americans. The reasons for these disparities likely include both genetic and environmental factors.

African Americans tend to develop hypertension at an earlier age than non-Hispanic whites, and their average blood pressures are much higher. African Americans have a higher risk of stroke and have strokes at younger ages. Survivors have more significant stroke-related disabilities. Some experts recommend that African Americans begin taking antihypertensive drugs when blood pressure reaches 130/80 rather than the typical 140/90 cutoff for hypertension.

A number of genetic and biological factors may contribute to CVD in African Americans. For instance, a higher

sensitivity to dietary sodium may lead to greater blood pressure elevation in response to a given amount of sodium. African Americans may also experience less dilation of blood vessels in response to stress (see Chapter 10).

Genetics also plays a large role in the tendency to develop diabetes, another important CVD risk factor that is more common in non-Hispanic blacks and Hispanics than in non-Hispanic whites. However, the prevalence of diabetes varies among those with different Hispanic backgrounds; for example, the rate of diabetes among Mexican Americans is nearly twice that of people who trace their background to South America.

Racial and ethnic groups other than non-Hispanic whites are more likely to be poor, and low income is associated with reduced access to health care and healthy dietary options for CVD prevention. Associated with low income is low educational attainment, which often means less access to information about preventive health measures, such as diet and stress management. Populations with low incomes tend to smoke more, consume more salt, and exercise less than those with higher incomes. Residents of low-income neighborhoods also experience longer delays between the onset of heart attack symptoms and reaching a hospital.

Discrimination may also play a role in CVD. Physicians and hospitals may treat the medical problems of non-whites differently from those of whites. Discrimination, low income, and other forms of deprivation may also increase stress, which is linked to hypertension and CVD. Lack of insurance coverage and less-advanced medical technologies in hospitals that serve minority and low-income neighborhoods may also play a role.

All Americans, regardless of background, are advised to have their blood pressure checked regularly, exercise on a regular basis, eat a healthy diet, manage stress, and avoid tobacco products. Tailoring your lifestyle to any risk factors especially relevant for you can also help. Discuss your particular risk profile with your physician to help identify the lifestyle changes most appropriate for you.

Box icon: ©Rawpixel Ltd/Getty Images RF

Ask Yourself

QUESTIONS FOR CRITICAL THINKING AND REFLECTION

What risk factors do you have for cardiovascular disease? Which ones are factors you have control over, and which are factors you can't change? If you have risk factors you cannot change (such as a family history of CVD), were you aware that you can make lifestyle adjustments to reduce your risk? Do you think you will make them? Why or why not?

infections, has been found in sections of clogged, damaged arteries but not in sections of healthy arteries. This effect may be secondary to the inflammation that many infectious agents produce.

Gum disease has long been suspected to be linked to CVD. Gingivitis, the beginning stages of gum disease, occurs when bacteria accumulate on the teeth, causing gums to become inflamed and to bleed easily; thus both gum disease and CVD are inflammatory processes. The exact linkages are still unknown, but studies suggest a potential relationship between oral disease and CVD, so it makes sense to practice good oral hygiene. For recommendations on good dental self-care, visit the American Dental Association's consumer website: http://www.mouthhealthy.org.

PROTECTING YOURSELF AGAINST CARDIOVASCULAR DISEASE

You can take several important steps right now to lower your risk of developing CVD (Figure 11.5). Reducing CVD risk factors when you are young can pay off with many extra years of life and good health.

Eat a Heart-Healthy Diet

For most Americans, a dietary pattern for heart health emphasizes whole grains, a variety of fruits and vegetables, low-fat dairy products, nuts, legumes, fish, lean meats, and vegetable oils. Limit saturated and trans fats, sweets and sugar-sweetened beverages, sodium, and red meat. Specific guidelines for heart health include the following:

- *Fats:* Saturated fats should be limited to 7% of total daily calories, or 5–6% for adults who have elevated LDL. Trans fats should be avoided. The majority of fats in your diet should be unsaturated, from sources such as vegetable oils, fish, and nuts.

- *Fiber:* Studies have shown that a high-fiber diet is associated with a 40–50% reduction in the risk of heart attack and stroke. To get the recommended 25–38 grams of dietary fiber a day, eat whole grains, fruits, and vegetables. Good sources of fiber include oatmeal, some breakfast cereals, barley, legumes, and most fruits and vegetables.

- *Sodium and potassium:* Reducing sodium intake to recommended levels, while also increasing potassium intake, can help reduce blood pressure for many people. Limit sodium intake to no more than 2,300 mg/day for all Americans. Reducing sodium intake further, to 1,500 mg/day, is associated with even greater reductions in blood pressure.

- *Alcohol:* Moderate alcohol use may increase HDL cholesterol; it may also reduce stroke risk, possibly by dampening the inflammatory response or by affecting blood clotting. For most people under age 45, however, the risks of alcohol use probably outweigh any health benefit. Excessive alcohol consumption increases the risk of a variety of serious health problems, including hypertension, stroke, some cancers, liver disease, alcohol dependence, and injuries.

Do More

- Eat a diet rich in fruits, vegetables, whole grains, and low-fat or fat-free dairy products. Eat five to nine servings of fruits and vegetables each day.
- Eat several servings of high-fiber foods each day.
- Eat two or more servings of fish per week; try a few servings of nuts and soy foods each week.
- Choose unsaturated fats rather than saturated and trans fats.
- Be physically active; do both aerobic exercise and strength training on a regular basis.
- Achieve and maintain a healthy weight.
- Develop effective strategies for handling stress and anger. Nurture old friendships and family ties, and make new friends; pay attention to your spiritual side.
- Obtain recommended screening tests and follow your physician's recommendations.

Do Less

- Don't use tobacco in any form: cigarettes, spit tobacco, cigars and pipes, bidis, and clove cigarettes.
- Limit consumption of trans fats and saturated fats.
- Limit consumption of salt to no more than 2,300 mg of sodium per day (1,500 mg if you have or are at high risk for hypertension).
- Avoid exposure to environmental tobacco smoke.
- Avoid excessive alcohol consumption— no more than one drink per day for women and two drinks per day for men.
- Limit consumption of added sugars and refined carbohydrates.
- Avoid excess stress, anger, and hostility.

FIGURE 11.5 **Strategies for reducing your risk of cardiovascular disease.**

(left): ©Jessica Peterson/Rubberball Productions/Getty Images RF; (right): ©Vladyslav Starozhylov/Alamy Stock Photo RF

Exercise Regularly

You can significantly reduce your risk of CVD with a moderate amount of physical activity (see the box "How Does Exercise Affect CVD Risk?"). A formal exercise program can provide even greater benefits. The information in the chapters focused on exercise can help you create and implement a complete exercise program that meets your needs for fitness and prevention of chronic disease.

Avoid Tobacco

The number-one risk factor for CVD that you can control is smoking. If you smoke, quit or enroll in a stop-smoking program. If you don't smoke, don't start. If you live or work with people who smoke, encourage them to quit—for their sake and yours. If you find yourself breathing in smoke, take steps to prevent or stop this exposure.

Know and Manage Your Blood Pressure

If you have no CVD risk factors, have your blood pressure measured at least once every two years; yearly tests are recommended if you have other risk factors. If your blood pressure is high, follow your physician's advice on lowering it.

Know and Manage Your Cholesterol Levels

All people age 20 and over should have their cholesterol checked at least once every five years. The National Cholesterol Education Program recommends a fasting lipoprotein profile that measures total cholesterol, HDL, LDL, and triglyceride levels. After you know your baseline numbers, you and your physician can develop a treatment and lifestyle plan.

Develop Ways to Handle Stress and Anger

To reduce the psychological and social risk factors for CVD, develop effective strategies for handling the stress in your life. Shore up your social support network, and try some techniques described in Chapter 10 for managing stress and anger.

Ask Yourself

QUESTIONS FOR CRITICAL THINKING AND REFLECTION

Do you know what your blood pressure and cholesterol levels are? If not, is there a reason you don't know? Is there something preventing you from getting this information about yourself? How can you motivate yourself to have these easy but important health checks?

DIABETES

As described earlier, diabetes mellitus is both a major risk factor for cardiovascular disease and a leading cause of death among Americans. In diabetes, the process of metabolism is disrupted (Figure 11.6). The pancreas normally secretes insulin, which stimulates cells to take up glucose (blood sugar) to produce energy. Diabetes interferes with this process, causing a buildup of glucose in the bloodstream.

Types of Diabetes

About 29.1 million Americans (9.3% of the population) have one of two major forms of diabetes—more than double the number of people affected in 1995. About 5–10% of people with diabetes have the more serious form, known as *type 1 diabetes*. In this type of diabetes, the body's immune system, triggered by a viral infection or some other environmental factor, destroys the insulin-producing cells in the pancreas. The pancreas produces little or no insulin, so daily doses of insulin are required; without insulin, a person will lapse into a coma. Other medications to control blood sugar levels and other complications of the disease may also be necessary. Type 1 diabetes usually begins in childhood or adolescence and is not related to obesity.

The remaining 90–95% of Americans with diabetes have *type 2 diabetes*. This condition can develop slowly, and about 25% of affected individuals are unaware of their condition. In type 2 diabetes, the pancreas fails to produce enough insulin, cells are resistant to insulin, or both. This condition is usually diagnosed in people over age 40, although there has been a tenfold increase in type 2 diabetes in children in the past two decades. About one-third of people with type 2 diabetes must take insulin; others may take medications that increase insulin production or stimulate cells to take up glucose.

A third type of diabetes occurs in 2–10% of women during pregnancy. *Gestational diabetes* usually disappears after pregnancy, but 5–10% of women with gestational diabetes go on to have type 2 diabetes immediately after pregnancy. Women who had gestational diabetes during pregnancy have up to a 60% chance of developing diabetes within 10–20 years.

The term *prediabetes* describes blood glucose levels that are higher than normal but not high enough for a diagnosis of full-blown diabetes. According to a 2017 estimate from the American Diabetes Association, about 86 million Americans have prediabetes. Experts warn that most people with the condition will develop type 2 diabetes unless they adopt preventive lifestyle measures. People with prediabetes also face a significantly increased risk of CVD.

The major factors involved in the development of type 2 diabetes are age, obesity, physical inactivity, a family history of diabetes, and lifestyle. Excess body fat reduces cell sensitivity to insulin, and insulin resistance is usually a precursor of type 2 diabetes. Race and ethnicity also play a role. According to the Centers for Disease Control and Prevention, the rate of diagnosed diabetes cases is highest among Native Americans and Alaska Natives, followed by blacks, Hispanics, Asian Americans, and white Americans. About 26% of all Americans age 65 and older have diabetes, either diagnosed or undiagnosed.

THE EVIDENCE FOR EXERCISE
How Does Exercise Affect CVD Risk?

Regular exercise directly and indirectly benefits your cardiovascular health and can help you avoid a heart attack or stroke. The evidence comes from dozens of large-scale, population-based studies conducted over the past several decades. There is so much evidence about the cardiovascular health benefits of exercise, in fact, that physicians regard physical activity as a magic bullet against heart disease.

Physical activity has an inverse relationship with cardiovascular disease, meaning that the more exercise you get, the less likely you are to develop or die from CVD. Compared to sedentary individuals, people who engage in regular, moderate physical activity lower their risk of CVD by 20% or more. People who get regular, vigorous exercise reduce their risk of CVD by 30% or more. This positive benefit applies regardless of gender, age, race, or ethnicity.

Most studies focus on various aerobic endurance exercises, such as walking, running on a treadmill, or biking. The type of exercise performed is less important than the amount of energy expended during the activity. The greater the energy expenditure, the greater the health benefits.

Exercise affects heart health via many mechanisms, all of which are being studied. For example, exercise helps people lose weight and improve body composition. Weight loss can improve heart health by reducing the amount of stress on the heart. Changing body composition to a more positive ratio of fat to fat-free mass boosts resting metabolic rate. Exercise directly strengthens the heart muscle itself, and it improves the balance of fats in the blood by boosting HDL and reducing LDL and triglyceride levels.

Exercise improves the health and function of the endothelial cells—the inner lining of the arteries. These cells secrete nitric oxide, which regulates blood flow, improves nerve function, strengthens the immune system, enhances reproductive health, and suppresses inflammation. Exercise training also improves the function of sodium-potassium pumps, which regulate fluid and electrolyte balance and cellular communication throughout the body.

One of the clearest positive effects of exercise is on hypertension. Many studies, involving thousands of people, have shown that physical activity reduces both systolic and diastolic blood pressure. These studies showed that people who engaged in regular aerobic exercise lowered their resting blood pressure by 2–4%, on average. Lowered blood pressure itself reduces the risk of other kinds of CVD.

Even with limited evidence, there appears to be an inverse relationship between physical activity and stroke. That is, according to a handful of studies, the most physically active people reduced their risk of both ischemic and hemorrhagic strokes by up to 30%. Although this benefit appears to apply equally to men and women, there is not sufficient evidence that it applies equally across races or ethnicities.

Of course, exercise isn't possible for everyone and may actually be dangerous for some people. People with CVD or serious risk factors for heart disease should work with their physician to determine whether or how to exercise.

Keep these guidelines in mind as you strive to reduce CVD risk factors:

- **Set goals.** Target a behavior (such as exercising for 30 minutes per day).

- **Monitor yourself.** Self-monitoring increases your awareness of physical cues and behaviors and helps you identify the barriers to changing a behavior.

- **Schedule follow-up exercise sessions.** Multiple sessions are more effective than single sessions.

- **Get feedback from your health care provider.** Feedback can encourage healthy choices by giving you an external measuring stick you can use to monitor your progress.

- **Keep a positive outlook on your progress.** A feeling of accomplishment is very important in motivating you to initiate new behaviors and continue your efforts.

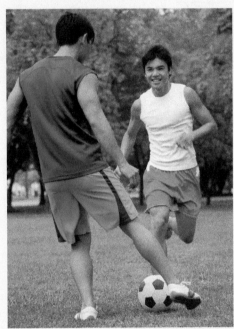

©Asia Images Group/Getty Images RF

SOURCES: Brawner, C. A., et al. 2017. Maximal exercise capacity is associated with survival in men and women. *Mayo Clinic Proceedings* 92(3): 383–390; Eckel, R. H., et al. 2014. 2013 AHA/ACC guideline on lifestyle management to reduce cardiovascular risk: A report of the American College of Cardiology/American Heart Association Task Force on Practice Guidelines. *Journal of the American College of Cardiology* 63(25_PA); Physical Activity Guidelines Advisory Committee. 2008. *Physical Activity Guidelines Advisory Committee Report, 2008.* Washington, DC: U.S. Department of Health and Human Services.

Box icon: ©Vstock LLC/Getty Images RF

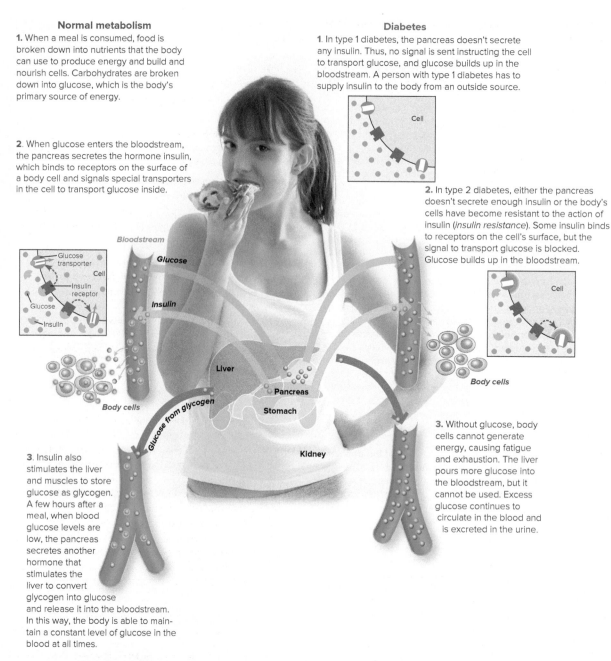

Normal metabolism

1. When a meal is consumed, food is broken down into nutrients that the body can use to produce energy and build and nourish cells. Carbohydrates are broken down into glucose, which is the body's primary source of energy.

2. When glucose enters the bloodstream, the pancreas secretes the hormone insulin, which binds to receptors on the surface of a body cell and signals special transporters in the cell to transport glucose inside.

3. Insulin also stimulates the liver and muscles to store glucose as glycogen. A few hours after a meal, when blood glucose levels are low, the pancreas secretes another hormone that stimulates the liver to convert glycogen into glucose and release it into the bloodstream. In this way, the body is able to maintain a constant level of glucose in the blood at all times.

Diabetes

1. In type 1 diabetes, the pancreas doesn't secrete any insulin. Thus, no signal is sent instructing the cell to transport glucose, and glucose builds up in the bloodstream. A person with type 1 diabetes has to supply insulin to the body from an outside source.

2. In type 2 diabetes, either the pancreas doesn't secrete enough insulin or the body's cells have become resistant to the action of insulin (*insulin resistance*). Some insulin binds to receptors on the cell's surface, but the signal to transport glucose is blocked. Glucose builds up in the bloodstream.

3. Without glucose, body cells cannot generate energy, causing fatigue and exhaustion. The liver pours more glucose into the bloodstream, but it cannot be used. Excess glucose continues to circulate in the blood and is excreted in the urine.

Labels on figure: Bloodstream; Glucose transporter; Cell; Insulin receptor; Glucose; Insulin; Glucose; Body cells; Glucose from glycogen; Liver; Pancreas; Stomach; Kidney; Cell; Cell; Body cells

FIGURE 11.6 **Diabetes mellitus.** During digestion, carbohydrates are broken down in the small intestine into glucose, a simple sugar that enters the bloodstream. The presence of glucose signals the pancreas to release insulin, a hormone that helps cells take up glucose; once inside a cell, glucose can be converted to energy. In diabetes, this process is disrupted, resulting in a buildup of glucose in the bloodstream.
©webphotographer/Getty Images RF

Warning Signs and Testing

Be alert for the warning signs of diabetes:

- Frequent urination
- Extreme hunger or thirst
- Unexplained weight loss
- Extreme fatigue
- Blurred vision
- Frequent infections
- Cuts and bruises that are slow to heal
- Tingling or numbness in the hands or feet
- Generalized itching with no rash

The best way to avoid complications is to recognize these symptoms and get early diagnosis and treatment. Because type 2 diabetes is often asymptomatic in the early stages, major health organizations now recommend routine screening for people over age 45 and anyone younger who is at high risk, including those who are obese.

Screening involves a blood test to check glucose levels after either a period of fasting or the administration of a set dose of glucose. A fasting glucose level of 126 mg/dl or higher indicates diabetes; a level of 100–125 mg/dl indicates prediabetes. If you are concerned about your risk for diabetes, talk with your physician about being tested.

Treatment

There is no cure for diabetes, but it can be managed successfully by keeping blood sugar levels within safe limits through diet, exercise, and, if necessary, medication. Blood sugar levels can be monitored with a home test; close control of glucose levels can significantly reduce the rate of serious complications.

Nearly 90% of people with type 2 diabetes are overweight when diagnosed, including 55% who are obese. An important step in treatment is to lose weight. Even a small amount of exercise and weight loss can be beneficial. Regular exercise and a healthy diet are often sufficient to control type 2 diabetes.

Prevention

It is estimated that 90% of cases of type 2 diabetes could be prevented if people adopted healthy lifestyle behaviors, including regular physical activity, a moderate diet, and modest weight loss. For people with prediabetes, lifestyle measures are more effective than medication for delaying or preventing the development of diabetes. Studies of people with prediabetes show that a 5–7% weight loss can lower diabetes onset by nearly 60%. Exercise (endurance and/or strength training) makes cells more

Wellness Tip Most cases of type 2 diabetes can be prevented through lifestyle measures such as regular physical activity and modest weight loss. For those who have type 2 diabetes, careful management to keep blood sugar levels within a healthy range through diet, exercise, and, if needed, medication can reduce the rate of complications from the disorder.

©Sean Prior/ Alamy Stock Photo RF

TIPS FOR TODAY AND THE FUTURE

Because cardiovascular disease and diabetes can develop slowly, beginning when you're young, it's important to develop healthy habits early in life.

RIGHT NOW YOU CAN
- Make an appointment to have your blood pressure, cholesterol, and glucose levels checked.
- List key stressors in your life, and decide what to do about the ones that bother you most.
- Plan to replace one high-fat, high-sugar item in your diet with one that is high in fiber. For example, replace a doughnut with a bowl of whole-grain cereal.

IN THE FUTURE YOU CAN
- Track your eating choices for one week, then compare them to the DASH eating plan. Make adjustments to bring your diet closer to the DASH recommendations.
- Sign up for a class in CPR. A CPR certification equips you with valuable lifesaving skills you can use to help someone who is choking, having a heart attack, or experiencing cardiac arrest.

sensitive to insulin and helps stabilize blood glucose levels; it also helps keep body fat at healthy levels.

A moderate diet to control body fat is perhaps the most important dietary recommendation for the prevention of diabetes. However, the composition of the diet may also be important. Studies have linked diets low in fiber and high in sugar, refined carbohydrates, saturated fat, red meat, and high-fat dairy products to increased risk of diabetes. Specific foods linked to higher diabetes risk include soft drinks, white bread, white rice, French fries, processed meats, and sugary desserts. Diets rich in whole grains, fruits, vegetables, legumes, fish, and poultry may be protective.

SUMMARY

- The major controllable risk factors for CVD are smoking, hypertension, unhealthy cholesterol levels, inactivity, overweight and obesity, and diabetes.

- Contributing factors for CVD that can be changed include high triglyceride levels, inadequate stress management, a hostile personality, depression, anxiety, lack of social support, poverty, and alcohol and drug use.

- Major risk factors for CVD that can't be changed are heredity, aging, being male, and ethnicity.

- Hypertension weakens the heart and scars and hardens arteries, causing resistance to blood flow. It is defined as blood pressure equal to or higher than 140 over 90.

COMMON QUESTIONS ANSWERED

Q I know what foods to avoid to prevent CVD, but are there any foods I should eat to help protect myself from CVD?

A The most important dietary change for CVD prevention is a negative one: cutting back on foods high in sugar and in saturated and trans fat. However, certain foods may be helpful. The positive effects of unsaturated fats, soluble fiber, and limited alcohol on heart health (alcohol for those over age 45) were discussed earlier in the chapter. Other potentially beneficial foods include those rich in the following:

• *Omega-3 fatty acids.* Found in fish, shellfish, and some nuts and seeds, omega-3 fatty acids reduce clotting and inflammation and may lower the risk of fatal arrhythmia.

• *Folic acid, vitamin B-6, and vitamin B-12.* These vitamins may affect CVD risk by lowering homocysteine levels; see Table 8.7 for a list of food sources.

• *Plant stanols and sterols.* Plant stanols and sterols, found in some types of trans-fat-free margarines and other products, reduce the absorption of cholesterol in the body and help lower LDL levels.

• *Soy protein.* Replacing some animal protein with soy protein can lower LDL cholesterol. Soy-based foods include tofu, tempeh, and soy-based beverages.

• *Calcium.* Diets rich in calcium may help prevent hypertension and possibly stroke by reducing insulin resistance and platelet aggregation. Low-fat and fat-free dairy products are rich in calcium; refer to Chapter 8 for other sources.

Q The advice I hear from the media about protecting myself from CVD seems to be changing all the time. What should I believe?

A Health-related research is now described in popular newspapers and magazines rather than just medical journals, meaning that more and more people have access to the information.

Researchers do not deliberately set out to mislead or confuse people. However, news reports may oversimplify the results of research studies, omitting some qualifications and questions the researchers present with their findings. In addition, news reports may not differentiate between a preliminary finding and a result that has been verified by a large number of long-term studies. And researchers themselves must strike a balance between reporting promising preliminary findings to the public, thereby allowing people to act on them, and waiting 10–20 years until long-term studies confirm (or disprove) a particular theory.

Although you cannot become an expert on all subjects, there are some strategies you can use to assess the health advice that appears in the media; see the box "Evaluating Sources of Health Information" in Chapter 1.

Q What's a heart murmur, and is it dangerous?

A A heart murmur is an extra or altered heart sound detectable during a routine medical exam. The source

---

• Atherosclerosis is a progressive hardening and narrowing of arteries that can lead to restricted blood flow and even complete blockage.

• Heart attacks, strokes, and congestive heart failure are the results of a long-term disease process; hypertension and atherosclerosis are usually involved.

• Reducing heart disease risk involves eating a heart-healthy diet, exercising regularly, avoiding tobacco, managing blood pressure and cholesterol levels, and managing stress and anger.

• The most common type of diabetes, a disorder of metabolism, is linked to older age and lifestyle factors, including inactivity and obesity; treatment can help reduce the rate of serious complications.

FOR FURTHER EXPLORATION

American Diabetes Association. Provides information, a free newsletter, and referrals to local support groups; the website includes an online diabetes risk assessment.

http://www.diabetes.org

American Heart Association. Provides information on hundreds of topics relating to the prevention and control of CVD. See especially "My Life Check--Life's Simple 7" for seven factors to ideal cardiovascular health.

http://www.heart.org

Centers for Disease Control and Prevention: Preventing or Managing High Cholesterol. Gives succinct advice on diet, weight, physical activity, smoking, and drinking alcohol, as well as links to other CDC websites.

http://www.cdc.gov/cholesterol/healthy_living.htm

Franklin Institute: The Heart: The Engine of Life. An online museum exhibit containing information on the structure and function of the heart, how to monitor your heart's health, and how to maintain a healthy heart.

https://www.fi.edu/heart-engine-of-life

Mayo Clinic. Gives reader-friendly definitions and descriptions of symptoms, tests, and treatments, and prepares you to discuss your health with an expert.

http://www.mayoclinic.org/diseases-conditions/heart-disease/basics/definition/con-20034056 is often a problem with one of the heart valves that separate the chambers of the heart. Congenital defects and certain infections can cause abnormalities in the valves. The most common heart valve disorder is mitral valve prolapse (MVP), which occurs in about 4% of the population. MVP is characterized by a "billowing" of the mitral valve, which separates the left ventricle and left atrium, during ventricular contraction. In some cases, blood leaks from the ventricle into the atrium. Most people with MVP have no symptoms; they have the same capability for exercising as people without MVP, and they also live as long.

MVP can be confirmed with echocardiography. Treatment is usually unnecessary, although surgery may be needed in the rare cases where leakage through the faulty valve is severe. Experts disagree over whether patients with MVP should take antibiotics prior to dental procedures, a precautionary step used to prevent bacteria, which may be dislodged into the bloodstream during some types of dental and surgical procedures, from infecting the defective valve. Most often, only those patients with significant blood leakage are advised to take antibiotics.

Although MVP usually requires no treatment, more severe heart valve disorders can impair blood flow through the heart. Treatment depends on the location and severity of the problem. More serious defects may be treated with surgery to repair or replace a valve.

Q How does stress contribute to cardiovascular disease?

A With stress, the brain tells the adrenal glands to secrete cortisol and other hormones and neurotransmitters, which in turn activate the sympathetic nervous system—causing the fight-or-flight response. This response increases heart rate and blood pressure so that more blood is distributed to the heart and other muscles in anticipation of physical activity. Blood glucose concentrations and cholesterol also increase to provide a source of energy, and the platelets become activated so that they will be more likely to clot in case of injury. Such a response can be adaptive if you're being chased by a hungry lion but may be more detrimental than useful if you're sitting at a desk taking an exam or feeling frustrated by a task given to you by your boss.

If you are healthy, you can tolerate the cardiovascular responses that take place during stress, but if you already have CVD, stress can lead to adverse outcomes such as abnormal heart rhythms, heart attacks, and sudden cardiac death. It has long been known that an increase in heart rhythm problems and deaths is associated with acute mental stress. For example, the rate of potentially life-threatening arrhythmias in patients who already had underlying heart disease doubled during the month after the September 11 terrorist attacks; this increase was not limited to people in proximity to Manhattan.

Because avoiding all stress is impossible, having healthy mechanisms to cope with it is your best defense. Instead of adopting unhealthy habits such as smoking, drinking, or overeating to deal with stress, try healthier coping techniques such as exercising, getting enough sleep, meditating, and talking to family and friends.

MedlinePlus: Blood, Heart and Circulation Topics. Provides links to reliable sources of information on cardiovascular health.

http://www.nlm.nih.gov/medlineplus/bloodheartandcirculation.html

National Heart, Lung, and Blood Institute. Provides information on a variety of topics relating to cardiovascular health and disease, including cholesterol, smoking, obesity, hypertension, and the DASH diet.

http://www.nhlbi.nih.gov/

National Stroke Association. Provides information and referrals for stroke victims and their families; the website has a stroke risk assessment.

http://www.stroke.org/site/PageNavigator/HOME

See also the listings for Chapters 9 and 10.

SELECTED BIBLIOGRAPHY

Akesson, A., et al. 2014. Low-risk diet and lifestyle habits in the primary prevention of myocardial infarction in men: A population-based prospective cohort study. *Journal of the American College of Cardiology* 64(13): 1299–1306.

American Heart Association. 2014. *Diet and Lifestyle Recommendations* (http://www.heart.org/HEARTORG/GettingHealthy/NutritionCenter/HealthyEating/The-American-Heart-Associations-Diet-and-Lifestyle-Recommendations_UCM_305855_Article.jsp).

American Heart Association. 2015. *Dental Health and Heart Health* (http://www.heart.org/HEARTORG/GettingHealthy/Dental-Health-and-Heart-Health_UCM_459358_Article.jsp).

American Heart Association. 2016. *Understand Your Risks to Prevent Heart Attack* (http://www.heart.org/HEARTORG/Conditions/HeartAttack/UnderstandYourRiskstoPreventaHeartAttack/Understand-Your-Risks-to-Prevent-a-Heart-Attack_UCM_002040_Article.jsp).

American Heart Association. 2017. *The Facts About High Blood Pressure* (http://www.heart.org/HEARTORG/Conditions/HighBloodPressure/GettheFactsAboutHighBloodPressure/The-Facts-About-High-Blood-Pressure_UCM_002050_Article.jsp).

American Heart Association. 2017. *Heart Attack Symptoms in Women* (http://www.heart.org/HEARTORG/Conditions/HeartAttack/WarningSignsofaHeartAttack/Heart-Attack-Symptoms-in-Women_UCM_436448_Article.jsp).

Bavry, A. A., and M. C. Limacher. 2014. Prevention of cardiovascular disease in women. *Seminars in Reproductive Medicine* 32(06): 447–453.

Benjamin, E. J., et al. 2017. Heart disease and stroke statistics—2017 update. *Circulation* 135. doi:10.1161/CIR.0000000000000485.

Bucholz, E. M., et al. 2016. Life expectancy after myocardial infarction, according to hospital performance. *New England Journal of Medicine* 375(14): 1332–1342.

Centers for Disease Control and Prevention. 2015. *Treating High Cholesterol* (http://www.cdc.gov/cholesterol/treating_cholesterol.htm).

Centers for Disease Control and Prevention. 2016. *Current Cigarette Smoking among Adults in the United States* (http://www.cdc.gov/tobacco/data_statistics/fact_sheets/adult_data/cig_smoking/index.htm).

Centers for Disease Control and Prevention. 2016. *Heart Disease Fact Sheet* (http://www.cdc.gov/dhdsp/data_statistics/fact_sheets/fs_heart_disease.htm).

Centers for Disease Control and Prevention. 2016. *High Blood Pressure Fact Sheet* (http://www.cdc.gov/dhdsp/data_statistics/fact_sheets/fs_bloodpressure.htm).

Centers for Disease Control and Prevention, National Center for Health Statistics. 2015. *Underlying Cause of Death 1999–2013* on CDC WONDER Online Database. Data are from the Multiple Cause of Death Files, 1999–2013, as compiled from data provided by the 57 vital statistics jurisdictions through the Vital Statistics Cooperative Program (http://wonder.cdc.gov/ucd-icd10.html).

Diabetes Prevention Program Research Group. 2015. Long-term effects of lifestyle intervention or metformin on diabetes development and microvascular complications over 15-year follow-up: The Diabetes Prevention Program Outcomes Study. *Lancet: Diabetes & Endocrinology* 3(11): 866–875.

Eckel, R. H., et al. 2014. 2013 AHA/ACC guideline on lifestyle management to reduce cardiovascular risk: A report of the American College of Cardiology/American Heart Association Task Force on Practice Guidelines. *Journal of the American College of Cardiology* 63(25_PA).

Goff, D. C., Jr., et al. 2014. 2013 ACC/AHA guideline on the assessment of cardiovascular risk: A report of the American College of Cardiology/American Heart Association Task Force on Practice Guidelines. *Journal of the American College of Cardiology* 63(25_PB).

Guan, W., et al. 2015. Race is a key variable in assigning lipoprotein(a) cutoff values for coronary heart disease risk assessment: The Multi-Ethnic Study of Atherosclerosis. *Arteriosclerosis, Thrombosis, and Vascular Biology* 35(4): 996–1001.

Heinl, R. E., et al. 2016. Comprehensive cardiovascular risk reduction and cardiac rehabilitation in diabetes and the metabolic syndrome. *Canadian Journal of Cardiology* 32(10S2): S349–S357.

Hernandez, D. C., et al. 2014. Social support and cardiovascular risk factors among black adults. *Ethnicity and Disease* 24(4): 444–450.

Jamal, A., et al. 2016. Current cigarette smoking among adults—United States, 2005–2015. *MMWR* 65: 1205–1211.

James, P. A., et al. 2014. Evidence-based guideline for the management of high blood pressure in adults: Report from the panel members appointed to the Eighth Joint National Committee (JNC 8). *JAMA* 311(5): 507–520.

Johnston, L. D., et al. 2017. *Monitoring the Future national survey results on drug use, 1975–2016: Overview, key findings on adolescent drug use.* Ann Arbor: Institute for Social Research, The University of Michigan.

Kones, R., and U. Rumana. 2015. Current treatment of dyslipidemia: A new paradigm for statin drug use and the need for additional therapies. *Drugs,* June 27.

Larsson, S. C., et al. 2015. Primary prevention of stroke by a healthy lifestyle in a high-risk group. *Neurology* 84(22): 2224–2228.

Micha, R., et al. 2017. Association between dietary factors and mortality from heart disease, stroke, and type 2 diabetes in the United States. *JAMA* 317(9): 912–924.

Miller, M., et al. 2011. Triglycerides and cardiovascular disease: A scientific statement from the American Heart Association. *Circulation* 123: 2292–2333.

Mozzafarian, D. 2016. Dietary and policy priorities for cardiovascular disease, diabetes, and obesity: A comprehensive review. *Circulation* 133(2): 187–225.

Stone, N. J., et al. 2014. 2013 ACC/AHA guideline on the treatment of blood cholesterol to reduce atherosclerotic cardiovascular risk in adults. A report of the American College of Cardiology/American Heart Association Task Force on Practice Guidelines. *Journal of the American College of Cardiology* 63(25_PA).

Tang, G., et al. 2015. Meta-analysis of the association between whole grain intake and coronary heart disease risk. *American Journal of Cardiology* 115(5): 625–629.

Tran, T. M., and N. M. Giang. 2014. Changes in blood pressure classification, blood pressure goals, and pharmacological treatment of essential hypertension in medical guidelines from 2003 to 2013. *International Journal of Cardiology Metabolic & Endocrine* 2: 1–10.

U.S. Department of Agriculture. 2015. *Scientific Report of the 2015 Dietary Guidelines Advisory Committee* (http://www.health.gov/dietaryguidelines/2015-scientific-report).

U.S. Department of Health and Human Services. 2016. *E-Cigarette Use Among Youth and Young Adults: A Report of the Surgeon General—Executive Summary.* Atlanta, GA: U.S. Department of Health and Human Services.

Willershausen, I., et al. 2013. Association between chronic periodontal and apical inflammation and acute myocardial infarction. *Odontology,* April 21.

Zwald, M. L., et al. 2017. Prevalence of low high-density lipoprotein cholesterol among adults, by physical activity: United States, 2011–2014. *NCHS Data Brief* No. 276. Hyattsville, MD: National Center for Health Statistics.

Name _____   Section _____   Date _____

LAB 11.1   Cardiovascular Health

Part I CVD Risk Assessment

Your chances of suffering a heart attack or stroke before age 55 depend on a variety of factors, many of which are under your control. To help identify your risk factors, circle the response for each risk category that best describes you.

1. Sex and Age

    (0) Female age 55 or younger; male age 45 or younger

    2 Female over age 55; male over age 45

2. Heredity/Family History

    (0) Neither parent suffered a heart attack or stroke before age 60.

    3 One parent suffered a heart attack or stroke before age 60.

    7 Both parents suffered a heart attack or stroke before age 60.

3. Smoking

    0 Never smoked

    (3) Quit more than 2 years ago and lifetime smoking is less than five pack-years*

    6 Quit less than 2 years ago and/or lifetime smoking is greater than five pack-years*

    8 Smoke less than 1/2 pack per day

    13 Smoke more than 1/2 pack per day

    15 Smoke more than 1 pack per day

4. Environmental Tobacco Smoke

    (0) Do not live or work with smokers

    2 Exposed to ETS at work

    3 Live with smoker

    4 Both live and work with smokers

5. Blood Pressure

    (If available, use the average of the last three readings.)

    0 120/80 or below

    1 121/81–130/85

    (3) Don't know blood pressure

    5 131/86–150/90

    9 151/91–170/100

    13 Above 170/100

6. Total Cholesterol

    0 Lower than 190

    1 190–210

    (2) Don't know total cholesterol

    3 211–240

    4 241–270

    5 271–300

    6 Over 300

7. HDL Cholesterol

    0 Over 60 mg/dl

    1 55–60

    (2) Don't know HDL

    3 45–54

    5 35–44

    7 25–34

    12 Lower than 25

8. Exercise

    (0) Exercise three times a week

    1 Exercise once or twice a week

    2 Occasional exercise less than once a week

    7 Rarely exercise

9. Diabetes

    (0) No personal or family history

    2 One parent with diabetes

    6 Two parents with diabetes

    9 Type 2 diabetes

    13 Type 1 diabetes

10. Body Mass Index (kg/m^2)

    0 <23.0

    (1) 23.0–24.9

    2 25.0–28.9

    3 29.0–34.9

    5 35.0–39.9

    7 ≥ 40

11. Stress

    0 Relaxed most of the time

    (1) Occasionally stressed and angry

    2 Frequently stressed and angry

    3 Usually stressed and angry

Scoring

Total your risk factor points. Refer to the list below to get an approximate rating of your risk of suffering an early heart attack or stroke.

Score	Estimated Risk
Less than 20	Low risk
20–29	Moderate risk
30–45	High risk
Over 45	Extremely high risk

*Pack-years can be calculated by multiplying the number of packs you smoked per day by the number of years you smoked. For example, if you smoked a pack and a half a day for 5 years, you would have smoked the equivalent of 1.5 × 5 = 7.5 pack-years.

LABORATORY ACTIVITIES

Part II Hostility Assessment

Are you too hostile? To help answer that question, Duke University researcher Redford Williams, M.D., has devised a short self-test. It's not a scientific evaluation, but it does offer a rough measure of hostility. Are the following statements true or false for you?

1. I often get annoyed at checkout cashiers or the people in front of me when I'm waiting in line.
2. I usually keep an eye on the people I work or live with to make sure they do what they should.
3. I often wonder how homeless people can have so little respect for themselves.
4. I believe that most people will take advantage of you if you let them.
5. The habits of friends or family members often annoy me.
6. When I'm stuck in traffic, I often start breathing faster and my heart pounds.
7. When I'm annoyed with people, I really want to let them know it.
8. If someone does me wrong, I want to get even.
9. I like to have the last word in any argument.
10. At least once a week, I have the urge to yell at or even hit someone.

According to Williams, five or more "true" statements suggest that you're excessively hostile and should consider taking steps to mellow out.

Using Your Results

How did you score?

(1) What is your CVD risk assessment score? Are you surprised by your score?

Are you satisfied with your CVD risk rating? If not, set a specific goal:

(2) What is your hostility assessment score? Are you surprised by the result?

Are you satisfied with your hostility rating? If not, set a specific goal:

What should you do next? Enter the results of this lab in the Preprogram Assessment column in Appendix B.

(1) If you've set a goal for the overall CVD risk assessment score, identify a risk area that you can change, such as smoking, exercise, or stress. Then list three steps or strategies for changing the risk area you've chosen.

Risk area:

Strategies for change:

(2) If you've set a goal for the hostility assessment score, begin by keeping a log of your hostile responses. Review the anger-management strategies in Chapter 10 and select several that you will try to use to manage your angry responses. Strategies for anger management:

Next, begin to put your strategies into action. After several weeks of a program to reduce CVD risk or hostility, do this lab again and enter the results in the Postprogram Assessment column of Appendix B. How do the results compare?

SOURCE: Adapted from from *Life Skills* by Virginia Williams and Redford Williams.

Credits

Online Supplements   369

Online Supplements

Connect with LearnSmart Fitness and Wellness Online Access for Fit & Well, 13th Edition

McGraw-Hill Connect is a digital teaching and learning environment that improves performance over a variety of critical outcomes. With Connect, instructors can deliver assignments, quizzes and tests easily online. Students can practice important skills at their own pace and on their own schedule.

HOW TO REGISTER

Using a <u>Print Book</u>?
To register and activate your Connect account, simply follow these easy steps:
1. **Go to the Connect course web address provided by your instructor or visit the Connect link set up on your instructor's course within your campus learning management system.**
2. **Click on the link to register.**
3. **When prompted, enter the Connect code found on the inside back cover of your book and click Submit. Complete the brief registration form that follows to begin using Connect.**

Using an <u>eBook</u>?
To register and activate your Connect account, simply follow these easy steps:
1. **Upon purchase of your eBook, you will be granted automatic access to Connect.**
2. **Go to the Connect course web address provided by your instructor or visit the Connect link set up on your instructor's course within your campus learning management system.**
3. **Sign in using the same email address and password you used to register on the eBookstore. Complete your registration and begin using Connect.**

Note: Access Code is for one use only. If you did not purchase this book new, the access code included in this book is no longer valid.

Need help? Visit mhhe.com/support